PROGRESS IN BRAIN RESEARCH

VOLUME 70

AGING OF THE BRAIN AND ALZHEIMER'S DISEASE

Recent volumes in PROGRESS IN BRAIN RESEARCH

Volume 46: Membrane Morphology of the Vertebrate Nervous System. A Study with Freeze-etch Technique, by C. Sandri, J. M. Van Buren and K. Akert — *revised edition* — 1982

Volume 53: Adaptive Capabilities of the Nervous System, by P. S. McConnell, G. J. Boer, H. J. Romijn, N. E. Van de Poll and M. A. Corner (Eds.) — 1980

Volume 54: Motivation, Motor and Sensory Processes of the Brain: Electrical Potentials, Behaviour and Clinical Use, by H. H. Kornhuber and L. Deecke (Eds.) — 1980

Volume 55: Chemical Transmission in the Brain. The Role of Amines, Amino Acids and Peptides, by R. M. Buijs, P. Pévet and D. F. Swaab (Eds.) — 1982

Volume 56: Brain Phosphoproteins, Characterization and Function, by W. H. Gispen and A. Routtenberg (Eds.) — 1982

Volume 57: Descending Pathways to the Spinal Cord, by H. G. J. M. Kuypers and G. F. Martin (Eds.) — 1982

Volume 58: Molecular and Cellular Interactions underlying Higher Brain Functions, by J.-P. Changeux, J. Glowinski, M. Imbert and F. E. Bloom (Eds.) — 1983

Volume 59: Immunology of Nervous System Infections, by P. O. Behan, V. ter Meulen and F. Clifford Rose (Eds.) — 1983

Volume 60: The Neurohypophysis: Structure, Function and Control, by B. A. Cross and G. Leng (Eds.) — 1983

Volume 61: Sex Differences in the Brain: The Relation Between Structure and Function, by G. J. De Vries, J. P. C. De Bruin, H. B. M. Uylings and M. A. Corner (Eds.) — 1984

Volume 62: Brain Ischemia: Quantitative EEG and Imaging Techniques, by G. Pfurtscheller, E. J. Jonkman and F. H. Lopes da Silva (Eds.) — 1984

Volume 63: Molecular Mechanisms of Ischemic Brain Damage, by K. Kogure, K.-A. Hossmann, B. K. Siesjö and F. A. Welsh (Eds.) — 1985

Volume 64: The Oculomotor and Skeletal Motor Systems: Differences and Similarities, by H.-J. Freund, U. Büttner, B. Cohen and J. Noth (Eds.) — 1986

Volume 65: Psychiatric Disorders: Neurotransmitters and Neuropeptides, by J. M. Van Ree and S. Matthysse (Eds.) — 1986

Volume 66: Peptides and Neurological Disease, by P. C. Emson, M. N. Rossor and M. Tohyama (Eds.) — 1986

Volume 67: Visceral Sensation, by F. Cervero and J. F. B. Morrison (Eds.) — 1986

Volume 68: Coexistence of Neuronal Messengers — A New Principle in Chemical Transmission, by T. G. M. Hökfelt, K. Fuxe and B. Pernow (Eds.) — 1986

Volume 69: Phosphoproteins in Neuronal Function, by W. H. Gispen and A. Routtenberg (Eds.) — 1986

Volume 70: Aging of the Brain and Alzheimer's Disease, by D. F. Swaab, E. Fliers, M. Mirmiran, W. A. van Gool and F. van Haaren (Eds.) — 1986

Volume 71: Neuronal Regeneration, by F. J. Seil, E. Herbert and B. Carlson (Eds.) — in preparation

PROGRESS IN BRAIN RESEARCH

VOLUME 70

AGING OF THE BRAIN AND ALZHEIMER'S DISEASE

Proceedings of the 14th International Summer School of Brain Research,
held at the Royal Netherlands Academy of Arts and Sciences,
Amsterdam, The Netherlands, 26–30 August, 1985

EDITED BY

D. F. SWAAB, E. FLIERS, M. MIRMIRAN, W. A. VAN GOOL and F. VAN HAAREN

Netherlands Institute for Brain Research
Meibergdreef 33, 1105 AZ Amsterdam ZO, The Netherlands

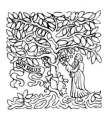

ELSEVIER
AMSTERDAM — NEW YORK — OXFORD
1986

Special regulations for readers in the USA:
This publication has been registered with the Copyright Clearance Center Inc. (CCC), Salem, Massachusetts. Information can be obtained from the CCC about conditions under which photocopying of parts of this publication may be made in the USA. All other copyright questions, including photocopying outside of the USA, should be referred to the publisher.
ISBN 0-444-80793-4 (volume)
ISBN 0-444-80104-9 (series)

Published by:
Elsevier Science Publishers B. V. (Biomedical Division)
P.O. Box 211
1000 AE Amsterdam
The Netherlands

Sole distributors for the USA and Canada:
Elsevier Science Publishing Company, Inc.
52 Vanderbilt Avenue
New York, NY 10017
USA

Library of Congress Cataloging in Publication Data
International Summer School of Brain Research (14th :
    1985 : Royal Netherlands Academy of Arts and Sciences)
    Aging of the brain and Alzheimer's disease.

    (Progress in brain research; v. 70)
    Includes bibliographies and index.
    1. Senile dementia—Etiology—Congresses.
2. Alzheimer's disease—Etiology—Congresses.   3. Brain—
Aging—Congresses.   4. Brain—Diseases—Congresses.
5. Senile dementia—Animal models—Congresses.
6. Alzheimer's disease—Animal models—Congresses.
I. Swaab, D. F. (Dick Frans) II. Title. III. Series.
[DNLM: 1. Aging—congresses.   2. Alzheimer's Disease—
congresses.   3. Brain—physiopathology—congresses.
4. Dementia, Senile—congresses.   W1 PR667J v.70 /

WT 150 I615 1985a]
QP367.P7   vol. 70 [RC524]   618.97'83   86–19787
ISBN 0-444-80793-4 (U.S.)

55,150

Printed in The Netherlands

List of Contributors

T. M. Abou-Nader, Department of Applied Biological Sciences, Massachusetts Institute of Technology, Cambridge, MA 02139, USA

R. T. Bartus, Department of Central Nervous System Research, Medical Research Division, Lederle Laboratories, American Cyanamid Company, Pearl River, NY 10965 and Department of Psychiatry, New York University School of Medicine, New York University, New York, NY 10016, USA

A. Björklund, Department of Histology, University of Lund, Biskopsgatan 5, S-223 62 Lund, Sweden

E. Braak, Department of Anatomy, Theodor Stern Kai 7, D-6000 Frankfurt am Main 70, FRG

H. Braak, Department of Anatomy, Theodor Stern Kai 7, D-6000 Frankfurt am Main 70, FRG

J. M. Candy, MRC Neuroendocrinology Unit, Newcastle General Hospital, Westgate Road, Newcastle upon Tyne NE4 6BE, UK

P. Chen, Queensland Institute of Medical Research, Bramston Terrace, Brisbane, Australia 4006

W.-G. Chou, Cancer Center, University of Rochester Medical School, Rochester, NY, USA

P. D. Coleman, Department of Neurobiology and Anatomy, School of Medicine and Dentistry, University of Rochester, 601 Elmwood Avenue, Rochester, NY 14642, USA

J. F. Coughlin, New England Deaconess Hospital, Boston, MA 02115, USA

J. A. Court, MRC Neuroendocrinology Unit, Newcastle General Hospital, Westgate Road, Newcastle upon Tyne NE4 6BE, UK

D. R. Crapper McLachlan, Departments of Physiology and Medicine, Faculty of Medicine, University of Toronto, Toronto, Ontario, Canada M5S 1A8

A. J. Cross, Department of Physiology, University of Manchester, Manchester M13 9PT, and Divisions of Psychiatry and Clinical Cell Biology, Clinical Research Centre, Harrow HA1 3UJ, UK

T. J. Crow, Department of Physiology, University of Manchester, Manchester M13 9PT, and Divisions of Psychiatry and Clinical Cell Biology, Clinical Research Centre, Harrow HA1 3UJ, UK

A. R. Damasio, Department of Neurology, University of Iowa, Iowa City, IA 52242, USA

P. Davies, Department of Pathology, Albert Einstein College of Medicine, Building F, Room 538, 1300 Morris Park Avenue, Bronx, NY 10461, USA

R. L. Dean, Department of Central Nervous System Research, Medical Research Division, Lederle Laboratories, American Cyanamid Company, Pearl River, NY 10965, USA

P. N. E. De Graan, Division of Molecular Neurobiology, Rudolf Magnus Institute for Pharmacology and Institute of Molecular Biology, University of Utrecht, Padualaan 8, 3584 CH Utrecht, The Netherlands

E. Donchin, Department of Psychology and Cognitive Psychophysiology Laboratory, University of Illinois at Urbana-Champaign, Champaign, IL 61820, USA

J. A. Edwardson, MRC Neuroendocrinology Unit, Newcastle General Hospital, Westgate Road, Newcastle upon Tyne NE4 6BE, UK

L. A. Farwell, Department of Psychology and Cognitive Psychophysiology Laboratory, University of Illinois at Urbana-Champaign, Champaign, IL 61820, USA

J. Figueiredo, Department of Central Nervous System Research, Medical Research Division, Lederle Laboratories, American Cyanamid Company, Pearl River, NY 10965, USA

S. Fisher, Department of Central Nervous System Research, Medical Research Division, Lederle Laboratories, American Cyanamid Company, Pearl River, NY 10965, USA

C. Flicker, Department of Psychiatry, New York University School of Medicine, New York University, New York, NY 10016, USA

E. Fliers, Netherlands Institute for Brain Research, Meibergdreef 33, 1105 AZ Amsterdam ZO, The Netherlands

D. G. Flood, Department of Neurology, School of Medicine and Dentistry, University of Rochester, 601 Elmwood Avenue, Rochester, NY 14642, USA

R. S. J. Frackowiak, MRC Cyclotron Unit, Hammersmith Hospital, Du Cane Road, London W12 0HS, UK

F. H. Gage, Department of Neuroscience, University of California at San Diego, La Jolla, CA, USA

W. H. Gispen, Division of Molecular Neurobiology, Rudolf Magnus Institute for Pharmacology and Institute of Molecular Biology, University of Utrecht, Padualaan 8, 3584 CH Utrecht, The Netherlands

K. G. Go, Department of Neurosurgery, University of Groningen, Oostersingel 59, 9713 EZ Groningen, The Netherlands

C. G. Gottfries, Department of Psychiatry and Neurochemistry, St. Jörgens Hospital, S-422 03 Hisings Backa, Sweden

J. Goudsmit, Virology Department, Academic Medical Center, Meibergdreef 9, 1105 AZ Amsterdam ZO, The Netherlands

J.-B. P. Gramsbergen, Department of Biological Psychiatry, University Psychiatric Clinic, Oostersingel 59, 9713 EZ Groningen, The Netherlands

I. Grundke-Iqbal, NYS Institute for Basic Research in Developmental Disabilities, 1050 Forest Hill Road, Staten Island, NY 10314, USA

J. M. Henry, Molecular Physiology and Genetics Section, Laboratory of Cellular and Molecular Biology, Gerontology Research Center, National Institute on Aging, Francis Scott Key Medical Center, Baltimore, MD 21224, USA

C. F. Hollander, Laboratoires MSD CHIBRET, Centre de Recherche, Département d'E.I.M., Route de Marsat, B.P. 134, 63203 RIOM Cedex, France

B. T. Hyman, Department of Neurology, University of Iowa, Iowa City, IA 52242, USA

K. Iqbal, NYS Institute for Basic Research in Developmental Disabilities, 1050 Forest Hill Road, Staten Island, NY 10314, USA

O. Isacson, Department of Histology, University of Lund, Biskopsgatan 5, S-233 62 Lund, Sweden

J. Jolles, Department of Clinical Psychiatry, State University of Limburg, P.O. Box 616, 6200 MD Maastricht, The Netherlands

J. A. Joseph, Lederle Laboratories of American Cyanamid, Pearl River, NY 10965, USA

J. Korf, Department of Biological Psychiatry, University Psychiatric Clinic, Oostersingel 59, 9713 EZ Groningen, The Netherlands

C. Kidson, Queensland Institute of Medical Research, Bramston Terrace, Brisbane, Queensland, Australia 4006

H. R. Lieberman, Departments of Brain and Cognitive Sciences and Applied Biological Sciences, E20–138, Massachusetts Institute of Technology, Cambridge, MA 02139, USA

R. E. Majocha, Department of Psychiatry, Harvard Medical School and Mailman Research Center, McLean Hospital, 115 Mill Street, Belmont, MA 02178, USA

H. J. Manz, Department of Pathology, Georgetown University Schools of Medicine and Dentistry, 3900 Reservoir Road, Washington, DC 20007, USA

C. A. Marotta, Department of Psychiatry and Program in Neuroscience, Harvard Medical School, Massachusetts General Hospital and Mailman Research Center, McLean Hospital, 115 Mill Street, Belmont, MA 02178, USA

S. Matthysse, Mailman Research Center, McLean Hospital, 115 Mill Street, Belmont, MA 02178, USA

G. A. Miller, Department of Psychology and Cognitive Psychophysiology Laboratory, University of Illinois at Urbana-Champaign, Champaign, IL 61820, USA

M. Mirmiran, Netherlands Institute for Brain Research, Meibergdreef 33, 1105 AZ Amsterdam ZO, The Netherlands

J. Mos, Duphar B.V., Department of Pharmacology, P.O. Box 2, 1380 AA Weesp, The Netherlands

A. E. Oakley, MRC Neuroendocrinology Unit, Newcastle General Hospital, Westgate Road, Newcastle upon Tyne NE4 6BE, UK

A. B. Oestreicher, Division of Molecular Neurobiology, Rudolf Magnus Institute for Pharmacology and Institute of Molecular Biology, State University of Utrecht, Padualaan 8, 3584 CH Utrecht, The Netherlands

J. M. Palacios, Preclinical Research, Sandoz Ltd., CH-4002 Basle, Switzerland

R. C. A. Pearson, Department of Human Anatomy, University of Oxford, South Parks Road, Oxford OX1 3QT, UK

E. K. Perry, Department of Pathology, Newcastle General Hospital, Westgate Road, Newcastle upon Tyne NE4 6BE, UK

R. H. Perry, Department of Pathology, Newcastle General Hospital, Westgate Road, Newcastle upon Tyne NE4 6BE, UK

T. J. Peters, Department of Physiology, University of Manchester, Manchester M13 9PT, and Divisions of Psychiatry and Clinical Cell Biology, Clinical Research Centre, Harrow HA1 3UJ, UK

C. E. Polak, Department of Psychology, University of Amsterdam, Weesperplein 8, 1018 XA Amsterdam, The Netherlands

M. Pontecorvo, Department of Central Nervous System Research, Medical Research Division, Lederle Laboratories, American Cyanamid Company, Pearl River, NY 10965, USA

G. H. M. Prenen, Department of Neurosurgery, University of Groningen, Oostersingel 59, 9713 EZ Groningen, The Netherlands

G. S. Roth, Molecular Physiology and Genetics Section, Laboratory of Cellular and Molecular Biology, Gerontology Research Center, National Institute on Aging, Francis Scott Key Medical Center, Baltimore, MD 21224, USA

E. M. Sajdel-Sulkowska, Department of Psychiatry, Harvard Medical School and Mailman Research Center, McLean Hospital, 115 Mill Street, Belmont, MA 02178, USA

M. V. Sofroniew, Anatomy School, Downing Street, Cambridge CB2 3DY, UK

R. S. Sohal, Department of Biology, Southern Methodist University, Dallas, TX 75275, USA

R. Spiegel, Clinical Research, Sandoz Ltd., CH-4002 Basle, Switzerland

D. F. Swaab, Netherlands Institute for Brain Research, Meibergdreef 33, 1105 AZ Amsterdam ZO, The Netherlands

R. D. Terry, Department of Neurosciences, University of California, San Diego, La Jolla, CA 92093, USA

M. F. A. Van Berkum, Departments of Physiology and Medicine, Faculty of Medicine, University of Toronto, Toronto, Ontario, Canada M5S 1A8

H. Van Crevel, Department of Neurology, Academic Medical Center, Meibergdreef 9, 1105 AZ Amsterdam ZO, The Netherlands

F. Van der Waals, Virology Department, Academic Medical Center, Meibergdreef 9, 1105 AZ Amsterdam ZO, The Netherlands

W. A. Van Gool, Netherlands Institute for Brain Research, Meibergdreef 33, 1105 AZ Amsterdam ZO, The Netherlands

F. Van Haaren, Netherlands Institute for Brain Research, Meibergdreef 33, 1105 AZ Amsterdam ZO, The Netherlands

G. W. Van Hoesen, Departments of Anatomy and Neurology, University of Iowa, Iowa City, IA 52242, USA

M. Ventosa-Michelman, Mailman Research Center, McLean Hospital, 115 Mill Street, Belmont, MA 02178, USA

R. S. Williams, Shriver Center, 200 Trapelo Road, Waltham, MA 02154, USA

H. M. Wisniewski, NYS Institute for Basic Research in Developmental Disabilities, 1050 Forest Hill Road, Staten Island, NY 10314, USA

L. S. Wolfe, Donner Laboratory of Experimental Neurochemistry, Montreal Neurological Institute, McGill University, Montreal, Canada H3A 2B4

S. B. Zain, Cancer Center, University of Rochester Medical School, Rochester, NY, USA

Preface

This book contains the proceedings of the 14th International Summer School of Brain Research organized by the Netherlands Institute for Brain Research and the University of Amsterdam in August 1985. According to tradition, the Summer School took place at the stately Trippenhuis. This building, which is situated in one of the oldest parts of Amsterdam, was built from 1660–1664 for the families of the brothers Louis and Hendrik Trip. From 1814 to 1885 it served as the 'Rijksmuseum', and since 1812 as the seat of the Royal Netherlands Academy of Sciences.

In such an environment it was easy to let one's mind wander back to the meeting of the International Association of Academies, held in Paris in 1901, where the anatomist Wilhelm His proposed that research into the nervous system should be placed on an international footing. Three years later this proposal resulted in the formation of the International Academies Committee, and in 1909 in the foundation of the Netherlands (Central) Institute for Brain Research. Soon after its installation, the Committee pointed out that "the time is not far distant when the study of the millions of brain cells will have to be divided amongst researchers in the way the astronomers have been obliged to divide the millions of stars into various groups". The success of the series of International Summer Schools of Brain Research has proven that such a division is not satisfactory for present-day neurosciences. Today's researchers do not merely study 'their' part of the brain in depth, but feel an increasing need to integrate their data in a broad international, multidisciplinary setting.

At the diamond jubilee of the Netherlands Institute for Brain Research, it seemed highly appropriate to select 'Aging of the Brain and Alzheimer's Disease' as the theme for our 14th Summer School. This topic appeared especially timely because it was felt, both internationally and in The Netherlands, to be a research field of considerable social and clinical relevance. Indeed, various organizations (e.g., ZWO, SOOM, Eurage, the Alzheimer Foundation) were trying to stimulate the interest of Dutch neuroscientists in this direction. We felt that the Summer School would contribute to this important initiative by bringing together a group of internationally well-known scientists in Amsterdam.

The authors have been requested to relate, whenever possible, (a) functional and morphological studies and (b) human clinical and animal experimental data. The question of whether or not the changes observed in aging are qualitatively different from those observed in Alzheimer's disease has also received attention.

The present book which has been compiled with the indispensable help of T. Eikelboom and W. Chen-Pelt contains a great number of the current central questions regarding brain aging and dementia, along with the strategies being followed in order to tackle such problems. We are very grateful for the enthusiasm with which a great number of scientists have agreed to contribute their knowledge and expertise to our endeavor.

We are under no illusion that the 14th International Summer School has answered all the questions in a field where disagreement continues over the nomenclature of the dementias, or whether or not 'normal' brain aging actually exists or even over the spelling of aging (ageing?). We think, however, that this extensive review will be of interest not only for those involved in fundamental research, but also for medical practitioners working in the field such as psychologists, neurologists, psychiatrists and geriatrists and may help us, neurobiologists, to formulate the right questions to ask ourselves (and our aging brains) while we have still got the time.

D. F. Swaab
E. Fliers
M. Mirmiran
W. A. Van Gool
F. Van Haaren

Amsterdam, December 1985

Acknowledgements

The organization of the 14th International Summer School of Brain Research was made possible by generous financial support from the C. N. van den Houten Fund. We are indebted in addition to all of the following for supplementary contributions:

Nederlandse Organisatie voor Zuiver-Wetenschappelijk Onderzoek (ZWO), 's-Gravenhage, The Netherlands

Koninklijke Nederlandse Akademie van Wetenschappen, Amsterdam, The Netherlands

Stimuleringsfonds Gerontologie, supported by Ministeries van Onderwijs en Wetenschappen; Sociale Zaken; Volkshuisvesting en Milieu; Welzijn, Volksgezondheid en Cultuur, Rijswijk, The Netherlands

Stichting Het Remmert Adriaan Laan-Fonds, Amsterdam, The Netherlands

Genootschap ter Bevordering van Natuur-, Genees- en Heelkunde, Amsterdam, The Netherlands

Dr. Saal van Zwanenbergstichting, Oss, The Netherlands

Fidia Research Laboratories, Abano Terme, Italy

I.B.M. Nederland N.V., Amsterdam, The Netherlands

Sandoz B.V., Uden, The Netherlands

Shell Nederland B.V., 's-Gravenhage, The Netherlands

Zeiss Nederland B.V., Weesp, The Netherlands

D. F. Swaab
E. Fliers
M. Mirmiran
W. A. Van Gool
F. Van Haaren

Contents

Section III — Etiological Factors and Animal Models

Section IV — Therapeutic Strategies

SECTION I

Diagnosis

D. F. Swaab, E. Fliers, M. Mirmiran, W. A. Van Gool and F. Van Haaren (Eds.)
Progress in Brain Research, Vol. 70.
© 1986 Elsevier Science Publishers B.V. (Biomedical Division)

CHAPTER 1

Clinical approach to dementia

H. Van Crevel

Department of Neurology, Academic Medical Center, Meibergdreef 9, 1105 AZ Amsterdam ZO, The Netherlands

Introduction

Dementia has devastating effects on patients and their relatives (Anonymous, 1950). Memory, intellect and personality are progressively impaired. This process is irreversible in most cases and often necessitates admission to an institution for chronic care. Moreover, dementia often leads to death from secondary complications (Barclay et al., 1985), and its main cause, Alzheimer's disease, has been called 'a major killer' (Katzman, 1976). Epidemiological data differ, but with 10% of the population aged 65 or older, and 5–10% of people over 65 demented, 0.5–1% of the population may be demented. The prevalence rises steeply with age, from 2% at 65 to 20% at 80. As the number of aged people in our population grows, the prevalence of dementia increases; this has been called 'an approaching epidemic' (Plum, 1979).

Definition of dementia

The definition of dementia is controversial (Fliers et al., 1983). Here it will be defined as an acquired syndrome of intellectual impairment produced by brain dysfunction (Cummings and Benson, 1983); the important point is that dementia is thus regarded as a syndrome and not as a nosological entity. Its onset is always gradual (except in posttraumatic and postanoxic cases, when it follows coma of acute onset). Its course is often progressive but can be stationary. Fortunately, it is now widely known that dementia may be revers-

ible, and the search for treatable causes is pursued with great energy, albeit with varying success.

Description of dementia

To define is not to describe: dementia produces many different clinical pictures. Although impairment of memory, deterioration of intellect and change of personality are essential features, many other characteristics may be present, depending on the cause and the stage of the process. For example, in Alzheimer's disease, amnesia is followed by focal signs such as spatial disorientation and dysphasia, while social behaviour remains relatively spared. But even within Alzheimer's disease, different clinical pictures occur, with different rates of progression (Mayeux et al., 1985). So-called typical features of one disease sometimes occur in other diseases. For example, myoclonus, characteristic of Creutzfeldt-Jakob disease, is sometimes seen in Alzheimer's disease.

Presentation of dementia

It is important to know that the presenting complaint in many cases is not 'dementia'. This is not only a diagnostic problem but also an obstacle to clinical research, as the records may not be filed under 'dementia'. The following presentations all occur in medical practice:
— as 'dementia?': the patient, or more often the family, are concerned that he/she may become demented;

— as psychiatric symptoms: anxiety, neurasthenic complaints, obsessional behaviour, paranoid ideas or depression;

— as various somatic complaints (Wells, 1977): frequent consultations for unrelated and often trivial somatic symptoms;

— as an acute problem (but not dementia): e.g. an infection, accident or stroke bring the patient to medical attention, after which dementia becomes apparent;

— as part of another disease (usually neurological), e.g. Parkinson's disease (Brown and Marsden, 1984), Huntington's disease, progressive supranuclear palsy, olivo-ponto-cerebellar atrophy, cerebral tumour.

Causes of dementia

Dementia has many causes (Wells, 1977; Cummings and Benson, 1983). Some, such as neurosyphilis, have become rare, while others (e.g. AIDS) are becoming more frequent. The main diagnostic groups are enumerated in Table I.

Alzheimer's disease, both presenile (AD) and senile (SDAT) is the most frequent cause of dementia, followed by multi-infarct dementia (MID) and combinations of the two (MIX).

TABLE I

Causes of dementia

Alzheimer's disease, presenile (AD) and senile (SDAT)
Multi-infarct dementia (MID)
Combinations of the two (MIX)
Toxic (prescribed drugs, alcohol)
Metabolic (e.g. vit. B_{12} deficiency)
Endocrine (e.g. hypothyroidism)
Infectious (e.g. neurosyphilis)
Inflammatory (e.g. vasculitis)
Posttraumatic and postanoxic
Genetic (e.g. Huntington)
Degenerative (e.g. Parkinson)
Cerebral tumours
Subdural haematoma
Hydrocephalus
Others

Together, these three constitute approximately 80% of all cases. The list of all causes is long: more than 50 are enumerated in Wells (1977). In practice, it is helpful to distinguish between 'dementia diseases' (in which dementia is the only or main problem, such as Alzheimer's disease), and 'diseases with dementia' (with obvious other symptoms and signs, but in which dementia may occur, such as Parkinson's disease).

The tasks of the clinician faced with dementia are:

I. diagnosis and prognosis;
II. treatment and care;
III. clinical research and teaching.

Diagnosis

Three questions

In the individual patient with possible dementia, the clinician should ask himself three questions:

(1) Does this patient have dementia or not? If yes:

(2) Does this patient have other neurological signs? These may provide clues to answer:

(3) What is the aetiology — single or multiple — of dementia in this patient? The emphasis should be on detecting treatable causes of dementia.

The conventional clinical approach, i.e. history and examination, followed by ancillary investigations, is applicable in dementia, but with special attention to mental status examination and observation of behaviour.

History and examination

The history is most important and should be taken not only from the patient but also from relatives or other witnesses. Important points are:

— the spontaneous complaint, with mode of onset and time course (slowly progressive or stepwise deterioration?);

— other symptoms (e.g. headache, seizures, gait disorder, incontinence, focal disturbances);

— depressive symptoms, now or in the past;

— previous medical and neurological history (head injury, stroke, hypertension);
— drugs (prescribed or not) and alcohol consumption;
— family history of dementia.

The history — and the way the patient presents it — may reveal disturbance of memory and impairment of cognition, and thus contribute to diagnosing the dementia syndrome (cf. question 1). Moreover, the history may provide clues as to its possible cause (cf. question 3). For example, gradual progression of dementia with intact personality is compatible with Alzheimer's disease; stepwise progression and a history of hypertension and/or strokes with MID; headache and/or seizures with subdural hematoma or cerebral tumour; gait disorder early in the course of dementia with normal pressure hydrocephalus. Both depression and drug intoxications — important treatable causes of dementia — may be diagnosed partly by the history; while hereditary causes of dementia may be ascertained by the family history.

The examination of a patient with dementia demands flexibility and patience, because the subject may be uncooperative and easily tired. It will be clear from the list of causes of dementia that the general physical (internal) examination should be thorough. The neurological examination (cf. question 2) may provide diagnostic pointers (cf. question 3) that save ancillary investigations, which is most important (see below).

Special attention should be paid to:
— consciousness (clouded consciousness precludes the diagnosis of dementia);
— dysphasia and apraxia;
— pseudobulbar signs (dysarthria, reflexes);
— involuntary movements (chorea, myoclonus) and ataxia;
— abnormalities of ocular fundus, pupils and eye movements;
— gait apraxia, marche à petit pas;
— signs of polyneuropathy.

These signs may raise the possibility of specific diseases. For example, dysphasia and apraxia may suggest Alzheimer's disease, whereas pseudobulbar signs and/or marche à petit pas is often found in MID. Other examples: the characteristic dysarthria and pupil signs of general paresis, vertical gaze paresis in progressive supranuclear palsy, chorea in Huntington's disease, ataxia in olivo-ponto-cerebellar atrophy, polyneuropathy in alcohol addiction, and gait apraxia in normal pressure hydrocephalus.

The value of primitive reflexes for the diagnosis of dementia is doubtful (Koller et al., 1982; Tweedy et al., 1982) and one should be aware of the neurological signs often found in normal aged people (Wolfson and Katzman, 1983).

The mental status examination (cf. question 1) is the most difficult and time-consuming part of the procedure, although many excellent descriptions are available (Wells, 1977; Cummings and Benson, 1983; Pearce, 1984). Not only the effects of age should be taken into account, but also previous educational and occupational level. Memory and orientation are tested, as well as intellect and knowledge. Signs of dysphasia, apraxia and agnosia are sought and visuospatial functions are examined. Mood and effect are evaluated, but distinguishing dementia from depression can be extremely difficult.

Observation of spontaneous behaviour (e.g. by the nursing staff) may change diagnostic first impressions, which is an advantage (as opposed to the well-known disadvantages) of clinical observation.

Psychiatric examination may be indicated if behaviour is abnormal. Early personality change occurs in Pick's disease, Huntington's disease and general paresis. Neuropsychological tests are of course invaluable, but are discussed elsewhere in this volume (Jolles, 1986).

Ancillary investigations

Ancillary investigations are usually necessary to establish the aetiology of dementia (cf. question 3), but their use generates problems. They should be performed only as indicated, and not in a 'battery' fashion (see below). An exhaustive list of all

tests that may be needed will not be given here (Cummings and Benson, 1983). The following groups of investigations are available:
— blood and urine tests and other tests for internal medical investigation, see NIA Task Force (1980);
— clinical neurophysiological procedures, e.g. electroencephalography (EEG);
— neuroradiological and nuclear medicine techniques, including computed tomography (CT);
— examination of the cerebrospinal fluid (CSF);
— 'chronography': observation over a period of time may be the best method of investigation in some cases.

Newer techniques, such as magnetic resonance imaging (MRI) and positron emission tomography (PET) will be presented in this volume by Frackowiak (1986).

The CT scan has been a diagnostic breakthrough in the field of dementia as elsewhere, and has rapidly made the highly unpleasant pneumencephalography (PEG) obsolete. In patients with possible dementia, CT may visualise:
— mass lesions (tumour, haematoma, abscess).
— infarct and focal atrophy (e.g. in Pick's disease).
— general atrophy i.e. dilated ventricles and widened sulci; in the interpretation, the age of the patient should be taken into account (Barron et al., 1976; Earnest et al., 1979; Zatz et al., 1982).
— hydrocephalus caused by obstruction of the CSF circulation.
— a variety of other abnormalities, such as leukencephalopathy.

However, dementia cannot be diagnosed by the CT scan. Although a statistical correlation is found between cerebral atrophy and cognitive dysfunction, e.g. in Alzheimer's disease, individual patients with that disease may have normal CT scans, while some normal subjects have cerebral atrophy. Perhaps, exact quantitative measurements may improve the diagnostic results of CT scanning (Damasio et al., 1983; Albert et al., 1984). At present, the greatest yield of CT scanning in the diagnosis of Alzheimer's disease is the exclusion of

other causes, e.g. subdural haematoma and cerebral tumour.

Differential diagnosis

The first question to be answered for the individual patient with possible dementia is: does this patient have dementia or not? The differential diagnosis of the dementia syndrome includes:
— normal aging and 'benign senescent forgetfulness' (Kral, 1962);
— 'pseudodementia' due to depression (Wells, 1979; Caine, 1981);
— confusional states (delirium);
— amnesic syndromes (Korsakoff's syndrome);
— focal neurological dysfunction, such as dysphasia due to left or spatial disorientation due to right hemisphere lesions.

With growing public medicalisation, many elderly people consult their doctors with fear of dementia (males especially seem often unable to remember names; Fisher, 1985). Early diagnosis in dementia will often turn out to be false-positive and memory disturbance is not enough for a diagnosis of dementia.

Depressive 'pseudodementia' is characterised by memory disturbance and cognitive impairment without cortical signs such as dysphasia. The onset is relatively sudden and progression rather rapid. There may have been previous depressions. The patient is distressed, aware of and concerned about the cognitive dysfunction, responding to questions typically with 'I don't know' (Wells, 1979). Information processing is slow, and the clinical picture is reminiscent of subcortical dementia, see below (Caine, 1981). However, dementia and depression can coexist and dementing illnesses can present as depression (Reding et al., 1985).

Delirium (acute confusional state) can be distinguished from dementia by its sudden onset, usually in the context of systemic illness — which should be sought energetically — or toxic exposure. The patient is incoherent, with a fluctuating level of consciousness and poor attention. Tremor, asterixis or myoclonus may be seen and behaviour is restless and anxious, often with evidence of hallucinations. In practice, 'acute dementia' is usually delirium (or aphasia). Properly treated, delirium usually abates. However, a disposition to delirium may be a sign of incipient dementia (NIA Task Force, 1980; Pearce, 1984).

'Subcortical' dementia

When dementia has been concluded to be present in a patient, then the second question is: does this patient have other neurological signs? In this context, the concept of 'subcortical' dementia should be considered. First described in progressive supranuclear palsy (Albert et al., 1974), its main features are forgetfulness, slow responses, apathy, and poor ability to use knowledge. Although this concept is controversial — the clinical distinction between 'cortical' and 'subcortical' dementia may be difficult and the pathological substrate may not be restricted to one or the other — yet it appears useful in clinical diagnosis, especially because most treatable causes of dementia have 'subcortical' characteristics (Cummings and Benson, 1983), see Table II.

As an example of subcortical dementia, Binswanger's subcortical arteriosclerotic encephalopathy should be mentioned. Clinically these patients, usually hypertensive and/or atherosclerotic, pre-

TABLE II

Cortical versus subcortical dementia

Characteristic	Cortical	Subcortical
Speech	normal	dysarthric
Language	aphasic	normal
Memory	amnesia	forgetfulness
Cognition	impaired	slowed
Posture Tone Movement Gait	all normal	may be abnormal

(Modified from Cummings and Benson, 1983)

sent with progressive dementia characterised by marked slowing of response and apathy (giving the impression of depression), and often accompanied by focal neurological signs due to small strokes. On CT scanning, patchy periventricular leukencephalopathy is shown, often combined with small deep infarcts. Possible therapeutic effects remain to be investigated (Rosenberg et al., 1979; Derix et al., 1986).

Strategy in aetiological diagnosis

The third question in diagnosis: what is the aetiology — single or multiple — of dementia in this patient? is answered mainly by using ancillary investigations. These tests are sometimes dangerous, often unpleasant, and usually expensive. Therefore, the diagnostic strategy — which tests to use and when, for what purpose — presents crucial problems. These are aggravated by:
— the great number of patients with dementia, with constraints on facilities and funds;
— the fact that these patients are aged and frail and often tolerate diagnostic procedures poorly;
— the fact that they cannot give 'informed consent' because of their mental state.

No attempt will be made here to propose which procedures should be selected in what patients. However, the general rules for diagnostic strategy are especially compelling in this situation. As explained by Wulff (1981), these can be summarised as follows:

(1) Avoid the 'minimax loss principle', which has the purpose to minimise the maximal loss. Also called the 'better safe than sorry' principle (safe for the doctor), it leads to major investigations to exclude remote diagnostic possibilities. Example: angiography in all patients with dementia to diagnose vasculitis.

(2) Also avoid a purely 'probabilistic' approach, in which the decision to investigate depends only on the probability of the disease. This does not take into account the possible benefit for the patient of the diagnosis in question, and ignores the loss of utility (costs) that the test itself may

cause. Example: brain biopsy in all patients suspected of Alzheimer's disease.

(3) In principle, apply decision analysis, with 'maximisation of expected utility' (Weinstein et al., 1980). The probabilities of diagnoses and the values of outcomes after possible treatment are taken into account, as well as the costs (in terms of morbidity) of diagnostic tests. From those data the expected utility of each diagnostic test is calculated. From all options — including no further investigation — that with the greatest expected utility is chosen. This approach is an aid, not a substitute for clinical reasoning. By making explicit the structure of problems, it facilitates discussion, highlights areas of ignorance, and clarifies the causes of controversy (Politser, 1981). By assigning values to outcomes — difficult as that may be, especially in dementia — it stresses the patient's interests. Decision analysis is at present limited in application by lack of numerical data, which may stimulate clinical research. Examples of this approach: serological tests for syphilis are justified in dementia, even though the probability of neurosyphilis is small, because the test is non-invasive, while the value is great if the diagnosis is made in time; CSF examination may be justified in immuno-compromised patients with dementia, because (though unpleasant) it is not dangerous and may lead to diagnosing cryptococcal meningitis, with therapeutic benefit.

How reliable is diagnosis?

Diagnosing the dementia syndrome is often difficult, with false-negative and false-positive diagnoses as a result. This is clear from the diagnostic delay, which is often years (false-negatives) and from follow-up studies (30% false-positives; Ron et al., 1979). As pointed out above, attempts at early diagnosis will raise the number of false-positives. The reliability of the diagnosis dementia as syndrome depends of course on the definition of dementia and on the patient population, but also on the clinical expertise, as shown by extreme examples (Hoffman, 1982).

Diagnosing the aetiology of dementia may be reliable in some instances, e.g. normal pressure hydrocephalus, if treatment with a CSF shunt results in obvious improvement. However, in most cases, the 'gold standard' of diagnosis is histopathological examination. Moreover, textbook tables are often of the 'a or b' kind (Alzheimer or Pick, Alzheimer or Creutzfeldt-Jakob, or even Alzheimer or non-Alzheimer; Sim, 1979) and are of little use in clinical practice, because the patient may have any of the numerous causes of dementia (Wells, 1977).

Although some authorities state that Alzheimer's disease can be diagnosed positively (Cummings and Benson, 1983), most clinicians are of the opinion that this diagnosis is made by exclusion, and requires pathological proof (Terry and Katzman, 1983). Practical problems are: the clinical heterogeneity in Alzheimer's disease (Mayeux et al., 1985), the changes of clinical features in different stages, the possibility of combinations with other dementing diseases, especially in the very old, and the lack of laboratory proof. Long survival and poor follow-up preclude histopathological verification in most cases. Even in well-studied series, the diagnosis may be found incorrect in some 20% (Sulkava et al., 1983). Recently, a consensus proposal for criteria of 'probable' and 'possible' Alzheimer's disease has been made (McKhann et al., 1984) which must still be tested.

The second most frequent cause of dementia, according to current opinion, is multi-infarct dementia (MID). This term was suggested after it had become clear that 'cerebral atherosclerosis' as such did not cause dementia (Hachinski et al., 1974). An 'ischaemic score' was developed, as criterion for the clinical diagnosis of MID (Hachinski et al., 1975), and later tested pathologically and modified (Rosen et al., 1980). However, though the 'ischaemic score' is a plausible aid to diagnose cerebral infarcts, it provides no proof of the causal relation between such infarcts and the dementia, and it does not exclude other causes. Combinations of MID and Alzheimer's disease (MIX) will look clinically like MID. Although the total volume of cerebral infarcts needed to cause dementia has been studied (Tomlinson et al., 1970), their localisation must also be relevant to dementia, and this clinical problem appears unsolved. Neither CT (Glatt et al., 1983) nor even pathological examination (Brust, 1983) has provided the definitive solution. To provoke further study, one could say that the clinician can only diagnose MIAD (many infarcts *and* dementia). The whole situation reminds one of the once popular diagnosis 'arteriosclerotic Parkinsonism'.

Treatment

Treatable causes

The search for treatable causes of dementia is a comparatively recent development and has been stimulated by the description of normal pressure hydrocephalus (Adams et al., 1965). Some of the most important are listed in Table III.

Depression may present as dementia, especially in the elderly ('pseudo-dementia') and is therefore usually included in this category. It may of course coexist with dementia, and cause further clinical deterioration (Reding et al., 1985). The same applies to the factors called 'secondary' in Table III, and these are stressed here to avoid overemphasis on distinguishing reversible from irreversible dementia (Larson et al., 1984). All clinicians should be aware of the metabolic encephalopathies of old age (Blass and Plum, 1983).

Three patient series have been described, focused on the detection of treatable causes of dementia (Marsden and Harrison, 1972; Freemon, 1976; Smith and Kiloh, 1981). They consisted of 106, 60 and 200 patients respectively, with mean ages of 61, 66 and 58 years, i.e. relatively young patients. All were hospital-based series, collected before CT was available (except for a few patients in the third series). The results were that 15, 30 and 8% of the patients had some treatable condition. However, the outcome for the treatable patients was not described fully in the papers. It can be concluded from the short remarks on that point that, with the exception of depression and chronic drug intoxication, the outcome was often poor. In another series (of 500 patients who were referred for CT scanning because of dementia, mean age 68 years) the same trend becomes apparent (Bradshaw et al., 1983). Though 42 tumours were found, only one of these was a meningioma and most of the others were gliomas and metastases, while not even all patients with hydrocephalus and subdural haematoma actually improved.

Many studies have been made of therapeutic response to a CSF shunt operation in normal pressure hydrocephalus. They will not be enumerated here, but our own experience confirms the general conclusion from the papers: only about

TABLE III

Treatable causes of dementia

Treatable causes (primary)	Treatable causes (secondary)	Treatable causes (neurosurgical)
Depression ('pseudodementia')	Poor nutrition	Some tumours, (meningioma, third
Toxins (drugs, alcohol)	Dehydration	ventricle cyst, acoustic neuroma)
Metabolic (vit. B_{12})	Cardiac failure	Subdural haematoma
Endocrine (hypothyroidism)	Hypoxaemia	Hydrocephalus (NPH)
Infection (neurosyphilis)	Anaemia	Glioma: treatable?
Vascular disease (MID?)	Electrolyte disturbance	
Others, rare	Intercurrent infection	
	Other medical	
	Psychological	

For discussion of the term 'secondary' see text.

half of the patients show worthwhile improvement: whereas complications — some fatal — occur in 10–40% (e.g. infection, subdural haematoma, seizures). This makes the decision 'to shunt or not to shunt' difficult. Again, a decision-analytic approach might be advantageous to the patient; it will then be necessary to quantitate the loss of value caused by dementia, compared to other risks.

How effective is treatment?

Nowadays it is often stated that 15, 20 or even more percent of patients with dementia have 'treatable' conditions. How effective is such treatment? This obviously depends on the specific causes discovered. If depression and chronic drug intoxication are excluded, the main 'treatable' groups left are cerebral tumours (mostly gliomas and metastases) and normal pressure hydrocephalus, with treatment mostly ineffective in the former and 50% effective in the latter. Of course, patients with hypothyroidism, vitamin B_{12} deficiency, neurosyphilis or meningioma may show dramatic response to treatment, but such cases are rare, at least in our experience. Whether MID can be arrested by antihypertensives and/or platelet anti-aggregants remains to be seen. Of course, this is not meant as a defeatist attitude, but as a realistic appraisal of the present situation. 'Treatable' does not always mean 'curable', and — after depressive pseudodementia and drug intoxication have been excluded — treatment appears disappointing except in a small proportion of patients. Proper studies of treatment in dementia are needed, and should be clear about diagnosis (on referral? on admission? at discharge? after follow-up?) and criteria for outcome (is the patient at home? independent? functioning at previous level?).

Management of 'untreatable' dementia

Neurologists cannot claim much credit for their contribution to the care for patients with 'untreatable' dementia. Nevertheless, some remarks should be made on this topic (Pearce, 1984). Too much emphasis on distinguishing between treatable and untreatable (or reversible and irreversible) can lead to neglect of factors that may be influenced (Larson et al., 1984).

The following points are of practical importance:
— activity should be stimulated and social isolation should be prevented; the influence of the environment merits further study;
— deafness should be corrected if possible, and the same holds for cataract;
— attention should be paid regularly to the secondary factors listed in Table III: poor nutrition, dehydration, cardiac failure, chronic hypoxaemia, anaemia, electrolyte disturbance, intercurrent infections, the regulation of diabetes, etc. (Blass and Plum, 1983);
— drugs should be avoided if possible (e.g. nocturnal confusion due to a distended bladder should not be treated with hypnotic drugs), as many drugs may cause confusion even in non-demented elderly people, e.g. digitalis, antihypertensives, hypnotics and sedatives, psychotropics, and anticholinergic drugs such as used in Parkinson's disease; on the other hand, anxiolytic or antipsychotic drugs may be necessary;
— the risks of anaesthesia for cerebral function should be realised;
— depression should be treated, if necessary with antidepressants;
— the relatives should be supported and the agonising decisions about keeping the patient at home or not should not be left to them alone.

Clinical research

It has been argued in this paper that clinical performance in dementia leaves little room for complacency. Diagnosis is unreliable, and treatment disappointing. Therefore, research — including clinical research — becomes all the more important. This will remain true also if progress is made at a more fundamental level. To quote Wulff (1981): "At present there is a need for more research which directly concerns the clinical decision process (assessment of diagnostic tests, therapeutic trials and studies of the natural history of diseases) in order that progress made in the laboratory may be exploited more rationally in clinical practice".

Examples of areas where clinicians, working together with other disciplines, could make useful contributions to the problem of dementia are:
— improvement and quantification of diagnostic methods; development of a positive test for the diagnosis of Alzheimer's disease would be important;
— study of diagnostic strategy, using the methods of decision analysis, to guarantee optimal — not maximal — usage of medical technology;
— further analysis of the pathophysiology of vascular dementia, and the relation with the site of the causative infarcts;
— better description of clinical pictures and their variation; valid measurement of the severity of dementia; longitudinal studies of natural history and prognostic factors;
— evaluation of treatment in 'treatable' forms of dementia, with well-defined criteria of outcome; the same in MID;
— study of the influence of the environment on 'untreatable' dementia, with due attention to patient selection and description, confounding factors and placebo effects;
— if new treatments are developed from basic research, clinical trials will have to be performed, and the design of these trials should be sound (Wulff, 1981; DerSimonian et al., 1982).

As to 'what to measure' in those trials, lessons have been learned from other crippling neurological conditions such as multiple sclerosis and Parkinson's disease: not what is simple to measure for the investigator, but what is of functional importance for the patient should be the final yardstick of therapeutic benefit.

Summary and conclusions

The dementia syndrome has many causes, some of which are treatable. In the diagnosis of dementia three questions should be answered: (1) Does this patient have dementia or not? If yes: (2) Does this patient have other neurological signs? These may provide clues to: (3) What is the aetiology — single or multiple — of dementia in this patient? The emphasis should be on detecting treatable causes. Clinical history and examination, including mental status examination, are all-important in the differential diagnosis, which includes normal aging, depression, delirium, amnesic syndromes and focal neurological dysfunction. The concept 'subcortical' dementia appears useful in the analysis of patients with dementia, as most treatable forms of dementia belong to this group. Ancillary investigations should not be used indiscriminately: neither 'minimax' nor purely 'probabilistic' strategies are permissible or feasible in dementia. The principle of decision analysis should be applied: 'maximisation of expected utility'. Both the diagnosis of the dementia syndrome and of its causes are rather unreliable. Alzheimer's disease is diagnosed by exclusion, no positive test being available yet. Multi-infarct dementia is a problematic concept which needs further research.

Treatable causes of dementia include: depression ('pseudodementia'), drug intoxications, metabolic, endocrine, infective and other conditions, and neurosurgical processes such as normal pressure hydrocephalus, subdural haematomas and cerebral tumours. However, too much emphasis on distinguishing between treatable and untreatable dementia may be harmful. Secondary factors — both medical and psychological — may be remediable, with partial improvement as a result. Though treatable causes of dementia are rightly stressed, the effects of such treatment appear disappointing, except in a small proportion of patients. However, symptomatic management of patients with dementia is important. Regular follow-up is mandatory. Clinicians, working together with other disciplines, could make useful contributions to the many problems of dementia, resulting in more reliable diagnosis and, hopefully, more effective treatment.

Acknowledgement

I wish to thank Dr. G. J. M. Walstra for our fruitful discussions about dementia.

References

Adams, R. D., Fisher, C. M., Hakim, S., Ojemann, R. G. and Sweet, W. H. (1965) Symptomatic occult hydrocephalus with 'normal' cerebrospinal fluid pressure: a treatable syndrome. *N. Engl. J. Med.*, 273: 117–126.

Albert, M. L., Feldman, R. G. and Willis, A. L. (1974) The 'subcortical dementia' of progressive supranuclear palsy. *J. Neurol. Neurosurg. Psychiat.*, 37: 121–130.

Albert, M., Naeser, M. A., Levine, H. L. and Garvey, A. J. (1984) Ventricular size in patients with presenile dementia of the Alzheimer's type. *Arch. Neurol.*, 41: 1258–1263.

Anonymous (1950) Death of a mind. *The Lancet*, i: 1012–1015.

Barclay, L. L., Zemcov, A., Blass, J. P. and Sansone, J. (1985) Survival in Alzheimer's disease and vascular dementias. *Neurology*, 35: 834–840.

Barron, S. A., Jacobs, L. and Kinkel, W. R. (1976) Changes in size of normal lateral ventricles during aging determined by computerized tomography. *Neurology*, 26: 1011–1013.

Blass, J. P. and Plum, F. (1983) Metabolic encephalopathies in older adults. In R. Katzman and R. Terry (Eds.), *The Neurology of Aging*, Davis, Philadelphia, pp. 189–220.

Bradshaw, J. R., Thomson, J. L. G. and Campbell, M. J. (1983) Computed tomography in the investigation of dementia. *Br. Med. J.*, 286: 277–280.

Brown, R. G. and Marsden, C. D. (1984) How common is dementia in Parkinson's disease? *The Lancet*, ii: 1262–1265.

Brust, J. C. M. (1983) Vascular dementia — still overdiagnosed. *Stroke*, 14: 298–300.

Caine, E. D. (1981) Pseudodementia. Current concepts and future directions. *Arch. Gen. Psychiat.*, 38: 1359–1364.

Cummings, J. L. and Benson, D. F. (1983) *Dementia: a Clinical Approach*, Butterworths, London.

Damasio, H., Eslinger, P., Damasio, A. R., Rizzo, M., Huang, H. K. and Demeter, S. (1983) Quantitative computed tomographic analysis in the diagnosis of dementia. *Arch. Neurol.*, 40: 715–719.

Derix, M., Hijdra, A. and Verbeeten, B. (1986) The dementia of subcortical arteriosclerotic encephalopathy, submitted.

DerSimonian, R., Charette, L. J., McPeek, B. and Mosteller, F. (1982) Reporting on methods in clinical trials. *N. Engl. J. Med.*, 306: 1332–1337.

Earnest, M. P., Heaton, R. K., Wilkinson, W. E. and Manke, W. F. (1979) Cortical atrophy, ventricular enlargement and intellectual impairment in the aged. *Neurology*, 29: 1138–1143.

Fisher, C. M. (1985) Vascular disease, senility and dementia. *The Lancet*, i: 173.

Fliers, E., Lisei, A. and Swaab, D. F. (1983) *Dementia. Some current concepts and research in The Netherlands.* A report at the request of the Netherlands Institute for Gerontology, Netherlands Institute for Brain Research, Amsterdam.

Frackowiak, R. S. J. (1986) Measurement and imaging of cerebral function in aging and dementia. In D. F. Swaab, E.

Fliers, M. Mirmiran, W. A. Van Gool and F. Van Haaren (Eds.), *Aging of the Brain and Alzheimer's Disease, Progress in Brain Research, this volume*, Elsevier Science Publishers, Amsterdam, pp. 69–85.

Freemon, F. R. (1976) Evaluation of patients with progressive intellectual deterioration. *Arch. Neurol.*, 33: 658–659.

Glatt, S. L., Lantos, G., Danziger, A. and Katzman, R. (1983) Efficacy of CT in the diagnosis of vascular dementia. *Am. J. Neuroradiol.*, 4: 703–705.

Hachinski, V. C., Lassen, N. A. and Marshall, J. (1974) Multiinfarct dementia. A cause of mental deterioration in the elderly. *The Lancet*, ii: 207–209.

Hachinski, V. C., Iliff, L. D., Zilhka, E., Du Boulay, G. H., McAllister, V. L., Marshall, J., Ross Russell, R. W. and Symon, L. (1975) Cerebral blood flow in dementia. *Arch. Neurol.*, 32: 632–637.

Hoffman, R. S. (1982) Diagnostic errors in the evaluation of behavioral disorders. *J. Am. Med. Assoc.*, 248: 964–967.

Jolles, J. (1986) Cognitive, emotional and behavioral dysfunctions in aging and dementia. In D. F. Swaab, E. Fliers, M. Mirmiran, W. A. Van Gool and F. Van Haaren (Eds.), *Aging of the Brain and Alzheimer's Disease, Progress in Brain Research, this volume*, Elsevier Science Publishers, Amsterdam, pp. 15–39.

Katzman, R. (1976) The prevalence and malignancy of Alzheimer disease. A major killer. *Arch. Neurol.*, 33: 217–218.

Koller, W. C., Glatt, S., Wilson, R. S. and Fox, J. H. (1982) Primitive reflexes and cognitive function in the elderly. *Ann. Neurol.*, 12: 302–304.

Kral, V. A. (1962) Senescent forgetfulness: benign and malignant. *Can. Med. Assoc. J.*, 86: 257–260.

Larson, E. B., Reifler, B. V., Featherstone, H. J. and English, D. R. (1984) Dementia in elderly outpatients: a prospective study. *Ann. Intern. Med.*, 100: 417–423.

Marsden, C. D. and Harrison, M. J. G. (1972) Outcome of investigation of patients with presenile dementia. *Br. Med. J.*, 2: 249–252.

Mayeux, R., Stern, Y. and Spanton, S. (1985) Heterogeneity in dementia of the Alzheimer type: evidence of subgroups. *Neurology*, 35: 453–461.

McKhann, G., Drachman, D., Folstein, M., Katzman, R., Price, D. and Stadlan, E. M. (1984) Clinical diagnosis of Alzheimer's disease: Report of the NINCDS–ADRDA Work Group under the auspices of Department of Health and Human Services Task Force on Alzheimer's Disease. *Neurology*, 34: 939–944.

NIA Task Force (1980) Senility reconsidered. Treatment possibilities for mental impairment in the elderly. *J. Am. Med. Assoc.*, 244: 259–263.

Pearce, J. M. S. (1984) *Dementia, a Clinical Approach*, Blackwell, Oxford.

Plum, F. (1979) Dementia: an approaching epidemic. *Nature*, 279: 372–373.

Politser, P. (1981) Decision analysis and clinical judgment: a re-evaluation. *Med. Decis. Making*, 1: 361–389.

Reding, M., Haycox, J. and Blass, J. (1985) Depression in patients referred to a dementia clinic. A three-year prospective study. *Arch. Neurol.*, 42: 894–896.

Ron, M. A., Toone, B. K., Garralda, M. E. and Lishman, W. A. (1979) Diagnostic accuracy in presenile dementia. *Br. J. Psychiat.*, 134: 161–168.

Rosen, W. G., Terry, R. D., Fuld, P. A., Katzman, R. and Peck, A. (1980) Pathological verification of ischemic score in differentiation of dementias. *Ann. Neurol.*, 7: 486–488.

Rosenberg, G. A., Kornfeld, M., Stovring, J. and Bicknell, J. M. (1979) Subcortical arteriosclerotic encephalopathy (Binswanger): computerized tomography. *Neurology*, 29: 1102–1106.

Sim, M. (1979) Early diagnosis of Alzheimer's disease. In A. I. M. Glen and L. J. Whalley (Eds.), *Alzheimer's Disease. Early Recognition of Potentially Reversible Deficits*, Churchill Livingstone, Edinburgh, pp. 78–85.

Smith, J. S. and Kiloh, L. G. (1981) The investigation of dementia: results in 200 consecutive admissions. *The Lancet*, i: 824–827.

Sulkava, R., Haltia, M., Paetau, A., Wikström, J. and Palo, J. (1983) Accuracy of clinical diagnosis in primary degenerative dementia: correlation with neuropathological findings. *J. Neurol. Neurosurg. Psychiat.*, 46: 9–13.

Terry, R. D. and Katzman, R. (1983) Senile dementia of the Alzheimer type. *Ann. Neurol.*, 14: 497–506.

Tomlinson, B. E., Blessed, G. and Roth, M. (1970) Observations on the brains of demented old people. *J. Neurol. Sci.*, 11: 205–242.

Tweedy, J., Reding, M., Garcia, C., Schulman, P., Deutsch, G. and Antin, S. (1982) Significance of cortical disinhibition signs. *Neurology (NY)*, 32: 169–173.

Weinstein, M. C., Fineberg, H.V. et al. (1980) *Clinical Decision Analysis*, Saunders, Philadelphia.

Wells, C. E. (1977) *Dementia*, 2nd edn., Davis, Philadelphia.

Wells, C. E. (1979) Pseudodementia. *Am. J. Psychiat.*, 136: 895–900.

Wolfson, L. I. and Katzman, R. (1983) The neurologic consultation at age 80. In R. Katzman and R. Terry (Eds.), *The Neurology of Aging*, Davis, Philadelphia, pp. 221–244.

Wulff, H. R. (1981) *Rational Diagnosis and Treatment. An Introduction to Clinical Decision-making*, 2nd edn., Blackwell, Oxford.

Zatz, L. M., Jernigan, T. L. and Ahumada, A. J., Jr. (1982) Changes on computed cranial tomography with aging: intracranial fluid volume. *Am. J. Neuroradiol.*, 3: 1–11.

Discussion

F. W. VREELING: You don't do biopsies of the brain of demented patients. Other clinicians are in favour of performing a biopsy. Could you explain to us why we are against it?

ANSWER: I said that in purely 'probabilistic' medicine, a biopsy would be indicated in suspected Alzheimer's disease. Decision analysis would not lead to biopsy, because there is some morbidity and no therapeutic gain. There are other situations where a biopsy is indicated. In addition, if effective treatment would become available for Alzheimer's disease, biopsy could become indicated.

E. MENA: Finding a quantifiable change in AD patients is important in being able to evaluate any potential treatment. Do you feel that a characteristic such as the rate of decline could be measured?

ANSWER: Some statistical data on rate of decline are available, but in the individual case the rate of progression is hard to predict; there are patients with Alzheimer's disease with 'plateaus' during which they do not deteriorate (Mayeux et al., 1985). This is one reason why control groups in clinical trials are necessary.

J. M. RABEY: Concerning the 'skepticism' about the evidence of a true vitamin B_{12} deficit induced dementia, I recently had the opportunity to treat a patient of 65 years old suffering from gait ataxia and dementia who was misdiagnosed first as 'probable Creutzfeldt-Jakob'. His MCV was 120, the B_{12} level was low. After being given B_{12} injections he improved mentally and physically. The psychodiagrams revealed better performance and he became a fair and independent salesman. So, I wouldn't underestimate the existence of the syndrome. I would like to know your opinion.

ANSWER: I am not 'skeptical' about this, and we look for vitamin B_{12} deficiency in all our patients with dementia; I only said that I have not encountered such a patient yet, but of course I don't question that they exist.

W. VAN TILBURG: For the diagnosis of dementia an evaluation of depressive symptoms is not sufficient. A complete psychiatric evaluation has to be done. Don't you think that your third patient demonstrates this?

ANSWER: Yes, I agree with you. The third patient I discussed was psychiatrically evaluated, though in practice this will not always be feasible.

References

Mayeux, R., Stern, Y. and Spanton, S. (1985) Heterogeneity in dementia of the Alzheimer type: evidence of subgroups. *Neurology*, 35: 453–461.

D. F. Swaab, E. Fliers, M. Mirmiran, W. A. Van Gool and F. Van Haaren (Eds.)
Progress in Brain Research, Vol. 70.
© 1986 Elsevier Science Publishers B.V. (Biomedical Division)

CHAPTER 2

Cognitive, emotional and behavioral dysfunctions in aging and dementia

J. Jolles

Department of Clinical Psychiatry, State University of Limburg, Box. 616, 6200 MD Maastricht, The Netherlands

Introduction

There has been extensive research into psychological dysfunctions in aging and senile dementia over the past 30 years. A number of papers have appeared on deficits in intellectual, memory, language, and several other cognitive functions. The research knowledge has been acquired generally in group comparison studies and — unfortunately — only very recently attempts have been made to use this knowledge for the assessment of individual patients. In addition, attempts to relate the psychological dysfunctions to the underlying cerebral substrate have been relatively scarce.

Assessment of the very early stages of senile dementia is important for several reasons. First of all, it is important to differentiate between 'normal' aging and various psychiatric and neurological diseases, in view of the possible intervention in the disease process by biological (drugs) and non-biological (training, psychotherapy) methods. Treatment in an earlier stage of the disease process can be expected to be more successful in view of the less pronounced structural changes. Secondly, when a person can be diagnosed as being in a (very) early stage of senile dementia, the 'profile' of behavioral, emotional, and cognitive deficits may give some clue as to a possible 'cause' of the disease(s) and its pathogenesis.

In this chapter the research on psychological dysfunctions in aging and dementia, focussing on cognitive and behavioral dysfunction is critically evaluated. Because of the fact that at present early assessment is difficult, this paper also tries to provide some information on the paradigms and methods that are used in the assessment of (senile) dementia and especially in (senile) dementia of the Alzheimer type. It also summarizes the present knowledge on the cerebral substrate involved in aging and dementia, as far as can be concluded from behavioral research in patients. The reader is referred to others for more extensive reviews on the psychological dysfunctions in aging (Botwinnick, 1977, 1981; Jolles and Hijman, 1983), memory (Craik, 1977; Russell, 1981), dementia (Miller, 1981) and psychological assessment in senile dementia (Jolles, 1985; Miller, 1984; Branconnier and DeVitt, 1984).

Cognitive functions in aging and dementia

Perceptual functions

Aging. Several experimental paradigms have been used to study perception in the aged, and the results, generally, point in the same direction. The effect of sensory stimulation seems to persist longer in the central nervous system (CNS) of the aged subject, leading to a less efficient response to subsequent stimulation. This notion evolved from experiments, which started in the forties, with the so-called 'critical flicker fusion' technique: a brief (e.g. 20 ms) light stimulus was presented, followed by others which were separated by a brief time interval of the same duration. When this time interval is progressively shortened, the sequence of light stimuli is 'fused' and the subject sees one steady light. Old people experience fusion at longer interstimulus intervals than young people. This indicates that stimuli are perceived for a longer period of time after discontinuation of the physical stimulus (e.g. Misiak, 1947). Similar findings were obtained with sounds and tactile stimuli (see Botwinnick, 1981 for references).

Other studies supporting the stimulus persistence theory either used the technique of 'backward masking' or that of 'stimulus enhancement': two (different) stimuli are presented, separated by a short time period. When the second stimulus is a masking stimulus, old people are inferior in the recall of the first stimulus (e.g. Kline and Szafran, 1975). When the second stimulus is an 'enhancing' stimulus (that is, when it adds information which is missing in the first), old people performed better than younger persons (Kline and Orme-Rogers, 1978). All the studies mentioned are thus in line with the notion that elderly people perceive the first stimulus for a longer time. Similarly, visual after-effects seem to be present for a longer time period in the old (Kline and Nestor, 1977). Neuropsychologically, a lack of inhibition of irrelevant information may underly this stimulus persistence.

Elderly subjects required more time to process visual input (Eriksen et al., 1970) and they have been found to be inferior in tasks in which parts of a complex visual figure have to be integrated to a meaningful whole (Hooper, 1958). In addition, figure-background discrimination is harder for the elderly than for the young (Axelrod and Cohen, 1961).

In conclusion, elderly people are inferior in tasks of simple and complex perception. This may partly be because stimuli, once perceived, are present for a longer period of time, partly because an efficient perception takes more time.

Dementia. Some perceptual deficits have been demonstrated in demented patients (Willanger and Klee, 1966). Visuospatial functions deteriorate as deduced from observations in visuoconstructive tasks in which the patient is required to copy drawings. These tasks are among the tests frequently used in the assessment of dementing patients (Strub and Black, 1981). Patients with senile dementia have difficulty in solving paper and pencil mazes; they also have an impaired appreciation of reflected space (such as mirrorview) (Botwinnick, 1981). Demented subjects may also experience a disintegration of the body scheme and they are impaired in tasks that require the subjects to fit together pictures of different parts of the human body (Miller, 1981).

Data are scarce with respect to the question whether deficits in simple sensory functions exist in dementia. Some studies suggest that elementary perceptual functions might stay intact longer than more complex functions in Alzheimer-type dementia (see Sulkava and Amberla, 1982).

Language functions

Aging. A large body of evidence suggests that verbal abilities do not deteriorate with age. Indeed, many authors have demonstrated that some verbal abilities in normal elderly subjects are superior to those of young controls (e.g. Goldstein and Shelly, 1975; Goldstein, 1980). Waugh and Barr (1980) thus demonstrated that normal elderly subjects are slightly faster than young normals in a naming latency task which assessed the speed of retrieval of words from the internal lexicon. A similar conclusion has been reached by others (Drachman and Levitt, 1972; Eysenck, 1975) in experiments using 'category instance fluency' tests for free and cued production of exemplars of specific categories. Word finding difficulties are seldom observed in normal aging, in contrast to difficulties with respect to finding names or episodes (see below, 'memory functions'). Several authors suggest that the fairly stable verbal IQ in 'normal' aging is a manifestation of the verbal functions which do not deteriorate with age (see below, 'intellectual functions' and Botwinnick, 1981).

Dementia. Language deficits are a frequently observed symptom in Alzheimer's disease (AD) (Strub and Black, 1977, 1981). Word naming deficits appear already fairly early in the disease process (Benson, 1979) and the nature and extent of the language deficits change with progression of the disease. Ernst et al. (1970) showed that their demented subjects had a general poverty of vocabulary in narrative speech in common, but many dementing subjects showed impairments in object naming. In other studies, age-matched controls also showed a relative impairment in naming, although demented patients were clearly inferior in this respect (Barker and Lawson, 1968; Lawson and Barker, 1968). A demonstration of the way in which an object could be used (confrontation naming) improved naming in the demented patients but had no effect in the control subjects. This may mean that the demented patients do not recognize the object and are, therefore, not able to find the correct word. Patients who are aphasic due to a focal lesion in the posterior parts of the neocortex may also be deficient in object naming but the aphasic, in contrast to the demented patient, characteristically gives the strong impression that he knows what the object is without being able to find the right word to describe it (Rockford, 1971). In experiments designed to assess word production in demented patients, Miller and Hague (1975) used a fluency task in which the subjects were required to produce words beginning with a certain letter. It appeared that these patients produce fewer words in a 5-min period than controls, but demented patients did not rely on a small set of commonly used words, as might have been expected. In other words, the data are not consistent with the hypothesis that the pattern of word use is different in aged versus demented people.

When AD progresses to later stages, verbal output becomes 'empty' and circumlocutory. Demented patients increasingly show repetitive elements in their speech. This repetitiveness may in some instances be a type of perseveration resulting from linking a word inappropriately to an object when the same word has been linked appropriately just before (Botwinnick, 1981). The lexicon becomes impoverished but there is evidence to suggest that syntactic processes are less affected (Irigaray, 1973). In addition to a deterioration of expressive language, receptive aspects of language are also impaired. At still later stages, the involuntary repetition of words spoken by others (echolalia) becomes more common. In the final stages of the disease global aphasia may be present, resulting in undirected babbling in which only syllables are uttered.

The clear-cut differences in language functions in aged versus demented subjects have led to proposals to use language tests in the clinical assessment of subjects suspected of incipient dementia. The use of 'category instance fluency' tests (Branconnier and DeVitt, 1984) and the 'Nelson adult reading' test (Nelson and McKenna, 1975) are examples of such a strategy.

Memory functions

On memory and memory dysfunctions

Since memory complaints are among the most frequently reported signs of decreasing abilities in both normal aged and dementing subjects, an enormous amount of research has been directed at establishing the nature of memory disorders in aging and dementia. Generally, different kinds of memory and memory disorders have been characterized (see Russell, 1981). In the clinic the term 'remote memory' is used to describe retrieval of information which has been acquired many years ago. The term 'recent memory', on the other hand, is used to describe retrieval of information which has been acquired some months, weeks, or only days ago. Much research has been centered around the concepts of 'short-term memory' or 'long-term memory' in the sixties, whereas a more recent trend in memory research asks the question 'how information is processed and used'.

An information processing type of theory states

that information from the environment is sensed by the sensory registers (visual, auditory, tactile, etc.) and passed on to a central processing unit. There is temporary storage in short-term memory (primary memory), and the information is then transferred to long-term storage (secondary memory or long-term memory) by a process of 'memory consolidation'. 'Retrieval' from storage in long-term memory makes the information available again. Recent trends in memory research discuss the importance of the strategies which subjects use to consolidate and retrieve information (encoding processes, rehearsal, use of mnemonic aids, active search, etc.).

A quantitative analysis of the temporal retention of verbal and non-verbal information has been used most extensively both in the laboratory and in the clinic to assess these different aspects of memory.

With respect to the methods of assessing retention, 'recognition' and 'recall' are direct and 'relearning' is indirect (Deese and Hulse, 1967). Tulving and Pearlstone (1966) have shown a distinction between what is in memory ('availability') and what can be retrieved from it ('accessibility'). Recall performance has frequently been shown to be correlated with the degree of initial storage but to be an insensitive indicator of availability (Hulicka and Weiss, 1965; Slamecka, 1967). Recognition performance, on the other hand, is a more sensitive measure of availability than recall (accessibility).

Aging. Memory complaints are frequently encountered in elderly people and several memory deficits can indeed be assessed by psychometric tests. An impairment in the accessibility or availability of new (and old) information is thus a cognitive deficit associated with normal aging. This memory impairment is what Kral (1962) calls 'benign senescent forgetfulness' (BSF), the inability to recall unimportant or minor details of an episode while the episode itself can be recalled. This deficit is not permanent and the information might be recalled on a different occasion.

Research of memory deficits in aging has shown that elderly subjects have an impaired sensory memory. This first stage in information processing lasts several hundred ms in healthy young subjects (e.g. Sperling, 1960). When very short stimulus durations (50 ms) were used, only two out of ten elderly subjects showed normal sensory memory as compared to nine out of nine controls (Walsh, 1975). With stimulus presentations of longer duration (100 ms), sensory memory was present, but to a lesser extent than in young persons (Salthouse, 1976).

The second stage in information processing is also very temporary in nature. It lasts several seconds and is conceived by some as a kind of working memory: short-term memory is more a temporary 'holding' and organizational process than a structured memory store (Craik, 1977). According to Botwinnick (1981) old and young subjects behave similarly in short-term memory tests as long as the number of items to be recalled does not exceed about four or five. However, in view of the fact that some authors define short-term memory as a type of memory that can retain seven items plus or minus two (Miller, 1956), older people may be somewhat impaired when compared to younger subjects.

The third stage in the processing of new information is the consolidation into long-term memory. An efficient consolidation requires some kind of organization of the information to be stored. The formation of new memories can be strengthened by rehearsal, mnemonic aids, imagery and other coding strategies, and it is especially the use of these strategies which seems to be impaired in the aged (Craik, 1977). Generally, elderly people are inferior in tasks involving acquisition and retrieval of new information. More specifically, some investigators found that aged subjects do not use memory search strategies spontaneously, even when the experimenter presents such a strategy (Arenberg and Robertson-Tchabo, 1977; Craik, 1977). It is only under some circumstances that the subjects can be encouraged to do so (Treat and Reese, 1976). These findings may indicate that old people are less able to (actively) manipulate and organize the content of short-term memory (Craik, 1977); there is an age-associated deficit in the use of cues which are important for encoding (consolidation) processes. A similar finding has been done with respect to retrieval processes. There is a preponderance of experimental evidence showing that an increase in age is associated with deterioration of recall performance while recognition is not affected (e.g. Schonfield and Stones, 1979; Erber, 1974). This observation has been interpreted in terms of a retrieval deficit which may be due to ineffective search (Branconnier and DeVitt, 1984) and/or to ineffective use of strategies (Jolles and Hijman, 1983).

An important parameter with respect to the formation of stable memories is the speed with which the information is presented and/or reproduced. Old subjects performed less well than younger subjects, when the presentation rate in a word-learning test was high. This age-associated deficit was also present when the time to respond was short. When the time limits were not so strict, age-associated deficits were not found (Arenberg, 1965; Kinsbourne and Berryhill, 1972). Another parameter which has been studied in relation to aging is the susceptibility to interference: some studies claim that older people are more susceptible than younger subjects, but others conclude that such age differences do not exist (see Craik, 1977).

Dementia. Memory research in dementing subjects has, generally, been aimed at defining some stage in which these patients might be specifically impaired as compared to 'benign senescent forgetfulness' and depression (e.g. Branconnier and DeVitt, 1984). Most of the research which has been carried out was concerned with the distinction between short-term and long-term memory.

There seems not to have been much research on sensory memory in demented patients, possibly because these experiments are difficult to conduct with these patients (Miller, 1981). One study used the 'backward masking paradigm' to measure iconic memory. Demented patients were inferior to non-demented controls in reporting the first stimulus, indicating that masking had occurred. According to Miller (1977), this could be due to a defect in attention or iconic memory, and/or an enhanced susceptibility to interference. According to the theory on stimulus persistence, there may have been a lack of inhibition of the first percept.

With respect to short-term memory, Inglis (1957, 1959) found that elderly psychiatric patients were slow to learn paired associates. Performance was inferior to that of controls in both recall and recognition. This is suggestive of a problem in acquisition rather than in retention (see Branconnier and DeVitt, 1984). Later experiments favored the hypothesis that short-term memory did not function properly (Inglis, 1960, but see Miller, 1981). Experiments in which a word list had to be learned give some clue as to the differential involvement of short-term and long-term memory: characteristically, the first and the last words of such a list are learned better than words in the middle of the list. Better retention of the last words in the list is ascribed to the fact that these words are still in short-term memory, while the superior recollection of the first words is ascribed to the fact that these are already transferred to long-term memory. Characteristically, demented patients do not show a better retention of the first and last words of a list. This finding may be taken to indicate that demented patients experience both a short-term and a long-term memory deficit (Miller, 1981).

Of course, the long-term memory deficit could be secondary to the impairment in short-term memory. This hypothesis has been tested by Miller (1972). He presented the words in the list at a slower rate, and found that control subjects performed better in this condition, as indicated by the number of words recalled from the beginning of the list. The demented patients did not benefit from the slower presentation rate. These findings were interpreted to show that the patients did not use the opportunity to increase the consolidation of short-term into long-term memory, indicating that the memory impairment in dementia has at least two components (involving STM and LTM). The notion that long-term memory is involved was supported by the finding that demented patients have appreciable difficulty in learning word lists which are longer than the memory span (i.e. the number of words that can be correctly recalled after a single presentation). Long-term memory is essential for this supra-span learning (Miller, 1972).

The performance deficits discussed above have been interpreted in different ways. Memory processes could be involved but the impairments could also be a secondary consequence of an attentional deficit or impaired sensory memory. Furthermore, a decreased ability in the use of coding strategies is also probable: this notion is supported by the fact that acoustically presented material was coded less efficiently by demented patients (Miller, 1972).

Word list learning experiments are also used to measure long-term memory. Experimentally, recall and/or recognition are tested after an interval in which distraction prevents the subject from rehearsing the words. It has been shown that demented patients perform badly in the delayed recall and delayed recognition condition (Miller, 1975). However, the patients are indistinguishable from controls in a 'partial information' condition in which the subjects were given the initial letters of the words as a cue. Similar findings have been observed in patients suffering from the amnesic syndrome (Warrington and Weiszkrantz, 1970). The data indicate that some trace has been formed which is too weak to get expressed unless extra cues are given which enhance it. Such an interpretation suggests that retrieval is also inferior in demented patients in addition to an improper memory consolidation (resulting in weak traces). Again, this may be due to a decreased or inefficient use of coding strategies (see above). According to Miller (1981) there is not a clear difference between aged and demented subjects in this respect, but it is known that both groups of subjects perform worse than younger controls. An alternative explanation for the partial information effect was given by

Warrington and Weiszkrantz (1970): successful performance would depend not only on the ability to recall the correct words but also on the ability to inhibit the recall of incorrect words. However, Miller (1978) tested this 'disinhibition hypothesis' and did not find data to support it. It was observed, however, that demented patients became progressively less able to recognize a correct word from several alternatives as the number of alternatives increased. That the choice between alternatives is difficult for these patients was also found in an experiment in which a single choice (yes/no) was compared to a forced choice between yes and no (two alternatives). The forced choice appeared to lead to better performance (Whitehead, 1975), possibly because a response is elicited also when the patient is insecure. The personality characteristic '(over)cautiousness' may prevent the elderly/dementing subject from responding in other choice situations. In other words, the elderly subject has a 'negative response bias'; he prefers to choose 'no' unless he is really sure that the answer has to be different.

Taken together, the memory studies indicate that demented patients are inferior to age-matched controls in several aspects of memory, especially those relating to the acquisition of new information (sensory memory, short-term memory and long-term memory; recent memory). With respect to remote memory, the issue is less clear. The commonly held belief that old people have a good preservation of remote memory may not be right. Clinical observations suggest that some 'childhood memories' can become dominant at the cost of other memories, indicated by many gaps in remote memory (Jolles and Hijman, 1983).

Intelligence

Aging. The question whether intelligence decreases with age has been extensively studied during the last decades. However, despite many studies, in which a gradual decrease in intelligence test scores was found with age, the matter is still controversial (Botwinnick, 1977, 1981). Traditionally, research into intelligence of aged (or demented) subjects has been performed according to the psychometric tradition, which uses standardized test batteries. An important parameter which has often been studied with the Wechsler Adult Intelligence Scale (WAIS), is the differential response on 'verbal' versus 'performal' subtests of this test battery. It has been demonstrated many times that the verbal IQ (VIQ) does not decline significantly until fairly old age in normal subjects whereas the performal IQ (PIQ) decreases more rapidly with age. Several interpretations have been offered to explain this differential response. A suggestion which has often been made takes speed factors into account. The inferior performance on performal subtests of the WAIS might be due to a general slowness in the subjects studied, as these tests tend to be timed, whereas the verbal subtests are not (Botwinnick, 1977; Miller, 1981). However, slowing becomes a less attractive explanation as scores on other intelligence tests (such as the Mill Hill Vocabulary Scale and Progressive Matrices) are also decreased though these tests are not timed (Miller, 1981). According to another explanation, the VIQ/PIQ discrepancy reflects the fact that the performance on visuo-constructive tasks determines the PIQ, indicating that a selective loss of visuo-constructive (or visuo-integrative) ability might underlie the intellectual deterioration. The most probable interpretation, however, refers to the fact that the verbal subtests measure well-practised and overlearned activities whereas the performal subtests measure the ability to deal with new tasks and the acquisition of new information (Botwinnick, 1977, 1981; Miller, 1981). The selective deficit of aging subjects on performal subtests of the WAIS may thus have to do with impaired memory or learning ability more than with anything else (Miller, 1981). In addition to speed, memory, verbal and perceptual factors, a factor called 'general ability' is an important determinant for the performance on intelligence tests. This indicates that educational level is important for the IQ score found, and explains the finding that the correlation between chronological age and intelligence is rarely as high as .50 (Botwinnick, 1981). Taken together, studies with intelligence tests have not provided unequivocal results with respect to the nature of the deficits in aging. The same applies for dementia.

Dementia. As the term 'dementia' implies a disturbance in cognitive functioning, many studies have addressed themselves to the determination of intellectual deficits in dementing subjects. As was evident from the foregoing discussion, intellectual changes become evident in the course of the illness. These clinical observations have been substantiated in experimental studies in which demented patients showed a lowered mean IQ (Miller, 1977) compared to age-matched controls. Unfortunately, research into the differential performance on 'verbal' versus 'performal' subtests of the WAIS has not yielded clear insights into the cognitive functions underlying the intellectual deterioration of dementing patients. The interpretational problems are similar to those encountered in the study of intellectual functioning in normal aged subjects. Thus, the performal IQ of demented patients is much more decreased than the verbal IQ, but it is not easy to characterize the underlying deficit as being due to general slowness, failing memory or problem solving ability, or other factors (Miller, 1981). Those authors who conceive of dementia as a disease process in which 'crystallized intelligence' (abilities which are well practised and overlearned) is relatively more preserved than 'fluid intelligence' (new activities which do not rely upon familiar or routine strategies), simply rephrase the findings in other terms and thus add little to our knowledge of what is happening in dementia (Miller, 1981). The findings, until now, do not indicate that there is more than a quantitative difference between normal aging and dementia of the Alzheimer type.

Recently, some attention has been given to the notion that the profile of scores on the WAIS subtests might be characteristic of a particular type of dementia (for review see Fuld, 1984). It has been suggested that such a profile might be of relevance for the clinical differentiation of AD from other dementing processes. Unfortunately, the results add little to our insight into the nature of the cognitive deficits in dementia.

Behavioral organization

Elderly people perform badly on those tasks which require the initiation, planning and evaluation of complex behavioral acts. This has been interpreted by some as a deficit in 'problem solving' (by Arenberg, 1965), by others as an impaired 'planning' or 'behavioral organization' (e.g. Luria, 1966, 1973). In addition, several studies have attributed the difficulties to 'inflexibility', defined in terms of 'giving up a selection procedure that once was effective but no longer is' (Heglin, 1956), or the 'inability to shift concepts' (Wetherick, 1965). Others have shown that elderly people generally are less able to discern relevant from irrelevant information: a redundancy of irrelevant information was found to be disruptive to problem solving behavior (Arenberg, 1965). In addition, there was less efficient use of environmental cues for an optimal plan of action. For instance, when asking for extra information regarding the problem to be solved, old subjects performed in a more haphazard fashion. Likewise, there was a lack of order in their information seeking (see Botwinnick, 1981 for references). Characteristically, they did not have explicit knowledge of their goal until very late (Jerome, 1962). Interestingly, certain personality characteristics which are often found in, and attributed to aged people, can be interpreted in terms of inflexibility, decreased concept shift and impaired ability to use (new) environmental information. This applies especially to trends towards introversion, conservatism and cautiousness, and to the reluctance in making decisions, especially when the outcome is uncertain (Botwinnick, 1981).

It will be clear that an inferior performance of elderly people on complex tests of memory, perception and other cognitive functions can be attributed to difficulties in behavioral organization/

problem solving ability, unless care is taken that instructions and procedure are really understood by the subject. Neuropsychologically, the deficits described (inflexibility, difficulty with concept shifts, deficient use of environmental information to guide one's own behavior) may be indicative of a primary deficit in the planning, control and evaluation of the behavior, and thus of frontal cortex involvement (Luria, 1966, 1973; Fuster, 1980; Jolles, 1985). For the frontal neocortex monitors and programs activity of the whole cortex and creates the necessary conditions for the integration of environmental information with memories, to make an optimal action plan and to monitor its outcome.

The nature of the deficits in planning and behavioral organization in (Alzheimer type) dementia, seem similar to those in 'normal' aging but are much more readily apparent. Unfortunately, only a few studies have been performed with AD patients (but see Lawson et al., 1967; Hibbard et al., 1975).

Motor functions

There has been a substantial amount of research on motor dysfunctions in aging. Welford (1977) in his comprehensive review of the literature, and his own research over the past 30 years, used an information processing model to describe the different aspects of motor functioning. In his view, the flow of information may be envisaged to pass through several discrete stages, such as (1) sensation (level of the senses), (2) perception (within CNS), (3) translation from perception to action (CNS), (4) effector control (CNS), and (5) motor output (level of peripheral nerves and muscles). Stages 3 and 4 refer to the integration of information from the senses, the generation of plans to use this information for an act, and the computation of the motor performance. This planning is a prerequisite in order to perform the planned action in a sequential order (Luria, 1973, 1966).

According to Welford (1977) the main limitations in motor performance which elderly people experience seem due to a combination of a reduced speed, and less efficient information processing in stages 3 and 4. He concluded that aged subjects are considerably slower in performing relatively large movements at maximum speed. This seems primarily due to peripheral (e.g. muscular) limitations. Most other movements are not limited by muscular factors but by the speed of the decisions that have to be made to guide movements. When decisions can be made beforehand, such as in simple reaction time tasks, and in simple repetitive movements, the change with age is relatively small. The performance on a new or complex task, however, is much slower; the extra time is needed for the planning of (the stages of) the motor act. In addition, elderly people pay more attention (and thus more time) to the signals presented before they act. This is especially the case when the relation between signal and response is not straightforward. The performance of elderly people becomes slower and less accurate when the subject has to choose between alternatives or when an extra judgement of spatial relations has to be made (see Welford, 1977). Clearly, such a complex motor task has the characteristics of a problem solving task as discussed above.

Thus, the performance on simple tasks which do not require a complex 'computation' of the motor act is relatively normal in aged people. The performance in complex motor tasks and in tasks requiring complex sensorimotor integration is inferior in old, compared to young people because of the extra time needed for decision making and planning of the movement to be performed. This is, once again, an indication for a planning deficit more than a deficit in motor performance per se.

Discussion

The performance in virtually all the cognitive functions which can be tested decreases with age. Elderly subjects are characterized by a deterioration in intellectual functioning, memory, language functions, problem solving and perception. It

seems that specific parameters are more involved than others. For instance, elderly people are not inferior in tasks in which they can rely on well-established skills and knowledge, whereas they perform poorly in tasks involving new information, especially in situations in which the planning of new activities or the active use of coding strategies in recent memory is important. In addition, trends towards inflexibility, cautiousness and conservatism are found, which are paralleled by 'stimulus persistence'. Finally, the speed of information processing seems to decrease with age.

With respect to AD, evidence has not been found to show that the pattern of cognitive deficits would be different from that seen in 'normal' aging (Jolles and Hijman, 1983), especially with respect to the earlier stages in the development of the dementia. Dementing subjects perform significantly inferiorly to age-matched controls on all functions tested, but there is not a different pattern in their deficits. Thus, more or less profound deterioration is found with respect to perception, memory, language, higher cognitive functions, planning, rate of information processing and other cognitive functions (Jolles and Hijman, 1983; Miller, 1981). In addition to the deficits seen in normal subjects, AD patients also deteriorate with respect to recognition memory and verbal IQ measures which stay at a fairly constant level in normal aging.

It is important to acknowledge that the major part of the studies described above reflects group comparison data. Unfortunately, this reduces the direct application of the results in clinical assessment of (individual) patients. Several investigators have proposed particular methods of investigation which are based upon the knowledge which has been described (see for instance Branconnier and DeVitt, 1984). There are several additional methodological problems. There are important differences between the studies with respect to the characteristics of the patient population described. Some studies do not clearly discern primary degenerative dementia from dementias of other origin. Furthermore, the progress of the disease (the stage) is often not described, which makes the comparison of different studies difficult, if at all possible. This indicates that future research in this field may benefit from a careful clinical diagnosis of the patients involved, and from the use of standardized classification systems such as DSM-III (Clayton and Martin, 1981). In addition, control groups of age-matched or other control subjects should also be assessed carefully, especially in view of differences in personality characteristics, which tend to confuse age-associated cognitive changes: for instance, some people over 65 years of age do not retire and remain active until high age. Other elderly people retire and become inactive (see Botwinnick, 1981; Miller, 1981); either because they want to, or because society isolates them. These social and personality factors will have a profound influence on psychological (coping) mechanisms and the social relations of these subjects, and thus on their cognitive functioning. In addition to the factors mentioned, the studies reviewed differ with respect to the age of the subjects but the brain of a subject aged 85 with incipient dementia can be expected to differ from that of a similar patient, aged 65! Future research must take these methodological points into consideration.

Differential diagnosis and stages in Alzheimer's disease

Differential diagnosis

Traditionally, (neuro)psychologists working in a psychiatric setting are frequently asked to assess whether a particular patient is dementing or not. It appears very difficult to differentiate early stages of senile dementia from depression. In the first place, early stages in dementia are very frequently accompanied by a depressed mood (Jolles and Hijman, 1983; Strub and Black, 1981). This depression is most probably a secondary consequence of the subjective feeling that there is cognitive deterioration (see for instance Strub and Black, 1981). There is evidence to suggest that the

major catecholaminergic pathways that are involved in depression (Van Praag, 1982) are also involved in the pathogenesis of AD (Rossor, 1982). There may thus be a common cerebral substrate in both depression and dementia. Secondly, profoundly depressed patients frequently display overt signs of dementia such as slowness, general inertia, disorientation and memory disturbances. The differentiation of depression and dementia based on clinical observation alone thus appears very difficult. A thorough neuropsychological investigation may be of importance in this respect. Preliminary results presented in Jolles (1985) suggest that neuropsychological methods and theory may contribute to the differentiation of depression and dementia.

With respect to the differentiation of 'normal' aging from senile dementia, it is very difficult to discriminate between BSF and incipient dementia. Very recently, some authors have proposed the use of some newer methods to accomplish this discrimination. Much emphasis is given to the differentiation between active recall and passive recognition in learning tasks, and to the use of verbal tasks such as the 'Nelson adult reading task' (Nelson and McKenna, 1975), 'category instance fluency' tests (Branconnier and DeVitt, 1984) and computer-aided tests based upon an information processing paradigm (see below and Poon, 1983; Jolles, 1985).

Clear differences seem to exist in the pattern of cognitive deficits seen in other types of dementia. For instance, the (pre)senile dementia of Pick's type shows pronounced behavioral disturbances such as inappropriate social behavior and bizarre behavior, and deficits in the planning and organization of behavior. These deficits are not accompanied by intellectual deterioration or amnesia and are characteristic for dysfunctions of the frontal lobe. This neuropsychological interpretation is in line with current knowledge on the cerebral substrate of Pick's disease which appears to be a fairly specific degeneration of frontal lobe areas (see Strub and Black, 1981).

A differentiation between primary degenerative

dementia (e.g. AD) and dementias of vascular origin can usually be made after careful examination of the pattern of cognitive deficits. Those dementias which depend primarily on vascular disorders ('multiinfarct dementia') seem to be characterized more often by focal deficits. For instance, a patient who has difficulty in object naming (anomia) without a concomitant impairment in object recognition or apraxia may be suffering from localized cerebral dysfunctions, as a result of cerebral vascular insufficiency in the left temporoparietal region. Likewise, a patient with modality-specific deficits for complex visual material and disorientation in space without a memory deficit for verbal material, almost certainly does not suffer from a primary degenerative dementia but may have had infarct(s) confined to right hemisphere structures. The interpretation proposed here may be problematic because of the fact that in primary degenerative dementia multiple small infarctions may accompany the degeneration of cortical tissue, such that the cognitive dysfunctions which are evident in a particular patient may result from both the infarctions and neuronal degeneration (Strub and Black, 1981; Jolles, 1985).

The progression of clinical signs of dementia

The signs and symptoms of AD have been described by many investigators and researchers. However, there are few detailed accounts of the symptomatic progression of the disease. Sjögren and coworkers (1952) have defined three clinically distinct stages. Stage I is characterized by — among others — incipient dementia, memory disturbances (including anomia) and spatial disorientation. In stage II, the dementia becomes more pronounced with marked disturbances in memory and disorientation with apraxia, agnosia, aphasia, etc. In the terminal stage (III) there is no cognitive activity left and only vegetative functions remain. Reisberg (1983) and Reisberg et al. (1982) describe the progression of symptoms in seven stages which range from 'normal' via 'early', 'middle' and 'late confusion' to 'early', 'middle' and 'late dementia'.

The classification proposed by Reisberg is appealing in its systematic description of cognitive and observational items that help in the characterization of the stage of the disease. It will be evident that a more systematic classification will be of much value both for clinical and scientific purposes.

The following account of the progression of the symptomatology of AD is based upon the work of Strub and Black (1981). They described a clear evolution of the successive stages in the temporal sequence of the disease:

Stage 1. Changes in social behavior and expressed emotions are among the very early signs of primary degenerative dementia. There is a lack of normal initiative and interest in family, work and other activities. Increased fatigue and restlessness are frequently noted in this stage, as well as depression and anxiety. Some patients are overly concerned with somatic complaints whereas others deny any problem. There is often an accentuation of previous personality traits super-imposed upon a background of euphoria or apathy. In other patients, personality changes are noted which are quite uncharacteristic of the premorbid personality (e.g. inappropriate or bizarre behavior). This applies especially to patients with extensive frontal lobe lesions such as those suffering from Pick's disease, Huntington's chorea or general paresis.

Cognitive changes such as memory deficits are the most frequently noted early signs of the disease process. The patient forgets names and recent events, and experiences increasing trouble in finding things around the house. Recent memory seems to be affected more than remote memory. In addition to memory, general problem solving ability deteriorates; this is most evident in new tasks in which the patient cannot rely upon well-established skills and routines. Furthermore, comprehension and the expression of complex ideas, abstract thinking and critical judgement deteriorate. More basic cognitive deficits also become evident, such as an impaired visuo-motor integrative ability. A routine neurological examination is usually normal in this stage.

Stage 2. The signs noted in stage 1 accentuate. The patient is less able to manage his personal and business affairs, because of failing memory and lack of initiative. Several language problems also become evident although they do not yet reach the level of clear-cut aphasia: speech remains fluent at first, but circumlocutions and paraphasias appear, and the patient experiences difficulties in word finding. The ability to express abstract thoughts decreases and there is an overall decrease in intellectual functioning. The restlessness already noted in stage 1 increases; patients become upset at night, and they tend to wander around. They may constantly be manipulating things in their hands. Emotionally, patients in this stage often retain sufficient insight into their condition to develop secondary anxiety and depression; the dementia may thus appear more severe than it is.

Stage 3. With further progression, the patients develop a clear aphasia, apraxia and agnosia. Spontaneous speech decreases further; there is a tendency to echo what is said (echolalia); there is greatly reduced comprehension and an inability to name objects. This anomia appears to be more than a simple problem in finding the correct word: the patient characteristically acts as if not recognizing the object and the failure therefore is a visual agnosia. An ideomotor apraxia develops, i.e. a difficulty with the execution of previously learned skilled movements, such as combing the hair. In addition, a so-called ideational apraxia develops, which is a total disruption in the ability to carry out a complex action composed of several relatively independent acts (such as taking a match from a box and lighting a cigarette). Inattention and distractibility become very common in this stage, as well as involuntary emotional outbursts. A number of primitive/infantile reflexes reappear and are now evident from neurological investigation. In addition, involuntary movements are noted, and urinary and fecal incontinence begins. In short, the patient experiences increasing difficulty in inhibiting natural reflexes. In some patients features of organic psychosis are prominent.

Stage 4. (terminal stage). The patient becomes uncommunicative, uttering only short phrases of undirected babbling. Emotions are involuntary, delusions appear and the patient finally gets completely apathetic and withdrawn. More neurological signs become apparent, including generalized seizures (in 22% of the patients during the last year of life) (Sjögren et al., 1952). Death usually results from pneumonia, aspiration or urinary infection (see Strub and Black, 1981 for more detailed account).

Stages in dementia: methodological issues

Alzheimer's disease can occur at any age, and the course of the illness is variable: some patients live only a few months after initial assessment, but 25–30% of the patients live over 10 years, and some live over 20 years (Corsellis, 1976). The average life span from diagnosis to death is slightly over seven years (Sjögren et al., 1952). It is important to determine whether the dementing process is similar in these individuals of different ages. Although the succession of stages seems to be identical in presenile versus senile forms of AD (e.g. Sulkava and Amberla, 1982), there is an increasing amount of research papers describing differences in either neurobiological variables (e.g. Rossor, 1982) or neuropsychological variables (Friedland et al., 1985).

Although similarities exist between different forms of primary progressive dementia (e.g. Alzheimer's disease versus Pick's disease), several differences are also evident.

The sequence emerging in senile dementia of Alzheimer's type is different from that noted in Pick's disease although the terminal stages may be similar (Strub and Black, 1981). Careful examination of the mental status of the patient is therefore very important for an early diagnosis of any dementia, as neurological signs develop only in the terminal stages. An extensive neuropsychological evaluation may therefore be the only means for an early diagnosis (Jolles, 1985).

In view of the temporal sequence in the

development of symptoms, there is quite some variation within the demented groups: of course patients in the first stages differ in quantitative and qualitative ways from those in the later stages.

Besides, there is a quite considerable variation due to personality characteristics, as premorbid personality tends to be exaggerated in the first stages. This may explain an important part of the individual differences within a group of patients that may be pathogenetically homogenous. Whereas Reisberg (1983) differentiates seven stages in the disease process and Strub and Black (1981) discern four stages, others differentiate only between 'mild', 'moderate' and 'severe' dementia, but the criteria used for the inclusion of a patient in the different groups are usually vague. This may be an important reason for the difficulty in comparing different studies on dementing patients. Of course, the differentiation between different types of dementia is of utmost importance for treatment and management of the patient at home or in a nursing home, but also for the assessment whether the memory complaints may be indicative of a relatively 'normal' senescent forgetfulness or the early sign of beginning dementia.

Stages in Alzheimer's disease: neuropsychological issues

It has been suggested that the stages in AD may be a behavioral parallel of similar stages in neuroanatomical degeneration (Jolles and Hijman, 1983). Interestingly, there is some experimental evidence in favor of such a notion.

Sulkava and Amberla (1982) in a study with the Luria-Christensen neuropsychological test battery found that different stages in the development of the disorder could be discriminated even at the later stages of dementia. Both presenile and senile AD patients deteriorate particularly in memory, higher cognitive, higher visual and motor functions and in orientation. Impressive and expressive speech were relatively spared. All functions deteriorated gradually during the disease process so that the differences between the various abilities and the

slope of the performance profile were preserved. All neuropsychological abilities tested had disappeared in the final phase (Sulkava and Amberla, 1982). According to these authors, the clearly definable course of progression of both the presenile and the senile form of AD affects different functions of the brain in a certain order: symptoms such as general lowering of activity, deterioration of short-term memory and deterioration of awareness appear at an early stage of the disease. Consequent behavioral dysfunctions are disorientation and paranoid delusions. Theoretically, this may indicate that ascending fibers from brain stem to cortex are affected (see below and Luria 1966, 1973). Apraxia, agnosia and aphasia which appear in the next phase are taken to be indicative of cortical dysfunctions. The same applies to the deterioration of logical reasoning and loss of control over behavior. In the advanced stages of the disease only some basic automatic functions may still be preserved, correlating to extensive neocortical degeneration (Sulkava and Amberla, 1982; Jolles and Hijman, 1983).

Methods for early assessment of age-associated cognitive decline

Psychometrics

Generally, standardized tests have increased our knowledge of the development of deficits in normal aging and dementia. Unfortunately, this knowledge has been obtained from groups of elderly subjects and patients as a whole but psychometric tests appear not sensitive and reliable enough to be used in early assessment of individual subjects (e.g. Russell, 1981). Psychometric tests have a number of advantages: they are standardized and published norms are generally available. In addition, they are easy to administer and there is usually a good reliability. A drawback of the psychometric approach is that the use of test scores as such does not allow the identification of cognitive deficits that underlie the performance changes. The traditionally used tests allow only a fairly crude estimation of the cognitive functions and, in addition, do not properly differentiate between different aspects of these functions. This is a consequence of the empirical, non-theoretical nature of these tests, which have been developed for other purposes than to be used with brain-damaged subjects. For example, the 'digit symbol' subtest of the 'Wechsler adult intelligence scale' (WAIS) is the most sensitive among the 11 subtests, showing the greatest difference between the performance of young and old adults (Botwinnick, 1981). However, it is not clear whether psychomotor slowing, poor learning or retrieval of the digit-symbol codes, poor visual motor coordination or all of the above are responsible for the poor performance of the aged subject (Poon, 1983). The psychometric test measures thus give a quantitative index of 'performance below the norm' without any clue as to the nature of the cognitive deficit and the underlying cerebral substrate.

A second drawback of the traditional psychometric tests is the relatively long time needed for the test administration, when compared to the amount of data the test battery yields. For instance, the administration of the WAIS takes several hours, and yields only 11 (subtest) scores when the tests are used in the classical way. These scores are usually converted into two scores for verbal IQ and performal IQ, and are often combined into the total IQ. Another test battery such as the 'Halstead Reitan neuropsychological test battery' (HRNTB; administration in 5–6 h), has the disadvantage that standard norms are available until 55 years of age but not for older subjects.

Apart from the use of standardized test batteries (HRNTB, WAIS, the Nebraska battery), several more specific psychometric tests are used for the determination of deficits in aging and dementia. This applies especially to the determination of aspects of memory processes (see Jolles and Hijman, 1983). Characteristically, the resulting quantitative data are used for the analysis of group differences (e.g. 'young' versus 'old' adults). Generally, the nature of the quantitative results does not enable their use in individual diagnosis,

especially in differentiating early dementia from other syndromes. More recently, there has been some development in the use of psychometric tests and test batteries in a less rigid and more qualitative way (e.g. Lezak, 1983; Goodglass and Kaplan, 1979). Proponents of such an approach make use of a combination of the quantitative results and more qualitative signs. Published data are not yet available on the use of this new approach in early diagnosis of senile dementia.

Information processing

Investigations of cognitive processes in the psychological laboratory have generally made use of an information processing paradigm. The strength of this approach is the theoretical framework. It is aimed at examining cognitive processes by analyzing behavior in quantifiable components and qualitative patterns. The information processing tasks characteristically are composed of subtasks, and reaction time measurements are used to probe into the different stages of information processing (e.g. Brand and Jolles, 1986; Poon, 1983).

The use of information processing tasks which are developed in the psychological laboratory and later adapted for use in clinical testing is still in its infancy. The 'Sternberg memory comparison task' (Sternberg, 1966, 1975) which has been used extensively in the laboratory, has been used in measuring the efficacy of drugs in clinical trials and in group comparison studies but not in individual psychodiagnosis. However, a recently developed 'paper-and-pencil' version appears to be a reliable and sensitive task which can be used in combination with clinical neuropsychological tests (Jolles and Gaillard, 1984). Data obtained with this test suggest that the intercept of the 'reaction time – setsize function' increases with age. This suggests that there is a decreased rate of memory search. However, there is an increased slope in those dementing subjects who are characterized by some aspects of frontal lobe dysfunctioning. This is suggestive of a fairly specific effect on search processes (Jolles, unpublished).

Other information processing paradigms have been recommended for use in geriatric psychopharmacology (Poon, 1983). These methods could also be important in the clinical assessment of subjects suspected of a developing dementia. According to Poon, these paradigms measure common behavioral complaints in community dwelling elderly as well as in elderly patient populations. A large amount of data has been obtained on speed, accuracy and the pattern of responses, especially with respect to the following functions: ability to attend and concentrate; ability to make decisions quickly; ability to acquire and retrieve new information; ability to retrieve familiar information (naming); ability to manipulate spatial information. It is important to note — again — that inferences are made with respect to aspects of cognitive functioning by the use of reaction time measurements. Poon (1983) recommends and describes the following procedures for use in geriatric assessment: (1) measurement of the alerting function to assess attention/arousal; (2) measurement of choice reaction time to assess decision making processes; (3) measurement of continuous recognition memory to assess retrieval from primary and secondary memory; (4) measurement of naming latency to assess retrieval from tertiary memory; and (5) measurement of mental rotation to assess spatial processing (a detailed description and rationale can be found in Poon, 1983).

It is of interest to note that several psychometric tests which have been in clinical use for several decades can be used as an information processing task: one example is the 'Stroop test' (see Lezak, 1983) which consists of three subtasks which measure: (1) the speed at which color names are read; (2) the speed at which colors are named; (3) the speed at which the color of printing ink is named when there is interference from the printed color name. An interference score can be calculated by subtracting the time scores on tasks 3 and 2. This is a relatively pure index which is not contaminated by a perceptual or motor component. A similar procedure can be performed with the 'trail making test' (see Lezak, 1983). The subtraction of time scores

gives a timed measure for the ease at which a concept shift is made (here shifting between letters and digits, Vink and Jolles, 1985).

Behavioral neurology

A different approach to assess cognitive functioning in geriatry has been presented by the neuropsychologist Luria (1966, 1973). He presented a model of brain–behavior relationships which served as a basis for an extensive neuropsychological investigation. His approach consists of a set of procedures which systematically assess different aspects of cognitive functioning (see Table I). Luria's

TABLE I

Luria's neuropsychological investigation according to Christensen (1975)

Motor functions
  of the hands, oral praxis, speech regulation of the motor act

Acoustico-motor organization
  perception and reproduction of pitch and of rhythmic structures

Higher cutaneous and kinesthetic functions
  cutaneous and muscle and joint sensation, stereognosis

Higher visual functions
  visual perception, spatial orientation, intellectual operations in space

Impressive speech
  phonemic hearing, word comprehension, simple and complex grammar

Expressive speech
  articulation, reflected speech, nominative speech, narrative speech

Writing and reading
  word analysis and synthesis, writing, reading

Arithmetical skill
  comprehension of number structure, arithmetical operations

Mnestic processes
  learning processes, retention and retrieval, logical memorizing

Intellectual processes
  thematic pictures and texts, concept formation, discursive intellectual activity

---

method which has become well known in the adapted version of Christensen (1975), is qualitative and flexible in nature. When needed, more than 250 simple tasks are given to the subject, ranging from tests for simple and complex motoracts via perceptual, language, and memory functions to tests for higher cognitive functions. Total administration time is 1–2 h. In essence, Luria's method is aimed at generating hypotheses concerning specific disabilities, and then testing these hypotheses by a proper choice of small tasks. For instance, with respect to memory functions, Luria differentiates between memory for visual forms ("draw the figures that you saw") and verbal material ("write the words you saw"). The learning performance is measured, as well as the sensitivity to interference by homogeneous material or heterogeneous material. In addition, the formation of a stable intention to memorize or to associate is measured in addition to several other aspects of memory function (Luria, 1976). Luria used his method originally to investigate brain-injured subjects, and the tests have provided important information in assessing the location of brain injuries and in planning rehabilitation programs. More recently, it appeared effective in assessing 'functional' psychiatric illness from 'organic' patients (Purish et al., 1978) and also in the assessment of AD (Ernst et al., 1970; Sulkava and Amberla, 1982).

Luria's investigation is essentially behavioral neurology. The administration of the tasks is systematic but non-structured. Its main advantage is the fact that the assessment schedule is based upon a theory of brain–behavior relationships. This allows for an interpretation with respect to the specific aspect or part of a 'functional system' which is affected. This approach gives rise to a wealth of data which has more coherence than the data which arise from a battery of standard psychometric tests. An important disadvantage of the procedure is its qualitative nature which necessitates extensive observer training and reduces the interobserver reliability. In addition, the lack of quantifiable data prohibits the use of the

paradigm in the assessment of treatment efficacy and cognitive decline in individual subjects. However, used in combination with psychometric tests and information processing tasks, it can provide important information on the selective nature of cognitive deficits in elderly subjects and AD. Recently, attempts have been directed at quantifying Luria's neuropsychological investigation. Unfortunately, the Luria-Nebraska battery (Golden et al., 1979) which is a structured and semi-quantitative test series, has lost the flexibility and richness of the original method. In addition, it has several other shortcomings (Adams, 1984).

Behavioral and cognitive testing; an integrated approach

Both the psychometric, the information processing and the behavioral neurological approach have their strengths and weaknesses. A combination of them may be fruitful in the early assessment of AD and related disorders. The assessment procedure used for this purpose in our clinic is a combination of a qualitative behavioral neurological investigation and quantitative methods derived from psychometrics and information processing paradigms. The procedure is, first, to get a qualitative impression on the total range of cognitive functions. When signs are present which may indicate a deficit, a more detailed investigation is performed in that direction: other qualitative tests are used in order to test the hypothesis that something is wrong and to find out the specific nature of the deficit. These tests are then followed by quantitative methods which 'measure' the deficit and relate it to existing norms. This approach has several advantages: (1) it is possible to make a profile of cognitive functioning in all its different aspects — for instance, it is fairly easy to indicate those aspects of cognition which do not show deficiencies; (2) many observations are done, increasing the reliability of the final interpretation; (3) the duration of the neuropsychological investigation has been decreased as a result of the relatively shorter duration of the qualitative tests;

(4) some kind of hypothesis testing is performed; the hypotheses are based upon a thorough knowledge of brain–behavior relationships; and (5) much emphasis is placed on 'pathognomonic signs' which are clear-cut signs that pathology is present. The psychometric tradition usually does not give attention to these signs.

The test series used in the assessment of early dementia in our clinic consists of the following tests and tasks: (1) the Luria-Christensen test battery; (2) 'fifteen word learning test' (which provides information on the use of active coding strategies, on consolidation versus retrieval, on the rate of retrieval, on sensitivity to interference; Luria, 1976; Brand and Jolles, 1986); (3) 'Utrecht memory comparison task' (rate of perception and motor output, rate of memory comparison; Jolles and Gaillard, 1984; Brand and Jolles, 1986); (4) 'Stroop interference task' (naming: retrieval of words and colornames, color-word interference; Lezak, 1983); (5) 'Utrecht trail making test' (rate of perception, retrieval of letters, flexibility towards concept shift; Vink and Jolles, 1985); (6) 'road map test' (left-right discrimination; evaluation; mental rotation; Lezak, 1983); and (7) 'symbol digit modalities test' (general speed of perception and motor output; Lezak, 1983). In addition to this test series many other tests are performed to better localize a specific deficit, if found. These tests are chosen from standard batteries (e.g. 'tapping test' from HRNTB or 'block design' from WAIS) or experimental tasks (e.g. an experimental task for the assessment of decision speed, a test for the assessment of tactile functions or the dichotic listening task).

Luria used a syndrome analysis to describe the profile of cognitive strengths and weaknesses of his subjects. Such a syndrome appeared specific to involvement of particular brain structures. For instance, an involvement of 'frontal areas' could be observed in many different functional systems, such as a perseveration in motor function, a proactive memory interference, a flat learning curve on a word learning test, an inability in concept shifting, etc. A similar syndrome analysis

appears to be important when test methods are used such as described in this paragraph.

In fact, a cognitive profile emerges which is a description of the cognitive strengths and weaknesses of a certain subject at a certain moment. Such a profile analysis is an attempt to simplify the picture which might otherwise contain too much information to be intelligible. Some examples of such an approach are given in Jolles (1985). The large amount of data gathered per individual subject appears to allow a fairly reliable description of individual cases.

The neuropsychology of aging and dementia

Similarities and differences between aging and AD

Neuropsychological research in aging and dementia has primarily focussed on memory processes although it is obvious that other cognitive functions are impaired as well. The quantity of research on memory may thus give the wrong impression that memory is the major function involved. There is an obvious need for further studies of information processing, language, perception and planning/organization/coding processes. There exists a parallel with biological research on aging and dementia, which focusses on the structure and function of the hippocampus (involved in memory function; Newcombe, 1980). The emphasis on memory and hippocampus tends to obscure the fact that other cognitive functions (information processing, language, perception, problem solving) and other brain areas (other neocortical and limbic/subcortical) are involved as well. The neuropsychological knowledge discussed so far does not provide any indication that there is more than a gradual difference between 'normal' aging and AD. Of course, when demented patients are compared to age-matched controls, the demented patients perform worse on all test parameters. But, generally, there is not a different pattern of cognitive deficits in aged and AD subjects. Thus, as pointed out in the preceding paragraphs, a relative deficit is seen in the areas of intelligence, language functions, memory, problem solving, perception, coding processes etc. This indicates that — on the basis of behavioral observation and neuropsychological tests alone — senile dementia might be considered 'exaggerated aging'. It is important to note that this is a controversial issue (see for instance Whitehouse et al., 1983). Several authors have proposed a similar view on the basis of (neuro)biological data (e.g. Terry and Wisniewsky, 1975), whereas others have stated that the cerebral processes underlying 'normal' aging are different from those underlying senile dementia.

The possible cerebral substrate underlying aging. Neuropsychologically, a clear pattern is visible in the cognitive deficits in normal aging. One common element refers to aspects of cognition which have been related to frontal lobe functioning: in this sense, stimulus persistence, proactive interference, lack of behavioral planning, deficient memory search and other deficits can be indicative of less efficient frontal lobe functioning (Luria, 1973, 1980; Fuster, 1980). Interestingly, morphological evidence is available to show that areas in the frontal lobes degenerate already in people aged 40–50 (Haug, 1985). With respect to memory consolidation, limbic areas must be involved on the hippocampal and diencephalic level (Newcombe, 1980; Luria, 1966). It remains to be seen whether a general decrease in the rate of information processing has to do specifically with the ascending fiber system, as would be hypothesized on the basis of Luria's model of brain– behavior relationships (1973, 1966).

The cerebral substrate possibly underlying AD: a neuropsychological hypothesis. The nature of the memory disorders which are associated with aging and dementia suggest that limbic/subcortical structures are involved, especially those involving the hippocampus. This notion evolves from the consideration that the memory deficits are modality-aspecific, and that there seems to be an impairment in the consolidation of new information. However, another important aspect of memory processes which is frequently overlooked, concerns the impairment in encoding processes; the search in memory is less effective, with a consequent impairment in active recall (with preservation of passive recognition); there is also less efficient planning and programming. These cognitive deficits in both aged and demented patients suggest that frontal neocortical structures may be involved. Likewise, the (relative) lack of inhibition, the stimulus persistence, the lack of flexibility, the deficits in planning (problem solving behavior) and other cognitive dysfunctions are in line with this notion.

The data which have been gathered by clinical and experimental neuropsychological research are suggestive of frontal cortex dysfunctions: this hypothesis is based upon the brain–behavior model of Luria (1973, 1976, 1966), who differentiated between three types of frontal syndromes (see also Fuster, 1980).

It may be the case that several dysfunctions which are found in the earlier stages of the dementing process are a result of cerebral dysfunctions in the medial zones of the frontal lobe. This applies especially to memory disturbances, confabulation tendencies, orientation disturbance and loss of flexibility. Similarly, the deficits in emotional control and impulsivity which are noted in these stages, may depend on basal/orbital and medial zones. In later stages, involvement of secondary cortical areas (lateral convex structures of the frontal lobe) may become apparent in disturbances in the organization and planning of the motor functions, perseverative tendencies, general inertia and adynamic speech regulation. This argument is described in Jolles and Hijman (1983) and is based upon Luria (1973, 1966) and Fuster (1980).

Parallel to the development of symptoms involving the tertiary (association) areas on the lateral aspect of the frontal neocortex, similar observations can be done with respect to cognitive functions which depend on proper functioning in the tertiary areas in the posterior neocortex. For instance the higher order integration between sensory modalities breaks down earlier than the cognitive functions which depend on secondary areas (e.g. language functions, figure background discrimination) or the primary projection areas. In fact, the temporal sequence of the development of cognitive deficits in AD suggest that there may be a gradual increase in the number of neocortical areas involved, the tertiary association areas degenerating before the secondary areas and the primary areas staying relatively intact until very late in the disease process. This is suggested by the fact that performance of simple motor acts is preserved (activity of the primary motor cortex) as is the use of syllables and phonemes (but not words) in undirected babbling, which severely demented patients are still capable of. Support for this view also comes from histological investigations in which it was found that several cortical areas are indeed relatively spared in the course of this disease (Brody and Vijayashankar, 1977; Hanley, 1974). In addition, it has been known for some time that there is a correlation between extent of cortical degeneration (senile plaques) and poor test performance (e.g. Blessed et al., 1968). If the notion that tertiary, secondary and primary cortical areas degenerate in that order is true, this degeneration is exactly the reverse of the ontogenetical development (primary projection areas develop before secondary, and these before tertiary areas; 'law of the hierarchical structure of the cortical zones', Luria, 1973, 1966). This would suggest that the processes underlying aging and dementia are reversed compared to those in ontogenesis. Several investigators address this interesting possibility (e.g. Heiman, 1985; De Ajuriaguerra et al., 1967).

With respect to the question "What are the very first signs of decreasing abilities in AD?", one is tempted to hypothesize that the cognitive deficits associated with neocortical degeneration are *secondary to* dysfunctions in the subcortical systems. The neuropsychological findings suggest that the very first symptoms of decreasing abilities might depend upon dysfunctions of ascending fibers and fronto-limbic connections. These symptoms seem to be evident especially in speed factors, general activity and aspects of memory processes. This neuropsychological hypothesis agrees with current neurobiological findings on the importance of cholinergic fibers originating in the basal forebrain (e.g. nucleus basalis of Meynert) and projecting onto the neocortex and hippocampus. However, it is not clear whether the degeneration of these subcortical fibers is itself secondary to degeneration of structures located deeper in the brain (as would be a prediction based upon neuropsychological data alone), or secondary to a corticofugal influence.

Summary and conclusions

Elderly subjects perform worse than young persons on virtually all cognitive and behavioral functions that are tested. Thus, performance decrements in intellectual functions, memory, perception, behavioral organization and motor functions have been noted. However, elderly people are not inferior in tasks in which they can rely on well-established skills and knowledge. With respect to AD, the pattern of cognitive deficits seems to be similar to that seen in 'normal' aging but the dementing subject is also characterized by deficiencies in verbal functions and recognition memory. Other forms of dementia such as multiinfarct dementia and Pick's disease appear to have another pattern of cognitive strengths and weaknesses. This knowledge of the age-associated cognitive decline and of deficits in the different forms of dementia has recently been used to propose the use of new methods in the assessment of early stages in dementia: most of the methods which until now have been used in the assessment of early stages of dementia have their drawbacks. It appears that the use of a *combination* of psychometric tests with techniques based upon information processing paradigms and behavioral neurology may be a fruitful approach. Future developments will almost certainly be in the direction of techniques that are more sensitive, and give more insight into the nature of the cognitive deficits. Information processing tasks such as those proposed by several authors (Poon, 1983; Branconnier and DeVitt, 1984; Jolles, 1985; Brand and Jolles, 1986) will contribute, provided that some relation is established between the cognitive functions and the underlying cerebral substrate, and provided that tasks will be constructed which have ecological validity.

With respect to the potential contributions of neuropsychology, several points deserve to be mentioned. In the first place, modern neuropsychology is a neuroscience discipline trying to relate behavioral and cognitive functions to the underlying cerebral substrate. A brain–behavior model presents a working hypothesis which is essential to relate aspects of behavior and cognition which would otherwise never have been known to contain common elements (see for instance the different aspects of frontal involvement). A contribution based on neuropsychological theory predicts that the development of stages in the behaviorally observable deficits in the AD may be a manifestation of an underlying degeneration of subsequently (1) ascending fibers, (2) hippocampus and sensory non-specific neocortical association areas and (3) neocortical sensory association areas (Jolles and Hijman, 1983). Another theoretical contribution concerns the findings that — based on neuropsychological investigation alone — there is no qualitative but only a quantitative difference between aging and AD (Jolles and Hijman, 1983) and between presenile and senile forms of AD (Sulkava and Amberla, 1982). Human neuropsychology may thus provide testable hypotheses which deepen our insight into the nature of the underlying disease and its cerebral substrate.

A second important aspect of neuropsychology concerns the implications which emerge from a better behavioral and cognitive description of the deficits: for instance, the old subject seems to lose the ability to retrieve information which was consolidated some time ago. A consolidation deficit appears especially in dementia. Might it be the case that the underlying deficit is really a decreasing ability to cope with environmental stimuli? This notion could motivate changes in society such that older people get more opportunities to engage in new activities and actively plan their own behavior. Presently, there is a tendency in exactly the opposite direction, to take the responsibility out of the hands of the elderly subjects. This is especially true in psychiatric institutions. Patient rehabilitation and training based upon neuropsychological theory would suggest that subjects be trained to compensate for lost capabilities. In this respect, much emphasis must be given to activate behavior planning as opposed to passive perception. The strategy of 'enriched' environments which is known to have an effect on cortical thickness and neuronal connections in animals might have similar effects in man. Analogous to the muscular dystrophy in a disused broken leg, there may be a brain atrophy because of lack of interaction of the organism with its environment (Jolles, 1985). This atrophy could — theoretically — be 'reversible' when assessed in the very early stages. Such a stimulation therapy — possible in combination with newly developed drugs — might be the treatment of choice in elderly people that are at risk of becoming demented.

References

Adams, K.M. (1984) Luria left in the lurch: unfulfilled promises are not valid tests. *J. Clin. Neuropsychol.*, 6: 455–458.

Arenberg, D. (1965) Anticipation interval and age differences in verbal learning. *J. Abnormal. Psychol.*, 10, 419–425.

Arenberg, D. and Robertson-Tchabo, E. A. (1977) Learning and aging. In J. E. Birren and K. W. Schaie (Eds.), *Handbook of the Psychology of Aging*, Van Nostrand Reinhold Co., New York, pp. 421–449.

Axelrod, S. and Cohen, L. D. (1961) Senescence and embedded figure performance in vision and touch. *Percept. Mot. Skills*, 12: 283–288.

Barker, M. G. and Lawson, J. S. (1968) Nominal aphasia in dementia. *Br. J. Psychiat.*, 114: 1351–1356.

Benson, D. F. (1979) Neurologic correlates of anomia. In H. Whitaker and H. A. Whitaker (Eds.), *Studies in Neurolinguistics, Vol. 2*. Academic Press, New York, pp. 293–327.

Blessed, G., Tomlinson, B. E. and Roth, M. (1968) The association between quantitative measures of dementia and of senile changes in the cerebral grey matter of aged subjects. *Br. J. Psychiat.*, 114: 797–811.

Botwinnick, J. (1977) Intellectual abilities. In J. E. Birren and K. W. Schaie (Eds.) *Handbook of the Psychology of Aging*, Van Nostrand Reinhold Co., New York, pp. 580–605.

Botwinnick, J. (1981) Neuropsychology of aging. In S. B. Filskov and T. J. Boll (Eds.), *Handbook of Clinical Neuropsychology*, Wiley, New York, pp. 135–171.

Branconnier, R. J. and DeVitt, D. R. (1984) Early detection of incipient Alzheimer's disease. In B. Reisberg (Ed.), *Alzheimer's Disease*, Free Press/Macmillan, New York, pp. 214–227.

Brand, N. and Jolles, J. (1986) Information processing in depression and anxiety. *Psychol. Med.*, 16, in press.

Brody, H. and Vijayashankar, N. (1977) Anatomical changes in the nervous system. In C. E. Finch and L. Hayflick (Eds.), *Handbook of the Biology of Aging*, Van Nostrand, New York, pp. 241–261.

Christensen, A. L. (1975) *Luria's Neuropsychological Investigation. Text*, Munxgaard, Copenhagen.

Clayton, P. J. and Martin, R. (1981) Classification of late life organic states and the DSM–III. In N. E. Miller and G. D. Cohen (Eds.), *Clinical Aspects of Alzheimer's Disease and Senile Dementia*, Raven Press, New York, pp. 47–60.

Corsellis, J. A. N. (1976) Aging and dementia. In W. Blackwood and J. A. N. Corsellis (Eds.), *Greenfield's Neuropathology*, Arnold, London, pp. 796–848.

Craik, F. I. M. (1977) Age differences in human memory. In J. E. Birren and K. W. Schaie (Eds.), *Handbook of the Psychology of Aging*, Van Nostrand Reinhold Co., New York, pp. 384–420.

De Ajuriaguerra, J., Boehme, M., Richard, J. and Tissot, R. (1967) Désintégration des notions du temps dans les démences dégénératives du grand âge. *Encéphale*, 56: 385–438.

Deese, J. and Hulse, S. H. (1967) *The Psychology of Learning*, 3rd edn., McGrawHill, New York.

Drachman, D. A. and Levitt, J. (1972) Memory impairment in the aged: storage versus retrieval deficit. *J. Exp. Psychol. (Gen.)*, 93: 302–308.

Erber, J. T. (1974) Age differences in recognition memory. *J. Gerontol.*, 29: 177–181.

Eriksen, C. W., Hamlin, R. M. and Breitmeyer, R. G. (1970) Temporal factors in visual perception as related to aging. *Percept. Psychophys.*, 7: 354–356.

Ernst, B., Dalby, M. A. and Dalby, A. (1970) Luria testing in demented patients. *Acta Neurol. Scand.*, Suppl. 43, 97–102.

Eysenck, M. W. (1975) Retrieval form semanctic memory as a function of age. *J. Gerontol.*, 30: 174–180.

Friedland, R. P., Budinger, T. F., Jagust, W. J., Koss, E., Derenzo, S., Huesman, R. H. and Yano, Y. (1985) Positron tomography and the differential diagnosis and pathophysiology of Alzheimer's disease. In W. H. Gispen and J. Traber (Eds.), *Senile Dementia of the Alzheimer type*, Springer, Berlin, pp. 124–133.

Fuld, P. A. (1984) Psychometric differentiation of the dementias. In B. Reisberg (Ed.), *Alzheimer's Disease*, Free Press/Macmillan, New York, pp. 201–210.

Fuster, J. M. (1980) *The Prefrontal Cortex*, Raven Press, New York.

Golden, C. J., Hammeke, T. A. and Purish, A. D. (1979) *The Luria-Nebraska Neuropsychological Battery Manual*, Western Psychological Services, Los Angeles.

Goldstein, G. (1980) Psychological dysfunction in the elderly. In J. O. Cole and J. E. Barrett (Eds.), *Psychopathology in the Aged*, Raven, New York, pp. 205–232.

Goldstein, G. and Shelley, C. M. (1975) Similarities and differences between psychological deficit in aging and brain damage. *J. Gerontol.*, 30: 448–455.

Goodglass, H. and Kaplan, E. (1979) Assessment of cognitive deficit in the brain-injured patient. In M. Gazzaniga (Ed.), *Handbook of Behavioral Neurobiology, Vol. 2 (Neuropsychology)*, Plenum Press, New York, pp. 3–22.

Hanley, T. (1974) Neuronal 'fall-out' in the aging brain: a critical review of the quantitative data. *Age Aging*, 3: 133–151.

Haug, H. (1985) Are neurons of the human cerebral cortex really lost during aging? A morphometric examination. In W. H. Gispen and J. Traber (Eds.), *Senile Dementia of the Alzheimer Type*, Springer, Berlin, pp. 150–163.

Heglin, H. J. (1956) Problem solving set in different age groups. *J. Gerontol.*, 11: 310–317.

Heiman, H. (1985) Clinical aspects of dementia syndrome. *Gerontopsychiatry*, 18: 2–5.

Hibbard, T. R., Migliaccio, J. N., Goldstone, S. and Lhamon, W. T. (1975) Temporal information processing by young and senior adults and patients with senile dementia. *J. Gerontol.*, 30: 326–330.

Hooper, H. E. (1958) *The Hooper Visual Organization Test Manual*. Beverly Hills, CA, Western Psychological Services.

Hulicka, I. M. and Weiss, R. L. (1965) Age differences in retention as a function of learning. *J. Consult. Psychol.*, 29: 125–129.

Inglis, J. (1957) An experimental study of learning and 'memory function' in elderly psychiatric patients. *J. Ment. Sci.*, 103: 796–803.

Inglis, J. (1959) Learning, retention and conceptual usage in elderly patients with memory disorder. *J. Abnorm. Soc. Psychol.*, 59: 210–215.

Inglis, J. (1960) Dichotic stimulation and memory disorder. *Nature*, 186: 181–182.

Irigaray, L. (1973) *Le Language des Déments*. Mouton, The Hague.

Jerome, E. A. (1962) Decay of heuristic processes in the aged. In C. Tibbets and W. Donahue (Eds.), *Social and Psychological Aspects of Aging*, Columbia University Press, New York, pp. 802–823.

Jolles, J. (1985) Early diagnosis of dementia: possible contributions from neuropsychology. In W. H. Gispen and J. Traber (Eds.), *Aging of the Brain*, Springer, Berlin, pp. 84–100.

Jolles, J. and Gaillard, A. W. K. (1984) A paper and pencil version of the Sternberg Memory Comparison task. Report No. 840901 of the Department of Psychiatry, State University Utrecht, The Netherlands.

Jolles, J. and Hijman, R. (1983) The neuropsychology of aging and dementia. *Dev. Neurol.*, 7: 227–250.

Kendrick, D. C., Parboosingh, R. C. and Post, F. (1965) A synonym learning test for use with elderly psychiatric patients: a validation study. *Br. J. Soc. Clin. Psychol.*, 4: 63–71.

Kinsbourne, M. and Berryhill, J. L. (1972) The nature of interaction between pacing and the age decrement in learning. *J. Gerontol.*, 27: 471–477.

Kline, D. W. and Nestor, S. (1977) The persistence of complementary after-images as a function of adult age and exposure duration. *Exp. Aging Res.*, 3: 191–201.

Kline, D. W. and Orme-Rogers, C. (1978) Examination of stimulus persistence as the basis for superior visual identification performance among old adults. *J. Gerontol.*, 33: 76–81.

Kline, D. W. and Szafran, J. (1975) Age differences in backward monoptic visual noise masking. *J. Gerontol.*, 30: 307–311.

Kral, V. A. (1962) Senescent forgetfulness: benign and malignant. *Can. Med. Assoc. J.*, 86: 257–260.

Lawson, J. S., McGhie, A. and Chapman, J. (1967) Distractibility in schizophrenia and organic cerebral disease. *Br. J. Psychiat.*, 113: 527–535.

Lawson, J. S. and Barker, M. G. (1968) The assessment of nominal dysphasia in dementia: the use of reaction-time measures. *Br. J. Med. Psychol.*, 41: 411–414.

Lezak, M. D. (1983) *Neuropsychological Assessment*, 2nd edn., Oxford University Press, New York, Oxford.

Luria, A. R. (1966, 1st edn.; 1980, 2nd edn.) *Higher Cortical Functions in Man.* Basic Books, New York.

Luria, A. R. (1973) *The Working Brain.* Penguin Books, Harmondsworth, UK.

Luria, A. R. (1976) *The Neuropsychology of Memory.* Winston, Washington DC.

Miller, E. (1972) Efficiency of coding and the short-term memory defect in presenile dementia. *Neuropsychologia*, 10: 133–136.

Miller, E. (1973) Short- and long-term memory in patients with presenile dementia (Alzheimer's disease). *Psychol. Med.*, 3: 221–224.

Miller, E. (1975) Impaired recall and the memory disturbance in presenile dementia. *Br. J. Soc. Clin. Psychol.*, 14: 73–79.

Miller, E. (1977a) *Abnormal Aging.* Wiley, Chichester.

Miller, E. (1977b) A note on visual information processing in presenile dementia: a preliminary report. *Br. J. Soc. Clin. Psychol.*, 16: 99–100.

Miller, E. (1978) Retrieval from long-term memory in presenile dementia: two tests of an hypothesis. *Br. J. Soc. Clin. Psychol.*, 17: 143–148.

Miller, E. (1981) The nature of the cognitive deficit in dementia. In N. E. Miller and G. D. Cohen (Eds.), *Clinical Aspects of Alzheimer's Disease and Senile Dementia*, Raven, New York, pp. 103–120.

Miller, E. (1984) Neuropsychological assessment. In D. W. K. Kay and G. D. Burrows (Eds.), *Handbook of Studies on

Psychiatry and Old Age.* Elsevier Biomedical Press, Amsterdam, pp. 455–469.

Miller, E. and Hague, F. (1975) Some characteristics of verbal behavior in presenile dementia. *Psychol. Med.*, 5: 255–259.

Miller, G. A. (1956) The magical number seven, plus or minus two: some limits on our capacity for processing information. *Psychol. Rev.*, 63: 81–97.

Misiak, H. (1947) Age and sex differences in critical flicker frequency. *J. Exp. Psychol.*, 37: 318–332.

Nelson, H. E. and McKenna, P. (1975) The use of current reading ability in the assessment of dementia. *Br. J. Soc. Clin. Psychol.*, 14: 259–267.

Newcombe, F. (1980) Memory: a neuropsychological approach. *Trends Neurosci.*, 3: 179–182.

Poon, L. W. (1983) Application of information-processing technology in psychological assessment. In T. Crook, S. Ferris and R. Bartus (Eds.), *Assessment in Geriatric Psychopharmacology*, M. Powley Ass. New Canaan, CT, pp. 187–201.

Purish, A. D., Golden, C. J. and Hammeke, T. A. (1978) Discrimination of schizophrenia and brain–injured patients by a standardized version of Luria's neuropsychological tests. *J. Consult. Clin. Psychol.*, 46: 1266–1273.

Reisberg, B. (1983) The brief cognitive rating scale and global deterioration scale. In T. Crook, S. Ferris and R. Bartus (Eds.), *Assessment in Geriatric Psychopharmacology*, Mark Powley Ass. New Canaan, CT, pp. 19–35.

Reisberg, B., Ferris, S. H. and Crook, T. (1982) Signs, symptoms and course of age-associated cognitive decline. In S. Corkin, K. I. Davis, J. H. Growdon, E. Usdin and R. J. Wurtman (Eds.), *Alzheimer's Disease: a Report of Progress in Research*, Raven Press, New York, pp. 177–181.

Rockford, G. (1971) A study of naming errors in dysphasic and in demented patients. *Neuropsychologia*, 9: 437–443.

Rossor, M. N. (1982) Neurotransmitters and CNS disease: dementia. *The Lancet*, II: 1200–1204.

Russell, E. W. (1981) The pathology and clinical examination of memory. In S. B. Filskov and T. J. Boll (Eds.), *Handbook of Clinical Neuropsychology*, Wiley, New York, pp. 287–319.

Salthouse, T. A. (1976) Age and tachistoscopic perception. *Exp. Aging Res.*, 2: 91–103.

Schonfield, D. and Stones, M. J. (1979) Remembering and aging. In J. F. Kihlstrom and F. J. Evans (Eds.), *Functional Disorders of Memory*, Erlbaum, Hillsdale, NJ, pp. 103–139.

Sjögren, T., Sjögren, H. and Lindgren, A. G. H. (1952) Morbus Alzheimer and morbus Pick; genetic, clinical and pathoanatomic study. *Acta Psychiat. Scand.*, Suppl. 82: 68–108.

Slamecka, N. J. (1967) Recall and recognition in list discrimination tasks as a function of the number of alternatives. *J. Exp. Psychol. (Gen)*, 74: 187–192.

Sperling, G. A. (1960) The information available in brief visual presentation. *Psychol. Monogr.*, 74: 498.

Sternberg, S. (1966) High-speed scanning in human memory. *Science*, 153: 652–654.

Sternberg, S. (1975) Memory scanning: new findings and current controversies. *Q. J. Exp. Psychol.*, 27: 1–32.

Strub, R. I. and Black, F. W. (1977) *The Mental Status Examination in Neurology.* Davis, Philadelphia.

Strub, R. I. and Black, F. W. (1981) Alzheimer's/senile dementia. In. R. I. Strub and F. W. Black (Eds.), *Organic Brain Syndromes*, F. A. Davis Co., Philadelphia, pp. 119–164.

Sulkava, R. and Amberla, K. (1982) Alzheimer's disease and senile dementia of Alzheimer type: a neuropsychological study. *Acta Neurol. Scand.*, 65: 541–552.

Terry, R. D. and Wisniewsky, H. M. (1975) Structural and chemical changes of the aged human brain. In S. Gershon and A. Raskin (Eds.) *Aging*, Raven Press, New York, pp. 127–141.

Treat, N. J. and Reese, H. W. (1976) Age, pacing and imagery in paired-associate learning. *Develop. Psychol.*, 12: 119–124.

Tulving, E. and Pearlstone, Z. (1966) Availability versus accessibility of information in memory for words. *J. Verbal Learning Behav.*, 5: 381–391.

Van Praag, H. M. (1982) Depression. *Lancet*, II: 1259–1264.

Vink, M. and Jolles, J. (1985) A new version of the trailmakingtest as an information processing task. *J. Clin. Neuropsychol.*, 7: 162.

Walsh, D. A. (1975) Age differences in learning and memory. In P. S. Woodruff and J. E. Birren (Eds.), *Aging*, D. Van Nostrand Co., New York.

Warrington, E. K. and Weiszkrantz, L. (1970) Amnesic syndrome: consolidation or retrieval? *Nature*, 228: 628–630.

Waugh, N. C. and Barr, R. A. (1980) Memory and mental tempo. In L. W. Poon, T. L. Fozard and L. S. Cermak (Eds.), *Directions in Memory and Aging*, Erlbaum, Hillsdale, NJ, pp. 251–260.

Welford, A. T. (1977) Motor performance. In J. E. Birren and K. W. Schaie (Eds.), *Handbook of the Psychology of Aging*, Van Nostrand Reinhold Co., New York, pp. 450–496.

Wetherick, N. E. (1965) Changing an established concept: a comparison of the ability of young, middle aged and old subjects. *Gerontologia*, 11: 82–95.

Whitehead, A. (1975) Recognition memory in dementia. *Br. J. Soc. Clin. Psychol.*, 14: 191–194.

Whitehouse, P. J., Hedreen, J. C. and Price, D. L. (1983) Aging and Alzheimer's disease, *Dev. Neurol.*, 7: 261–274.

Willanger, R. and Klee, A. (1966) Metamorphopsia and other visual disturbances with latency occurring in patients with diffuse cerebral lesions. *Acta Neurol. Scand.*, 42: 1–18.

Discussion

D. F. SWAAB: How long does it take to obtain a neuropsychological profile as you described from one patient, and how good are the chances to obtain a positive diagnosis of Alzheimer's disease?

ANSWER: Generally, the neuropsychological investigation takes 1 to 2.5 h depending on the patient's complaints and deficits. Deteriorated patients such as those with more advanced stages of AD cannot be subjected to psychometric tests. However, it is still possible to investigate such cases with behavioral neurological tests such as those described by Luria (see Jolles, 1986). It is possible to obtain a profile of cognitive functions. The validity and reliability of the profile thus obtained by behavioral neurology is increased, generally, by adding psychometric and information processing tests to the investigation in order to get more quantitative information on functions, studied qualitatively with the behavioral neurological procedure. The procedure described is able to find those patients who have been provisionally described as 'Alzheimer', but who appear to have a neuropsychological profile of deficits suggesting another disease (for example 'normal pressure hydrocephalus' (NPH)), alcoholic amnesia, depression or focal deficits related to multiinfarct dementia. With respect to the chances to obtain a positive diagnosis of AD: we do not have enough information yet on neuropathology in the patients we have seen, to answer that question.

J. M. RABEY: Could you give the neuropsychological profile of patients suffering from Parkinson's dementia and NPH as obtained through your methods?

ANSWER: The neuropsychological investigation has been given to six patients with mild Parkinson's disease. The profile of strengths and weaknesses was suggestive of deficits in motor functions (especially 'dynamic organization') and complex behavioral planning. Particularly interesting were findings with respect to defective initiation of motor patterns and motor integration. None of these patients had a profile suggestive of dementia: knowledge was usually completely intact although several of them were inferior with respect to mobilising this knowledge (which again may be a characteristic of a planning deficit). NPH patients are among the slowest subjects that we have tested with our methodology (even more than AD patients). When given the time, their performance appeared not to be due to general cognitive deficits. A group of NPH patients given a shunt dramatically improved in speed factors and in other cognitive functions such as concept shifting. This improvement was still present 6 months after the operation (Vanneste and Hijman, 1986).

W. VAN TILBURG: Is the distinction between cortical and subcortical dementia useful from a neuropsychological point of view? Has it some validity?

ANSWER: The answer to this question is yes *and* no. Neuropsychological theory and practice have committed themselves especially to the higher cognitive functions, 'localized' in the neocortex. It is of importance for neuropsychology and for workers in this field that attention is given to subcortical structures and their role in the cerebral mechanisms that underly both complex and more elementary aspects of behavior. It is relevant to know that subcortical dementia is a classification derived from clinical observation by neurologists (Cummings and Benson, 1984); it only states that patients show slowness without higher cortical deficits such as aphasia, agnosia and apraxia. In those cases a neuropsychological investigation often shows minor signs of language dysfunctions and other performance deficits.

With respect to the distinction between cortical and subcortical dementia: this dichotomy seems to suggest that in 'subcortical dementias' there is no involvement of the neocortex and vice versa for the cortical dementias. In my opinion there are many arguments to conclude that such a statement is not true. For example, it seems very probable that subcortical structures are involved in the early stages in AD, and that in fact cortical degeneration may be secondary to subcortical dysfunctions. Furthermore, several subcortical dementias may be characterized by the fact that the subcortical dysfunctions inhibit the efficient use of information which is stored cortically.

E. DONCHIN: I was struck by the contrast between your presentation which illustrated the ability of the psychologist to give very detailed descriptions of behavior and Dr. Van Crevel who reported that there are very few actions that the neurologist can take. If so, what would the neurologist do with all the information you provide?

ANSWER: A relevant part of the information on cognitive and behavioral functions in aging and dementia has been obtained in experimental studies, often using a group-comparison design. This is why we know a lot on 'average aging' and 'average AD'. It is a difficult story as to how to relate this knowledge to diagnosis and care of individual patients. This is — in my opinion — an important area of work for the neuropsychologist: to bridge the gap between theory and practice and to translate the existing knowledge into assessment procedures that will allow a differentiation of patients that the neurologists' methods are not sensitive for. The neuropsychologist may be able to (1) provide the neurologist with hypotheses on the nature of the disease process and (2) give information on cognitive functions and other psychological processes: information that may be important for an optimal choice of treatment strategies and other interventions.

D. A. M. TWISK: The psychological tests you derived from experimental psychology (like the Sternberg paradigm) usually do require extensive training on behalf of the patient. Do the modified tests you use also require a training session in clinical practice?

ANSWER: We do not use a training session and we do not need them. The original Sternberg tasks as such cannot be used in the clinic: they have been experimentally used in group comparison studies and are not applicable for individual diagnosis. We have developed clinically applicable tasks that can be used for this purpose. The tasks concern paper and pencil tasks which appear to give results which are essentially similar to those found by Sternberg and others with computer-aided apparatus. In addition, new complex tasks were developed such as the facial recognition task which also follows the 'additive factor method' proposed by Sternberg (1975). The time needed per task is about 3–4 min for the paper and pencil tasks and 6–9 min for the computer tasks (including a short training).

L. BLOMERT: You showed that Alzheimer patients of moderate severity showed language deficits of the following kind: empty speech, circumlocutory speech, paraphasias, anomia. The same profile states that these patients have no syntactic deficits. How is this possible in the light of the already mentioned language disturbances?

ANSWER: The notion that both receptive and expressive lexical aspects of language are deteriorating rapidly in advanced stages of AD, while confrontation naming is only minimally affected and syntactic processes are not affected, has been put forward by L. Irigaray (1973). Branconnier and DeVitt (1974) suggest that there is a breakdown of a conceptual network (category generation) while the lexicon remains intact (confrontation naming) and give some experimental evidence in favor of this notion.

R. S. SOHAL: Your data seem to imply that AD is merely an accelerated form of aging. Is that correct?

ANSWER: When you state your question in this form: no. As a neuropsychologist, looking at behavior and performance on psychometric and other tests, I observe that the pattern of deficits in aging and in Alzheimer type dementia is similar although the performance decrement is much greater in the early and late stages in AD. Consequently, my statement was that aging and AD do not seem to differ when seen from the behavioral point of view. That does not imply that 'AD is merely an accelerated form of aging'. Such a statement can only be based upon a combination of arguments from the neurobiological, the clinical and the behavioral point of view.

J. E. PISETSKY: Can the neuropsychological tests be used for basal standards and tests which show changes with medications? No tests have been sensitive enough to show changes.

ANSWER: In principle they can. Presently, the tests that are used for treatment evaluation are standard psychometric tests that are often not usable for repeated testing. Generally, these tests are not very sensitive. I favor the use of tests based upon experimental cognitive psychology (originally developed in the psychological laboratory) because timed measures are usually more sensitive and do allow repeated testing. The other neuropsychological tests described are useful as basal standards provided that they give quantitative (numerical) results.

References

Branconnier, R. J. and DeVitt, D. R. (1974) Early detection of incipient Alzheimer's disease. In B. Reisberg (Ed.), *Alzheimer's Disease*, Raven Press, New York, pp. 214–227.

Cummings, J. L. and Benson, D. F. (1984) Subcortical dementia: review of an emerging concept. *Arch. Neurol.*, 41: 874–879.

Irigaray, L. (1973) *Le Langage des Déments*, Mouton, The Hague.

Jolles, J. (1986) Cognitive, emotional and behavioral dysfunctions in aging and dementia. In D. F. Swaab, E. Fliers, M. Mirmiran, W. A. Van Gool and F. Van Haaren (Eds.), *Aging of the Brain and Alzheimer's Disease, Progress in Brain Research*, this volume, pp. 15–39.

Sternberg, S. (1975) Memory scanning: new findings and current controversies. *Quart. J. Exp. Psychol.*, 27: 1–32.

Vanneste, J. A. L. and Hijman, R. (1986) Non tumoral aquaduct stenosis and normal pressure hydrocephalus in the elderly. *Neurol. Neurosurg. Psychiat.*, 49: 529–535.

D. F. Swaab, E. Fliers, M. Mirmiran, W. A. Van Gool and F. Van Haaren (Eds.)
Progress in Brain Research, Vol. 70.

CHAPTER 3

Interrelations among the lesions of normal and abnormal aging of the brain

R. D. Terry

Department of Neurosciences, University of California, San Diego, La Jolla, CA 92093, USA

Normal aging

Before one can discuss the organic aspects of the normal aged brain, he must establish an acceptable level of clinical and cognitive normalcy for the elderly, although rigorous definition is not readily at hand. We must first accept the notion that that which is common is not necessarily normal. For example, although upper respiratory infections in children are very common in the winter months in colder countries and may involve 75% of 12-year olds during a cold February, it is not normal to have these symptoms. Also, although the histologic evidence of carcinoma of the prostate is to be found in the great majority of 80-year-old men, that must not be regarded as normal either. The cold and the indolent prostate carcinoma are common, but not normal. It is also common to accept as normal, and I believe erroneously, the elderly person with mild forgetfulness, some difficulty in word finding, diminished ability to solve problems, etc. But, however frequent, these too should not be accepted as normal. As examples of elderly normal, one might better think of Pablo Casals, or Picasso, or Rebecca West — all active, stimulating, imaginative and productive people into old age. Such is the fortunate future for about one-third of those reaching 80. Another third display so-called benign senescent forgetfulness, while the final third become frankly demented (Katzman, 1985). A prospective study of a large group of independent, community-living people in their 80's revealed that those who scored four or five errors on a modified 'blessed mental status' test went on at yearly examinations to show a significant further decline of cognitive ability, while those who had tested at zero to one error remained that way during the next several years (Katzman, 1985). This would indicate that benign senescent forgetfulness is not altogether benign.

Neuropathology of normal aging

At this time of the century in the United States, it is quite difficult to collect a large series of normal autopsy specimens from patients who had been thoroughly tested and found to be cognitively intact on all counts. What one can say in this regard about the series to be described is that the great majority had been so tested, while some individuals were accepted on faith since they came from independent community situations and had no historical evidence of any level of dementia. Most of these untested subjects were below age 50. Furthermore, all specimens were histologically intact with only a few lesions (plaques and tangles) in the hippocampus and entorhinal areas and far fewer plaques and no tangles in the neocortex.

In accordance with many series, our own, which consisted of 50 specimens, demonstrated a steady decline in weight of fixed brain as a function of age between 20 and 100 years (Terry et al., 1986,

42

submitted). The negative slope was almost 7 g per year, and accelerated somewhat beyond age 70. Although it is conceivable that some of this loss may be from extracellular fluid, we must assume that most of it is due to a loss of parenchymal elements; that is, both cells and myelin. Miller et al. (1980) have reported that there is a change in the ratio between gray matter and white, which first falls from 1.28 to 1.13 and then rises to 1.55 at old age.

Although Brody (1955) reported a nearly 50% loss of cortical neurons in the course of normal aging and emphasized the loss of small cells, our own findings on this series of cases provide quite different conclusions. We counted cells in histologic sections of midfrontal, superior temporal and inferior parietal areas with an image analysis apparatus, which to our satisfaction counted almost all glia as smaller than 40 mμ^2 in cross section, while neurons were almost always larger than this size (Terry et al., 1981). Neuron-specific staining, of course, would make these data even more precise. We found with cresyl violet preparations, that in the course of normal aging there is a significant increase in the number of glia, a significant decrease in the number of large neurons (greater than 90 mμ^2), but an equally increased number of small neurons, that is, those measuring between 40 and 90 mμ^2 in cross-sectional area of their perikarya. We conclude that some large neurons shrink into the smaller size class, but there is no significant regression of total neurons to be found in these three neocortical areas in normal aging (Terry et al., 1986, submitted).

Neuropathology of Alzheimer's disease

In Alzheimer's disease, there is an additive significant loss of brain tissue, and this involves both neocortex and cerebral white matter, septum, amygdaloid, and hippocampus. The weight loss, however, does not regress as a function of age, with which there is no correlation. Brain weight correlates significantly with the concentration of plaques in the neocortex if normals are included.

Counting neuroectodermal cells in three areas of the neocortex revealed population changes which are distinctly different from those of normal aging. Comparing groups of age-matched normal specimens with 70- to 90-year-old specimens of senile dementia of the Alzheimer type (SDAT), we found in the latter a major loss of large neurons in all three areas, but no change of small neurons in temporal or parietal areas (Terry et al., 1981), and a barely significant decrement in the midfrontal region (Terry, unpublished data). The number of glial cells did not change, but there was an increased proportion of fibrous astrocytes among the glia (Schechter et al., 1981). These changes are, of course, in addition to those of normal aging, so that a comparison of elderly SDAT patients with young (20–55 y) normals, reveals a difference of about 55% as to large neurons. Alzheimer's disease specimens aged 50 to 70 display a great percentage loss of large neurons plus a significant loss of small neurons, the latter in the superior temporal and inferior parietal areas, as compared with 50- to 70-year-old normals. The younger patients had the more severe disease (Terry et al., 1986, in preparation).

These cell counts were done with a semi-automated, computerized image analysis apparatus on the side of a sulcus in an area 600 micra wide along the pia through the full thickness of the cortical ribbon. This thickness is variable to some degree in disease and to a lesser extent as a function of age. The numbers cited, therefore, cannot be referred to directly as cell density. Since the cortical thickness, including molecular layer, is measured in each counted area, the cell density can be calculated. This recalculation does not change the conclusions as to statistical significance.

The neocortex is not the only area from which neurons are lost in Alzheimer's disease. Significant neuronal decreases have been found among the hippocampal pyramids (Ball, 1977), the entorhinal cortex (Hyman et al., 1984), the amygdaloid nucleus (Herzog and Kemper, 1980), the basal nucleus of Meynert (Whitehouse et al., 1982), and the locus ceruleus (Bondareff et al., 1982). The decreased number of neurons in each of these areas implies an associated loss of neurotransmitters, receptors and function. Decreased somatostatin might be the result of loss of large neurons in the neocortex (Morrison et al., 1983). Glutamate (Greenamyre et al., 1985) and M_2-muscarinic (Mash et al., 1985) receptors are reported to be diminished in the neocortex. Cholinergic activity in the neocortex comes in large part from the susceptible neurons of the basal nucleus (Whitehouse et al., 1981), and norepinephrine arises in the affected locus ceruleus (Perry et al., 1981). In some systems, however, the change in transmitter concentration in the target area is greater than the loss of cell bodies where the transmitter or its synthetic enzyme originate (Candy et al., 1983). This bespeaks either or both of two possibilities: (1) a dying back and consequent disconnection phenomenon, or (2) a metabolic decrease in formation of the synthetic enzyme prior to death of the cell; that is, a loss of so-called luxury function (Oldstone et al., 1977).

Possible causes of cell loss in Alzheimer's disease

The causes of neuronal loss in Alzheimer's disease are, of course, still unknown, but a number of possibilities can be suggested. Clearly, inheritance must play a role, especially in view of the fact that 5 or 10% of Alzheimer patients come from families with the dominant inheritance pattern, and another 30 to 50%, or perhaps more, have more affected relatives than statistically expected, although not in any simple Mendelian pattern (Heston et al., 1981; Breitner and Folstein, 1984). Nevertheless, it has to be admitted that studies of DNA to date have failed to reveal abnormalities in affected specimens (Spector and Kornberg, 1985). An endogenous neurotoxin such as a neurotransmitter analog might be formed by some error in synthesis; but analog transmitters have not been reported. Immunologic abnormalities have been suggested, but have not been demonstrated to be cytopathic (Miller et al., 1981). The suggestion of a deficient trophic factor (Appel, 1981) begs this

question as to cause, since these trophic factors are synthesized by target cells, and so one must ask what causes this still hypothetical failure and then start the questions all over. Abnormal oxidation and peroxidation might well have a significant role in both normal and abnormal aging, but there is no specific evidence here regarding Alzheimer's disease. It might be pointed out in this regard that lipofuscin, which is at least partially caused by peroxidation, is not increased beyond normal in SDAT (Mann and Sinclair, 1978). Lipofuscin seems to be a symbol of peroxidation, rather than the mechanism through which free radicals damage cells. Both conventional and unconventional virus have also been suggested as possible etiologic factors, and the latter, in the form of prions, has attracted much recent attention (Prusiner, 1982). Nevertheless, Alzheimer's disease has not been transmitted in the laboratory or the operating room as far as we know (Goudsmit et al., 1980). Furthermore, scrapie-associated filaments, which are characteristic of the transmissible spongy encephalopathies, have not been found in Alzheimer's disease (Merz et al., 1984). Finally, there might be an exogenous toxin such as aluminum. This and some of the other possibilities are to be discussed elsewhere in this book.

Microscopic lesions in Alzheimer's disease

The dendritic arbor of pyramidal cells has been reported to be markedly deficient in hippocampal and neocortical areas in Alzheimer's disease (Scheibel, 1978). This shrinkage of the arbor involves not only the dendrites themselves, but also their spines. On the other hand, in normal aging the arbor is actually increased according to some reports (Buell and Coleman, 1979), and decreased in others (Scheibel, 1978). It is not at all impossible that both processes are going on simultaneously even in adjacent cells in the course of normal aging. At any rate, dendritic shrinkage might well be a step toward cell death, and certainly reduces synaptic contacts.

There are three widespread lesions which are

characteristic of Alzheimer's disease, the first two being essential to the diagnosis. First is the neurofibrillary tangle, made up of paired helical filaments (PHF) (Kidd, 1963), and found in large and medium size neurons especially in neocortex, hippocampus, parahippocampus, amygdaloid, innominata, septum, and mesencephalic raphe. The second is the neuritic or senile plaque made up of an array of mostly presynaptic, swollen neurites containing large numbers of lamellar lysosomes, degenerating mitochondria, and paired helical filaments, all surrounding an extracellular core of amyloid (Terry et al., 1964). These are found in the same regions with tangles, but in the neocortex they are in higher concentration in superficial layers, while tangles are more common in the deeper levels (Rogers and Morrison, 1985). Neurites in plaques have been found so far to contain cholinergic activity (Struble et al., 1982), somatostatin (Armstrong et al., 1985; Morrison et al., 1985), substance P (Armstrong et al., 1985), tyrosine hydroxylase (Kitt et al., 1984), and neuropeptide Y (Dawbarn and Emson, 1985). It has not been shown that a single plaque contains more than one transmitter, but it does seem likely. Tangles are largely alone in the entorhinal cortex and in the basal nucleus of Meynert. The concentration of plaques correlates strongly with mental status tests when one includes normals as well as Alzheimer cases (Blessed et al., 1968). More variable is the third lesion — amyloid infiltrates in the walls of small arteries of leptomeninges and cortex. The former is the more common, but neither is invariably present in Alzheimer's disease, nor does the intensity of this change, which is called amyloid or congophilic angiopathy, correlate with the concentration of plaques and tangles in any given area.

The fact that both plaques and tangles are commonly found in most normal elderly specimens has been conceptually troublesome to all observers. Of course, their quantity in the normal is very different from that in Alzheimer's at every age. In the normal aged specimen, plaques are rare in the neocortex, and tangles exquisitely so. A somewhat larger number may be found in the hippocampal pyramids, but not great numbers even here. A few tangles may also be found in the superficial layers of the normal aged entorhinal cortex, which is apparently particularly susceptible. The reasons for this regional susceptibility of hippocampal and entorhinal neurons are entirely unknown. If, as suggested above, Alzheimer's disease is due to an essential genetic factor plus a second environmental or additional endogenous factor, it is difficult to believe that almost everyone carries this gene. Perhaps only the second factor is enough to induce the changes in these particularly susceptible neurons. That, however, would imply that if the dose of the second factor is great enough, less susceptible cells could be affected.

In 1967, we suggested that the plaque may be related to the tangle because the latter interferes with axoplasmic and dendritic flow (Suzuki and Terry, 1967). Diminished supply of substrates and other important metabolites might well cause dystrophic change in the terminals, manifested by swelling, abnormal mitochondria and increased numbers of lysosomes just as we find in the plaque. The PHF themselves would proceed toward the terminals, as do the components of normal neurofibers, albeit at a slower rate. The cellular elements of the plaque are largely these dystrophic, presynaptic terminals. A few dendritic terminals are involved, but not many. On the basis of morphologic evidence, we also proposed some years ago that the earliest changes in the neuropil of Alzheimer's disease were these dystrophic changes of the terminals, and that the extracellular amyloid came later (Terry and Wisniewski, 1970).

Protein from leptomeningeal vascular amyloid has been isolated and sequenced, and was found to be a 4 000-dalton polypeptide unique among proteins catalogued to date (Glenner and Wong, 1984). Subsequently, it has very recently been reported that this sequence is present in the amyloid of the plaque core and also in isolated neurofibrillary tangles (Kidd et al., 1985). This last point conflicts with several previous reports concerning monoclonal and polyclonal antibodies, made against isolated paired helical filaments, and which do not cross-react with the core of the plaques nor with the vascular amyloid. Some of these antibodies do cross-react with normal neurofilament protein (Anderton et al., 1982), while others do not (Ihara et al., 1983), and this leads to the impression that the protein of the tangle is partially conserved and partially modified from normal neurofilaments. On the other hand, the four-kilodalton protein sequence is not apparently related to that of neurofilaments (Glenner and Wong, 1984).

If we assume that the protein of tangle, plaque core and intramural amyloid are indeed identical, despite conflicting evidence, then it would seem very likely that they all come from the same source. Since proteins are not synthesized in the extracellular space, the core of the plaques cannot be the origin. This leaves three possibilities: (1) an extra cerebral source connected to the brain by the blood stream, (2) the neuron, and (3) glia. If the material comes from the blood stream and is first deposited in the walls of the arterioles, then amyloid angiopathy ought to be present in all cases where plaques are found and ought, probably, to be correlated as to intensity with the concentration of plaques. In fact, amyloid angiopathy is not invariably found in association with Alzheimer's disease, and when it is, it is more often found in the leptomeninges than in the parenchyma, and neither is correlated as to intensity with the concentration of plaques in any given region. On the other hand, if the abnormal protein is first synthesized in the neurons as paired helical filaments and then moves into the plaque as the neurites deteriorate in the neuropil, then the number of plaques might be expected to increase as the number of tangles declines. This does seem to be the case, especially in patients above the age of

80, where tangles are often very rare relative to the number of plaques (Terry et al., 1982). Glia were suggested as the source of the amyloid in the plaque core some years ago (Terry et al., 1964), but have not apparently been discussed in relation to either PHF or vascular amyloid. The morphologic differences among these three fiber types could be otherwise resolved on physico-chemical bases.

Summary and conclusions

In summary, the major lesions of Alzheimer's disease are tangles, plaques, amyloid angiopathy, and neuronal loss, as well as a variety of neuropharmacologic deficiencies. The sequence of events might be that the genetic factor plus a second factor induce the synthesis of an abnormal protein which, perhaps on a core of aluminum-silicate filaments, forms PHF which in aggregate make neurofibrillary tangles. These on the one hand kill the cells and their processes causing deficiencies of transmitters and receptors, while on the other hand, the abnormal fibers leave the dying neuron, pass into the extracellular space to form the core of the plaque, and subsequently infiltrate the vessel walls. Another hypothesis is that an abnormal substrate is formed elsewhere and is transported to the brain via the blood stream. It passes through the vessel wall and is processed in the mural cells to be deposited as amyloid. It also gains the parenchyma to be deposited, again perhaps on aluminum-silicate filaments, as amyloid. Clumps of the latter induce focal degeneration of neurites to form the plaque. This sequence does not explain the neurofibrillary tangle which might be an independent process. In either case, clinical symptoms are the result of the pharmacologic abnormalities, which in turn are caused by death and degeneration of neurons and their axons and dendrites.

References

Anderton, B. H., Breinburg, D., Downes, M. J., Green, P. J., Tomlinson, B. E., Ulrich, J., Wood, J. N. and Kahn, J. (1982) Monoclonal antibodies show that neurofibrillary tangles and neurofilaments share antigenic determinants. *Nature (Lond.)*, 298: 84–86.

Appel, S. H. (1981) A unifying hypothesis for the cause of amyotrophic lateral sclerosis, Parkinsonism, and Alzheimer disease. *Ann. Neurol.*, 10: 499–505.

Armstrong, D. M. and Terry, R. D. (1985) Substance P immunoreactivity within neuritic plaques. *Neurosci. Lett.*, 58: 139–144.

Armstrong, D. M., LeRoy, S., Shields, D. and Terry, R. D. (1985) Somatostatin-like immunoreactivity within neuritic plaques. *Brain Res.*, 338: 71–79.

Ball, M. J. (1977) Neuronal loss, neurofibrillary tangles and granulovacuolar degeneration in the hippocampus with aging and dementia. A quantitative study. *Acta Neuropathol.*, 37: 111–118.

Blessed, G., Tomlinson, B. E. and Roth, M. (1968) The association between quantitative measures of dementia and of senile changes in the cerebral grey matter of elderly subjects. *Br. J. Psychiat.*, 114: 797–811.

Bondareff, W., Mountjoy, C. Q. and Roth, M. (1982) Loss of neurons of origin of the adrenergic projection to cerebral cortex (nucleus locus ceruleus) in senile dementia. *Neurology*, 32: 164–168.

Breitner, J. C. S. and Folstein, M. F. (1984) Familial nature of Alzheimer's disease. *N. Engl. J. Med.*, 311: 192.

Brody, H. (1955) A study of aging in the human cerebral cortex. *J. Comp. Neurol.*, 102: 511–556.

Buell, S. J. and Coleman, P. D. (1979) Dendritic growth in the aged human brain and failure of growth in senile dementia. *Science*, 206: 854–856.

Candy, J. M., Perry, R. H., Perry, E. K., Irving, D., Blessed, G., Fairbairn, A. F. and Tomlinson, B. E. (1983) Pathological changes in the nucleus of Meynert in Alzheimer's and Parkinson's diseases. *J. Neurol. Sci.*, 54: 277–289.

Dawbarn, D. and Emson, P. C. (1985) Neuropeptide Y-like immunoreactivity in neuritic plaques of Alzheimer's disease. *Biochem. Biophys. Res. Commun.*, 126: 189–294.

Glenner, G. G. and Wong, C. W. (1984) Alzheimer's disease: initial report of the purification and characterization of a novel cerebrovascular amyloid protein. *Biochem. Biophys. Res. Commun.*, 120: 885–890.

Goudsmit, J., Morrow, C. H., Asher, D. M., Yanagihara, R. T., Masters, C. L., Gibbs, C. J., Jr. and Gajdusek, D. C. (1980) Evidence for and against the transmissibility of Alzheimer disease. *Neurology*, 30: 945–950.

Greenamyre, J. T., Penney, J. B., Young, A. B., D'Amato, C. J., Hicks, S. P. and Shoulson, I. (1985) Alterations in L-glutamate binding in Alzheimer's and Huntington's disease. *Science*, 227: 1496–1499.

Herzog, A. G. and Kemper, T. L. (1980) Amygdaloid changes in aging and dementia. *Arch. Neurol.*, 37: 625–629.

Heston, L. L., Mastri, A. R. and Anderson, V. E. (1981) Dementia of the Alzheimer type. Clinical genetics, natural history, and associated conditions. *Arch. Gen. Psychiat.*, 38: 1085–1090.

Hyman, B. T., Van Hoesen, G. W., Damasio and A. R., Barnes, C. L. (1984) Alzheimer's disease: cell-specific pathology isolates the hippocampal formation. *Science*, 225: 1168–1170.

Ihara, Y., Abraham, C. and Selkoe, D. J. (1983) Antibodies to paired helical filaments in Alzheimer's disease do not recognize normal brain proteins. *Nature*, 304: 727–730.

Katzman, R. (1985) Aging and age-dependent disease: cognition and dementia. In *America's Aging: Health in Older Society*, Committe on an Aging Society, Institute of Medical/National Research Council, National Academy Press, Washington, D.C., pp. 129–152.

Kidd, M. (1963) Paired helical filaments in electron microscopy in Alzheimer's disease. *Nature (Lond.)*, 197: 192–193.

Kidd, M., Allsop, D. and Landon, M. (1985) Senile plaque amyloid, paired helical filaments and cerebrovascular amyloid in Alzheimer's disease are all deposits of the same protein. *Lancet*, 1: 278.

Kitt, C. A., Price, D. L., Struble, R. G., Cork, L. C., Walker, L. C., Mobley, W. C., Bechen, W. M., Joh, T. H. and Wainer, B. H. (1984) Transmitter specificity of neurites in senile plaques of aged monkeys. *Trans. Soc. Neurosci.*, abstract 82.2.

Mann, D. M. A. and Sinclair, K. G. A. (1978) The quantitative assessment of lipofuscin pigment, cytoplasmic RNA and nucleolar volume in senile dementia. *Neuropathol. Appl. Neurobiol.*, 4: 129–135.

Mash, D. C., Flynn, D. D. and Potter, L. T. (1985) Loss of M_2-muscarine receptors in the cerebral cortex in Alzheimer's disease and experimental cholinergic denervation. *Science*, 228: 1115–1117.

Merz, P. A., Rohwer, R. G., Kascsak, R., Wisniewski, H. M., Somerville, R. A., Gibbs, C. J. Jr. and Gajdusek, D. C. (1984) Infection-specific particle from the unconventional slow virus diseases. *Science*, 225: 437–440.

Miller, A. E., Neighbour, A., Katzman, R., Aronson, M. and Lipkowitz, R. (1981) Immunologic studies in senile dementia of the Alzheimer type: evidence for enhanced suppressor cell activity. *Ann. Neurol.*, 10: 506–510.

Miller, A. K. H., Alston, R. L. and Corsellis, J. A. N. (1980) Variation with age in the volumes of grey and white matter in the cerebral hemispheres of man: measurements with an image analyser. *Neuropathol. Appl. Neurobiol.*, 6: 119–132.

Morrison, J. H., Benoit, R., Magistretti, P. J. and Bloom, F. E. (1983) Immunohistochemical distribution of pro-somatostatin-related peptides in cerebral cortex. *Brain Res.*, 262: 344–351.

Morrison, J. H., Rogers, J., Scherr, S., Benoit, R. and Bloom, F. E. (1985) Somatostatin immunoreactivity in neuritic plaques of Alzheimer's patients. *Nature*, 308: 90–92.

Oldstone, M. B. A., Holmstoen, J. and Welsh, R. M., Jr. (1977) Alterations of acetylcholine enzymes in neuroblastoma cells persistently infected with lymphocytic choriomeningitis virus. *J. Cell Physiol.*, 91: 459–472.

Perry, E. K., Tomlinson, B. E., Blessed, G., Perry, R. H., Cross, A. J. and Crow, T. J. (1981) Neuropathological and biochemical observations on the noradrenergic system in Alzheimer's disease. *J. Neurol. Sci.*, 51: 279–287.

Prusiner, S. B. (1982) Novel proteinaceous infectious particles cause scrapie. *Science*, 216: 136–144.

Rogers, J. and Morrison, J. H. (1985) Quantitative morphology and regional and laminar distributions of senile plaques in Alzheimer's disease. *J. Neurosci.*, 5: 2801–2808.

Schecter, R., Yen, S-H. C. and Terry, R. D. (1981) Fibrous astrocytes in senile dementia of the Alzheimer type. *J. Neuropathol. Exp. Neurol.*, 40: 95–101.

Scheibel, A. B. (1978) Structural aspects of the aging brain: spine systems and the dendritic arbor. In R. Katzman, R. D. Terry and K. L. Bick (Eds.), *Alzheimer's Disease: Senile Dementia and Related Disorders, Aging, Vol. 7*, Raven Press, New York, pp. 353–373.

Spector, R. and Kornberg, A. (1985) Search for DNA alterations in Alzheimer's disease. *Neurobiol. Aging*, 6: 25–28.

Struble, R. G., Cork, L. C., Whitehouse, P. J. and Price, D. L. (1982) Cholinergic innervation in neuritic plaques. *Science*, 216: 413–415.

Suzuki, K. and Terry, R. D. (1967) Fine structural localization of acid phosphatase in senile plaques in Alzheimer's presenile dementia. *Acta Neuropathol.*, 8: 176–284.

Terry, R. D. and Wisniewski, H. M. (1970) The ultrastructure of the neurofibrillary tangle and the senile plaque. In G. E. W. Wolstenholme and M. O'Connor (Eds.), *Ciba Foundation Symposium on Alzheimer's Disease and Related Conditions*, J. & A. Churchill, London, pp. 145–168.

Terry, R. D., Gonatas, K. and Weiss, M. (1964) Ultrastructural studies in Alzheimer's presenile dementia. *Am. J. Pathol.*, 44: 269–297.

Terry, R. D., Peck, A., DeTeresa, R., Schechter, R. and Horoupian, D. S. (1981) Some morphometric aspects of the brain in senile dementia of the Alzheimer type. *Ann. Neurol.*, 10: 184–192.

Terry, R. D., Davies, P., DeTeresa, R. and Katzman, R. (1982) Are both plaques and tangles required to make it Alzheimer's disease? *J. Neuropathol. Exp. Neurol.*, 41: 364, abstract.

Whitehouse, P. J., Price, D. L., Clark, A. W., Coyle, J. T. and DeLong, M. R. (1981) Alzheimer's disease: evidence for selective loss of cholinergic neurons in the nucleus basalis. *Ann. Neurol.*, 10: 122–126.

Whitehouse, P. J., Price, D. L., Struble, R. G., Clark, A. W., Coyle, J. T. and DeLong, M. R. (1982) Alzheimer's disease and senile dementia: loss of neurons in the basal forebrain. *Science*, 215: 1237–1239.

Discussion

H. VAN CREVEL: How constant is the topological distribution of Alzheimer's changes? This is interesting because of the clinical heterogeneity.

ANSWER: By the time of death, most cases display global cognitive changes, and the autopsy findings reflect this broad effect. The concentration of plaques in mid frontal, superior temporal and inferior parietal cortex correlate closely with each other, and are approximately equal in each case for the most part.

C. G. GOTTFRIES: Is there a reduced number of neurons in the substantia nigra in brains from patients with AD/SDAT?

ANSWER: Usually not.

K. IQBAL: Comment: I would like to emphasize that there are *no* similarities between the amino acid sequence of the brain amyloid 4KDa polypeptide and neurofilament polypeptide(s).

ANSWER: I agree with your comment.

E. FLIERS: If indeed the amyloid core in plaques would be derived from some component in the blood (via congophilic angiopathy) then a close anatomical relationship between plaques and blood vessels might be expected. Are there any indications for such a relationship?

ANSWER: Many, but not all plaques are closely related to capillaries. In general, there is no correlation as to intensity or topography between the amyloid-infiltrated vessels and the plaques.

P. D. COLEMAN: Have you ever seen amyloid angiopathy in vessels clearly identified as capillaries?

ANSWER: Some vessels, especially in area 17, appear in the light microscope to be of capillary size and yet affected by amyloid. This is rare.

J. E. PISETSKY: If cells die and Wallerian degeneration occurs, what happens to the axis cylinders and myelin sheaths? Is Alzheimer's a white matter disease?

ANSWER: When the neuron dies, its axon and the surrounding myelin degenerate. This is secondary degeneration. Alzheimer's disease is not a primarily demyelinating disorder or primarily one of white matter.

W. VAN TILBURG: Do your findings confirm the results of research from Cambridge University (Bondareff et al., 1982) about the occurrence of two types of Alzheimer's disease to be distinguished from each other by the degree of cell loss in the locus ceruleus and in the neocortex?

ANSWER: Most autopsied Alzheimer cases show loss of pigmented neurons in the locus ceruleus. I do not believe that this represents a fundamentally different disease. I do not know of extensive correlation between the number of neurons in the ceruleus and in the neocortex.

H. B. M. UYLINGS: (1) You mentioned that the number of neurons calculated was not a density variable, but that these cells were measured in columns with a width and depth; they are thus expressed in terms of density.

(2) Did you measure one column per cortical area or did you measure several columns per cortical area? Did you find differences in columnar heterogeneity in control aged and SDAT groups?

(3) The smallest group of profiles you have measured contains both glial cells and neuronal gaps. Does the fraction of neuronal gaps change in the different comparisons you made between the SDAT and aged groups and between the different age groups?

ANSWERS: (1) The columns were 600 μ wide and through the full cortical thickness. The latter is variable from case to case.

Therefore the cell numbers are cited as such, not number per unit area. It is not a true density measure.

(2) A single column, 5 fields each of 120 μ or 600 μ total width by full thickness of cortex was counted in each area — frontal, temporal and parietal.

(3) The smallest category of 5–40 μ contains very few neurons recognizable as such — less than 5%.

C. A. MAROTTA: What neurons are lost in AD?

ANSWER: SDAT cortex loses 35–46% of neurons larger than 90 μ, but no loss of small neurons 40–90 μ. Therefore the total neuron loss is less than 20%, but these lost cells are the ones with the most RNA.

References

Bondareff, W., Mountjoy, C. Q. and Roth, M. (1982) Loss of neurons of origin of the adrenergic projection to cerebral cortex (nucleus locus ceruleus) in senile dementia. *Neurology*, 32: 164–168.

D. F. Swaab, E. Fliers, M. Mirmiran, W. A. Van Gool and F. Van Haaren (Eds.)
Progress in Brain Research, Vol. 70.
© 1986 Elsevier Science Publishers B.V. (Biomedical Division)

CHAPTER 4

Age-related changes in Down syndrome brain and the cellular pathology of Alzheimer disease

R. S. Williams* and S. Matthysse

Shriver Center, 200 Trapelo Road, Waltham, MA 02154, USA and Mailman Research Center, McLean Hospital, 115 Mill Street, Belmont, MA 02178, USA

Introduction

Down syndrome (DS) is one of the most common identifiable causes of mental retardation, affecting 1 or 2 per 1 000 live births (Hook, 1981). Approximately 95% of cases result from meiotic non-disjunction of chromosome 21. The genetic material responsible for the DS phenotype has been localized to a relatively short band of the long arm (q 22) of chromosome 21 (Summitt, 1981).

The neuropathological basis for mental retardation and delayed motor development in DS is not yet known with certainty. The range of brain weights of persons with DS is more variable and the mean is lower, but most are within two standard deviations of the normal population (Solitare and Lamarche, 1967). The smallness of the brain is roughly proportional to the smaller stature of DS individuals, but the cerebellum and hippocampal formation may be disproportionately small (Crome et al., 1966; Sylvester, 1983). Cytometric studies have given conflicting results (Cragg, 1975), but three have reported a decrease in the density of cortical neurons of approximately 50% (Colon, 1972; Ross et al., 1984; Wisniewski et al., 1984). The deficiency of neocortical neurons may affect small local circuit neurons preferentially (Ross et al., 1984). The density of pyramidal neurons in the hippocampus (Ball and Nutall,

1980) and large neurons of the nucleus basalis (Casanova et al., 1985) are reduced also in cases of DS, and this difference is not apparently age related. Cytopathological studies with Golgi methods suggest a decrease in dendritic branching and spine density, and altered dendritic spine morphology of pyramidal neurons in the neocortex (Marin-Padilla, 1976; Takashima et al., 1981; Suetsugu and Mehraein, 1980). Although Golgi studies imply that the density of axospinous synapses is reduced, Cragg (1975) and Petit et al. (1984) found no change in synaptic density in electronmicrographs from DS cortex.

In DS precocious age-related degenerative changes of the skin, hair and lens of the eye are encountered commonly. Mortality studies in institutionalized populations demonstrate a higher rate of deaths for DS cases over the age of 50 years than for retarded individuals without DS (Richards and Sylvester, 1969). In 1929, Struwe noted that the youngest case in his collection of brains with cortical neuritic plaques (NP), associated presumably with Alzheimer disease (AD), was a 37-year-old person with DS. Many subsequent studies have confirmed that the neuropathological changes characteristic of AD (viz. NP, neurofibrillary tangles [NFT] composed of paired helical filaments and granulovacuolar change) are present by the fourth decade in virtually all cases of DS, and increase in severity with advancing age (Ropper and Williams, 1980; Price et al., 1982).

---

* Correspondence should be addressed to Dr. R. S. Williams.

The relatively high prevalence of DS and the uniformly precocious appearance of the neuropathological changes of AD provide a unique opportunity to test theories about the pathogenesis of AD. It is important first to identify the similarities and differences between conventional AD, and AD in older persons with DS (DS/AD). In this review, these comparisons will be discussed in light of the available literature and our experience with 23 cases studied neuropathologically.

Materials and methods

Patient material

Twenty-seven cases of DS over age 30 years were autopsied at the Massachusetts General Hospital from 1960–1985. Adequate histological material (two or more tissue blocks from various regions of the cerebral cortex) and clinical data were available in 23 cases. A preliminary report of these findings has appeared elsewhere (Ropper and Williams, 1980). All patients had been confined to an institution for several decades prior to death. Their records included information about the perinatal and early developmental history, results of chromosomal studies and other laboratory tests, results of psychometric tests, annual reports of physical and neurological status and annual assessments of their behavior, self-help and vocational skills. In 20 cases trisomy 21 was confirmed by chromosomal analysis; in three cases the diagnosis was based on the typical clinical phenotype. One of the latter (age 73 years) had typical DS phenotype and was carried clinically as DS in the institutional records. Review of the records postmortem, however, revealed that a single karyotype analysis was performed in the 1960's, which was reported to be normal. Although he may have been a mosaic, he will be referred to hereafter as 'pseudo-DS' (Summitt, 1981).

The records were scrutinized for evidence of neurological or psychiatric symptoms developing in later life. When possible, families and direct care staff were questioned to clarify further the level of functioning near the time of death. A recent decline in self-help, communication or vocational skills; a striking change in mood, social skills or memory capacity; the appearance of epilepsy, myoclonus or impaired motor performance in the absence of alternative neuropathological diagnoses; were considered as possible clinical evidence for dementia of Alzheimer type (DAT).

Fixation

All brains were fixed in 4% formaldehyde. For the Golgi studies, the interval from death to tissue fixation ranged from 3–20 h. The interval between primary fixation in formalin and post-fixation in rapid Golgi solution was 1–4 days.

Histology

Tissue blocks had been taken from a variety of neocortical and brain stem areas and from the hippocampus, but no standard protocol had been followed over the years. Histological sections were prepared from blocks embedded in paraffin, sectioned at a thickness of 10 microns, and stained for cells (cresyl violet, hematoxylin and eosin) and axonal fibers (luxol fast blue, Bodian silver).

In four cases of DS (ages 31, 31, 57 and 64 years), small blocks of neocortex (areas 4, 9 and 22 in the classification of Brodmann), hippocampal formation and cerebellum were prepared successfully for rapid Golgi impregnations (Williams et al., 1978). Golgi blocks were embedded in 30% low-viscosity nitrocellulose and cut serially at a thickness of 100–150 microns. The morphology of Golgi-impregnated neurons in these four cases was compared to that of two younger cases of DS with trisomy 21 (ages 6 and 25 years), one case of DS with 18–21 translocation (age 6 years), four cases of senile dementia of Alzheimer type (SDAT) (ages 70, 78, 88 and 88 years) and 13 persons (controls) who died without neurological disease (ages 16, 27, 35, 36, 37, 37, 39, 61, 72, 75, 79, 80 and 91 years).

Morphometry

A computer-assisted planimeter was used to count the density of neuritic plaques (NP) and neurofibrillary tangles (NFT) in Bodian-stained sections of the hippocampal formation, including the dentate gyrus, cornu ammonis (CA 1–4) and subiculum complex. Counts were expressed as the number of NP and NFT per mm². No correction was made for the size of NP, which varied from 79.4–174.6 microns (mean 132.3, ±38.4 SD) in diameter, or for section thickness (microtome setting, 10 microns). Formal counts of NP and NFT density were not done in neocortex, because blocks had not been obtained in a consistent way and direct comparisons were not possible.

A computer-assisted semi-automatic microscope was used to measure the size- and shape-related geometric parameters of granule cell dendrites in the hippocampal dentate gyrus (for details see Williams and Matthysse, 1983). Size-related parameters included the number of stem segments and subordinate segments (all daughter segments beyond the stem, including terminal segments), and their mean individual and aggregate (total dendritic) length. In contrast to most mammals (Cajal, 1968), we found that about 50% of granule cells in the Golgi-impregnated human dentate gyrus have small basal dendrites in addition to the larger apical dendritic ensemble. Measures of size-related parameters included both. The shape of the apical dendrites is typically an ellipsoidal cone. Shape-related parameters were measured relative to an 'ideal axis' of symmetry, computed as the unit vector in the direction of the vector sum of all a cell's branches. We have found that three of the shape-related parameters best describe the characteristic 'wineglass' shape of granule cell dendrites. These include: (1) the angle between the daughter segments ('daughter angle'), (2) the angle between the ideal axis and the plane that contains tangents to the parent and two subordinate branch points ('planar angle'), and (3) the ratio of the ellipsoidal cross sections of the dendrites ('planarity'). Basal dendrites were excluded from the analysis of shape-related parameters.

Some dendrites of nearly all cells were cut at the edge of the tissue, and we did not attempt to find and reconstruct the missing segments from adjacent sections. Rather we labeled each terminus as a 'cut' or 'natural', and computed the percentage of cut ends for each cell.

The density of spines on terminal segments in the outer half of the molecular layer was also measured. All visible spines were counted along a 40–100 micron segment measured with the computer-assisted microscope, and the density was expressed as the number of spines per micron.

Dendritic morphometry and spine density were measured with a 65 × oil immersion objective (N.A. 1.25). Cells with dendrites judged to be incompletely impregnated or obscured by adjacent dendrites, astrocytes or blood vessels, and cells with their somas near the edge of the tissue section were excluded from analysis. Once a cell was judged appropriate for measurement, it was included or excluded based on a coin toss in an effort to additionally minimize selection bias (Buell and Coleman, 1979). Ten cells were selected in this manner from each case. The slides were coded so the examiner was not aware of the case diagnosis. The study of dendrite morphometry included all seven cases of DS, three cases of SDAT and 13 controls. The 70-year-old case of SDAT had too few granule cells impregnated for morphometric analysis.

Results

Clinical

Five of the 23 DS cases who died after age 30 years were found to have progressive neurological illness in later life compatible with DAT and not attributable to other acquired illness (Table I). Their ages at death were 49, 49, 50, 57 and 64 years. In all five, there was a progressive loss of interest in usual entertainments, and a decline in self-help and vocational skills. Three developed

TABLE I

Frequency of pathological changes of Alzheimer disease and clinical dementia in 23 cases of Down syndrome over the age of 30 years

Age (years)	Number of cases	NP/NFT neocortex	NP/NFT hippocampus	DAT
30–39	5	5/5	1/2	0/5
40–49	4	4/4	1/2	2/4
50–59	8	8/8	5/5	2/8
60–73[a]	6	5/6	5/6	1/6
Totals	23	22/23	12/15	5/23

[a] Includes case of pseudo-Down syndrome.
NP, neuritic plaques; NFT, neurofibrillary tangles; DAT, dementia of Alzheimer type.

epileptic seizures and two had polymyoclonus. Communication skills were lost progressively, and the last months of life were characterized by a helpless, bed-ridden condition. The exact time when neurological deterioration began could not be judged with certainty, but the interval from initial neurological consultation to death varied from 3–8 years.

Three cases died with neurological dysfunction and acquired illnesses that confounded attempts to evaluate retrospectively whether they also had DAT. These illnesses included stroke, renal failure and severe idiopathic hydrocephalus. Fourteen cases had no clinical evidence for neurological or behavioral change in later life.

Routine histology

NP and NFT were either absent or encountered rarely as isolated lesions in the older controls. NP and NFT appeared more abundant in limbic regions of the neocortex, and especially severe in the entorhinal cortex and cornu ammonis in all four cases of SDAT. In two out of four cases of SDAT, NP were not found in the dentate molecular layer.

All but one of the 23 DS cases over age 30 had NP and NFT in one or more areas of the neocortex (Table I). The exception was the case of pseudo-DS. The apparent density of neocortical NP and NFT was low in three younger cases (ages 31, 31 and 48 years), and varied widely between cases and cortical fields in the older cases. In general, the relative densities appeared to increase by decade, and were highest in those cases with clinical dementia and severe cortical atrophy. The severity of nerve cell loss and gliosis in neocortex also seemed more prominent in cases with clinical dementia.

Fourteen of the DS cases over age 30 had adequate sections of the hippocampal formation. Values for the density of NP and NFT, and qualitative estimates of the severity of nerve cell loss (+ to + + +) are given in Table II. (No changes of AD were found in the three cases of DS, ages 6, 6 and 25 years.) No NP or NFT were found in two cases, ages 31 and 48 years. Although there was wide individual variation, the histological

TABLE II

Correlation between age, histological changes of Alzheimer disease in the hippocampus[a] and clinical state in 15 cases of Down syndrome over the age of 30 years

Age (years)	NP (mm²)	NFT (mm²)	Cell loss	Clinical
31	0.8	0.9	0	—
31	0	0	0	—
48	0	0	+	—
49	16.5	4.2	+	DAT
50	20.4	20.5	+ +	hydrocephalus
55	12.9	11.5	0	—
57	9.5	12.9	+	stroke
57	32.0	23.9	+ +	DAT
58	22.2	31.5	0	—
60	5.2	10.5	0	—
60	27.9	10.1	+ +	—
63	19.5	73.7	+ + +	—
64	40.0	35.5	+ + +	DAT
64	28.0	60.2	+ + +	—
71	0	0	0	pseudo-DS

[a] Hippocampus: subiculum, cornu ammonis and dentate gyrus. NP, neuritic plaques; NFT, neurofibrillary tangles; DAT, dementia of Alzheimer type; pseudo-DS, pseudo-Down syndrome.

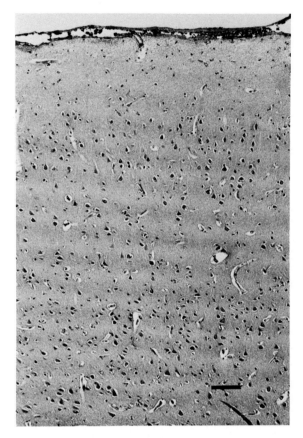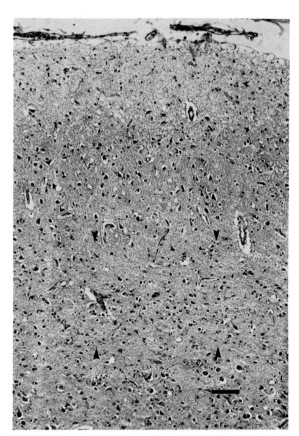

Fig. 1(a and b). On the left is a low power photomicrograph of the outer layers of the entorhinal cortex of a 31-year-old person with Down syndrome. Histological changes of Alzheimer disease are not present, and the size and density of cortical neurons is comparable to that of age-matched controls. On the right at the same magnification is the entorhinal cortex of a 57-year-old case of Down syndrome with severe histological changes of Alzheimer disease. Nerve cells in layer two are shrunken, and there is severe nerve cell loss in layers three and four (arrowheads). The density of astrocytic nuclei is increased, and the neuropil of layers one and two has a spongiform appearance. H&E, bar = 100 µm.

changes of AD in the hippocampus increased in relative severity with age in DS. The greatest degree of apparent cell loss and gross atrophy was found in the three cases over age 60 years, only one of whom was demented clinically. When evident, nerve cell loss was always greater in CA 1–2, subiculum and the adjacent entorhinal cortex than in CA 3–4 or the dentate gyrus (Fig. 1). NFT were seen primarily in CA 1–2 and 4 and the subiculum. NP were seen primarily in the outer layers of CA 1–2, the neuropil of CA 4, subiculum and the molecular layer of the dentate gyrus. The width of the molecular layer of the dentate gyrus decreased with age, and, in the cases of DS over age 50, there was severe atrophy with spongiosis and glial reaction in the outer two-thirds of the dentate molecular layer (Fig. 2). In contrast, there was no apparent change in the thickness or density of granule cells in the dentate gyrus. The histological and topographic features of AD were qualitatively similar in older DS and SDAT, but were generally more severe in DS whether or not there was clinical DAT.

In this retrospective study spanning 25 years, relatively few cases had adequate sections of the nucleus basalis, locus ceruleus and dorsal tegmental

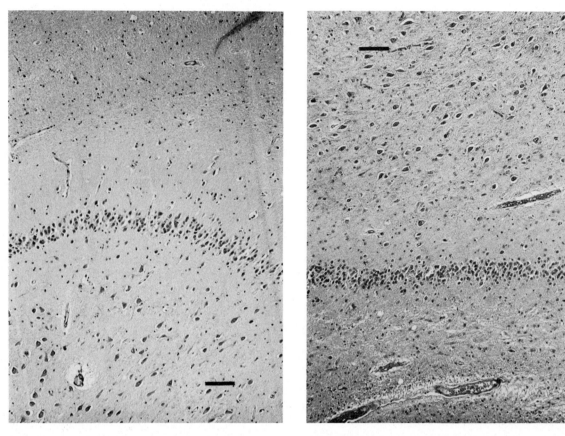

Fig. 2(a and b). On the left is a low power photomicrograph of the dentate gyrus from a 31-year-old person with Down syndrome and no changes of Alzheimer disease in the hippocampus. The plexiform molecular layer is relatively thick and contains few nerve cells. Granular neurons are closely packed into a prominent narrow band. A second narrower cell-sparse zone separates the granule cell layer from the large polymorphic neurons of the hilar region (CA 4) below. On the right is the dentate gyrus from a 57-year-old case of Down syndrome with severe changes of Alzheimer disease. The appearance and relative density of granule cells is little changed, but there is atrophy, gliosis and spongiform change in the outer two-thirds of the molecular layer (arrowheads). H&E, bar = 100 μm.

area. When sections through these nuclei were present, the severity of nerve cell loss and gliosis was generally proportional to the severity of AD changes in the cortex and the degree of clinical dementia.

The 73-year-old man with 'pseudo-DS' was of special interest. He was examined frequently in the 5 years before he died. His physiognomy was typically DS-like, and the staff assumed he had trisomy 21. He was well spoken, and had a keen memory until near the time of death. No changes of DAT were apparent. To our surprise, there were no signs of AD at autopsy.

This paradox prompted the more careful search

of the files that disclosed an apparently normal karyotype performed in the 1960's. Unfortunately, more modern methods of chromosomal analysis were never done.

Golgi impregnations

Satisfactory impregnations of neocortex were obtained in six cases of DS (ages 6, 6, 25, 31, 31 and 64 years), and all four cases of SDAT. Five cases of DS (ages 6, 6, 25, 31 and 64 years) and three cases of SDAT had satisfactory Golgi impregnations of the cerebellum. Seven cases of DS and four cases of

SDAT had satisfactory Golgi impregnations of the cornu ammonis and subiculum. Seven cases of DS and three cases of SDAT had satisfactory impregnations of the dentate gyrus.

In DS cases between ages 6–31 years, the dendrites of pyramidal and polymorphic neurons of the neocortex and hippocampus, and Purkinje and basket-stellate neurons in the cerebellum were well developed and qualitatively spine-rich, comparable to those of young adult controls. A wide variety of non-pyramidal neurons were impregnated in neocortex and hippocampus, but they were relatively few in number. Granule and Golgi-Lugaro cells of the cerebellum were also seldom impregnated. The apical dendrites of pyramidal neurons of the subiculum fasciculated into prominent bundles. The proximal segments and apical shafts of pyramidal and polymorphic neurons in CA 3–4 had typical 'spiny excrescences', which presumably participate in glomerular synapses with the mossy fiber terminals of the axons of dentate granule cells (Fig. 3) (Cajal, 1968; Braak, 1974; Amaral, 1978). Dentate granule cells had wineglass-shaped apical dendrites that ascended

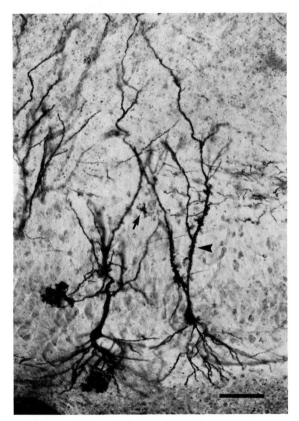 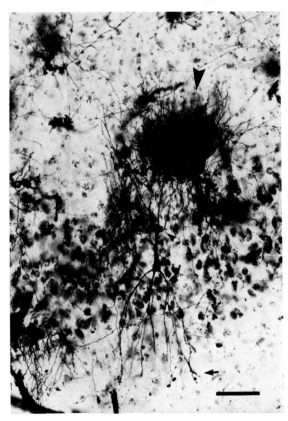

Fig. 3(a and b). On the left is a typical pyramidal neuron from region CA 3 of the hippocampus from a 31-year-old person with Down syndrome and no changes of Alzheimer disease. The proximal portions of the apical and basal dendrites are covered densely with spiny excrescences (arrowhead). A spicular mossy fiber terminal is impregnated to the left of the apical dendrite (arrow). On the right is a pyramidal neuron from region CA 3 of the hippocampus of a 64-year-old person with Down syndrome and Alzheimer disease. The apical dendrites are partly obscured by reactive fibrous astrocytes (large arrowhead). The cytoplasm of unimpregnated neurons contains abundant lipofuscin and is stained darkly with osmium and silver chromate. The proximal dendrites are relatively smooth and spiny excrescences are largely absent (small arrowhead). Varicose degenerative changes are evident in the terminal segments of the basal dendrites (arrow). Rapid Golgi, bar = 100 μm.

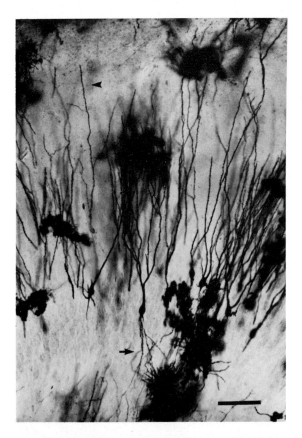
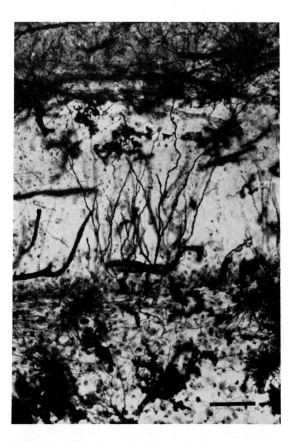

Fig. 4(a and b). On the left are typical granule cells from the dentate gyrus of a 6-year-old case of Down syndrome. The apical dendrites ascend into the molecular layer and bifurcate repeatedly into an ellipsoidal cone. In the younger cases of Down syndrome, the dendrites are exceptionally long, and subordinate segments are relatively straight and spine-rich. Terminal segments usually end abruptly at the hippocampal fissure (arrowhead). Many granule cells of the human dentate gyrus also have basal dendrites in the cellular layer, which may extend into the hilus below (arrow). Basal dendrites are not organized into any characteristic shape. On the right are two granule cells from the dentate gyrus of a 25-year-old case of Down syndrome. The molecular layer is thinner, and the dendrites are not as long. Subordinate and terminal segments are often more tortuous in their course through the molecular layer toward the hippocampal fissure (arrowhead). Rapid Golgi, bar = 100 μm.

into the molecular layer (Fig. 4). About half of the granule cells also had 1–3 basal dendrites that meandered through the granule cell layer and occasionally entered CA 4. Protoplasmic astrocytes had normal appearing irregular, richly bifurcating processes that resembled a bushy plant.

In the 57- and 64-year-old cases of DS, and in the four cases of SDAT, the dendrites of pyramidal neurons in neocortex and subiculum seemed to have fewer branches. These were thinner and relatively spine-poor when compared to nondemented elderly controls. Many had varicose

degenerative changes that affected terminal segments primarily (Fig. 3). Fascicles of pyramidal cell apical dendrites were no longer apparent in the outer layers of subiculum and CA 1. Spiny excrescences were absent or greatly diminished on the dendrites of neurons in CA 3–4, and mossy fiber terminals were seldom seen (Fig. 3). The dendrites of granule cells were thinner, more irregular in caliber and tortuous in their course through the molecular layer (Fig. 5). Spine density was greatly reduced, and long spine-free segments were axon-like in their silhouetted Golgi appear-

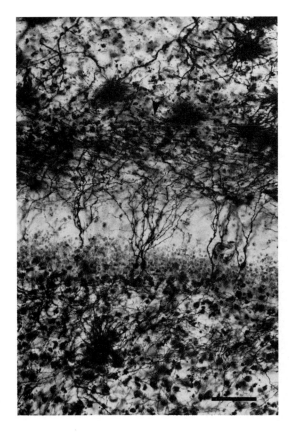 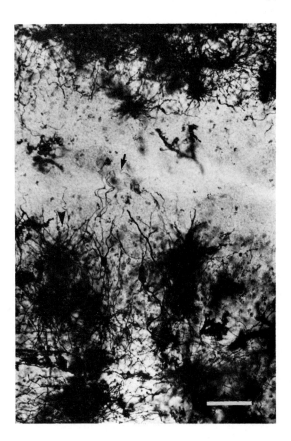

Fig. 5(a and b). On the left are dentate granule cells from a 68-year-old patient with dementia of Alzheimer type. Apical dendrites are thinner, more irregular in contour, and terminal segments course irregularly through the truncated molecular layer. Many reactive astrocytes, and coherent fascicles of astrocytic processes are present in the outer molecular layer near the hippocampal fissure (arrowhead). On the right are granule cells from the dentate gyrus of a 64-year-old case of Down syndrome and Alzheimer disease. Several reactive astrocytes are impregnated nearby (arrowhead). One terminal segment branches richly in the vicinity of a neuritic plaque (arrow). Rapid Golgi, bar = 100 μm.

ance (Fig. 6). Normal Golgi-impregnated proto-plasmic astrocytes were few in number, and large fibrous astrocytes with long, thin unbranched processes predominated (Figs. 3 and 5). In contrast to the findings in cerebral cortex, cerebellar neurons in the 64-year-old DS and in all four cases of SDAT remained well developed, and spiny cerebellar neurons appeared normally spine-rich, as compared to older controls.

In cases with the most severe histological changes of AD in Golgi impregnations, NP (which presumably contained abundant amyloid fibrils) appeared as orange globules scattered in the outer layers of the neocortex and hippocampus (Fig. 7).

The cytoplasm of some cells within the NP, presumably microglia and astrocytes, was speckled with osmium and/or silver salts. In favorable sections, Golgi-impregnated neurites and glial processes were clustered around the NP (Figs. 7 and 8). These processes often branched excessively, encapsulating and occasionally penetrating the NP, and most were distorted in appearance with varicosities and appendages. They were not like any dendrites or axon terminals encountered normally in the hippocampus. Although most of these neurites had the appearance of aberrant axons, some were confirmed to be dendrites branching from nearby Golgi-impregnated neurons.

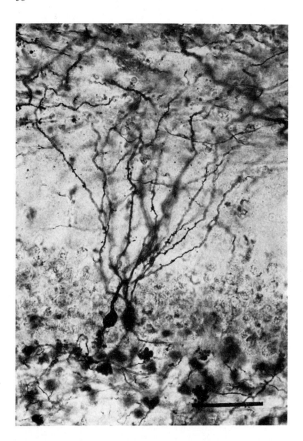
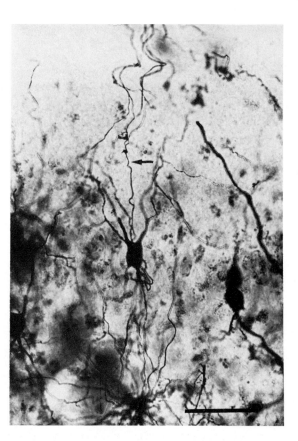

Fig. 6(a and b). Higher power view of the same two cells illustrated in Fig. 5 to show the details of dendritic morphology. Dendrites are abnormally thin, and sometimes axon-like in appearance (arrow). Spines are greatly reduced in number, and large stretches of dendrites may be spine free. Rapid Golgi, bar = 100 μm.

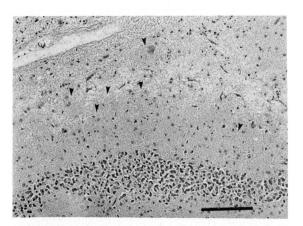
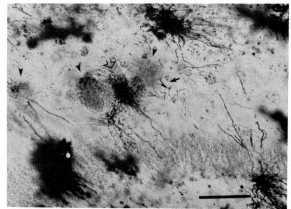

Fig. 7(a and b). On the left is an H&E section of the dentate gyrus from a 64-year-old case of Down syndrome. The molecular layer is thin, glial nuclei are increased, and there is spongiform change near the hippocampal fissure. Many neuritic plaques are evident (arrowheads). On the right a rapid Golgi impregnation from the same case, neuritic plaques with dense amyloid cores stand out prominently in the molecular layer (arrowheads). A reactive fibrous astrocyte is impregnated between two of them (open arrow). In the center (arrow), contiguous neurites branch richly around and within a plaque. Bar = 100 μm.

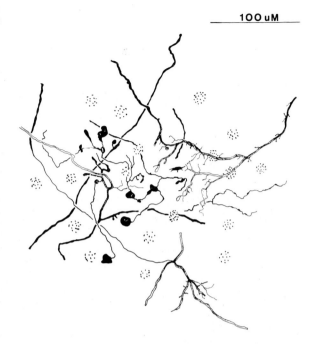

100 uM

Fig. 8. A camera lucida drawing of a neuritic plaque from a 64-year-old case of Down syndrome. The unimpregnated nuclei of glial cells and macrophages can be seen lightly in the background. A variety of aberrant neurites converge upon the neuritic plaque. The parent trunks are relative smooth and axon-like in appearance, but most have abnormal varicose or globular expansions. The one on the right has a number of spine-like appendages, and may be the terminal dendrite of a granule cell.

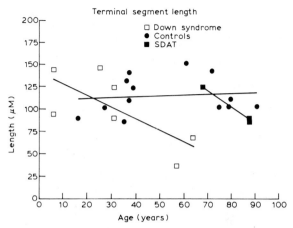

Fig. 10.

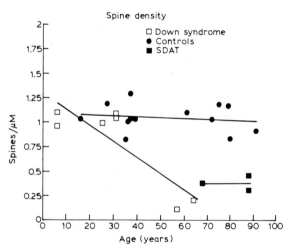

Fig. 11.

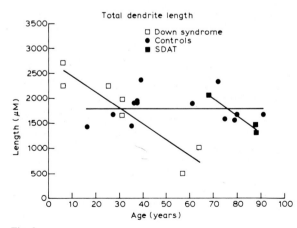

Fig. 9.

Figs. 9–11. Age-related changes in total dendritic length (Fig. 9), terminal segment length (Fig. 10) and spine density (Fig. 11) are illustrated graphically for seven cases of Down syndrome, three cases of senile dementia of Alzheimer type and 13 controls without neurological disease. The points of each of the three groups were fitted with regression lines. There is no significant age-related change in mean values for the 13 controls. In Down syndrome, mean values are highest at age 6, join the normal curve in the 3rd and 4th decades, and decline sharply in later life (respective r values -0.919, -0.718 and -0.869; $p < 0.001$, < 0.05 and < 0.01). In the three cases of senile dementia of Alzheimer type, spine densities are reduced but values for dendritic length are within the range for non-demented, age-matched controls.

TABLE III

Age-related changes in the density of neuritic plaques in the dentate molecular layer, and the size and spine density of granule cell dendrites in Down syndrome

Age and sex		6yM[a]	6yM	25yM	31yM	31yM[b]	57yM[b]	64yM[b]	r
Postmortem delay (h)		12	6	12	3	20	10	6	
NP density/mm^2		0	0	0	0	2.41	33.32	35.51	
% cut ends		4.9	10.3	12.1	10.6	6.8	0	1.8	−0.657
Total	X	2244.21	2689.54	2249.27	1968.98	1641.29	488.47	1018.72	−0.919
dendrite	SD	860.77	1368.49	786.60	508.67	447.79	188.94	339.47	
length (μm)	n	10	10	10	10	10	10	10	
Subordinate	X	85.68	110.47	111.86	112.85	74.71	35.49	54.01	−0.752
segment	SD	68.08	90.31	86.93	100.14	57.08	33.52	47.40	
length (μm)	n	234	208	167	177	164	104	165	
Terminal	X	93.85	142.88	146.24	122.73	89.04	37.16	67.97	−0.718
segment	SD	68.17	97.80	90.41	69.18	58.21	35.51	52.10	
length (μm)	n	133	109	97	95	104	68	104	
Number of	X	24.22	22.00	18.00	19.80	20.60	10.40	16.80	−0.822
subordinate	SD	11.56	12.33	6.13	4.69	6.82	4.18	8.16	
segments	n	10	10	10	10	10	10	10	
Spine	X	1.09	0.95	0.99	1.08	1.03	0.11	0.20	−0.869
density	SD	0.11	0.22	0.16	0.18	0.11	0.07	0.14	
(No./μm)	n	10	10	10	10	10	10	10	

[a], 18–21 translocation; [b], with Alzheimer disease; r, correlation coefficient; NP, neuritic plaques; X, mean; SD, standard deviation; n, number.

Morphometric analysis of granule cell dentrites in seven cases of DS revealed age-related changes in values for size-related parameters (Table III, Figs. 9 and 10). The mean values for total segment number and length were higher in the two 6-year-old cases of DS than in any of the controls 16 years and older. Values for all size-related parameters in young adult DS (age 25–31 years) were similar to controls, but these values fell sharply in later life as the changes of AD became severe. The dendritic changes were not as severe in the three cases of SDAT in which adequate numbers of granule cells were impregnated (Table IV, Figs. 9 and 10). Differences in segment length and number in patients with DS/AD were even more pronounced when the percentage of cut ends was considered. Mean values for cut ends were 11.77% ($\pm$5.08 SD)

for controls, 11.67% ($\pm$1.24 SD) for SDAT, 9.48% ($\pm$2.73 SD) for DS without AD, and only 2.87% ($\pm$2.88 SD) for DS/AD.

There were no significant differences in values for shape-related geometric parameters between DS and controls, or in association with the dendritic changes of DS/AD and SDAT. Dendrites appeared abnormal at a glance in cases of DS/AD and SDAT, as mentioned above, because of small size, slender and irregular segment contour or low spine density (Figs. 5 and 6). Nevertheless, the characteristic shape of an ellipsoidal cone was preserved.

Discussion

In this study we have examined the morphology of selected neurons in Golgi impregnations of the

TABLE IV

The density of neuritic plaques in the dentate molecular layer and the size and spine density of granule cell dendrites in senile dementia of Alzheimer type

Age and sex		68yF	88yM	88yM
Postmortem delay (h)		10	12	8
NP density/mm^2		4.85	0	0
% cut ends		9.6	11.9	12.8
Total dendrite length (μm)	X	2065.24	1287.57	1465.18
	SD	666.38	446.89	723.67
	n	10	10	10
Subordinate segment length (μm)	X	85.14	70.98	80.48
	SD	76.23	44.66	61.66
	n	208	148	142
Terminal segment length (μm)	X	124.48	87.14	90.94
	SD	76.89	44.31	62.52
	n	119	87	86
Number of subordinate segments	X	23.00	16.80	16.20
	SD	6.83	7.28	4.84
	n	10	10	10
Spine density (No./μm)	X	0.38	0.31	0.46
	SD	0.13	0.10	0.11
	n	10	10	10

precentral and dorsolateral prefrontal cortex, hippocampal formation and cerebellum in seven cases of DS between ages 6 and 64 years. No changes pertinent to the cognitive and motor impairments of DS were evident. For example, in our younger cases of DS we did not find striking alterations of the morphology of dendritic spines, or apparent reduction in the numbers of dendrites or dendritic spines of neocortical pyramids at a qualitative level. This is at variance with some published reports (Marin-Padilla, 1976; Suetsugu and Mehraein, 1980; Takashima et al., 1981). Two other recent reports have also emphasized an apparent reduction of the numbers of small, presumably local circuit neurons in the neocortex of young DS cases (Ross et al., 1984, Wisniewski et al., 1984). A wide variety of neocortical a-spiny and sparsely spiny local circuit neurons were examined in our younger cases of DS, and no qualitative morphologic abnormalities were apparent. However, the rapid Golgi method we employ generally impregnates pyramidal neurons of cerebral cortex preferentially, and local circuit neurons seldom account for more than 10% of those present. In general, no conclusions can be made regarding relative neuron numbers in rapid Golgi impregnations, and we did not attempt to estimate neuron numbers directly. The morphology of Purkinje and stellate-basket cell dendrites in the cerebellum also appeared comparable to that of controls.

Some differences in dendritic geometry were evident in the hippocampus of younger DS cases at a quantitative level. The overall size (total segment number and length) was greater in the first decade than in the third or fourth. If one assumes that our cases of DS are representative, this suggests that granule cell dendrites are more robust in DS children, and that they are pruned to lower average values in young adults (Table III, Fig. 9). This may be true of normal children too, but our youngest control was 16 years old. A similar pattern of more exuberant early growth followed by pruning and slower growth later in life has been reported for granule cell dendrites in rodents (Duffy and Teyler, 1978; Williams et al., 1982) and monkeys (Duffy and Rakic, 1983). We have not yet examined younger controls and have an unfortunate 20-year hiatus between ages 40–60 years. Hence, the normal pattern of growth for this class of dendrites is not yet firmly established in the human dentate gyrus.

There is no apparent correlation ($r < 0.20$) between advancing age and granule cell dendritic size in our controls from the second to the tenth decades (Fig. 9). By contrast, Buell and Coleman (1979) reported a progressive increase in the size of the dendrites of small pyramids in the human parahippocampal gyrus from the fifth to the tenth decades, and lower values in patients with SDAT. Uemura (1985) has also recently confirmed continued growth of pyramidal dendrites in the monkey subiculum. Neurons of different classes and/or of different brain regions may therefore differ in their patterns of age-related dendritic morphology.

The most striking differences in dendritic morphology were encountered in DS/AD and SDAT. The cytopathological changes in Golgi impregnations of the neocortex and hippocampus were essentially those of dendritic degeneration and reactive gliosis. There may also have been a significant degree of nerve cell death (Ball and Nutall, 1980; Terry and Katzman, 1983), but we did not measure cell density directly. The degenerative changes encountered in the apical dendrites of granule cells in the dentate gyrus probably resulted largely from loss of afferents from the entorhinal cortex and medial septal nucleus. Basal dendrites seemed less affected. By extrapolation from anatomical and pathological studies in animals, the entorhinal cortex may be the principal source of excitatory (glutamate/aspartate) afferents to the outer two-thirds of the dentate molecular layer (Caceres and Steward, 1983), and the medial septal nucleus may be the principal source of cholinergic inputs to the hippocampus (Mesulam et al., 1984). Although a substantial number of granule cells appeared to survive, despite deafferentation of their dendrites, the density of Golgi-impregnated mossy fiber efferents from granule cells to CA 3–4 also appeared to be reduced. This conclusion is suggested by the apparent reduction in the amount of postsynaptic membrane specializations (spiny excrescences) on pyramidal and polymorphic neurons in CA 3–4 in our cases of DS/AD. Neuritic alterations in Golgi impregnations confirm and enlarge upon observations using other methods, which suggests that the hippocampus in AD is effectively isolated from its principal afferent zones and efferent targets (Kemper, 1978; Hyman et al., 1984).

Evidence for aberrant neuritic growth in the vicinity of NP, comparable to that reported previously by Probst et al. (1983) and Ferrer et al. (1983) in AD, was encountered primarily in the hippocampus in our cases of DS/AD and in SDAT

(Figs. 7 and 8). Exuberant growth of more normal looking dendrites away from NP, as reported by Scheibel and Tomiyasu (1978), was not encountered.

Severe degenerative changes of pyramidal neurons of cerebral cortex and Purkinje cells of the cerebellum have been reported by others in Golgi studies of AD (Scheibel et al., 1975, 1976; Scheibel and Tomiyasu, 1978; Mehraein et al., 1975). This extreme degree of apparent neuronal degeneration was seldom seen in our Golgi impregnations, probably because tissue blocks were placed promptly into Golgi fixative. When tissue fixed in formalin for long periods (months to years in the cited reports) is prepared later for Golgi histology, the processes of many neurons are impregnated incompletely and may be mistakenly interpreted as severely degenerated (Buell, 1982; Williams, 1983).

Our observations in routine cell and fiber stains are in accord with previous reports that the neuropathological changes in DS/AD are not different qualitatively from cases of AD with normal karyotype (Struwe, 1929; Owens et al., 1971; Ellis et al., 1974; Ball and Nutall, 1979, 1981; Mann et al., 1984). These changes begin by the fourth decade in DS, and increase in overall severity with advancing age. A number of studies published recently confirm also comparable and significant reductions in the concentration of choline acetyltransferase and noradrenalin (Yates et al., 1980–83), reductions in nerve cell density in the nucleus basalis and locus ceruleus (Price et al., 1982; Mann et al., 1984; Rogers et al., 1985), and cross-reactivity with antibodies to paired helical filaments (Rasool and Selkoe, 1985); in DS cases over 40 and in patients with AD. Although the neuropathological changes of AD are qualitatively similar in older DS and SDAT, in our cases they are in general more severe quantitatively in DS, whether or not DS cases appeared to be demented clinically.

Despite the fact that the neuropathological changes of AD begin before age 40 years in virtually all cases of DS and increase in severity with advancing age, relatively few of those dying after age 40 have a clinical history consistent with DAT. The impression is that there is a relatively long asymptomatic or 'latent' period between the presumed onset of AD changes in the brain in the fourth decade, until the onset of clinically evident DAT in the fifth decade or later. A similar latent period may be encountered in AD in the general population, in view of the fact that up to 50% of elderly non-demented controls have substantial numbers of NP and NFT at autopsy (Tomlinson et al., 1968; Peress et al., 1973; Wilcox and Esiri, 1982). Once clinical symptoms are evident in DS/AD, the tempo of decline is often atypically rapid. Unlike typical SDAT, DS/AD is also associated more often with polymyoclonus and clinical seizures (Veall, 1974; Dalton and Crapper, 1977; Ropper and Williams, 1980; Lott, 1982; Lott and Lai, 1982; Wisniewski et al., 1985).

The latent period before the onset of clinical dementia in older DS persons may be more apparent than real. The more subtle early changes of DAT are masked by pre-existent mental retardation. A recent survey at the Shriver Center (unpublished) identified 16 of 62 persons with DS over 40 years old who have developed some neurological abnormality suggestive of DAT. It is probable, however, that a proportion of these will be found ultimately to have other neurological diseases, to which older DS cases are also susceptible.

The literature on neuropsychological changes in older DS patients is controversial (Nakamura, 1961; Francis, 1970; Dalton et al., 1974; Dalton and Crapper, 1977; Wisniewski et al., 1978, 1985; Eisner, 1983; Miniszek, 1983; Thase et al., 1984; Berry et al., 1985). In part, the inconclusive nature of these studies stems from the wide range of functional capacity present normally in individuals with DS, from the wide range of tests employed and from the fact that most were not longitudinal studies in which the same individuals were examined sequentially in time. In one such study, Dalton et al. (1974) found a significantly impaired performance only on delayed visual matching tasks in older DS patients. When examined 3 years later

(Dalton and Crapper, 1977), 4 of 11 of their older DS patients had deteriorated to such an extent that they could not be re-examined. By contrast, 5 of the 11 actually improved their performance over the 3-year period, suggesting that they had not initially been prepared adequately for the task. Prospective examination of larger cohorts of DS cases at risk for DAT will be necessary to determine whether, in addition to a long latency, there is also a 'threshold' phenomenon for the development of clinical DAT.

There have been important recent advances in our understanding of the biochemical pathology and selective vulnerability of specific nerve cell classes in AD (Terry and Katzman, 1983). However, it is still not yet known whether AD is an acquired neurological disease, an inevitable consequence of aging in an organ comprised of metabolically active postmitotic cells, or an hereditary neurodegenerative disorder (Berg, 1985). The nearly complete association between trisomy 21 and the neuropathological changes of AD after age 30 years has been cited as further evidence for the role of genetic factors in the pathophysiology of AD (Heston et al., 1981; Heyman et al., 1983; Schweber, 1985; Weinreb, 1985; Foncin et al., 1985). It is not yet clear whether this genetic factor lessens the vitality of selected neuronal classes, as in Huntington disease, or whether it lessens the host's resistance to an environmental pathogen or pathogens, which are as yet undefined (Gadjusek, 1985).

Summary and conclusions

Twenty-three cases of Down syndrome between the ages of 31 and 73 years were studied neuropathologically. All but one had histological changes of Alzheimer disease in the neocortex. The exception was a 73-year-old man with Down phenotype and normal karyotype. Eighty-six per cent had histological changes of Alzheimer disease in the hippocampus, and the severity of these changes generally increased with advancing age. Only five of these twenty-three cases were demented clini-

64

cally. In four cases of Down syndrome aged 31–64 years, rapid Golgi impregnations revealed age-related degeneration of the dendrites of neocortical and hippocampal pyramids, and granule cells of the dentate gyrus. Excessively branched aberrant neurites were observed in neuritic plaques. Cytopathological changes in cortical neurons in cases of Down syndrome with Alzheimer disease were qualitatively similar to, but generally more severe than those encountered in four cases of senile dementia of Alzheimer type (ages 78–88 years). Quantitative analysis of the numbers and lengths of segments, and spine densities of granule cell dendrites in these four older and three younger cases of Down syndrome revealed higher values in the first four decades, which were comparable to controls. Lowest values occurred in the sixth and seventh decades. Values for controls, by contrast, did not change significantly from the second through the tenth decades. We conclude that the dendritic morphology of cortical neurons in young adults with Down syndrome is not strikingly different from age-matched controls until the fourth decade when histological changes of Alzheimer disease invariably begin. At the time of death, decades later, the histological changes of Alzheimer disease are severe, yet only a relatively small percentage exhibit clinical dementia. Presumably there is in Down syndrome a latency of up to several decades from the onset of the neuropathological changes of Alzheimer disease and recognizable clinical symptoms, and death may occur from other causes prior to clinical expression. A comparable-'incubation period' may occur also in the general population at risk for Alzheimer disease.

Acknowledgements

We thank Mrs. L. Hassinger for excellent technical help, and Dr. E.D. Bird who provided material through the Brain Tissue Resource Center at McLean Hospital, Belmont, MA. This study was supported by Grants MH 34079 and MH/NS 31862.

References

Amaral, D. G. (1978) A Golgi study of cell types in the hilar region of the hippocampus in the rat. *J. Comp. Neurol.*, 182: 851–914.

Ball, M. J. and Nutall, K. (1980) Neurofibrillary tangles, granulovacuolar degeneration, and neuron loss in Down syndrome: quantitative comparison with Alzheimer dementia. *Ann. Neurol.*, 7: 462–465.

Ball, M. J. and Nutall, K. (1981) Topography of neurofibrillary tangles and granulo-vacuoles in hippocampi of patients with Down's syndrome: quantitative comparison with normal aging and Alzheimer's disease. *Neuropathol. Appl. Neurobiol.*, 7: 13–20.

Berg, L. (1985) Does Alzheimer's disease represent an exaggeration of normal aging? *Arch. Neurol.*, 42: 737–739.

Berry, P., Groeneweg, G., Gibson D. and Brown, R. I. (1985) Mental development of adults with Down syndrome. *Am. J. Ment. Defie.*, 89: 252–256.

Braak, H. (1974) On the structure of the human archicortex: I. The cornu ammonis, a Golgi and pigment architectonic study. *Cell Tiss. Res.*, 152: 349–383.

Buell, S. J. (1982) Golgi-Cox and rapid Golgi methods as applied to autopsied human brain tissue; widely disparate results. *J. Neuropathol. Exp. Neurol.*, 41: 500–507.

Buell, S. J. and Coleman, P. D. (1979) Dendritic growth in the aged human brain and failure of growth in senile dementia. *Science*, 206: 854–856.

Caceres, A. and Steward, O. (1983) Dendritic reorganization in the denervated dentate gyrus of the rat following entorhinal cortical lesions: a Golgi and electron microscopic analysis. *J. Comp. Neurol.*, 214: 387–403.

Casanova, M. F., Walker, L. C., Whitehouse, P. J. and Price, D. L. (1985) Abnormalities of the nucleus basalis in Down's Syndrome. *Ann. Neurol.*, 18: 310–313.

Colon, E. J. (1972) The structure of the cerebral cortex in Down's syndrome: a quantitative analysis. *Neuropaediat.*, 3: 362–376.

Cragg, B. G. (1975) The density of synapses and neurons in normal, mentally defective and aging human brains. *Brain*, 98: 81–90.

Crome, L., Cowie, V. and Slayer, E. (1966) A statistical note on the cerebellar and brain-stem weight in mongolism. *J. Ment. Defic. Res.*, 10: 69–72.

Dalton, A. J. and Crapper, D. R. (1977) Down's syndrome and aging of the brain. In: P. Mittler (Ed.), *Research to Practice in Mental Retardation: Biomedical Aspects*, University Park Press, Baltimore, pp. 391–400.

Dalton, A. J., Crapper, D. R. and Scholotterer, G. R. (1974) Alzheimer's disease in Down's syndrome; visual retention deficits. *Cortex*, 10: 366–377.

Duffy, C. J. and Teyler, T. J. (1978) Development of

potentiation in the dentate gyrus of rat: physiology and anatomy. *Brain Res. Bull.*, 3: 425–430.

Duffy, C. J. and Rakic, P. (1983) Differentiation of granule cell dendrites in the dentate gyrus of the rhesus monkey: a quantitative Golgi study. *J. Comp. Neurol.*, 214: 224–237.

Eisner, D. A. (1983) Down's syndrome and aging: is senile, dementia inevitable? *Psychol. Rep.*, 52: 119–124.

Ellis, W. G., McCulloch, J. R. and Corley, C. L. (1974) Presenile dementia in Down's syndrome: ultrastructural identity with Alzheimer's disease. *Neurology*, 24: 101–106.

Ferrer, I., Aymami, A., Rovira, A. and Grau-Veciana, J. M. (1983) Growth of abnormal neurites in atypical Alzheimer's disease with the Golgi method. *Acta Neuropathol.*, 159: 167–170.

Foncin, J. F., Salmon, D., Supino-Viterbo, V., Feldman, R. G., Macchi, G., Mariotti, P., Scopetta, C., Caruso, G. and Bruni, A.C. (1985) Démence présénile d'Alzheimer transmise dans une famille étendue. *Rev. Neurol.*, 141: 194– 202.

Francis, S. H. (1970) Behavior of low-grade institutionalized mongoloids: changes with age. *Am. J. Ment. Defic.*, 75: 92–101.

Gadjusek, C. D. (1985) Hypothesis; interference with axonal transport of neurofilament as a common pathogenetic mechanism in certain diseases of the central nervous system. *N. Engl. J. Med.*, 312: 714–719.

Heston, L. L., Mastri, A. R., Anderson, V. E. and White, J. (1981) Dementia of Alzheimer type: clinical genetics, natural history and associated conditions. *Arch. Gen. Psychiat.*, 38: 1085–1090.

Heyman, A., Wilkinson, W. E., Hurwitz, B. J., Schmechel, D., Sigmon, A. H., Weinberg, T., Helmes, M. J. and Swift, M. (1983) Alzheimer's disease: genetic aspects and associated clinical disorders. *Ann. Neurol.*, 14: 507–515.

Hook, E. B. (1981) Down syndrome frequency in human populations and factors pertinent to variation rates. In: F. F. de la Cruz and P. S. Gerald (Eds.), *Trisomy 21 (Down Syndrome)*, *Research Perspectives.*, University Park Press, Baltimore, pp. 3–68,

Hyman, B. T., Van Hoesen, G. W., Damasio, A. R. and Barnes, C. L. (1984) Alzheimer's disease: cell-specific pathology isolates the hippocampal formation. *Science*, 225: 1168–1170.

Kemper, T. L. (1978) Senile dementia: a focal disease of the temporal lobe. In: K. Nandy (Ed.), *Senile Dementia: A Biomedical Approach.* Elsevier/North-Holland, Amsterdam, pp. 105–113.

Lott, I. T. (1982) Down's syndrome, aging and Alzheimer's disease: A critical review. *Ann. NY Acad. Sci.*, 396: 15–27.

Lott, I. T. and Lai, F. (1982) Dementia in Down's syndrome: observations from a neurological clinic. *Appl. Res. Ment. Retard.*, 3: 233–239.

Mann, D. M. A., Yates, P. O. and Marcyniuk, B. (1984) Alzheimer's presenile dementia, senile dementia of Alzheimer type and Down's syndrome in middle age from a continuum of pathological changes. *Neuropathol. Appl. Neurobiol.*, 10: 185–207.

Marin-Padilla, M. (1976) Pyramidal cell abnormalities in the motor cortex of a child with Down's syndrome. A Golgi study. *J. Comp. Neurol.*, 167: 63–82.

Mehraein, P., Yamada, M. and Tarnowska-Dziduszko, E. (1975) Quantitative study on dendrites and dendritic spines in Alzheimer's disease and senile dementia. In: G. W. Kreutzberg (Ed.), *Advances in Neurology, Vol. 12*, Raven Press, New York, pp. 453–458.

Mesulam, M-M., Mufson, E. J., Levey, A. I. and Wainer, B. H. (1984) Atlas of cholinergic neurons in the forebrain and the upper brainstem of the Macaque based on monoclonal choline acetyltransferase immunocytochemistry and acetylcholinesterase histochemistry. *Neuroscience*, 12: 669–686.

Miniszek, N. A. (1983) Development of Alzheimer disease in Down syndrome individuals. *Am. J. Ment. Defic.*, 87: 377–385.

Nakamura, H. (1961) Nature of institutionalized adult mongoloid intelligence. *Am. J. Ment. Defic.*, 66: 456–458.

Owens, D., Dawson, J. C. and Losin, S. (1971) Alzheimer's disease in Down's syndrome. *Am. J. Ment. Defic.*, 75: 606–612.

Peress, N. S., Kane, W. C. and Aronson, A. M. (1973) Central nervous system findings in a tenth decade autopsy population. In D. H. Ford (Ed.), *Neurobiological Aspects of Maturation and Aging, Progress in Brain Research, Vol. 40*, Elsevier Scientific Publ. Co., Amsterdam, pp. 473–483.

Petit, T. L., Le Boutillier, J. C., Alfano, D. P. and Becker, L. E. (1984) Synaptic development in the human fetus: a morphometric analysis of the normal and Down's syndrome neocortex. *Exp. Neurol.*, 83: 13–23.

Price, D. L., Whitehouse, P. J., Struble, R. G., Coyle, J. T., Clarke, A. W., DeLong, M. R., Cork, L. C. and Hedreen, J. C. (1982) Alzheimer's disease and Down syndrome. *Ann. NY Acad. Sci.*, 396: 145–164.

Probst, A., Basler, V., Bron, B. and Ulrich, J. (1983) Neuritic plaques in senile dementia of Alzheimer type. A Golgi analysis in the hippocampal region. *Brain Res.*, 268: 249–254.

Rasool, C. G. and Selkoe, D. J. (1985) Sharing of specific antigens by degenerating neurons in Pick's disease and Alzheimer's disease. *N. Engl. J. Med.*, 312: 700–705.

Richards, B. W. and Sylvester, P. E. (1969) Mortality trends in mental deficiency institutions. *J. Ment. Defic. Res.*, 13: 276–292.

Rogers, J. D., Brogan, D. and Mirra, S. S. (1985) The nucleus basalis of Meynert in neurological disease: a quantitative morphological study. *Ann. Neurol.*, 17: 163–170.

Ropper, A. H. and Williams, R. S. (1980) Relationship between plaques, tangles and dementia in Down syndrome. *Neurology*, 30: 639–644.

Ross, M. H., Galaburda, A. M., Kemper, T. L. (1984) Down's

syndrome: is there a decreased population of neurons? *Neurology*, 34: 909–916.

Scheibel, A. B. and Tomiyasu, U. (1978) Dendritic sprouting in Alzheimer's presenile dementia. *Exp. Neurol.*, 60: 1–8.

Scheibel, M. E., Lindsay, R. D., Tomiyasu, U. and Scheibel, A. B. (1975) Progressive dendritic changes in aging human cortex. *Exp. Neurol.*, 47: 392–403.

Scheibel, M. E., Lindsay, R. D., Tomiyasu, U. and Scheibel, A. B. (1976) Progressive dendritic changes in the aging human limbic system. *Exp. Neurol.*, 53: 420–430.

Scheibel, M. E., Tomiyasu, U. and Scheibel, A. B. (1977) The aging human Betz cell. *Exp. Neurol.*, 56: 598–609.

Schweber, M. (1985) A possible unitary genetic hypothesis for Alzheimer's disease and Down's syndrome. In: G. Smith (Ed.), *Molecular Structure of the Number 21 Chromosome and Down Syndrome. Ann. NY Acad. Sci.*, 450: 223–238.

Solitare, G. B. and Lamarche, J. B. (1967) Brain weight in the adult mongol. *J. Ment. Defic. Res.*, 11: 79–84.

Struwe, F. (1929) Histopathologische Untersuchungen über Entstehung und Wesen der senilen Plaques. *Z. Neurol. Psychiat.*, 122: 291–307.

Suetsugu, M. and Mehraein, P. (1980) Spine distribution along the apical dendrites of pyramidal neurons in Down's syndrome. *Acta Neuropathol.*, 50: 207–210.

Summitt, R. L. (1981) Chromosome 21 specific segments that cause the phenotype of Down syndrome. In: F. F. de la Cruz and P. S. Gerald (Eds.), *Trisomy 21 (Down Syndrome) Research Perspectives*. University Park Press, Baltimore, pp. 225–235.

Sylvester, P. E. (1983) The hippocampus in Down's syndrome. *J. Ment. Defic. Res.*, 27: 227–236.

Takashima, S., Becker, L. E., Armstrong, D. M. and Chan, F. (1981) Abnormal neuronal development in the visual cortex of the human fetus and infant with Down's syndrome. *Brain Res.*, 225: 1–21.

Terry, R. D. and Katzman, R. (1983) Senile dementia of the Alzheimer type. *Ann. Neurol.*, 14: 497–506.

Thase, M. E., Tigner, R., Smeltzer, D. J. and Liss, L. (1984) Age-related neuropsychological deficits in Down's syndrome. *Biol. Psychiat.*, 19: 571– 585.

Tomlinson, B. E., Blessed, G. and Roth, M. (1968) Observations on the brains of non-demented old people. *J. Neurol. Sci.*, 7: 331–356.

Uemura, E. (1985) Age-related changes in the subiculum of the

Macaca mulatta: dendritic branching pattern. *Exp. Neurol.*, 87: 412–427.

Veall, R. M. (1974) The prevalence of epilepsy among mongols related to age. *J. Ment. Defic. Res.*, 18: 99–106.

Weinreb, H. J. (1985) Fingerpoint patterns in Alzheimer's disease. *Arch. Neurol.*, 42: 50–53.

Wilcox, G. K. and Esiri, M. M. (1982) Plaques, tangles and dementia; a quantitative study. *J. Neurol. Sci.*, 56: 343–356.

Williams, R. S. (1983) Letter to the editor. *J. Neuropathol. Exp. Neurol.*, 42: 210–211.

Williams, R. S. and Matthysse, S. (1983) Morphometric analysis of granule cell dendrites in the mouse dentate gyrus. *J. Comp. Neurol.*, 215: 154–164.

Williams, R. S., Ferrante, R. J. and Caviness, V. S. Jr. (1978) The Golgi-rapid method in clinical neuropathology: the morphological consequences of suboptimal fixation. *J. Neuropathol. Exp. Neurol.*, 37: 13–33.

Williams, R. S., Matthysse, S. and Hassinger, L. (1982) Quantitative analysis of dendritic development in the dentate gyrus of the mouse. *Soc. Neurosci. Abstr.*, 8: 326.

Wisniewski, K. E., Howe, J., Williams, D. G. and Wisniewski, H. M. (1978) Precocious aging and dementia in patients with Down's syndrome. *Biol. Psychiat.*, 13: 619–627.

Wisniewski, K. E., Laure-Kamionowska, M. and Wisniewski, H. M. (1984) Evidence of arrest of neurogenesis and synaptogenesis in brains of patients with Down's syndrome. *N. Engl. J. Med.*, 311: 1187–1188.

Wisniewski, K. E., Dalton, A. J., McLachlan, D. R. C., Wen, G. Y. and Wisniewski, H. M. (1985) Alzheimer's disease in Down's syndrome. *Neurology*, 35: 957–961.

Yates, C. M., Simpson, J., Maloney, A. F. J., Gordon, A. and Reid, A. H. (1980) Alzheimer-like cholinergic deficiency in Down's syndrome. *Lancet*, II: 979.

Yates, C. M., Ritchie, I. M., Simpson, J., Maloney, A. F. J. and Gordon, A. (1981) Noradrenalin in Alzheimer-type dementia and Down syndrome. *Lancet*, II: 39–40.

Yates, C. M., Simpson, J., Gordon, A., Maloney, A. F. J., Allison, Y., Ritchie, I. M. and Urquhart, A. (1983) Catecholamines and cholinergic enzymes in pre-senile and senile Alzheimer-type dementia and Down's syndrome. *Brain Res.*, 280: 119–126.

Y Cajal, S. R. (1968) *The Structure of Ammons Horn.* (Translated by L. M. Kraft), C. C. Thomas, Springfield, IL, pp. 32–57.

Discussion

J. DELABAR: Have you observed any partial trisomy among the cases with Down's syndrome and AD signs?

ANSWER: Only one of our cases, age 6, was due to 18–21 translocation. That case, of course, had no changes of AD.

R. RAVID: Is there any sex linkage between Down's syndrome

and Alzheimer disease? Were there cases with Alzheimer pathology in patients below 30 years of age?

ANSWER: Our cases were a nearly equal mix of the sexes. I am not aware of sex-related differences in the severity of AD in DS. None of the cases below age 31 had changes of AD.

G. S. ROTH: In your last two slides, despite the lack of age effect in the control, those normal subjects over 60 years of age seem to show the same negative regression as demented counterparts. Do you attach any significance to this?

ANSWER: There were too few cases at the lower and upper age extremes and none in the 40–60-years age range, to draw firm conclusions.

D. F. SWAAB: Are the Alzheimer changes specific for Down's syndrome or are such changes also met in other cases of mental retardation where precocious aging might be expected (i.e. microencephalics)?

ANSWER: In the limited studies done so far, and in my experience in the neuropathology of the elderly retarded, only Down's syndrome cases seem at greater risk of AD.

H. B. M. UYLINGS: Have you seen in all your demented cases only granule cells with the dramatic changes in dendritic diameter? In the four demented cases we (J.P. De Ruiter and H.B.M. Uylings) have examined we did not observe those cells, or only rarely, in our rapid Golgi preparations.

ANSWER: Yes, when neuropathological changes of Alzheimer disease were severe, dendrites were usually thin and more irregular in contour, more tortuous in their course, and spine poor. The change was not confined to dentate granule cells and was seen also in neocortical and hippocampal pyramids. However, there is great variation from cell to cell, region to region, and case to case, and only five such cases were examined.

E. DONCHIN: How do you diagnose dementia in Down's syndrome subjects?

ANSWER: In this retrospective study, dementia was defined as loss of language or functional skills, changes in behavior or the appearance of neurological signs (e.g. seizure, myoclonus) in later life in the absence of neurological illness other than AD, as defined neuropathologically.

D. F. Swaab, E. Fliers, M. Mirmiran, W. A Van Gool and F. Van Haaren (Eds.)
Progress in Brain Research, Vol. 70.
© 1986 Elsevier Science Publishers B.V. (Biomedical Division)

CHAPTER 5

Measurement and imaging of cerebral function in ageing and dementia

R. S. J. Frackowiak

MRC Cyclotron Unit, Hammersmith Hospital, Du Cane Road, London W12 0HS, UK

Introduction

There has been considerable interest in the measurement of cerebral energy metabolism in the dementing diseases since such measurements became possible in man in the 1940's (Kety and Schmidt, 1945, 1948a). The original interest was due to the prevalent pathogenic theories relating to chronic cerebrovascular insufficiency as a cause of dementia, not fully revised until the seminal work of the Newcastle pathologists in the late 1960's (Tomlinson et al., 1970). Concomitant with the change in pathological emphasis from chronic ischaemic to degenerative processes, techniques became available for the regional mapping of cerebral blood flow in man (Lassen and Ingvar, 1963). It had been shown that flow and energy consumption in the cerebral hemisphere were coupled in normal man under resting conditions and so regional flow information was taken to reflect regional cerebral metabolism, albeit indirectly. The search for diagnostic patterns of flow abnormalities and for structural-pathophysiological correlations in ageing and the various types of dementia became a principal goal of research.

As patterns of metabolic dysfunction were identified, the relationship of changes in normal ageing to pathological processes became a field of primary interest. This was paralleled by the elaboration of sophisticated techniques for measuring cerebral flow and glucose metabolism in animals with a very high degree of regional precision, using autoradiographic techniques (Sokoloff, 1984). Various animal models of ageing, have subsequently been studied (Smith et al., 1980; Ohata et al., 1981).

Anatomical localisation in human studies advanced dramatically with the application of tomographic reconstruction techniques to imaging by transmitted (X-ray) or emitted (γ-ray) radiation. With X-ray computed tomography (CT) the main thrust of research has been clinical and oriented diagnostically. The differentiation between the degenerative and vascular dementias has occupied the majority of workers and, as a result, much effort has also been expended on defining structural changes in the brain that accompany normal as well as abnormal ageing.

The advent of tomography to radioisotope imaging has resulted in the elaboration of sophisticated techniques, using positron-emitting isotopes of biologically important elements such as carbon, oxygen and nitrogen, designed to quantitate various physiological and biochemical functions (Phelps et al., 1982; Phelps and Mazziotta, 1985). Positron-emission tomography (PET) has developed into a technique for applying quantitative tracer methodology to investigate cerebral function regionally in man. In terms of dementia and ageing, studies have to-date concentrated on re-examining the significance of disturbed energy metabolism, though more recently investigations of specific neurotransmitter pathways in certain dementing diseases have also commenced. The eventual aim of research with these functional imaging tools must be the elucidation of pathophysiological mechanisms and to some degree this has been a feature of some studies already (see below). There are also diagnostic and predictive features in functional images which are becoming identified in certain specific dementing illnesses.

Most recently, the techniques of nuclear magnetic resonance (NMR) imaging and, hopefully in the near future, NMR spectroscopy are being applied to investigations of the dementias (Besson et al., 1985). The former represents an apparently safe technique sensitive to structural changes which involve alterations in cerebral water or fat content. NMR imaging appears to be providing new information concerning the extent of white matter disease in certain varieties of dementing illness (Bradley et al., 1984). The application of NMR spectroscopy to topical measurements in the human brain in vivo is in its infancy (Pritchard et al., 1983). In the near future it seems unlikely that information on more than high energy phosphates and pH will be readily available. However, the possibility of recognising changes in amino acid concentrations of possible significance for neurotransmission using proton, as opposed to phosphorus spectroscopy is conceivable (Gadian, 1982).

In summary it can be said that imaging and measurement of cerebral metabolism and blood flow continues to occupy clinical research for the following reasons. It allows the localisation of areas of dysfunction in vivo with increasing precision, which permits a study of the natural history of the diseases in functional terms which can then be correlated to specific structures. This localisation of in vivo pathophysiology may have clinical implications in terms of prognosis and in pointing towards new, possibly fruitful areas of investigation. However, it seems reasonable to suggest that the thrust of new research must now progress beyond isolated studies of energy metabolism towards more fundamental questions concerning the delineation of possible specific neuronal populations affected in dementia. The measurement of physiological, biochemical and pharmacological variables in

absolute units also presents a unique opportunity to monitor the effects of therapeutic intervention objectively. Disturbances of other aspects of metabolism, e.g. amino acid turnover and protein metabolism, analysis of receptor function, transmitter storage and release and the selective marking and function of glial as well as neuronal elements in the brain are further areas which may become amenable to study. Metabolic imaging and measurement with PET will be at the forefront of such clinically oriented research in man. It is also clear that many of the insights into the mechanisms underlying the degenerative dementias are, and will continue to come from in vitro metabolic studies, molecular biology and genetics and in work with animal models, testing infective and other theories of pathogenesis.

The remainder of this chapter will review the work of the last 40 years into the changes of cerebral energy metabolism and blood flow that accompany human ageing and dementia.

Normal ageing

Hemispheric measurements

Studies of cerebral blood flow in the brain of man began with Kety and Schmidt who developed a technique for measuring the mean flow per hemisphere (Kety and Schmidt, 1945, 1948a). Extension of the method to include arteriovenous substrate or metabolite differences permits the measurement of mean uptake or release rates into or from the brain. The initial studies dating from the late 1940's showed a mean cerebral blood flow (CBF) of 52 ml/100 g/min with an oxygen consumption (CMR_{O_2}) of 3.5 ml/100 g/min and an arteriovenous oxygen difference ($A-V_{O_2}$) of 6.6 vol% corresponding to a fractional oxygen extraction (OER) of 0.37. The effects of hyperoxia and hypoxia as well as hyper- and hypocapnia were studied (Kety and Schmidt, 1946, 1948b). Relative anoxia caused by inhalation of 10% oxygen gas led to a significant fall in arterial oxygen content, compensating hyperventilation and hypocapnia.

Under these circumstances, CBF rose with evidence of peripheral vasodilation but CMR_{O_2} remained constant. Hyperoxia caused by inhalation of 100% oxygen gas resulted in a rise in oxygen content of arterial blood, no change in P_{CO_2}, a fall in CBF with again no change in CMR_{O_2}. There was evidence of vasoconstriction in the cerebral vasculature with an increase in vascular resistance. Hypercapnia under normoxic conditions resulted in respiratory acidosis, an increase in CBF, a marked fall in OER to 0.29 but no change in CMR_{O_2}. The increase in CBF was accompanied by a marked fall in cerebrovascular resistance.

Thus in these early experiments, the evidence was clear that homeostatic mechanisms served to maintain a constant cerebral oxygen consumption. In the case of altered oxygen content, blood flow rose or fell to maintain a constant oxygen delivery (CBF × arterial oxygen content). However, if oxygen delivery was compromised, by interference with blood flow homeostasis, oxygen extraction rose or fell appropriately, thus maintaining energy metabolism and, hence, function.

One of the observations made by Kety and Schmidt in their paper relating to the effects of hyperventilation and anoxia (1948b) remains pertinent to all subsequent studies. They noted that despite constant CMR_{O_2} mental changes were observed in their subjects. They speculated that "derangement of higher functions may occur from subtle or complex biochemical changes" and that their description in terms of CMR_{O_2} alone was as inadequate as predicting the fidelity of a radio by its power requirements.

Investigation of changes in CBF and CMR_{O_2} associated with increasing age has occupied many subsequent researchers. Kennedy (1967; Kennedy and Sokoloff, 1957) investigated children with the nitrous oxide (Kety-Schmidt) technique and showed in nine normal children with a mean age of 6 years that CBF averaged 106 ml/100 mg/min — twice that of normal young men. CMR_{O_2} averaged 5.2 ml O_2/100 ml/min, an increase of 50%. The fractional oxygen extraction was therefore considerably lower than in early adulthood (0.31 cf. 0.37).

This finding raises important questions. What is the nature of the $CBF:CMR_{O_2}$ couple and what determines its setting, as measured with the OER? Why is the metabolism of childrens' brains higher than that of young adults — is this a finding of physiological significance, or an artefact?

In terms of ageing, Kety reviewed in 1956 the 16 studies employing the nitrous oxygen technique to that date that had produced information on this subject. The studies quoted gave data from groups of subjects numbering 4 to 19, of mean ages ranging from 6 to 93. CBF seemed to decline with age, the largest decrease occurring in children and teenagers in whom average CBF in four groups of increasing age was 104, 90, 68 and 60 ml/100 g/min. By the twenties, CBF stabilised out at between 52 and 65 ml/100 g/min, remaining in the fifties until subjects of mean age 68 and 93 were reported with mean CBF of 43 and 39 ml/100 g/min, respectively. Kety commented that from young adulthood to old age there appeared to be a 25% reduction in CBF. The decline in CMR_{O_2} was less pronounced and of the order of 20%. However, this latter figure was greatly biased by very low values in the groups of mean age 68 and 93. Finally, Kety demonstrated that these pooled results suggested a small increase of $A-V_{O_2}$ with age. The problem with these data is that the nitrous oxide technique had undergone modifications so that not all the results were strictly comparable and the various age groups were represented by a greater or lesser number of subjects. Nevertheless there was a hint that the process of ageing was associated with some decline in metabolic and flow parameters, which were not exactly parallel and were associated with a gradual resetting of the flow:metabolism couple such that the proportion of oxygen extracted by the brain gradually increased.

A major problem with these studies was that the ageing populations were not adequately selected for normality and a disease-free state. Indeed some subjects had hypertension and various other diseases since many subjects were drawn from hospitalised populations. As a result of this, a major study was undertaken at NIMH in which selection criteria for normality were strictly defined (Dastur et al., 1963). Correlations were made with ageing in subjects who were apparently completely normal and in those with asymptomatic general medical disorders including hypertension or peripheral vascular disease. Sokoloff summarised the results in 1966 at the Association for Research into Nervous and Mental Diseases (Sokoloff, 1966). In these studies, there was no appreciable difference in CBF between young and old (62 cf. 58 ml/100 g/min), though elderly normal people with asymptomatic disease showed a significant fall in CBF to 52 ml/100 g/min. CMR_{O_2}, however, was unchanged in all these groups (3.5, 3.3 and 3.2 ml/100 g/min, respectively). There was therefore a tendency for the $A-V_{O_2}$ to increase between the completely normal and the elderly with asymptomatic disease (5.7, 5.88 and 6.35 vol% respectively). Sokoloff made the observation that 'arteriosclerotic' subjects had significant reductions in CBF and cerebral venous P_{O_2} (i.e. increased OER) but that there was an absence of significant decline in oxygen consumption. The conclusions of this study were that decreases in CBF and CMR_{O_2} were not an inevitable consequence of chronological ageing per se.

One further, more remarkable, observation of this study related to glucose consumption, which was also measured. Cerebral glucose consumption (CMR_G) was significantly reduced in normal aged subjects and those with asymptomatic disorders compared with the normal young subjects. This implies a change in the normal stoichiometry of oxygen and glucose metabolism in the ageing brain. Thus the oxygen:glucose molar ratio was measured as 4.9 in the young, 5.7 in the elderly and 5.3 in those with asymptomatic disorders. The low figure for the young compared to the expected value of close to 6 is surprising and makes interpretation of this part of the study difficult. It is likely that the precision of making glucose measurements was not adequate to permit these comparisons of metabolic rates with sufficient accuracy.

Regional blood flow

Regional measurement of CBF represented a major advance in studying the cerebral circulation. It became clear that quite marked changes in the distribution of CBF could subtend similar mean hemispheric values. Thus, methods for measuring regional CBF (rCBF) gave insight into the distribution of flow and how this altered with age or physiological stimulation (Lassen et al., 1978). Various regional techniques evolved, from the intraarterial [85]Kr technique with intraoperative external detection over the exposed brain (Lassen and Munck, 1955; Ingvar and Lassen, 1961) to the use of ^{133}Xe as an indicator gas (Glass and Harper, 1963) given subsequently by inhalation (Mallett and Veall, 1963, 1965; Veall and Mallett, 1966) and intravenous injection (Thomas et al., 1979). ^{15}O-labelled water ($H_2{}^{15}O$) was also used by intravenous injection and detection with external heavily collimated detectors (Ter-Pogossian et al., 1969, 1970). A problem with reviewing the results of these studies lies in the use of various techniques, of varying validity and with a multitude of ways of computing flow in terms of the recorded activity clearance data from the brain (Betz, 1972). In general these studies have not resolved the problem whether normal ageing is inevitably associated with decreased perfusion and/or metabolism. However, a number of interesting qualitative observations, notably from Copenhagen and Lund, demonstrated regional alterations in perfusion in response to discrete physiological stimuli. Thus, alterations of rCBF in response to hand movement (execution as well as mental planning of the action), speech, memorising, reasoning and listening have been demonstrated (Risberg and Ingvar, 1973; Orgogozo and Larsen, 1979; Roland et al., 1980a,b). Complex motor movements have been shown to be associated with increases in rCBF over the appropriate motor cortex and also over the supplementary motor area.

These studies have been most stimulating, but major limitations should always be borne in mind in their interpretation. The method of external detection of single photon emitting isotopes from heterogenously perfused tissue of uncertain composition and physical dimensions is fraught with assumptions. Nevertheless consistent results have been obtained from a number of laboratories. Secondly, a major extrapolation has been made from the normal coupling of hemispheric CBF and CMR_{O_2} in the resting individual to regional measurements. Thus, it has been assumed that a change in rCBF means a local change in $rCMR_{O_2}$ and, hence, function. This has defied formal proof because not until the introduction of ^{15}O-labelled oxygen ($^{15}O_2$) did measurements of CMR_{O_2} become possible regionally (Ter-Pogossian et al., 1969, 1970). Unfortunately technical difficulties prevented the use of ^{15}O compounds to make such measurements with any precise degree of regionality until the introduction of positron tomography.

A further problem relates to the correlation between metabolic activity and clinically measured function. It has been tacitly assumed by many workers that the two are linearly related or at least correlated by some simple relationship. Formal evidence of such close regional metabolism:function coupling has been provided by Sokoloff in experimental animals using the deoxyglucose method of measuring glucose consumption (see Sokoloff, 1984). Thus changes in dorsal horn CMR_G in the lumbar spinal cord on ipsilateral sciatic nerve stimulation have been shown in the rat. Many other examples have now been published.

Ageing in animal models

A number of recent publications have attempted to study the process of metabolic ageing of the brain with reference to animal models. Local glucose metabolism from 47 cerebral structures have been measured in young, middle-aged and elderly rats (Smith et al., 1980). Decreases associated with ageing were found in caudate-putamen, parietal cortex and visual and auditory structures. The decreases were not progressive after middle age,

suggesting that the elderly group was self-selecting for maintained metabolism on the basis of a survival effect. Studies have been extended to young age groups, with increases of rCBF noted in the youngest rats and a suggestion that the rise occurs in those regions still immature at the time of the earliest measurements. In middle ages, rCBF remains constant and then in certain regions (mostly parietal and posterior structures) shows a progressive fall (Ohata et al., 1981). The interesting observation in this study is that rCBF and $rCMR_G$ do not appear to follow the same time course during development and maturation. Thus $rCMR_G$ falls at a time in early development when rCBF is constant or rising. The significance of these observations or their relevance to man is as yet unclear.

Positron tomographic studies

PET studies in normal ageing have concentrated on attempts at defining the normal regional changes in cerebral metabolism and haemodynamics and also on describing the regional metabolic response of the brain to normal physiological stimuli. In relation to energy metabolism, the picture remains surprisingly confused, given the great increase in both quantitative and spatial accuracy afforded by PET technology. A considerable part of the confusion may be ascribed to technical factors, as measurements have been made pari passu with rapid technical advances in their precision. Such factors as appropriate correction of tissue attenuation by measurement, method of introduction of the labelled molecule, blood sampling techniques, awareness of resolution effects on the sampling or region of interest size during measurement and modelling problems, have all required painstaking solution.

Energy metabolism

Measurements of energy metabolism and its relationship to regional blood flow have been the most informative and have been performed most extensively using the steady-state oxygen inhalation technique (Frackowiak et al., 1980; Lammertsma and Jones, 1983; Lammertsma et al., 1983). The conceptual and operational simplicity of this model, adequate biological validation (Rhodes et al., 1981; Baron et al., 1981), as well as statistical (Lammertsma et al., 1982) and theoretical characterisation (Lammertsma et al., 1981) have made this method most productive in terms of clinical research. A number of publications have suggested a decline in grey matter rCBF with age which just reaches statistical significance at the 5% level (Frackowiak, 1982; Frackowiak and Lenzi, 1982; Lenzi et al., 1983). White matter rCBF is unchanged with age. Of interest has been the observation of much greater variability in regional perfusion in younger than in older subjects, suggesting either a higher degree of anxiety, altered patterns, or rates of breathing and more variation in P_{a,CO_2} in the young, or alternatively a damping down of physiological vascular responsiveness in the elderly. These observations have been replicated independently (Pantano et al., 1984) and have been carried out on subjects considered normal on grounds of history, social functioning and simple clinical examination to exclude hypertension and clinically obvious vascular and neurological disease. The population may therefore represent a mixture of completely normal and asymptomatic elderly individuals by the NIMH criteria (Sokoloff, 1966).

The findings with respect to $rCMR_{O_2}$ have shown no such relationship with age in either the Hammersmith (Frackowiak, 1982) or Orsay (Pantano et al., 1984) data. In both, the slope of the $rCMR_{O_2}$ (grey) to age relationship was 0.02 ml O_2/100 ml/min and not significantly different from zero. This is of interest in that it implies that the $A–V_{O_2}$ increases with age. Metabolism is maintained despite a modest fall in flow. The actual change in rOER with age, though showing an upward trend, is not statistically significant. However, before final comments about rOER can be made, its measurement with the steady-state oxygen inhalation technique must be repeated with CBV correction (Frackowiak et al., 1984). If rOER

does indeed rise with age, albeit by a small amount, and this occurs in the face of normal vascular reactivity in terms of P_{a,CO_2} and autoregulation which has been demonstrated in the elderly (Simard et al., 1971), a likely conclusion is that this resetting of the flow:metabolism couple represents a gradual decline in cerebral capillary density. The latter may occur from subclinical vascular occlusion at capillary level or indeed as part of a vascular degeneration. It is possible that the mechanism underlying the setting of the baseline flow:metabolism couple, which increases from the very young to old, may have a morphological basis in terms of capillary density.

The measurement of CMR_G has provided much less consistent results. Thus Kuhl et al. (1982a) reported a decline in CMR_G and compared this to the Hammersmith CMR_{O_2} data (Kuhl et al., 1984b), suggesting that the brains of elderly subjects use energy substrates other than glucose. Some evidence for such a hypothesis had already been suggested by Gottstein et al. (1971) using arteriovenous Kety-Schmidt techniques. On the other hand, studies from NIH (Duara et al., 1983, 1984) and Brookhaven (DeLeon et al., 1984) suggest no decline in CMR_G. It is important to understand that the coefficient of variation of the latter studies is of the order 20–25% (compared with that of CMR_{O_2} studies of 8%). This makes the demonstration of a significant, though small negative relationship difficult. There appear to be technical problems which require solution before a definitive data set is produced, the most important of which seems to be attenuation correction.

Some preliminary studies combining CMR_{O_2}, CMR_G and CBF measurements at one session have been reported (Baron et al., 1982; Rhodes et al., 1983; Wise et al., 1983b), though the author is only aware of unpublished results from Hammersmith in normal subjects. Preliminary findings include the observation of a tight coupling of CMR_G and CBF regionally in the brain with a fractional glucose extraction (GER) averaging about 12%. The relationship between CMR_{O_2} and CMR_G, i.e. the stoichiometry of the oxidative respiration of glucose, is likewise uniform throughout the brain. Only normal subjects up to the age of 50 have been studied and no significant changes with age have been demonstrated in this as yet small group of adults.

Physiological stimulation

The effects of physiological stimulation on cerebral glucose metabolism in normal man have been studied extensively. States of sensory deprivation (Mazziotta et al., 1982b), audiovisual stimulation and deprivation (Phelps et al., 1981; Mazziotta et al., 1982a) and responses to graded stimuli have been explored. There appears to be a progressive increase in $rCMR_G$ with increasing complexity of visual stimulus in the occipital cortex. Indeed the cortical hypermetabolic responses (averaging 5–20%) bear a good topographical relationship to the expected sites whatever the type of stimulus. This applies to lateralisation as well as anatomical cortical locus. There have also been preliminary communications of patterns of hypermetabolism in subcortical structures in response to auditory stimuli (Mazziotta and Phelps, 1984). The most important implication of these results is that changes in magnitude and symmetry of local metabolism of glucose can be brought about by differences in the way, and conditions under which baseline measurements are made (Mazziotta et al., 1982a,b).

A disappointment in all this work has been the apparent inability to use the true quantitative nature of the PET measurements themselves to describe the effects of stimulation. Many of the reports present their results in terms of ratios of CMR_G — either right/left, anterior/posterior, lobe/lobe or local/global ratios. As has already been intimated, this may be due to camera resolution and implementation and analysis problems of measurements with ^{18}FDG. The field awaits a study which will show a clear correlation between a graded physiological stimulus and an increase in CMR_G measured in absolute units. It is possible that physiologically the response is not linear, but in any event it should be detectable and describable.

Ischaemia and ageing

The normal protective mechanisms against cerebral ischaemia — the haemodynamic and oxygen carriage reserves — have been clearly delineated in man in pathological states over the last 5 years (Frackowiak, 1985). Our recent normal studies with measurement of CBV demonstrate no change of CBF/CBV (which is the reciprocal of the cerebral red cell transit time and a measure of perfusion pressure) with age. This is further evidence that any decline in CBF with normal ageing does not constitute a part of a chronic ischaemic process. The ageing process seems to be associated with diffuse small changes in flow and possibly metabolism, with no specific focal emphasis.

Structure-function relationships

The relationship between structural and functional abnormalities in normal ageing have been studied with combined CT and PET scan analysis by the group from New York/Brookhaven (De-Leon et al., 1984). Structural cortical changes were observed with no decline in CMR_G and the authors suggest that the normal ageing brain undergoes structural change without metabolic correlation. The problem with the study is that the positron tomograph used has poor resolution in comparison with the CT scanner and there are deficiencies in the implementation of the ^{18}FDG technique. The scatter of values for young adults is between 3 and 5 mg/100 g/min, indicating a very large coefficient of variation. This provocative paper requires confirmation before the interpretation of results can be unequivocally accepted.

Dementia

Hemispheric studies

The application of the nitrous oxide technique to patients that would now be classified demented was complicated in the early days by inclusion of various clinical conditions classified together under the term 'chronic brain syndrome'. Many of the original studies included patients with end-stage psychiatric disease, large strokes, severe cerebral deterioration from uncontrolled hypertension and such like. Nevertheless, the studies were uniform in demonstrating a marked decrease in CBF and CMR_{O_2} which appeared to correlate well with cognitive abilities (see Lassen, 1959). Thus, Fazekas and colleagues (1952) assembled a large number of patients and showed a CMR_{O_2} of 2.4 ml $O_2/100$ ml/min in normal elderly subjects, 2.2 in those with normal mental status, but recent or old cerebral infarcts, 2.0 in those with vascular disease and mental change and 2.1 in those with vascular disease and depressed consciousness. They reported that the mean hemispheric $A–V_{O_2}$ in the various clinical groups were all within 0.7 ml% of one another (i.e. within 0.05 on the OER scale). Thus from the earliest reports it was equally clear that in global terms, chronic ischaemic processes were not important in the production of mental deterioration. That is not to say that acute ischaemic events do not lead to progressive stepwise, mental deterioration. Indeed Shenkin et al. (1953) demonstrated quite clearly that elderly subjects exhibiting arteriosclerosis and hypertension were found to have significant reductions in CBF and CMR_{O_2}.

As patient groups were progressively better defined, these observations were further confirmed. Lassen et al. (1957) made the fascinating observation of a progressive decline in CMR_{O_2} (from 3.6 to 1.6 ml $O_2/100$ g/min) in 19 patients which correlated with mental status measured by semi-quantitative psychological tests such as the block-pattern test, as well as with a global clinical evaluation of the degree of dementia. Lassen et al. (1960) also made the observation that the demented patients all had normal oxygen saturation of the cerebral venous blood, implying no change in oxygen extraction.

Regional blood flow

In the 1960's interest turned to regional CBF measurement, the definition of diagnostic patterns of flow reduction and the differentiation of vascular from degenerative dementias ante mortem. Initially, reports appeared suggesting significant decreases in rCBF in patients with vascular dementia, but not in those with primary degenerative disease. Thus, O'Brien and Mallett (1970) reported an rCBF of 45.3 ml/100 g/min for cortex in degenerative dementia as opposed to 34.9 ml/100 g/min in 'secondary' or vascular dementia. Similar results were obtained by Hachinski et al. (1975) and quoted by Simard et al. (1971). The reasons for this intriguing finding are still unclear and have not found support in the subsequent PET studies (see below).

Regional disturbances were extensively reported by the Copenhagen group in 1971 (Simard et al., 1971) and emphasis was put on the diminution of rCBF predominantly in fronto-temporal regions, especially in Alzheimer's disease. The decline in rCBF was of the order 23%. Cerebral reactivity was investigated in 15 demented patients and normal vasomotor function was demonstrated in all. This was taken as further evidence that dementia in the patients with vascular disease was not caused by long-standing diminished blood flow, but by the accumulation of tissue damage due to acute infarctions.

Ingvar has written much about changes in regional CBF patterns in relation to neuropsychiatric syndromes (see Ingvar, 1974). He has described generalised reductions of rCBF in Alzheimer's disease and reported a patient who failed to show normally observed increases in frontal rCBF when solving Raven's matrices. However, movements of the contralateral arm were still capable of producing clear-cut increases of normal type in the sensorimotor cortex. The implication is that cerebral areas concerned with planning and ideation have impaired activation, whereas apparently lower order, primary functions remain preserved till a much later stage of the disease.

In chronic schizophrenia, the same author has described the reversal of the so-called, normal 'hyperfrontal pattern' of rCBF distribution described by him (Ingvar, 1979). It has been subsequently difficult to demonstrate this pattern convincingly with the improved spatial resolution of PET (Mazziotta et al., 1982c; DeLeon et al., 1984; Duara et al., 1984). The pattern may to some extent have been an artifact of the delivery of isotope into the anterior (carotid) circulation and the effect of placement of external detectors such that a considerably greater axial thickness of cortex was visualised over the convexity of the frontal lobe, with comparatively less contamination by white matter. In any event, the marked hypofrontility of chronic schizophrenics has been seen and constitutes an observation of presumed pathological significance.

A detailed analysis and extensive conclusions based on non-invasive rCBF measurement using ^{133}Xe have been reported by Yamaguchi et al. (1980) (see also Obrist et al., 1970; Lavy et al., 1978). The inhalation route was used to administer isotope and 16 detectors were used to analyse clearance curves. The authors report a decline in rCBF in dements exceeding that in normal volunteers. Alzheimer's disease was associated with bilateral symmetrical reduction of rCBF (F_1) which correlated with atrophy on X-ray CT scanning and duration and severity of dementia. Patchy reductions were seen in patients with vascular dementia who also exhibited some impairment of CO_2 reactivity. Behavioural activation failed to elicit normal rCBF increases. Some of the conclusions do not seem entirely justified by the methods or the patient numbers, and classification of patients is questionable (e.g. a group with Alzheimer's disease plus multi infarct dementia is described, the diagnosis being effected ante mortem). However, this paper demonstrates the limits of the possible with external non-tomographic detection techniques of measuring blood flow using single-photon emitters.

Regional metabolism

The only paper using clearance methods to add regional metabolic information to the blood flow data is that of Grubb et al. (1977) who used ^{15}O-labelled water and molecular oxygen to obtain a crude degree of regionality to their washout data. Patients with dementia had significant decreases in rCBF and $rCMR_{O_2}$ but the measurements were not useful in distinguishing patients with cerebral atrophy from those with normal-pressure hydrocephalus. The values for rCBF obtained in normals and dements of the atrophic type (presumably of degenerative aetiology), were 54 ml/100 ml/min in normals compared with 34 ml/100 ml/min in dements and for $rCMR_{O_2}$ 3.6 and 2.4 ml O_2/100 ml/min, respectively. Of therapeutic interest was the observation that reducing the intracranial pressure acutely by removal of cerebrospinal fluid failed to alter cerebral energy metabolism.

Down's syndrome

Other amenting states have also been sporadically reported in the literature. Lassen et al. (1966) reported a CMR_{O_2} that was essentially identical in a group of patients with Down's syndrome and a group of normal subjects. A problem with this study is that all subjects were anaesthetised at examination. A group of subnormal children whose demented state was secondary to severe neurological disease at, or soon after birth, had by contrast a decreased CMR_{O_2}. It was held by the authors that anaesthesia probably affected the brains of subject and patient groups uniformly.

Positron tomography in dementia

Positron tomography was applied to the study of dementing illnesses quite early. The first quantitative report relating to cerebral energy metabolism posed questions concerning the possible influence of ischaemic processes regionally, the regional distribution of pathophysiology and its time course, and indirectly, the diagnostic potential of the imaging technique itself (Frackowiak et al., 1981). Subsequently all the findings have been corroborated by workers using ^{18}FDG to look at glucose metabolism (Benson et al., 1983; Friedland et al., 1983b, 1984a; Foster et al., 1983; Chase et al., 1984). Unfortunately, this method, without a flow technique, is unable to give information about energy balance and, without an independent measure of oxygen metabolism, is unable to distinguish aerobic from purely glycolytic metabolism of glucose. However, no group has published data on combined PET measurements of CMR_{O_2} and CMR_G in demented patients yet.

Energy metabolism

The principal findings have been a progressive decline of grey matter $rCMR_{O_2}$ and rCBF with increasing severity of dementia (Frackowiak et al., 1981). This phenomenon is also seen in white matter, which distinguishes the process fundamentally from normal ageing. Those with mild or moderate dementia demonstrated a 20% decrease in metabolism on average, and those with severe dementia a 40% decline, compared to normal age-matched subjects. There was no correlation between grey rCBF or $rCMR_{O_2}$ and clinico-pathological type of dementia. Thus, patients with vascular disease had the same $rCMR_{O_2}$ as those with degenerative dementia as a group. There was a correlation with severity but not type of disease.

The relationship between rCBF and $rCMR_{O_2}$ was unchanged in any of the groups of patients studied. Thus the rOER was the same whether patients were moderately or severely affected and of degenerative or vascular type. This was true not only for grey matter but also regionally throughout the brain. This observation extends the previously documented, coupled decline of hemispheric CBF and CMR_{O_2} in dementia onto a regional basis in the same way as rCBF measurements extended our understanding of hemispheric CBF values. It is now clear that there is not a heterogeneity of ischaemic and non-ischaemic areas in the brain subtending the coupled hemispheric decline, but that this is a diffuse generalised phenomenon. All the patients were studied at a time well removed from any acute neurological event, thus acute ischaemic episodes were not visualised in those patients with vascular dementia. It has been extensively shown that such acute events are associated with an initial severe rise in rOER,

followed soon after by a fall, before recoupling occurs with time (Wise et al., 1983a).

More recently we have shown that certain rare patients with severe occlusive neck artery disease can present with a pathophysiological picture indicating severe haemodynamic compromise of a chronic nature (Gibbs et al., 1984). Such patients, who may present clinically with transient ischaemic attacks or mild strokes, have a focally reduced rCBF/rCBV ratio (indicating focal reduction of perfusion pressure and depleted haemodynamic reserve) as well as a focal increase in rOER to levels between 50 and 70%. This indicates a considerable decrease in oxygen carriage reserve, but to levels insufficient to cause ischaemia. If perfusion were to fall further, for physiological as well as pathological reasons in such compromised patients, acute ischaemia and infarction might supervene. These patients are in a chronic state of pathophysiological compromise, in which homeostatic mechanisms which normally hold ischaemia at bay are almost exhausted (Frackowiak, 1985). This pathophysiological pattern represents, prima facie, an opportunity for preventive treatment of such patients with effective revascularisation operations. A further observation is that in patients with occlusive neck vessel disease, the ipsilateral and frequently contralateral hemisphere shows coupled low, or low normal CBF and CMR_{O_2}, even if presentation has been with TIA alone. This may reflect a degree of subclinical partial infarction, thus possibly representing a stage in the development of vascular dementia.

Patterns of physiological dysfunction

The regional distribution of pathophysiology in terms of $rCMR_{O_2}$ (confirmed by subsequent reports of $rCMR_G$) follows a progressive course in dementia. Initially the brunt of the disease is symmetrically distributed in temporo-parietal regions (Frackowiak et al., 1981). There have been reported individual case studies of a very asymmetrical onset in patients with apparent Alzheimer's disease (Ferris et al., 1981; Friedland et al., 1984a).

These suffer because of the lack of numerical data to support the images and the difficulty of making the differential diagnosis between Alzheimer and vascular dementia in individual (especially early) cases. Group data are therefore more reliable. As the dementia progresses and becomes severe, the frontal areas show a profound decline in metabolism, with comparatively little further decline in the temporo-parietal region. The impairment of metabolism does in fact affect all cortical regions, but is much less pronounced in primary motor and sensory regions (which includes the visual cortex). The caudate-putamen is frequently also relatively spared in degenerative disease. There is some evidence from studies of CMR_G that a low frontal pattern is present in patients suffering from 'subcortical' dementias, e.g. progressive supranuclear palsy (D'Antona et al., 1985).

The resolution of the PET cameras will dictate the diagnostic potential of these patterns. To date, instruments with a resolution over 1 cm^3 are able to show a 'diagnostic pattern' in only advanced cases. There remains a considerable overlap with normal subjects in the early stages of the disease, which interests the clinician most. Only in few cases have such patterns been verified by pathological data and it remains far from proven that such patterns are, or can be, better or more accurate at diagnosing dementing disease than a good clinical assessment. There is, however, hope that with instruments of improved resolution much more differential diagnostic information will become available.

Attempts have also been made to correlate specific clinically defined dysfunctions (e.g. aphasia, apraxia) to focal metabolic depression (Frackowiak et al., 1981; Foster et al., 1983; Chase et al., 1984). We were able to show that a decline in the 'appropriate' anatomical area was always found but that depression in other and contralateral areas was also present. In addition, direct correlations between severity of dysfunction and metabolic rate were not found. This is undoubtedly due in part to resolution factors. Likewise, the site and size of region of interest sampling are likely to influence results if inadequate appreciation of the limitations imposed by the grosser spatial resolution of early generation machines is not appreciated. Indeed, some of the reported and remarkable correlations between focal, clinically defined dysfunction and $rCMR_G$ are flawed by an inadequate attention to such considerations. When further studies with improved resolution characteristics are reported, some of these correlations will bear re-examination. In addition, the hierarchical derangement of inter-lobular connections and the examination of the different ways in which a dysphasia, or other focal deficit, can be produced in terms of the distribution of regional dysfunction will become the focus of much investigative attention.

Diagnostic potential of PET

A number of publications have attempted to derive diagnostic criteria for recognising Alzheimer's disease, some combining PET, CT and NMR scanning in a multiparametric approach to the problem (Friedland et al., 1984a; DeLeon et al., 1983: Benson et al., 1983). Claims that metabolic abnormalities antedate CT- or NMR-detectable changes have been made (Friedland et al., 1984a). The specificity of these changes remains to be defined. One report has noted changes in cerebral glucose metabolism in a patient with Creutzfeldt-Jacob disease (Friedland et al., 1984b). Temporal lobe hypometabolism with hemispheric asymmetry was noted and the authors mention the similarity of the pattern of dysfunction to that seen in Alzheimer's disease. They also make a rather ambitious extrapolation to suggest that this constitutes evidence for the possibility that Alzheimer's disease is caused by a slow infectious prion.

Other functional measurements in dementia

Protein synthesis

The study of cerebral metabolism in dementia has been extended to that of methionine metabolism by Bustany and colleagues at Orsay (Bustany et al., 1983, 1985). Of interest is the similarity of the temporo-parietal decrease in 'protein synthesis', and also the demonstration of profound decreases in frontal synthesis the more severe the degree of dementia. This technique appears quite sensitive, in that a 20% decline in synthetic rate correlates with just detectable clinical features of dementia. There is no correlation with CT abnormalities and certain regions showing a depression of 'protein synthesis' up to 70% apparently show no structural changes on CT. These results are of major interest, in that they indicate metabolic and functional derangement before structural change becomes apparent in vivo with X-ray CT. However, the quantitative technique remains incompletely reported and is in use currently in only one centre, though groups in Stockholm, Uppsala and Sendai have used ^{11}C-methionine in human imaging. Further corroborative studies must be awaited before the significance of these findings is entirely clear.

Cholinergic system

The use of labelled acetylcholine precursors has also attracted recent attention. Friedland has described the body distribution and cerebral autoradiographic characteristics of positron-labelled choline and phosphorylcholine showing a 0.2% uptake into the brain, with a rapid uptake and washout phase (Friedland et al., 1983a). The Uppsala group has synthesised and labelled a number of choline analogs, attempting to dissect out the unique acetylation step so that information can be obtained specifically on the cholinergic system in dementia (Eckernas, S.-A., personal communication). Reports on these studies are eagerly awaited.

Other cognitive disorders

There have been studies with PET techniques in allied cognitive disorders. Thus in first time, acute onset, drug-free schizophrenics, no difference in the values or patterns of cortical rCBF and $rCMR_{O_2}$ from normal were observed (Sheppard et al., 1983). At best there was a suggestion of a laterality deficit. In chronic schizophrenics Farkas has shown no metabolic differences between patients and normal subjects in mean CMR_G terms, though a significant decrease in front/occipital ratios was found in the patients (Farkas et al., 1984). The authors' interpretation is that this demonstrated 'hypofrontality'. No difference between treated and drug-free patients was found. Subsequent reports from the same group demonstrate a 25% increase in the CMR_G of the basal ganglia with medication (Brodie et al., 1984). The report unfortunately fails to mention the method of attenuation correction or data analysis used.

Autism has also been the subject of study, the group from Bethesda reporting generalised increases of about 20% in CMR_G in 10 autistic adults (Rumsey et al., 1985). However, a recent report from our laboratory failed to find this increase in CMR_G, and concurrent CBF and CMR_{O_2} measurements revealed a maintained and normal relationship, region for region, between these variables (Herold et al., 1985). It is likely that implementation strategies relating to attenuation correction are responsible for the Bethesda result.

Huntington's disease has been studied extensively by Kuhl and colleagues at UCLA (Kuhl et al., 1982b, 1984). Very interesting structural-metabolic correlations have been found. These authors have clearly demonstrated a decline in basal ganglion $rCMR_G$ prior to any structural change of the same region on CT. In addition, asymptomatic individuals at-risk have been noted to show low basal ganglion $rCMR_G$. Clinical follow-up is now in progress to see if these subjects go on to develop the disease. If studies can confirm the correlation, the predictive nature of this measurement will be potentially very useful.

More recently, CMR_G has been investigated in the dementia of progressive supranuclear palsy of Steele-Richardson-Olszewski by the Orsay group (D'Antona et al., 1985). A decline in frontal and basal ganglion CMR_G has been observed. The same group has also shown a markedly decreased uptake of ^{76}Br-labelled spiperone in the caudate-putamen and frontal regions (Baron et al., 1985).

The suggestion is that there is degeneration of neurons which are innervated by the nigrostriatal pathway (and hence exhibit D-2 receptors) in this disease. In addition, given the paucity of D-2 receptors in the frontal cortex, there is also a suspicion that 5-HT receptor bearing neurons may be involved at that site, (spiperone is a D-2 and a weak 5-HT antagonist). These receptor studies are likely to expand rapidly as investigators begin to look at basic mechanisms such as receptor function and transmitter-specific neuronal mapping, which may give further clues to the underlying pathogenesis and treatment of the dementing disorders.

Summary and conclusions

The problems of energy metabolism, a crude and indirect non-specific marker of neuronal damage have largely been answered in dementia as indicated above. It remains to be seen whether any of this knowledge can be applied in a diagnostic sense. Of therapeutic import is the demonstration that vasodilator drugs have no physiological basis for their use in the management of these disorders, but that certain highly selected and rare patients with obstructive vascular disease as a cause of dementia may benefit from reconstructive vascular surgery.

As to the future, the application of tracer techniques to clinical research of the dementing illnesses is in a rapidly expanding phase. Some examples of ligands imaging dopaminergic pathways have been mentioned in relation to progressive supranuclear palsy and the preliminary investigations of possible cholinergic pathway markers. The question of the specificity of the cholinergic dysfunction in Alzheimer's disease could be answered by performing studies of dopaminergic, 5-HT, opiate, benzodiazepine and other transmitter systems. This is already a possibility as ^{18}F-DOPA, ^{11}C-ketanserine, ^{11}C-diprenorphine, ^{11}C-carfentanyl and ^{11}C-flunitrazepam have all been synthesised. Similarly, it should be possible to evolve strategies for investigating the activity of specific enzymes in vivo with the production of appropriate positron-labelled substrates in a manner analogous to the use of ^{18}FDG to measure the activity of hexokinase. The scope of such metabolic and functional measurements is therefore large. The major advantage of providing a quantitative and objective means for monitoring the effects of any therapeutic regimen should also be remembered.

References

Baron, J. C., Steinling, M., Tanaka, T., Cavalheiro, E., Soussaline, F. and Collard, P. (1981) Quantitative measurement of CBF, oxygen extraction fraction (OEF) and CMR_{O_2} with ^{15}O continuous inhalation technique and positron emission tomography (PET): experimental evidence and normal values in man. *J. Cereb. Blood Flow Metabol.*, 1: S5–S6.

Baron, J. C., Lebrun-Grandie, P., Collard, P., Crouzel, C., Mestalan, G. and Bousser, M. G. (1982) Non invasive measurement of blood flow, oxygen consumption and glucose utilisation in the same brain regions in man by positron emission tomography: concise communication. *J. Nucl. Med.*, 23: 391–399.

Baron, J. C., Maziere, B., Loc'h, C., Sgouropoulos, P., Bonnet, A. M. and Agid, Y. (1985) Progressive supranuclear palsy: loss of striatal dopamine receptors demonstrated in vivo by positron tomography. *Lancet*, i: 1163–1164.

Benson, D. F., Kuhl, D. E., Hawkins, R. A., Phelps, M. E.,

Cummings, J. L. and Tsai, S. Y. (1983) The fluorodeoxyglucose ^{18}F scan in Alzheimer's disease and multi-infarct dementia. *Arch. Neurol.*, 40: 711–714.

Besson, J. A. O., Corrigan, F. M., Iljon Foreman, E., Eastwood, L. M., Smith, F. W. and Aschroft, G. W. (1985) Nuclear magnetic resonance (NMR). II. Imaging in dementia. *Br. J. Psychiat.*, 146: 31–35.

Betz, E. (1972) Cerebral blood flow: its measurement and regulation. *Physiol. Rev.*, 52: 595–630.

Bradley, W. G., Waluch, V., Brant-Zawadzki, M., Yadley, R. A. and Wycoff, R. R. (1984) Patchy, periventricular white matter lesions in the elderly: a common observation during NMR imaging. *Non-invas. Med. Imag.*, 1: 35–41.

Brodie, J. D., Christman, D. R., Corona, J. F., Fowler, J. S., GomezMont, F., Jaeger, J., Micheels, P. A., Rotrosen, J., Russel, J. A., Volkow, N. D., Wikler, A., Wolf, A. P. and Wolkin, A. (1984) Patterns of metabolic activity in the treatment of schizophrenia. *Ann. Neurol.*, 15, Suppl.: S166–S169.

Bustany, P., Henry, J. F., Sargent, T., Zarifian, E., Cabanis, E.,

Collard, P. and Comar, D. (1983) Local brain protein metabolism in dementia and schizophrenia: in vivo studies with ^{11}C-L-methionine and positron emission tomography. In W.-D. Heiss and M. E. Phelps (Eds.), *Positron Emission Tomography of the Brain*, Springer-Verlag, New York, pp. 208–211.

Bustany, P., Henry, J. F., De Rotrou, J., Signoret, P., Cabanis, E., Zarifian, E., Ziegler, M., Derlon, M., Crouzel, L., Soussaline, F. and Comar, D. (1985) Correlations between clinical state and positron emission tomography measurement of local brain protein synthesis in Alzheimer's disease, Parkinson's disease, schizophrenia, gliomas. In T. Greitz et al. (Eds.), *The Metabolism of the Human Brain Studied with Positron Emission Tomography*, Raven Press, New York, pp. 241–249.

Chase, T. N., Foster, L. N., Fedio, P., Brooks, R., Mansi, L. and DiChiro, G. (1984) Regional cortical dysfunction in Alzheimer's disease as determined by positron emission tomography. *Ann. Neurol.*, 15, Suppl.: S170–S174.

D'Antona, R., Baron, J. C., Samson, Y., Serdaru, M., Viader, F., Agid, Y. and Cambier, J. (1985) Subcortical dementia: frontal cortex hypometabolism detected by positron tomography in patients with progressive supranuclear palsy. *Brain*, 108: 785–800.

Dastur, D. K., Lane, M. H., Hansen, D. B., Kety, S. S., Butler, R. N., Perlin, S. and Sokoloff, L. (1963) Effects of aging on cerebral circulation and metabolism in man. In R. N. Butler and S. W. Greenhouse (Eds.), *Human Aging*. US Public Health Service Publication No. 986: pp. 59–76.

DeLeon, M. J., Ferris, S. H., George, A. E., Reisberg, B., Christman, D. R., Kricheff, I. I. and Wolf, A. P. (1983) Computed tomography and positron emission transaxial tomography evaluations of normal aging and Alzheimer's disease. *J. Cereb. Blood Flow Metabol.*, 3: 391–394.

DeLeon, M. J., George, A. E., Ferris, S. H., Christman, D. R., Fowler, J. S., Gentes, C. I., Brodie, J., Reisberg, B. and Wolf, A. P. (1984) Positron emission tomography and computed tomography assessments of the aging human brain. *J. Comput. Assist. Tomogr.*, 8: 88–94.

Duara, R., Margolin, R. A., Robertson-Tchabo, E. A., London, E. D., Schwartz, M., Renfrew, J. W., Koziarz, B. J., Sundaram, M., Grady, C., Moore, A. M., Ingvar, D. H., Sokoloff, L., Weingartner, H., Kessler, R. M., Manning, R. G., Channing, M. A., Cutler, N. R. and Rapoport, S. I. (1983) Resting cerebral glucose utilisation as measured with positron emission tomography in 21 healthy men between the ages of 21 and 83 years. *Brain*, 106: 761–775.

Duara, R., Grady, C., Haxby, J., Ingvar, D., Sokoloff, L., Margolin, R. A., Manning, R. G., Cutler, N. R. and Rapoport, S. I. (1984) Human brain glucose utilisation and cognitive function in relation to age. *Ann. Neurol.*, 16: 702–713.

Farkas, T., Wolf, A. O., Jaeger, J., Brodie, J. D., Christman, D. R. and Fowler, J. S. (1984) Regional brain glucose metabolism in chronic schizophrenia. *Arch. Gen. Psychiat.*, 41: 293–300.

Fazekas, J. F., Alman, R. W. and Bessman, A. N. (1952) Cerebral physiology of the aged. *Am. J. Med. Sci.*, 223: 245.

Ferris, S. H., DeLeon, M. J., Wolf, A. P., Farkas, T., Christman, D. R., Reisberg, B., Fowler, J. S., MacGregor, R., Goldman, A., George, A. E. and Rampal, S. (1981) Positron emission tomography in the study of aging and senile dementia. *Neurobiol. Aging*, 1: 127–131.

Foster, N. L., Chase, T. N., Fedio, P., Patronas, N. J., Brooks, R. A. and DiChiro, G. (1983) Alzheimer's disease: focal cortical changes shown by positron emission tomography. *Neurology*, 33: 961–965.

Frackowiak, R. S. J. (1982) Human regional cerebral blood flow and oxygen metabolism studied with oxygen-15 and positron emission tomography. MD Thesis, University of Cambridge, pp. 1–209.

Frackowiak, R. S. J. (1985) Pathophysiology of human cerebral ischaemia: studies with positron tomography and 15-oxygen. In L. Sokoloff (Ed.), *Brain Imaging and Brain Function*, Raven Press, New York, pp. 139–162. *Res. Publ. Assoc. Res. Nerv. Ment. Dis.*, 63: 139–162.

Frackowiak, R. S. J. and Lenzi, G. L. (1982) Physiological measurement in the brain: from potential to practice. In P. J. Ell and B. L. Holman (Eds.), *Computed Emission Tomography*, OUP, Oxford, pp. 188–210.

Frackowiak, R. S. J., Lenzi, G. L., Jones, T. and Heather, J. D. (1980) Quantitative measurement of regional cerebral blood flow and oxygen metabolism in man using ^{15}O and positron emission tomography: theory, procedure and normal values. *J. Comput. Assist. Tomogr.*, 4: 727–736.

Frackowiak, R. S. J., Pozzilli, C., Legg, N. J., DuBoulay, G. H., Marshall, J., Lenzi, G. L. and Jones, T. (1981) Regional cerebral oxygen supply and utilisation in dementia: a clinical and physiological study with oxygen-15 and positron tomography. *Brain*, 104: 753–778.

Frackowiak, R. S. J., Wise, R. J. S., Gibbs, J. M., Jones, T. and Leenders, N. (1984) Oxygen extraction in the ageing brain. *Monogr. Neurol. Sci.*, 11: 118–122.

Friedland, R. P., Mathis, C. A., Budinger, T. F., Moyer, B. R. and Rosen, M. (1983a) Labelled choline and phosphorylcholine: autoradiography: concise communication. *J. Nucl. Med.*, 24: 812–815.

Friedland, R. P., Budinger, T. F., Ganz, E., Yano, Y., Mathis, C. A., Koss, B., Ober, B. A., Huesman, R. H. and Derenzo, S. E. (1983b) Regional cerebral metabolic alterations in dementia of the Alzheimer type: positron emission tomography with [^{18}F]fluorodeoxyglucose. *J. Comput. Assist. Tomogr.*, 7: 590–598.

Friedland, R. P., Budinger, T. F., Brant-Zawadzki, M. and Jagust, W. J. (1984a) The diagnosis of Alzheimer-type dementia. A preliminary comparison of positron emission tomography and proton magnetic resonance. *J. Am. Med. Assoc.*, 252: 2750–2752.

Friedland, R. P., Prusiner, S. B., Jagust, W. J., Budinger, T. F. and Davis, R. L. (1984b) Bitemporal hypometabolism in Crentzfeldt-Jacob disease measured by positron emission tomography with [^{18}F]-2-fluorodeoxyglucose. *J. Comput. Assist. Tomogr.*, 8: 978–981.

Gadian, D. G. (1982) *Nuclear Magnetic Resonance and its Application to Living Systems.* Clarendon Press, Oxford.

Gibbs, J. M., Wise, R. J. S., Leenders, K. L. and Jones, T. (1984) Evaluation of cerebral perfusion reserve in patients with carotid artery occlusion. *Lancet*, i: 310–314.

Glass, H. I. and Harper, A. M. (1963) Measurement of regional blood flow in cerebral cortex of man through intact skull. *Br. Med. J.*, i: 593.

Gottstein, U., Muller, W., Berghoff, W., Gartner, H. and Held, K. (1971) Zur Utilisation von nicht-veresterten Fettsäuren und Ketonkorpen im Gehirn des Menschen. *Klin. Wschr.*, 49: 406–411.

Grubb, R. L., Raichle, M. E., Gado, M. H., Eichling, J. O. and Hughes, C. P. (1977) Cerebral blood flow, oxygen utilisation and blood volume in dementia. *Neurology*, 27: 905–910.

Hachinski, V. C., Iliff, L. D., Zilkha, E., DuBoulay, G. H., McAllister, V. L., Marshall, J., Ross-Russell, R. W. and Symon, L. (1975) Cerebral blood flow in dementia. *Arch. Neurol.*, 32: 632–637.

Herold, S., Frackowiak, R. S. J., Rutter, M. and Howlin, P. (1985) Regional cerebral blood flow, oxygen metabolism and glucose metabolism in young autistic adults. *J. Cereb. Blood Flow Metabol.*, 5: S189–S190.

Ingvar, D. H. (1974) Regional cerebral blood flow in organic dementia and in chronic schizophrenia. *Triangle*, 13: 17–23.

Ingvar, D. H. (1979) Hyperfrontal distribution of the cerebral grey matter flow in resting wakefulness: on the functional anatomy of the conscious state. *Acta Neurol. Scand.*, 60: 12–25.

Ingvar, D. H. and Lassen, N. A. (1961) Quantitative determinations of regional cerebral blood flow in man. *Lancet*, ii: 806.

Kennedy, C. (1967) The cerebral metabolic rate in mentally retarded children. *Arch. Neurol.*, 16: 55–58.

Kennedy, C. and Sokoloff, L. (1957) An adaptation of the nitrous oxide method to the study of the cerebral circulation in children: normal values for cerebral blood flow and cerebral metabolic rate in childhood. *J. Clin. Invest.*, 36: 1130–1137.

Kety, S. S. (1956) Human cerebral blood flow and oxygen consumption as related to aging. *Res. Publ. Assoc. Res. Nerv. Ment. Dis.*, 35: 31–45.

Kety, S. S. and Schmidt, C. F. (1945) The determination of cerebral blood flow in man by the use of nitrous oxide in low concentrations. *Am. J. Physiol.*, 143: 53.

Kety, S. S. and Schmidt, C. F. (1946) Effects of active and passive hyperventilation on cerebral blood flow, cerebral oxygen consumption, cardiac output and blood pressure of normal young man. *J. Clin. Invest.*, 24: 839–844.

Kety, S. S. and Schmidt, C. F. (1948a) The nitrous oxygen method for the quantitative determination of cerebral blood flow in man: theory, procedure and normal values. *J. Clin. Invest.*, 27: 476–483.

Kety, S. S. and Schmidt, C. F. (1948b) The effect of altered arterial tensions of carbon dioxide and oxygen on cerebral blood flow and cerebral oxygen consumption of normal young men. *J. Clin. Invest.*, 27: 493–499.

Kuhl, D. E., Metter, E. J., Riege, W. H. and Phelps, M. E. (1982a) Effects of human aging on patterns of local cerebral glucose utilisation determined by the [^{18}F]fluorodeoxyglucose method. *J. Cereb. Blood Flow Metabol.*, 2: 163–171.

Kuhl, D. E., Phelps, M. E. and Markham, C. E. (1982b) Cerebral metabolism and atrophy in Huntington's disease determined by ^{18}FDG and computed tomographic scan. *Ann. Neurol.*, 12: 425–434.

Kuhl, D. E., Metter, E. J., Riege, W. H. and Markham, C. H. (1984a) Patterns of cerebral glucose utilisation in Parkinson's disease and Huntington's disease. *Ann. Neurol.*, 15: S119–S125.

Kuhl, D. F., Metter, E. J., Riege, W. H. and Hawkins, R. A. (1984b) The effect of normal aging on patterns of local cerebral glucose utilisation. *Ann. Neurol.*, 15, Suppl.: S133–S137.

Lammertsma, A. A. and Jones, T. (1983) The correction for the presence of intravascular oxygen-15 in the steady state technique for measuring regional oxygen extraction in the brain. 1. Description of the method. *J. Cereb. Blood Flow Metabol.*, 3: 416–424.

Lammertsma, A. A., Jones, T., Frackowiak, R. S. J., Lenzi, G. L. and Pozzilli, C. (1981) A theoretical study of the steady state model for measuring regional cerebral blood flow and oxygen utilisation using oxygen-15. *J. Comput. Assist. Tomogr.*, 5: 544–550.

Lammertsma, A. A., Heather, J. D., Jones, T., Frackowiak, R. S. J. and Lenzi, G. L. (1982) A statistical study of the steady state model for measuring regional cerebral blood flow and oxygen utilisation using oxygen-15. *J. Comput. Assist. Tomogr.*, 6: 566–573.

Lammertsma, A. A., Wise, R. J. S., Heather, J. D., Gibbs, J. M., Leenders, K. L., Frackowiak, R. S. J., Rhodes, C. G., Jones, T. (1983) The correction for the presence of intravascular oxygen-15 in the steady state technique for measuring regional oxygen extraction ratio in the brain. 2. Results in normal subjects and brain tumour and stroke patients. *J. Cereb. Blood Flow Metabol.*, 3: 425–431.

Lassen, N. A. (1959) Cerebral blood flow and oxygen consumption in man. *Physiol. Rev.*, 39: 183–238.

Lassen, N. A. and Munck, O. (1955) The cerebral blood flow in man determined by the use of radioactive Krypton. *Acta Physiol. Scand.*, 33: 30–38.

Lassen, N. A. and Ingvar, D. H. (1963) Regional cerebral blood flow measurement in man. *Arch. Neurol.*, 9: 615–622.

Lassen, N. A., Munck, O. and Tottey, E. R. (1957) Mental function and cerebral oxygen consumption in organic dementia. *Arch. Neurol. Psychiat. (Chic.)*, 77: 126–133.

Lassen, N. A., Feinberg, I. and Lane, M. H. (1960) Bilateral studies of cerebral oxygen uptake in young and aged normal subjects and in patients with organic dementia. *J. Clin. Invest.*, 39: 491–500.

Lassen, N. A., Christensen, M. S., Høedt-Rasmussen, K. and Stewart, B. M. (1966) Cerebral oxygen consumption in Down's Syndrome. *Arch. Neurol.*, 15: 595–602.

Lassen, N. A., Ingvar, D. H. and Skinhøj, E. (1978) Brain function and blood flow. *Sci. Am.*, 239: 50–59.

Lavy, S., Melamed, E., Bentin, S., Cooper, G. and Rinot, Y. (1978) Bihemispheric decreases of regional cerebral blood flow in dementia: correlation with age-matched normal controls. *Ann. Neurol.*, 4: 445–450.

Lenzi, G. L., Gibbs, J. M., Frackowiak, R. S. J. and Jones, T. (1983) Measurement of cerebral blood flow and oxygen metabolism by positron emission tomography and the ^{15}O steady-state technique: aspects of methodology, reproducibility and clinical application. In P. L. Magistretti (Ed.), *Functional Radionuclide Imaging of the Brain*, Raven Press, New York, pp. 291–304.

Mallett, B. L. and Veall, N. (1963) Investigation of cerebral blood flow in hypertension using radioactive Xenon and inhalation and extracranial recording. *Lancet*, i: 1081–1082.

Mallett, B. L. and Veall, N. (1965) The measurement of regional cerebral clearance rates in man using Xe-133 inhalation and extracranial recording. *Clin. Sci.*, 29: 179–191.

Mazziotta, J. C. and Phelps, M. E. (1984) Human sensory stimulation and deprivation: positron emission tomographic results and strategies. *Ann. Neurol.*, 15, Suppl.: S50–S60.

Mazziotta, J. C., Phelps, M. E., Carson, R. E. and Kuhl, D. E. (1982a) Tomographic mapping of human cerebral metabolism: auditory stimulation. *Neurology*, 32: 921–937.

Mazziotta, J. C., Phelps, M. E., Carson, R. E. and Kuhl, D. E. (1982b) Tomographic mapping of human cerebral metabolism: sensory deprivation. *Ann. Neurol.*, 12: 435–444.

Mazziotta, J. C., Phelps, M. E., Miller, J. and Kuhl, D. E. (1982c) Tomographic mapping of human cerebral metabolism: normal unstimulated state. *Neurology*, 31: 503–516.

O'Brien, M. D. and Mallett, B. L. (1970) Cerebral cortex perfusion rates in dementia. *J. Neurol. Neurosurg. Psychiat.*, 33: 497–500.

Obrist, W. D., Chivian, E., Cronqvist, S. and Ingvar, D. H. (1970) Regional cerebral blood flow in senile and presenile dementia. *Neurology*, 20: 315–322.

Ohata, M., Sundaram, U., Fredericks, W. R., London, E. D. and Rapoport, S. I. (1981) Regional cerebral blood flow during development and ageing of the rat brain. *Brain*, 104: 319–332.

Orgogozo, J. M. and Larsen, B. (1979) Activation of the supplementary motor area during voluntary movement in man suggests it works as a supramotor area. *Science*, 206: 847–850.

Pantano, P., Baron, J.-C., Lebrun-Grandie, P., Duquesnoy, N., Bousser, M.-G. and Comar, D. (1984) Regional cerebral blood flow and oxygen consumption in human ageing. *Stroke*, 15: 635–641.

Phelps, M. E. and Mazziotta, J. C. (1985) Positron emission tomography: human brain function and biochemistry. *Science*, 228: 799–809.

Phelps, M. E., Mazziotta, J. C., Kuhl, D. E., Nuwer, M., Packwood, J., Metter, J. and Engel, J. Jr. (1981) Tomographic mapping of human cerebral metabolism: visual stimulation and deprivation. *Neurology*, 31: 517–529.

Phelps, M. E., Mazziotta, J. C. and Huang, S.-C. (1982) Study of cerebral function with positron computed tomography. *J. Cereb. Blood Flow Metabol.*, 2: 113–162.

Pritchard, J. W., Alger, J. R., Behar, K. L., Petroff, O. A. C. and Shulman, R. G. (1983) Cerebral metabolic studies in vivo by ^{31}P-NMR. *Proc. Natl. Acad. Sci. USA*, 80: 2748–2751.

Rhodes, C. G., Lenzi, G. L., Frackowiak, R. S. J., Jones, T. and Pozzilli, C. (1981) Measurement of CBF and CMR_{O_2} using the continuous inhalation of $C^{15}O_2$ and $^{15}O_2$: experimental validation using $C^{15}O_2$ reactivity in the anaesthetised dog. *J. Neurol. Sci.*, 50: 381–389.

Rhodes, C. G., Wise, R. J. S., Gibbs, J. M., Frackowiak, R. S. J., Hatazawa, J., Palmer, A. J., Thomas, D. G. T. and Jones, T. (1983) In vivo disturbance of the oxidative metabolism of glucose in human cerebral gliomas. *Ann. Neurol.*, 14: 614–626.

Risberg, J. and Ingvar, D. H. (1973) Patterns of activation in the grey matter of the dominant hemisphere during memorising and reasoning. *Brain*, 96: 737–756.

Roland, P. E., Larsen, B., Lassen, N. A. and Skinhøj, E. (1980a) Supplementary motor area and other cortical areas in organisation of voluntary movements in man. *J. Neurophysiol.*, 43: 118–136.

Roland, P. E., Skinhøj, E., Lassen, N. A. and Larsen, B. (1980b) Different cortical areas in man in organisation of voluntary movements in extrapersonal space. *J. Neurophysiol.*, 43: 137–150.

Rumsey, J. M., Duara, R., Grady, C., Rapoport, J. L., Margolin, R. A., Rapoport, S. I. and Cutler, N. (1985) Brain metabolism in autism: resting cerebral glucose utilisation as measured with positron emission tomography (PET). *Arch. Gen. Psychiat.*, 42: 448–455.

Shenkin, H. A., Novak, P., Goluboff, B., Soffe, A. M. and Bortin, L. (1953) The effects of aging, arteriosclerosis and hypertension upon the cerebral circulation. *J. Clin. Invest.*, 32: 459–465.

Sheppard, G., Gruzelier, J., Manchada, R., Hirsch, S. R., Wise, R., Frackowiak, R. and Jones, T. (1983) ^{15}O positron emission tomographic scanning in predominantly never-treated acute schizophrenic patients. *Lancet*, ii: 1448–1452.

Simard, D., Olesen, J., Paulson, O. B., Lassen, N. A. and Skinhøj, E. (1971) Regional cerebral blood flow and its regulation in dementia. *Brain*, 94: 273–288.

Smith, C. B., Goochee, C., Rapoport, S. I. and Sokoloff, L.

(1980) Effects of ageing on local rates of cerebral glucose utilisation in the rat. *Brain*, 103: 351–365.

Sokoloff, L. (1966) Cerebral circulatory and metabolic changes associated with aging. *Res. Publ. Assoc. Nerv. Ment. Dis.*, 41: 237–251.

Sokoloff, L. (1984) Metabolic probes of central nervous system activity in experimental animals and man. *Magnus Lecture Series*, 1: 1–97. Sinauer Assoc. Inc., Sunderland, MA.

Ter-Pogossian, M. M., Eichling, J. O., Davis, D. O., Welch, M. J. and Metzger, J. M. (1969) The determination of regional cerebral blood flow by means of water labelled with radioactive oxygen-15. *Radiology*, 93: 31–40.

Ter-Pogossian, M. M., Eichling, J. O., Davis, D. O. and Welch, M. J. (1970) The measure in vivo of regional cerebral oxygen utilisation by means of oxyhaemoglobin labelled with radioactive oxygen-15. *J. Clin. Invest.*, 49: 381–391.

Thomas, D. J., Zilkha, E., Redmond, S., DuBoulay, G. H., Marshall, J., Ross-Russell, R. W. and Symon, L. (1979) An intravenous ^{133}Xe clearance technique for measuring cerebral blood flow. *J. Neurol. Sci.*, 40: 53–63.

Tomlinson, B. E., Blessed, G. and Roth, M. (1970) Observations on the brains of demented old people. *J. Neurol. Sci.*, 11: 205–242.

Veall, N. and Mallett, B. L. (1966) Regional cerebral blood flow determination by ^{133}Xe inhalation and external recording: the effect of arterial recirculation. *Clin. Sci.*, 30: 353–369.

Wise, R. J. S., Bernardi, S., Frackowiak, R. S. J., Legg, N. J. and Jones, T. (1983a) Serial observations on the pathophysiology of acute stroke: the transition from ischaemia to infarction as reflected in regional oxygen extraction. *Brain*, 106: 197–222.

Wise, R. J. S., Rhodes, C. G., Gibbs, J. M., Hatazawa, J., Frackowiak, R. S. J., Palmer, A. J. and Jones, T. (1983b) Disturbance of oxidative metabolism of glucose in recent human cerebral infarcts. *Ann. Neurol.*, 14: 627–637.

Yamaguchi, F., Meyer, J. S., Yamamoto, M., Sakai, F. and Shaw, T. (1980) Non invasive regional cerebral blood flow measurements in dementia. *Arch. Neurol.*, 37: 410–418.

Discussion

E. A. VAN ROYEN: Will there be any role for single photon emission tomography (SPECT) in the diagnosis of Alzheimer disease?

ANSWER: The reply depends on the ability of single photon radiochemists to produce a specific marker of Alzheimer-disease-process affected nervous tissue and for such a marker to produce a visually recognisable diagnostic pattern. Blood flow markers are too non-specific, even with the depth information available to SPECT. Blood flow tells us the general metabolic state of the tissue (assuming the absence of uncoupling pathology such as ischaemia or vascular occlusive disease) and this can be affected by any number of diseases amongst which is included Alzheimer's disease.

H. VAN CREVEL: You found with positron emission tomography (PET) that oxygen extraction rate (OER) is normal in multiinfarct dementia (MID) between ischaemic events. You also showed impressive ischaemic lesions shown by nuclear magnetic resonance (NMR) in patients without dementia. Do you understand this?

ANSWER: The normal OER in MID between acute ischaemic events is not surprising in that it reflects recoupling of flow and metabolism in infarcted brain. The absence of permanent low OER regions of uncoupling as seen following some larger infarcts presumably indicates the smaller size or degree of infarction. The clinical picture is probably the result of an accumulation of such events. The NMR scanner is very sensitive to structural change involving water content, therefore especially so in white matter. I think the low attenuation periventricular areas and their presumed counterparts on NMR represent areas of subcortical arteriosclerotic change which is not clinically manifest, therefore the subject appears normal. Nevertheless, such subjects frequently are hypertensive or have a significant risk profile or indeed present with other manifestations of vascular disease, e.g. late onset epilepsy.

D. F. Swaab, E. Fliers, M. Mirmiran, W. A. Van Gool and F. Van Haaren (Eds.)
Progress in Brain Research, Vol. 70.
© 1986 Elsevier Science Publishers B.V. (Biomedical Division)

CHAPTER 6

The endogenous components of the event-related potential — a diagnostic tool?

E. Donchin, G. A. Miller and L. A. Farwell

Department of Psychology and Cognitive Psychophysiology Laboratory, University of Illinois at Urbana-Champaign, Champaign, IL, USA

Introduction

Goodin et al. (1978b) reported that a brain response, labeled the P300, is elicited with a substantially delayed latency in demented patients. Briefly described, they presented their subjects with a series of tones and recorded from the surface of the scalp an electrical response of the brain to these tones, using a technique requiring extensive computer analysis. This response takes the form of a sequence of peaks and troughs and is known as the 'event-related brain potential' (ERP). Goodin et al. (1978b) selected one specific peak, the P300, which is positive in polarity and which occurs at least 300 ms following the eliciting tone. This interval, the 'latency' of P300, is of particular interest because it seems to be useful as a tool in mental chronometry. There is considerable evidence that the latency of P300 increases with age (Ford et al., 1979; Pfefferbaum et al., 1980a, 1984a; Brown et al., 1983; Mullis et al., 1985; Picton et al., 1984). Goodin et al. (1978a,b) provided additional support for this thesis. However, the more striking aspect of their results was that the latency of the P300 was extraordinarily long only in the demented subjects, not in subjects showing very similar overt symptoms due to depression rather than dementia. These data implied that the P300 may serve as a tool in differential diagnosis.

The degree to which the increase in P300 latency is indeed a specific indicator of senile dementia has proven somewhat controversial (Brown et al., 1982; Pfefferbaum et al., 1984b; Slaets and Fortgens, 1984; Polich et al., 1986). It so happens that increases in P300 latency do tend to occur in association with other pathologies (Roth et al., 1979; Baribeau-Braun et al., 1983). Furthermore, conflicting results have been reported by other investigators (Slaets and Fortgens, 1984). However this matter is resolved, there is an aspect of Goodin et al.'s (1978b) contribution that is noteworthy and on which we wish to focus this review of the role that cognitive psychophysiology can play in the study of aging. We refer to the theory-based, rather than nosological, foundation of the study.

The nosological approach is a rather common, and in many cases beneficial, procedure for developing diagnostic applications of psychophysiological and other measures (see for example Halliday, 1978). The starting point for a nosological study is the availability of groups of clinically diagnosed patients as well as an adequate control group of non-patients. The strategy is empirical. Given that the studied groups are known to be proper representatives of the diagnostic classes of interest, then any measure that discriminates between the groups is potentially useful. This approach has, for example, been of great benefit in developing a diagnostic measure for multiple sclerosis based on the latency of brain responses elicited by moving checkerboards (Halliday et al.,

1973). However, the success of the nosological approach is contingent on the specificity of the deficit and the certainty with which patients can be diagnosed clinically.

Matters have proven considerably more complex when the same approach has been applied in the analysis of components of the ERP which are not simple, obligatory, perceptual responses (exogenous components) but reflect higher-order processes (endogenous components). Consider, for example, the P300, with which this paper is primarily concerned. Evidence has accumulated in the past two decades that the P300 is smaller in amplitude, and generally longer in latency, in most nosological groups investigated. Low amplitude P300 has been reported for the mentally retarded (N. Squires et al., 1979), for the schizophrenic (Pfefferbaum et al., 1984b), for the depressed (Roth et al., 1981; Pfefferbaum et al., 1984b), for the alexic (Neville et al., 1979), and for the alcoholic (Porjesz and Begleiter, 1982), to name but a few. Thus, to observe a difference between any nosological group and a control group does not necessarily imply that the primary diagnostic criterion according to which the groups were constructed is indeed responsible for the observed difference in the dependent measure. There may well be a non-specific deficit that the group studied shares with many other diagnostic groups.

The nosological approach can be substantially enriched if its empirical observation of differences can be augmented by a theoretical understanding of the functional significance of the psychophysiological observations and of the underlying neurophysiology. The choice of the latency of the P300 as a measure for examination in dementia has been driven by the extensive evidence that this latency can serve as an index of mental timing that is not contaminated by motor factors (Donchin, 1975, 1981; Kutas et al., 1977; McCarthy and Donchin, 1979, 1981; Donchin and McCarthy, 1980). Within this conceptual framework, Goodin et al.'s (1978a,b) work assumes increased value, because it goes beyond asserting merely that a group of demented patients are deviant on yet another

measure. Rather, the data are interpreted as supporting an assertion about the nature of the deficit in a manner that specifies directions for further study. A similar use of the theory presented by Donchin and associates to account for variance in P300 latency has been made by Ford et al. (1979), who inferred from an analysis of the P300 latency in a test of short-term memory that elderly subjects are slowed, in such a test, by motor rather than by cognitive factors.

Our purpose in this chapter is to introduce the conceptual foundations of the theory-based approach to the use of ERPs, in contrast to the nosological approach. In the course of this review we will survey currently available information on the P300 that is recorded in aged subjects. We will conclude this chapter with the description of a series of studies of P300 in aged subjects conducted in our laboratory that serves to illustrate our approach to the use of ERPs in cognitive psychophysiology.

The status of P300 in psychological theory

As is well known, the ERP is a sequence of voltage oscillations, recorded from the scalp, that are time-locked to an event. It is extracted from the electroencephalographic record by means of 'signal averaging' (see Regan, 1972, or Callaway et al., 1978, for a technical introduction to ERPs; Hillyard and Kutas, 1983, for a review of current cognitive research with ERPs; and Coles et al., 1986, for a general treatment of this methodology). The ERP is generally parsed into different 'components'. Components are defined in terms of their polarity (positive or negative voltage), latency (temporal relationship to the event), and topography (variation in voltage with electrode location on the scalp), as well as by their relationship to experimental variables. Components can be quantified using simple magnitude measures or through the application of more elaborate techniques such as 'principal component analysis' (PCA) and 'vector analysis' (Gratton et al., 1983; see also Gratton et al., 1986). Component labels are generated by a polarity descriptor and a characteristic latency descriptor. Thus, the P300 is a positive ERP component with a modal latency of 300 ms. In some cases, as with 'contingent negative variation' (CNV) and 'slow wave' (SW), the latency descriptors are omitted.

The assumptions and the model underlying our study of ERPs have been presented elsewhere (Donchin, 1979, 1981). In brief, we assume that the voltages we record at the scalp are the result of synchronous activation of neuronal ensembles whose geometry allows their individual fields to summate to a field whose strength can affect scalp electrodes (Galambos and Hillyard, 1981). As explained above, it is useful to parse the ERP into a set of components. The component, in our scheme of things, is characterized by its consistent response to experimental manipulations (see Donchin et al., 1978, for a discussion of components). We further assume that each component is a manifestation at the scalp of an intracranial processing entity. We are not implying that each ERP component corresponds to a specific neuroanatomical entity or that the activity manifested by the component corresponds to a distinct neural process. Rather, we assume that a consistent information processing need, characterized by its eliciting conditions, activates a collection of processes which, for perhaps entirely fortuitous reasons, have the biophysical properties that generate the scalp-recorded activity. As a working hypothesis, we postulate that ERP components are manifestations of functional processing entities that play distinct roles in the algorithmic structure of the information processing system. In other words, we believe that it is possible to describe in detail the transformations that the processing entity applies to the information stream. The goal of cognitive psychophysiology, within this framework, is to provide such detailed descriptions. This may be achieved by developing comprehensive descriptions of the conditions governing the elicitation and attributes of the components (the 'antecedent' conditions). These descriptions can be used to support theories that attribute certain functions to the 'subroutine' manifested by a component. In turn, the theories should lead to predictions regarding the consequences of the elicitation of the 'subroutines', predictions which can be tested empirically.

The ensemble of ERP components is rich in members, from the early brain stem potentials through general components such as N100, P200, N200, P300, the 'slow wave', and several event-preceding negativities. Each of these merits a detailed review, and with respect to each some work pertaining to aging has been done. However, both because our own work has focused on the P300, and because the scope of this chapter must be limited, we will restrict ourselves to the P300 component.

The most commonly used experimental context in the study of the P300 is the oddball paradigm (Donchin et al., 1978). The subject is presented with a series of stimuli that can be classified into one of two categories. The instructions are either to count, or to respond in some other manner, to items from one of the categories. An alternate response (which may be 'ignore') is required to elements from the other category. It is typically the case that occurrences in one of the categories are rare (the 'oddball'). There is an abundance of evidence that rare events elicit a large P300, whose amplitude tends to be inversely related to the subjective probability of the eliciting stimulus. However, probability is neither a necessary nor a sufficient condition for the elicitation of a P300. The task relevance of events is at least as important a determinant of the amplitude of P300 (Donchin, 1981). Fig. 1 presents an example of ERPs elicited in young and elderly subjects in four different oddball tasks (Marshall et al., 1983, described in detail in the section below on: P300 and working memory in the elderly). The P300 is the positive deflection (downward in the Fig.) between 300 and 600 ms post stimulus. Note the comparatively large P300s in the 'target' conditions, which are either rare, task-relevant, or both, and the smaller and longer-latency P300s in the elderly subjects.

In any usage of the ERP, or of a specific

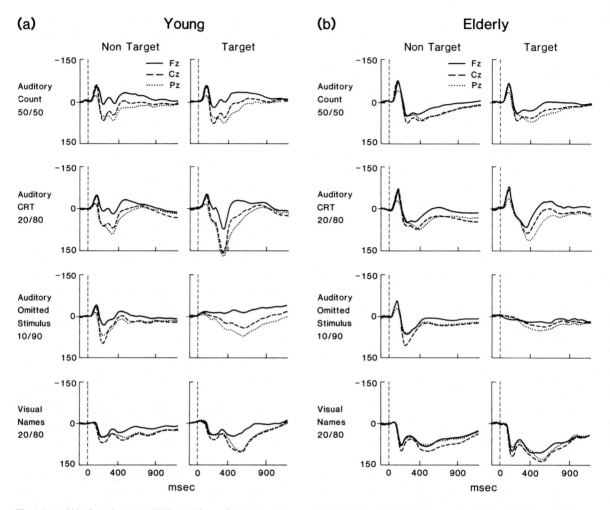

(a)   **Young**

(b)   **Elderly**

Fig. 1 (a and b). Grand average ERP waveforms for (a) 19 young and (b) 53 elderly subjects in four oddball tasks. Stimuli presented in Bernoulli series with the probabilities indicated. ERPs recorded at Fz, Cz, and Pz. Note the P300, a positive deflection (downward in the Fig.) between 300 and 600 ms post stimulus, larger in the 'target' conditions.

component of the ERP, these complex waveforms need to be converted in some manner into summarizing measures. The two attributes of the P300 which are generally quantified in this manner are the 'amplitude' and the 'latency' of the component. We place these terms in quotes because there is a need to distinguish between the use of these terms as referents to conceptual attributes and their use as referents to self-evident features of the waveform. In most studies, 'latency' refers to the interval between stimulus onset and the peak of the wave which is identified with the

P300. This is a self-evident feature which can be measured with relative ease. Conceptually, however, this feature is taken as a function of the interval between the event eliciting the P300 and the occurrence of the information processing manifested in P300. This conceptual latency can be represented by many different measures. The onset of the positive deflection, for example, is as obvious a measure of latency as is the peak of the positivity. The choice of the peak derives from the larger reliability with which it can be measured. Such choices in measurement must be made in any investigation. Yet it must be remembered that these are in many ways arbitrary choices. As the different measures are not perfectly correlated, it is conceivable that studies will conflict because they have used different features of the waveform to represent the conceptual attributes.

With this caveat in mind, it is possible to discuss the data that have accumulated to date, mostly from samples of young adults, regarding the behavior and possibly the functional significance of the P300. Detailed reviews can be found elsewhere (Pritchard, 1981; Hillyard and Kutas, 1983; Donchin, in press). Here, we shall only note that the amplitude can be interpreted as a measure of the activation of the intracranial processor whose activity is manifested by the P300 (Donchin et al., 1973; Donchin, 1981). The amplitude appears to increase with the task relevance and the improbability of the eliciting event (Pritchard, 1981). The relationship between task relevance and P300 amplitude has led to an extensive series of studies assessing the degree to which P300 can be used as a measure of 'mental workload' (Isreal et al., 1980; Kramer et al., 1983; Sirevaag et al., 1984; see also Gopher and Donchin, 1986).

The latency of the P300, on the other hand, has been shown to depend on the duration of information processing activities that must precede the elicitation of the P300. In the main, an entire class of variables that are known to either retard or to speed up reaction time also have a similar effect on P300 latency (Ritter and Vaughan, 1969; Kutas et al., 1977; Ragot and Renault, 1981; McCarthy, 1984). However, it turns out that there is a set of variables known to have a very large effect on reaction time that do not seem to affect, or at most have a microscopic effect, on P300 latency (McCarthy and Donchin, 1981; Duncan-Johnson and Donchin, 1981, 1982; Magliero et al., 1984; Coles et al., 1985). In the main, the variables that affect both P300 latency and reaction time are clearly associated with the evaluation of stimulus and response contingencies. Those variables that affect primarily RT and do not affect P300 latency appear to be related primarily to motor processes.

It is this distinction and the functional interpretation it implies that underlie the use of P300 latency in studies of aged subjects.

P300 in healthy and demented adults: basic findings

A number of studies have investigated the relationship between P300 latency and aging. The consensus of these studies seems to be that, in adults, P300 latency in both the auditory and visual modalities increases with age. A number of studies comparing groups of young vs. elderly adults have found longer latencies in the elderly (e.g., Ford et al., 1979, 1982a; Pfefferbaum et al., 1980a, 1984a). Several studies have indicated that P300 increases linearly in latency from early adulthood through old age, with a slope of between 1 and 2 ms/year (e.g., Syndulko et al., 1982, 1.1 ms/year; Brown et al., 1983, 1.12 ms/year; Picton et al., 1984, 1.36 ms/year; K. Squires et al., 1980, 1.64 ms/year; Goodin et al., 1978a, 1.8 ms/year). Some studies have found that the slope of the P300 latency curve increases with age. Beck et al. (1980) found twice the slope in the 63–79 years age range as in the 28–63 age range (1.6 vs. 0.8 ms/year). Brown et al. (1983) fitted the latency/age function with a curvilinear first- and second-degree orthogonal polynomial, indicating a positively accelerating function. Mullis et al. (1985) fitted data on 108 subjects aged 8 to 90 years with a similar function (the function included decreasing latencies with age in subjects between 8 and 22 years).

Although the increase of P300 latency with age appears to be a robust observation, this finding has not been accepted without controversy. Some investigators have failed to observe such an increase in P300 latency with age. Podlesny and Dustman (1982) found no age effects on P300 latency in visually signaled simple and choice-reaction time tasks. Snyder and Hillyard (1979) report a constant latency, with age, of P300 elicited by visual targets or novel visual stimuli. Michalewski et al. (1982) and Picton et al. (1984) found no significant increase with age in P300 latency in response to an omitted stimulus. Moreover, researchers have found a considerable variability in P300 latency within different age groups. Typically, the range of latency within each age group has been as large or nearly as large as the range across groups. Thus, no particular latency range specifically identifies a particular age group, although Goodin et al. (1978b) did report that their demented patients fell outside the normal range for the elderly.

Results on age-related changes in P300 amplitude are less clear than those relating to latency. Some investigators report decreases in P300 amplitude with age (Goodin et al., 1978a; Podlesny and Dustman, 1982; Brown et al., 1983; Picton et al., 1984; Podlesny et al., 1984; Mullis et al., 1985), while others report that P300 amplitude remains constant with age (Beck et al., 1980; Pfefferbaum et al., 1980a, 1984a; Ford et al., 1982b).

Several studies have found changes in the scalp distribution of P300 with age (Smith et al., 1980; Pfefferbaum et al., 1980b, 1984a; Picton et al., 1984). The P300 is parietally maximal in younger subjects but seems to shift frontally with age. Wickens et al. (1985; see also Braune et al., 1985; Strayer et al., 1985) report a study of 60 subjects ranging in age from 20 to 64 years, in which the amplitude of P300, averaged over three scalp recording sites — Fz (frontal), Cz (central), and Pz (parietal) — did not change with age. However, the difference between Pz amplitude and Fz amplitude decreased significantly. Both an increase in Fz amplitude and a decrease in Pz amplitude with advancing age contributed to this result.

As mentioned above, it has been proposed (Goodin et al., 1978b; K. Squires et al., 1979, 1980) that prolonged P300 latency may be a clinically useful tool in the differential diagnosis of dementia. The initial studies of P300 latency and dementia, as well as several subsequent studies (Syndulko et al., 1982; Brown et al., 1982; Polich et al., 1986) used a two-stimulus oddball paradigm, with the subjects required to count, or otherwise respond to, the rare events. All of these studies found prolonged P300 latency in demented patients. Polich et al. (1986) also reported a

positive correlation between P300 latency and the degree of cognitive impairment.

Pfefferbaum and colleagues (Pfefferbaum et al., 1984a,b) conducted an extensive study comparing 135 normal controls ranging in age from 18 to 90 with demented patients as well as non-demented, cognitively impaired patients, schizophrenics, and depressives. Both auditory and visual modalities were employed. Both rare target (subjects responded with a button press) and rare non-target (no response required) as well as frequent stimuli were included. P300s were elicited by both types of rare stimuli.

This study found that dements did exhibit significantly prolonged P300 latencies when compared with normal subjects for both target and non-target rare stimuli in both auditory and visual modalities. However, schizophrenics also showed significantly prolonged P300s. Non-demented, cognitively impaired patients and depressives seemed to exhibit somewhat longer P300 latencies than normals, but did not show as great an effect as the demented patients. Latency variability was significantly greater in demented patients and also in schizophrenics.

Amplitude effects were also observed in this study. Demented patients showed significantly diminished P300 amplitude for almost all conditions. Schizophrenics and depressives who were not under medication appeared to show a similar but less pronounced effect. Both demented and schizophrenic patients also were slower than controls in RT.

This important study illustrates the difficulties in attempting to employ ERPs to distinguish clinically defined populations. Although significant relationships were found, the lack of specificity of the effects makes application of these results in differential diagnosis problematic at best.

Moreover, not all studies have found P300 latency differences in demented patients. In a study of 42 demented elderly patients, 29 non-demented elderly patients, and 10 healthy young controls, Slaets and Fortgens (1984) found no significant difference in P300 latency between demented and non-demented patients performing an auditory oddball counting task.

Of course, in considering this seemingly conflicting literature, it is necessary to note that all too often studies designed as putative replications of previous work differ in important details. The pattern of ERPs one obtains in any experimental paradigm is enormously sensitive to subjects' perception of the task and the range of strategies that are employed by the subjects. It is crucial, therefore, that investigators take pains to ensure that when they claim to replicate a study they have indeed done so in the formal sense of the word 'replicate'. Thus, for example, if an original study reports a pattern of results that was obtained when a sequence of stimuli was randomly selected, then any study that imposes constraints on the stimulus sequence is, by definition, not a replication. Failure to confirm the original results in such cases is not entirely surprising. It is in such a context that one must, for example, evaluate the implication of Pfefferbaum et al.'s (1984b) failure to replicate Goodin et al. (1978b).

We cannot resolve the dispute regarding P300 and dementia in this chapter. Clearly, more data are needed. To be useful, such data must be obtained consistently and reliably. Yet methodological purity, while necessary, is not sufficient to ensure the utility of the results. There remains a need for a theoretical framework within which it may be possible to make more sense of the data. Although Goodin et al. (1978a,b) proceeded from a theoretical interpretation of P300 latency, their procedure was largely nosological. Subjects were classified according to age and medical history, and differences between the groups were sought. The debate in the literature boils down to a dispute about the degree to which groups labeled clinically do indeed show a consistent pattern of ERPs. However, the importance of the issue depends on the degree to which one accepts that the groups compared are indeed comparable and the procedures used with the different groups commensurate. This approach assigns much weight to standard classification and diagnostic criteria, or

to chronological age. We are not persuaded that this is a good strategy. Indeed, in our own work with the aged, which we will now discuss in some detail, we found it impossible to organize the results in a meaningful way by relying on standard tests and commonly used diagnostic criteria. We were forced to rely on our theory of the functional significance of the P300, and it was this theoretical approach that allowed us to organize the data (Marshall et al., 1983; Farwell et al., 1985).

P300 and working memory in the elderly

The study reviewed in this section was undertaken in the context of an investigation designed originally to use P300 latency in an attempt to identify the locus of mental slowing in the aged. The intent was to determine the stages of processing at which P300 latency is particularly lengthened in the elderly. As the study depended on our ability to run elderly subjects in oddball paradigms, we began, merely as a feasibility study, by asking a group of elderly subjects to participate in several variations of the oddball paradigm. We chose the following four tasks:

(1) 'Count': the subject counted one of two easily discriminable, equally probable tones (1000 and 1500 Hz). At the end of each block of 100 trials, the subject reported the number of target stimuli. This task provided a pure assessment of the target effect of P300, uncontaminated by rareness factors or overt response demands.

(2) 'Choice-reaction time' (CRT): the second oddball task required a choice-reaction time response. Two tones (1000 Hz, 20% probability, and 1500 Hz, 80%) corresponded to two microswitches, one under each thumb. This task highlighted the probability effect, holding task relevance and motor demands constant.

(3) 'Omitted stimuli': in this task, one of the two classes of 'stimuli' was actually the non-occurrence of a tone. Thus, the tone was omitted on 10% of the trials. A 1000 Hz tone occurred on the remaining trials. The subject was asked to count the number of omitted stimuli. Such a paradigm

facilitates study of endogenous components (such as P300) without troublesome overlap from exogenous components.

(4) 'Names': male (20%) and female (80%) names appeared on a computer-controlled video display, and the subject was asked to count the number of male names. This provided an assessment of P300 in a second modality.

Fifty-three generally healthy individuals (38 females) living in the community, aged 60 through 82, were paid for participating in each of the four studies. In the main, the results indicated that these subjects yielded an orderly data set in which rare stimuli elicited a clear and 'normal-looking' P300, albeit with a somewhat longer latency than we have observed in young adults. Perusal of the data, however, revealed one striking phenomenon. In about one-sixth of these individuals the P300 appeared to be absent. The remarkable aspect of these data was that the P300 was absent or very small in all four tasks for this subset of subjects. This was especially surprising as, in general, it is very easy to observe a P300 in such experiments, as we found in hundreds of young adults we have run in similar studies. Occasionally, a subject will show no P300, or a very small P300, in some experimental condition. However, invariably these subjects will produce a perfectly normal P300 in another experimental paradigm. Yet, here we had individuals who seemed to perform the tasks normally and yet had little, if any, P300.

To test the reliability of these observations, we repeated the four oddball tests with half of the original sample ($n = 27$). Nine of these were among the subjects who displayed very low P300s (averaged across the four rare or target conditions), nine were those with the highest P300s, and nine were randomly chosen from the remaining subjects. In addition, we ran a sample of unselected young adults ($n = 19$, 18–30 years) through the same tasks. It turned out that the low-P300 elderly subjects whose ERPs were consistent in lacking a P300 across tasks were also quite consistent across time. Test-retest correlations for P300 amplitude to target stimuli for the four tasks were as follows:

'count', 0.51; CRT, 0.73; 'omitted stimuli', 0.44; 'name', 0.66.

Our comparison of 19 young adults with the full elderly sample yielded findings consistent with those recorded in other laboratories, reviewed earlier. There was a highly significant P300 latency difference between our aged (539 ms) and young (455 ms) groups, averaged across tasks and target/non-target. This is a slowing of 1.77 ms/year, close to values found by other investigators.

On the average, P300 amplitude was also found to be lower in the elderly. Across tasks and conditions, the aged group's P300 was only 63% as large as that of the young group. (Note that this finding was not consistent across subjects: the average of the elderly subjects' P300 amplitude includes those elderly individuals who exhibited little or no P300, as well as those with a more normal response.) Young subjects also showed a larger enhancement to target stimuli than did the elderly. P300s to target stimuli were 49% larger than P300s to non-target stimuli in the young subjects but only 37% larger in the elderly.

Reaction time data were obtained in the 20/80 auditory choice-RT oddball task. While the target/non-target P300 latency effect in the elderly group was 20 ms (463 vs. 443), the RT effect was more than twice as large (434 vs. 385). Under the additive factors model, the extra delay in RT indicates that the RT effect reflects not only a delay in stimulus categorization (the P300 effect) but an additional delay in response selection and execution (by 'response selection and execution' we refer specifically to motor processes).

Thus, our preliminary data appeared to display a latency pattern that was consistent with the literature. Yet we had a subset of subjects with especially small, and in some cases entirely absent, P300. It was obviously necessary, if these data were to be interpretable as more than an empirical curiosity, that we determine what, if anything, functionally distinguished the low-P300 subjects from the rest of the sample. The standard operating procedure when one is confronted with individuals who consistently deviate from some norm is to assess what other variables may distinguish this group from the others. We tried a variety of metrics in the attempt to differentiate the two groups. Medical records were examined, data on educational background were collected, and numerous psychometric, sensory, and other tests were administered to the subjects. The exercise proved futile. None of these conventional approaches could serve to characterize the subjects who had no P300. It seemed that the only way in which these subjects differed from the norm is in the size of their P300s.

As we despaired of making sense of the data using the standard empirical approach, there remained one other possibility. We had tried a wide range of clinical tests, for none of which was there an a priori basis to believe that it would predict a reduction in P300 amplitude. This state of affairs was a reflection of the fact that we had no theoretical framework from which to derive predictions regarding the effect that the given values of any of these measures of individual attributes will have on the amplitude of the P300. An alternate approach would begin from a theory of the P300 and ask what subject attributes should correlate with its presence. In other words, if the P300 is a manifestation of a subroutine with some specific information processing mission, then one should be able to predict what functional difference should appear in subjects in whom this subroutine appears to be abnormally quiescent. In the next section we review briefly the evidence supporting a hypothesis concerning the functional significance of the P300. This theoretical structure led to an experiment yielding data that do indeed indicate a difference in the information processing system of the subjects with and those without the P300.

The functional significance of P300

Our attempt to identify the manner in which the low-P300 subjects differed from the subjects who displayed a normal P300 was guided by the proposition that the P300 is a manifestation of the processes associated with the updating of a cognitive schema or model (Donchin, 1981). This model of the P300 had developed within the context of a more general theory, proposed by several authors, ranging from Sokolov (1969) to Baddeley (1974, 1981), which assumes that some aspects of the information in memory are more readily available to processing than others. The more readily available segment is shaped by the tasks performed by the organism and can be viewed as a model of the current environment, or as a scratch pad in which currently important information is kept. This 'neuronal model' of the current context and its associated representations, to use Sokolov's term, appears equivalent, at least in part, to the concept of 'working memory'. In adopting this concept in the interpretation of the P300, we need concentrate on only one aspect of this 'working memory', namely that the system must continually update and revise this model. If 'working memory', or the 'neuronal model', is to be useful in the performance of the current task under current circumstances, then, even as tasks and circumstances change, so must the model change. Thus, it is plausible to assume that, if such a 'working memory' exists, there must be a set of processes that maintain it. In other words, regardless of our view of the organization and processes that characterize 'working memory', we have to assume that its representations are continually revised. A context-updating process must be included in any system that is context-sensitive. We suggest that it is this updating process which is manifested by the P300.

We are assuming here that the system maintains an activated representation of its schema and that this representation is utilized whenever action is required. Mismatches between actual inputs and schema-based expectations generally drive the organism to action which is, in some sense, reflected by the complex of activities referred to as the 'orienting response'. Thus, for example, whenever a mismatch is detected between the schema and an input, it is necessary that this very fact be registered in the schema. Repeated mismatches between expectations and events must be capable of forcing a revision of the schema. Otherwise, the schema will soon fail to be a realistic representation of the environment. That such updating and revision do occur is evidenced by the process of 'habituation'.

Several studies showing that variables which affect P300 amplitude also influence the strength of a representation in 'working memory' support this view. The effect of stimulus probability on the P300 has been modeled by K. Squires et al. (1976) as a result of the summation of decaying traces of past occurrences of each stimulus. This model implies that the amplitude of the P300 elicited by a task-relevant event depends on the interval between repetitions of that event. Presumably, the time period between repetitions of task-relevant events influences the strength of the representation available in 'short-term memory' (STM). If the representation is weak, more updating must be done following target presentation. From these studies, then, it may be inferred that P300 amplitude is related to the amount of updating which is required by a task-relevant event.

Also consistent with this hypothesis are the results of a study by Heffley et al. (1978). In this study, target and non-target stimuli were presented while subjects monitored a continuously moving display. Target probability and the interval between stimuli ('inter-stimulus interval', ISI) were manipulated. At the longer ISIs (6 s), target probability had no effect on P300 amplitude. All stimuli elicited large P300s. It is only when the ISI was shortened to approximately 2000 ms that low-probability stimuli elicited larger P300s than high-probability stimuli. This is consistent with the STM updating hypothesis of P300. With long ISIs, all targets regardless of probability will need updating of their representation because of the longer interval between repetitions. At the short ISIs, only rare targets need updating upon presentation. Frequent targets are most likely to occur while the previous occurrence is still held in STM.

Karis et al. (1984) report a study that demonstrates rather clearly the effects that the elicitation of a P300 has on the representations created by the eliciting stimuli. They employed the von Restorff paradigm. The subject was instructed to recall a series of words, and a deviant item (an 'isolate') was embedded in the series. Von Restorff (1933), the Gestalt psychologist who created this paradigm, demonstrated that the isolates were better recalled by subjects than were comparable non-deviant items. This enhanced recall of the isolates is the von Restorff or isolation effect.

As the isolates are both rare and task-relevant, they are apt to elicit a P300. The context-updating model of the P300 predicts that the larger the P300 elicited by an isolate the better it will be recalled. To test this hypothesis, Karis et al. (1984) examined the relationship between the amplitude of the P300 elicited by an isolate and whether or not it was subsequently recalled. Subjects were presented with word lists in which isolates were presented with a larger or smaller font than the other words, ERPs were recorded for each word, and after each list of 15 words subjects were asked to recall as many words as possible. The main experimental hypothesis was that isolated words recalled in the subsequent test should elicit larger P300s when initially presented than isolated words not recalled later.

Striking individual differences were found in the degree to which subjects showed the von Restorff effect. These differences were surprising, because this effect has always been described as very robust. Some subjects reported using a rote memorization strategy and showed a large von Restorff effect (i.e., recalled proportionately more isolates), though their overall recall was quite poor. For these subjects, isolates that were recalled did elicit larger P300s on their original presentation than non-recalled isolates. Other subjects, however, showed a very different pattern. They were good memorizers and used elaborate memorization strategies. These subjects showed no von Restorff effect; that is, they recalled the non-isolates as well as they recalled the isolates. In these subjects P300 amplitude was unrelated to recall.

These data are consistent with the suggestion that P300 amplitude is a manifestation of an updating process in 'working memory'. The data confirm that representation of a word in 'working memory' is affected, in some manner, when a P300 is elicited. The change in the representation aids recall in rote memorizers. All subjects produced equally large P300s, and we believe the same updating process occurred in all our subjects. If no further processing occurs, as in our group of rote memorizers, then P300 amplitude will be related to recall. However, if cognitive activity continues after the initial processing reflected by P300, then this additional activity may obscure the relationship between P300 and recall. When, for example, subjects link words together as part of an elaborate memorization strategy, the recall of any individual word becomes less dependent on its initial encoding and more dependent on its relationships to other words.

We will not review here subsequent work in the Cognitive Psychophysiology Laboratory in which the validity of this finding was confirmed (see Fabiani et al., 1985, 1986; Klein et al., 1984). Suffice it to say that we conclude from the work reviewed here and from other work that the amplitude of the P300 is proportional to the degree of activation of a process invoked when 'working memory' is updated and organized. We proceed now to illustrate how this conceptual interpretation of the P300 can be used in illuminating the difference, discussed above, between elderly subjects in whom the P300 is abnormally small and other subjects.

The low-P300 subjects and recall

The striking finding that a group of elderly subjects consistently lacked a P300 led us to a further investigation of the relationship between P300 and memory in the aged. We noted that the low-P300 subjects performed the oddball task as well as the other subjects. Comparing the low-P300 group with the high-P300 group revealed no differences in reaction time. The low-P300 subjects were 12 ms faster in mean RT than the high-P300 subjects for the rare stimuli (452 vs. 464 ms) and 38 ms slower

on the frequent stimuli (412 vs. 374 ms); neither difference is statistically significant. Nor were the groups different in P300 latency or response accuracy.

If P300 is, as we believe, a manifestation of an intracranial process that is associated with the specific information processing task of updating representations in 'working memory', then it is possible that subjects who lack a P300 will show a deficit in performing tasks that depend on the viability of those short-term representations. For this reason, we designed a task that was intended to determine the subject's ability to maintain the status of 'working memory'. Two years after the initial oddball testing, we presented this new task to the subjects who had been originally recalled for the reliability retest. (Not all subjects were available for further testing by this time; nine high-P300 subjects and seven low-P300 subjects were fully tested.)

The memory test was patterned after the Hebb-Corsi test used by Milner (1978) and her colleagues in evaluating the effects of severe temporal lobe damage on memory. We designed a somewhat simpler task than the original Hebb-Corsi test, one in which it would be possible to record ERPs to each stimulus. On each trial, the subject was presented with a digit followed by a second digit 1000 ms later. The subject was instructed to indicate by a button press whether or not the pair had appeared previously in that trial block. In each of four blocks of 60 trials, one specific pair was repeated approximately every three trials. All other pairs were different. Reaction time and error rate served as dependent variables.

In accord with our theory, we found significant differences in performance between the high- and low-P300 subjects. Both groups were able to accomplish the task with high accuracy (88% for the 'lows', and 93% for the 'highs'; not significantly different). The low-P300 subjects, however, were significantly slower in RT to the non-repeating digit pairs; that is, they were slow to report that a pair had not been seen before. Mean RTs to non-repeating pairs for the high-P300 and low-P300 groups respectively were 850 and 1009 ms. Spearman rank-order correlation between RT to non-repeating digit pairs and P300 amplitude in the original oddball study, for the high and low groups combined, was -0.49 ($p < 0.05$). The non-parametric Jonckheere test yields a significance level of $p < 0.025$ for these data.

The low-P300 subjects were somewhat slower (658 ms) than the high-P300 subjects (591 ms) on the repeating pairs (the one pair in each block that was repeated about every third trial). This difference between groups was not significant. A possible explanation for this differential deficit is that, for the low-P300 group, recall was impaired, whereas recognition was spared.

In order to test the reliability of these results, a new sample ($n = 32$) of elderly subjects was recruited and tested on the auditory choice-reaction time and visual names oddball tasks and in the memory paradigm. The essential findings of the first study were replicated.

Of the 32 new subjects, five had little or no P300, and eight were classified as high-P300 subjects. (Classification was by visual inspection of waveforms for the oddball tasks, blind to task performance results.) Once again, the low-P300 subjects did not differ from the high-P300 subjects on RT or accuracy in the oddball or memory tasks. (In auditory oddball CRT, low-P300 subjects were trivially faster than high-P300 subjects for the frequent stimuli — 432 vs. 435 ms — and slightly slower for the rare stimuli — 508 vs. 475 ms; neither difference is statistically significant.)

Like the initial group, the new low-P300 subjects were about 160 ms slower than the high-P300 subjects in RT to the non-repeating digit pairs in the memory task. (With the smaller sample size in the replication study, this difference fell short of statistical significance when analyzed using statistics that collapse all RTs for each subject to a single point — mean or median. An analysis of these data utilizing more powerful statistics is in progress.) The low-P300 subjects also appeared to be somewhat slower on the repeating pairs in some blocks. (This second group of subjects had pre-

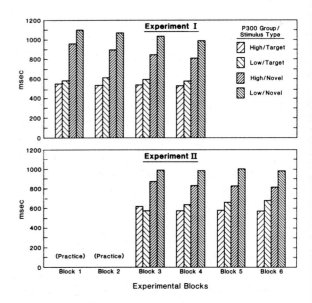

Fig. 2. Median reaction times for nine high-P300 and seven low-P300 elderly subjects to 'target' (repeating) and 'non-target' (non-repeating) digit pairs. (Blocks 1 and 2 in Experiment II were practice blocks; RTs not recorded.)

viously been presented with two practice blocks of the memory task in a screening study.) Again, as in the original study, the slowness of the low-P300 subjects was much more marked on the novel pairs than on the pairs they had already seen in that trial block (the repeating or target pairs). Fig. 2 presents the median reaction times, following the onset of the second digit in a pair, for the high-P300 and low-P300 subjects, for each block of each of the two experiments.

Summary and conclusions

In summary, we found that elderly subjects who lack a P300, but are otherwise normal, are slower in indicating that an item is novel; we interpret this as indicating that they are slower either in searching 'working memory' or in reporting the results of such a search, when the search is unaided by cues provided by the externally presented stimuli. The specificity of this finding is underscored by the fact that the high- and low-P300 subjects were equally fast in the choice-RT oddball task, which does not require the short-term maintenance of a memory set. Thus, an exceptionally low characteristic P300 reflects a deficit specific to recall from 'working memory', rather than a generalized deficit so often seen in special populations. These data support the interpretation of P300 as a manifestation of the updating of 'working memory' and suggest that it is useful to examine the deterioration of memory performance in the elderly and the demented in terms of specific properties such as the maintenance of 'working memory'.

In the previous section we saw an example of the power of theory-driven research. Beginning with a hypothesis about the functional significance of the P300 as a manifestation of a process invoked in the updating of 'working memory' made possible the design and implementation of a systematic series of experiments. This resulted in the discovery of a specific cognitive deficit that was predicted on the basis of a specific ERP deficit in a particular population. It is our view that such a theory-driven approach will prove to be a fruitful way to apply the knowledge and methods of psychophysiology in the clinical realm. Formulation and testing of hypotheses about information processing functions, their implementation by neural tissue, and the manifestations of this neural activity in psychophysiological measures such as ERPs may provide a key to unraveling the specific deficits in brain functioning which underlie dementia and other mental disorders.

Acknowledgements

The research reported here was supported principally by NIA grant 1R01 AG03151–03, and also by AFOSR Contract No. F49620-79-C-0233, Al Fregly, Project Manager. Theodore R. Bashore, Noel K. Marshall, Ron D. Chambers, Frank Morrell, Leyla DeToledo-Morrell, and Thomas Hoeppner were collaborators during various phases of the project. Kay Strayer's assistance in the execution of the project is greatly appreciated. The authors also wish to acknowledge the subjects who made this work possible.

References

Baddeley, A. D. (1981) The concept of working memory: a view of its current state and probable future development. *Cognition*, 10: 17–23.

Baddeley, A. D. and Hitch, G. J. (1974) Working memory. In G. A. Bower (Ed.), *The Psychology of Learning and Motivation: Vol. 8*, Academic Press, New York.

Baribeau-Braun, J., Picton, T. W. and Gosselin, J.-Y. (1983) Schizophrenia: a neurophysiological evaluation of abnormal information processing. *Science*, 219: 874–876.

Beck, E. C., Swanson, C. and Dustman, R. E. (1980) Long latency components of the visually evoked potential in man: effects of aging. *Exp. Aging Res.*, 6: 523–542.

Braune, R., Wickens, C. D., Strayer, D. and Stokes, A. (1985) Age-dependent changes in information processing abilities between 20 and 60 years. In R. W. Swezey (Ed.), *Proceedings of the Human Factors Society's 29th Annual Meeting.* Baltimore, MD, pp. 226–230.

Brown, W. S., Marsh, J. T. and LaRue, A. (1982) Event-related potentials in psychiatry: differentiating depression and dementia in the elderly. *Bull. Los Angeles Neurol. Soc.*, 47: 91–107.

Brown, W. S., Marsh, J. T. and LaRue, A. (1983) Exponential electrophysiological aging: P3 latency. *Electroencephalogr. Clin. Neurophysiol.*, 55: 277–285.

Callaway, E., Tueting, P. and Koslow, S. H. (Eds.) (1978) *Event-related Brain Potentials in Man.* Academic Press, New York.

Coles, M. G. H., Gratton, G., Bashore, T. R., Eriksen, C. W. and Donchin, E. (1985) A psychophysiological investigation of the continuous flow model of human information processing. *J. Exp. Psychol. Hum. Percept. Perform.*, 11: 529–553.

Coles, M. G. H., Gratton, G., Kramer, A., Miller, G. A. and Porges, S. W. (1986) Principles of signal acquisition and analysis. In M. G. H. Coles, E. Donchin and S. W. Porges (Eds.), *Psychophysiology: Systems, Processes and Applications — A Handbook*, Guilford Press, New York, pp. 183–221.

Donchin, E. (1975) On evoked potentials, cognition and memory. *Science*, 190: 1004–1005.

Donchin, E. (1978) The use of the scalp distribution as a dependent variable in event-related potential studies: excerpts of preconference correspondence. In D. Otto (Ed.), *Multidisciplinary Perspectives in Event-related Brain Potential Research*, (EPA-600/9-77-043), U.S. Government Printing Office, Washington, D.C., pp. 501–510.

Donchin, E. (1979) Event-related brain potentials: A tool in the study of human information processing. In H. Begleiter (Ed.), *Evoked Brain Potentials and Behavior*, Plenum, New York, pp. 13–75.

Donchin, E. (1981) Surprise!...Surprise?, *Psychophysiology*, 18: 493–513.

Donchin, E. (1986) Hypothetical constructs, intervening variables, and ERP components. In *Proceedings of the IIIrd Annual Carmel Conference*, in press.

Donchin, E. and McCarthy, G. (1980) Event-related brain potentials in the study of cognitive processes. In C. Ludlow and M. E. Doran-Quine (Eds.), *Proceedings of Symposium on Neurological Bases of Language Disorders in Children: Methods and Direction for Research*, NINCDS Monograph No.22, U.S. Government Printing Office, Washington, D.C., pp. 109–128.

Donchin, E., Kubovy, M., Kutas, M., Johnson, R., Jr. and Herning, R. I. (1973) Graded changes in evoked response (P300) amplitude as a function of cognitive activity. *Percept. Psychophys.*, 14: 319–324.

Donchin, E., Ritter, W. and McCallum, C. (1978) Cognitive psychophysiology: the endogenous components of the ERP. In E. Callaway, P. Tueting and S. H. Coslow (Eds.), *Event-related Brain Potentials in Man*, Academic Press, New York, pp. 349–411.

Duncan-Johnson, C. and Donchin, E. (1981) The relation of P300 latency to reaction time as function of expectancy. In H. H. Kornhuber and L. Deecke (Eds.), *Motivation, Motor and Sensory Processes of the Brain: Electrical Potentials, Behavior and Clinical Use. Progress in Brain Research, Vol. 54*, Elsevier, Amsterdam, pp. 717–722.

Duncan-Johnson, C. C. and Donchin, E. (1982) The P300 component of the event-related brain potential as an index of information processing. *Biol. Psychol.*, 14: 1–52.

Fabiani, M., Karis, D. and Donchin, E. (1985) Effects of strategy manipulation on P300 amplitude in a von Restorff paradigm. *Psychophysiology*, 21: 588–589.

Fabiani, M., Karis, D. and Donchin, E., (1986) P300 and recall in an incidental memory paradigm. *Psychophysiology*, 23: 298–308.

Farwell, L. A., Chambers, R. D., Miller, G. A., Coles, M. G. H. and Donchin, E. (1985) A specific memory deficit in elderly subjects who lack a P300. *Psychophysiology*, 22: 589.

Ford, J. M., Roth, W. T., Mohs, R. Hopkins, W. and Kopell, B. S. (1979) Event-related potentials recorded from young and old adults during a memory retrieval task. *Electroencephalogr. Clin. Neurophysiol*, 47: 450–459.

Ford, J. M., Duncan-Johnson, C. C., Pfefferbaum, A. and Kopell, B. S. (1982a) Expectancy for events in old age: stimulus sequence effects on P300 and reaction time. *J. Gerontol.*, 37: 696–704.

Ford, J. M., Pfefferbaum, A., Tinklenberg, J. R. and Kopell, B. S. (1982b) Effects of perceptual and cognitive difficulty on P3 and RT in young and old adults. *Electroencephalogr. Clin. Neurophysiol.*, 54: 311–321.

Galambos, R. and Hillyard, S. A. (1981) Electrophysiological approaches to human cognitive processing. *Neurosci. Res. Prog. Bull.*, 20: 145–265.

Goodin, D., Squires, K., Henderson, B. and Starr, A. (1978a) Age-related variations in evoked potentials to auditory stimuli in normal human subjects. *Electroencephalogr. Clin. Neurophysiol.*, 44: 447–458.

Goodin, D. S., Squires, K. C. and Starr, A. (1978b) Long latency event-related components of the auditory evoked potential in dementia. *Brain*, 101: 635–648.

Gopher, D. and Donchin, E. (1986) Workload — an examination of the concept. In K. Boff and L. Kaufman (Eds.), *Handbook of Perception and Human Performance, Vol. 2*, Wiley and Sons, New York, in press.

Gratton, G., Coles, M. G. H. and Donchin, E. (1983) Filtering for spatial distribution: a new approach (Vector filter). *Psychophysiology*, 20: 443–444.

Gratton, G., Coles, M. G. H. and Donchin, E. (1986) A multivariate approach to the analysis of scalp distribution of event related potentials: vector analysis, manuscript submitted for publication.

Halliday, A. M., McDonald, W. I. and Mushin, J. (1973) Visual evoked response in diagnosis of multiple sclerosis. *Br. Med. J.*, 4: 661–664.

Halliday, A. M. (1978) Clinical applications of evoked potentials. In W. B. Matthews and G. H. Glaser (Eds.), *Recent Advances in Clinical Neurology*, Churchill Livingstone, Edinburgh, pp. 47–73.

Heffley, E., Wickens, C. D. and Donchin, E. (1978) Intramodality selective attention and P300: a reexamination in a visual monitoring task. *Psychophysiology*, 15: 269–270.

Hillyard, S. A. and Kutas, M. (1983) Electrophysiology of cognitive processing. In M. R. Rosenzweig and L. W. Porter (Eds.), *Annual Review of Psychology, Vol. 34:* 33–61.

Isreal, J. B., Wickens, C. D., Chesney, G. L. and Donchin, E. (1980) The event-related brain potential as an index of display-monitoring workload. *Hum. Fact.*, 22: 211–224.

Karis, D., Fabiani, M. and Donchin, E. (1984) 'P300' and memory: individual differences in the von Restorff effect. *Cogn. Psychol.*, 16: 177–216.

Klein, M., Coles, M. G. H. and Donchin, E. (1984) People with absolute pitch process tones without producing a P300. *Science*, 223: 1306–1309.

Kramer, A., Wickens, C. D. and Donchin, E. (1983) An analysis of the processing demands of a complex perceptual-motor task. *Hum. Fact.*, 25: 597–622.

Kutas, M., McCarthy, G. and Donchin, E. (1977) Augmenting mental chronometry: The P300 as a measure of stimulus evaluation time. *Science*, 197: 792–795.

Magliero, A., Bashore, T. R., Coles, M. G. H. and Donchin, E. (1984) On the dependence of P300 latency on stimulus evaluation processes. *Psychophysiology*, 21: 171–186.

Marshall, N. K., Bashore, T. R., Miller, G. A., Coles, M. G. H.

and Donchin, E. (1983) ERP consistency in young adult and elderly subjects. *Psychophysiology*, 20: 422.

McCarthy, G. (1984) Stimulus evaluation time and P300 latency. In E. Donchin (Ed.), *Cognitive Psychophysiology: ERPs and the Study of Cognition, The Carmel Conferences, Vol. I*, Lawrence Erlbaum, Hillsdale, NJ, pp. 254–301.

McCarthy, G. and Donchin, E. (1979) Event-related potentials — manifestations of cognitive activity. In F. Hoffmeister and C. Muller (Eds.), *Bayer-Symposium VII, Brain Function in Old Age*, Springer-Verlag, New York, pp. 318–335.

McCarthy, G. and Donchin, E. (1981) A metric for thought: a comparison of P300 latency and reaction time. *Science*, 211: 77–80.

Michalewski, H. J., Patterson, J. V., Bowman, T. E., Litzleman, D. K. and Thompson, L. W. (1982) A comparison of the emitted late positive potential in older and young adults. *J. Gerontol.*, 37: 52–58.

Milner, B. (1978) Clues to the cerebral organization of memory. In P. A. Buser and A. Rougeul-Buser (Eds.), *Cerebral Correlates of Conscious Experiences*: Elsevier/North Holland, Amsterdam, pp. 139–153.

Mullis, R. J., Holcomb, P. J., Diner, B. C. and Dykman, R. A. (1985) The effects of aging on the P3 component of the visual event-related potential. *Electroencephalogr. Clin. Neurophysiol.*, 62: 141–149.

Neville, H. J., Snyder, E., Knight, R. and Galambos, R. (1979) Event related potentials in language and non-language tasks in patients with alexia without agraphia. In D. Lehmann and E. Callaway (Eds.), *Human Evoked Potentials*, Plenum, New York, pp. 269–283.

Pfefferbaum, A., Ford, J., Roth, W. T. and Kopell, B. S. (1980a) Age differences in P3-reaction time associations. *Electroencephalogr. Clin. Neurophysiol.*, 49: 257–265.

Pfefferbaum, A., Ford, J., Roth, W. T. and Kopell, B. S. (1980b) Age-related changes in auditory event-related potentials. *Electroencephalogr. Clin. Neurophysiol.*, 49: 266–276.

Pfefferbaum, A., Ford, J. M., Wenegrat, B., Roth, W. and Kopell, B. (1984a) Clinical application of the P3 component of event-related potentials. I. Normal aging. *Electroencephalogr. Clin. Neurophysiol.*, 59: 85–103.

Pfefferbaum, A., Ford, J. M., Wenegrat, B., Roth, W. and Kopell, B. (1984b) Clinical application of the P3 component of event-related potentials. II. Dementia, depression, and schizophrenia. *Electroencephalogr. Clin. Neurophysiol.*, 59: 104–124.

Picton, T. W., Stuss, D. T., Champagne, S. C. and Nelson, R.F. (1984) The effects of age on human event-related potentials. *Psychophysiology*, 21: 312–325.

Podlesny, J. A. and Dustman, R. E. (1982) Age effects on heart rate, sustained potential, and P3 responses during reaction-time tasks. *Neurobiol. Aging*, 3: 1–9.

Podlesny, J. A., Dustman, R. E. and Shearer, D. E. (1984) Aging and respond-withhold tasks: effects on sustained

potentials, P3 responses and late activity. *Electroencephalogr. Clin. Neurophysiol.*, 58: 130–139.

Polich, J., Ehlers, C. L., Otis, S., Mandell, A. and Bloom, F.E. (1986) P300 latency reflects the degree of cognitive decline in dementing illness. *Electroencephalogr. Clin. Neurophysiol.*, 63: 138–144.

Porjesz, B. and Begleiter, H. (1982) Evoked brain potential deficits in alcoholism and aging. *Alcoholism Clin. Exp. Res.*, 6: 53–63.

Pritchard, W. S. (1981) Psychophysiology of P300. *Psychol. Bull.*, 89: 506–540.

Ragot, R. and Renault, B. (1981) P300 as a function of S-R compatibility and motor programming. *Biol. Psychol.*, 13: 289–294.

Regan, D. (1972) *Evoked Potentials in Psychology, Sensory Physiology and Clinical Medicine*, Chapman and Hall, London.

Ritter, W. and Vaughan, H. G., Jr. (1969) Averaged evoked responses in vigilance and discrimination: a reassessment. *Science*, 164: 326–328.

Roth, W. T., Horvath, T. B., Pfefferbaum, A., Tinklenberg, J. R., Mezzich, J. E. and Kopell, B. S. (1979) Late event-related potentials and schizophrenia. In H. Begleiter (Ed.), *Evoked Brain Potentials and Behavior, Vol. 2, Downstate Series of Research in Psychiatry and Psychology*, Plenum, New York, pp. 499–515.

Roth, W. T., Pfefferbaum, A., Kelly, A. F., Berger, P. A. and Kopell, B. S. (1981) Auditory event-related potentials in schizophrenia and depression. *Psychiat. Res.*, 4: 199–212.

Sirevaag, E., Kramer, A., Coles, M. G. H. and Donchin, E. (1984) P300 amplitude and resource allocation. *Psychophysiology*, 21: 598–599, abstract; extended paper in preparation.

Slaets, J. P. J. and Fortgens, C. (1984) On the value of P300 event-related potentials in the differential diagnosis of dementia. *Br. J. Psychiat.*, 145: 652–656.

Smith, D. B. D., Michalewski, H. J., Brent, G. A. and Thompson, L. W. (1980) Auditory averaged evoked potentials and aging: factors of stimulus, task and topography. *Biol. Psychol.*, 11: 135–151.

Snyder, E. and Hillyard, S. A. (1979) Changes in event-related potentials in older persons. In F. Hoffmeister (Ed.), *Bayer-Symposium VII: Brain Function in Old Age*, Springer-Verlag, Berlin, pp. 112–125.

Sokolov, E. N. (1969) The modeling properties of the nervous system. In M. Cole and I. Maltzman (Eds.), *Handbook of Contemporary Soviet Psychology*, Basic Books, New York, pp. 671–704.

Squires, K., Goodin, D. and Starr, A. (1979) Event related potentials in development, aging and dementia. In D. Lehmann and E. Callaway (Eds.), *Human Evoked Potentials*, Plenum, New York, pp. 383–396.

Squires, K. C., Wickens, C. D., Squires, N. K. and Donchin, E. (1976) The effect of stimulus sequence on the waveform of the cortical event-related potential. *Science*, 193: 1142–1146.

Squires, K. C., Chippendale, T. J., Wrege, K. W., Goodin, D. W. and Starr, A. (1980) Electrophysiological assessment of mental function in aging and dementia. In L. Poon (Ed.), *Aging in the 1980s*, American Psychological Association, Washington, D.C., pp. 125–134.

Squires, N., Galbraith, G. and Aine, C. (1979) Event-related potential assessment of sensory and cognitive deficits in the mentally retarded. In D. Lehmann and E. Callaway (Eds.), *Human Evoked Potentials*, Plenum, New York, pp. 397–413.

Strayer, D., Wickens, C. D. and Braune, R. (1985) Mental chronometry and aging: an additive factors/psychophysiological approach. *Psychophysiology*, 22: 615–616.

Syndulko, K., Hansch, E. C., Cohen, S. N., Pearce, J. W.,

Goldberg, Z., Montana, B., Tourtelotte, W. W. and Potvin, A. R. (1982) Long-latency event-related potentials in normal aging and dementia. In J. Courjon, F. Mauguière and M. Revol (Eds.), *Clinical Applications of Evoked Potentials in Neurology*, Raven, New York, pp. 279–285.

Von Restorff, H. (1933) Uber die Wirkung von Bereichsbildungen im Spurenfeld. *Psychol. Forsch.*, 18: 299–342.

Wickens, C. D., Braune, R., Stokes, A. and Strayer, D. (1985) Individual differences and age-related changes: refinement and elaboration of an information processing performance battery with aviation relevant task structures. Final Report. *University of Illinois Engineering Psychology Research Laboratory Technical Report EPL-85-1/NAMRL-85-1*, February.

Discussion

D. F. SWAAB: Is the P300 after all a diagnostic tool for early diagnosis of Alzheimer's disease?

ANSWER: As I reviewed in the written version of my presentation, there is controversy regarding the utility of the P300 as a diagnostic tool even for the later phases of the disease. The literature is based on the proposal by Goodin et al. (1978b) that P300 latency can be used to differentiate the depressed from the demented patients. Even those who accept these data will not claim that the P300 can be used for early detection of Alzheimer. Of course, this depends a bit on what one calls "early" in this context. Let me note, however, that as far as I can tell Goodin's data were obtained in a very competent manner and were analyzed properly. Most of the studies (Pfefferbaum et al., 1984a,b) that have failed to replicate the results were sufficiently different in detail not to constitute proper replications. However, note that these remarks are made from the perspective of a cognitive psychophysiologist. I am not competent to judge the clinical validity of the diagnoses that Goodin et al. have used in constructing their various groups. My own view is that there is persuasive evidence to suggest that P300 can be developed into a useful tool in differential diagnosis but that much more orderly work is needed. As for early detection of Alzheimer, my belief is that the ERPs are a tool worth considering, but that no adequate work has been done to date, for reasons I enumerate in my paper. It would be folly not to examine this promising tool. It is quite evident that there is at present almost no useful tool for early detection of Alzheimer. Indeed, until pathologists get the brain there is no definite diagnosis of Alzheimer. As the ERPs do provide an in vivo window on neural activity and as they are very sensitive to cognitive function, they are a candidate source for diagnostic tools. However, as I note in the paper, such tools are unlikely to be developed within the standard "nosological" paradigm of clinical research.

J. M. RABEY: You described two groups of individuals which display a markedly reduced P300. In the people with perfect pitch the absence of the P300 is associated with improved recognition of tones. (Klein et al., 1984) In the elderly who lack a P300 you report a deficient ability to recognize stimuli. How do you reconcile this contradiction?

ANSWER: Actually, the two observations are consistent with our theoretical interpretation of the functional significance of the P300. In both cases we are witnessing a reduced utilization of a process which is associated with the maintenance, and updating of working memory. The subjects with perfect pitch do not engage in this updating activity because they apparently maintain a permanent tonal template and their auditory comparisons do not utilize working memory. The elderly who have a small P300 have a poorer ability to update and organize working memory. In their case the consequence is a recall deficit. Note that there was one critical difference between the two groups. The students who lacked a P300 in response to an acoustic stimulus, displayed a substantial P300 when instructed to make visual discriminations. Thus, they have the tool manifested by the P300; they just don't use it for auditory comparisons. The elderly who did not display a P300 appeared not to have the tool at their disposal as their P300 were consistently small in a variety of paradigms using different modalities and tasks.

References

Goodin, D. S., Squires, K. C. and Starr, A. (1978b) Long latency event-related components of the auditory evoked potential in dementia. *Brain*, 101: 635–648.

Klein, M., Coles, M. G. H. and Donchin, E. (1984) People with absolute pitch process tones without producing a P300 *Science*, 223: 1306–1309.

Pfefferbaum, A., Ford, J. M., Wenegrat, B., Roth, W. and Kopell, B. (1984a) Clinical application of the P3 component of event-related potentials. I. Normal aging. *Electroencephalogr. Clin. Neurophysiol.*, 59: 85–103.

Pfefferbaum, A., Ford, J. M., Wenegrat, B., Roth, W. and Kopell, B. (1984b) Clinical application of the P3 component of event-related potential. II. Dementia, depression, and schizophrenia. *Electroencephalogr. Clin. Neurophysiol.*, 59: 104–124.

SECTION II

Alterations in the brain

D. F. Swaab, E. Fliers, M. Mirmiran, W. A. Van Gool and F. Van Haaren (Eds.)
Progress in Brain Research, Vol. 70.
© 1986 Elsevier Science Publishers B.V. (Biomedical Division)

CHAPTER 7

The current status of the cortical cholinergic system in Alzheimer's disease and Parkinson's disease

J. M. Candy[a], E. K. Perry[b], R. H. Perry[b], J. A. Court[a], A. E. Oakley[a] and J. A. Edwardson[a]

[a]*MRC Neuroendocrinology Unit and* [b]*Department of Pathology, Newcastle General Hospital, Westgate Road, Newcastle upon Tyne NE4 6BE, UK*

Introduction

The seminal observations of the deleterious effects of cholinergic antagonists on memory in man (Drachman and Leavitt, 1974), and a deficit in the cortical cholinergic system in Alzheimer's disease (Davies and Maloney, 1976; Perry et al., 1977a,b; White et al., 1977), where loss of memory is one of the early cardinal features of the disease, led to the formulation of a cholinergic hypothesis of memory.

Furthermore, the existence of a correlation between the loss of choline acetyltransferase (ChAT) activity and the severity of the dementia in Alzheimer's disease (Perry et al., 1978), suggested the existence of an important functional relationship between reduced activity of the cholinergic system and cognitive impairment. This relationship has recently been reinforced by the finding of a marked decrease in cortical ChAT activity in cognitively impaired Parkinsonian patients (Perry et al., 1983; Perry et al., 1985), which correlated with the severity of the dementia (Perry et al., 1985). Attention has also recently been focussed on neuropathological changes in the nucleus of Meynert, in the basal forebrain, in Alzheimer's disease and Parkinson's disease, as this nucleus appears to be the source of the cortical cholinergic afferents. In the last few years, major advances have been made in understanding the neuroanatomical relationships between the nucleus of Meynert and its cortical cholinergic projections, in animals and also

in the neurochemical, pharmacological and electrophysiological characteristics of cortical cholinergic receptors. The changes that occur in this system in Alzheimer's and Parkinson's diseases will therefore be considered in the light of these recent advances and their therapeutic implications discussed.

Cognitive and cortical neuropathological features of Alzheimer's and Parkinson's diseases

The cognitive changes in both Alzheimer's disease and Parkinson's disease are characterised by symptoms of dementia. While in both the presenile (onset before 65 years) and senile forms of Alzheimer's disease progressive dementia is invariably present, in Parkinson's disease the presence and degree of the dementia is variable. Alzheimer's disease presents clinically with a progressive loss of memory and a deterioration in other specific cognitive functions (see McKhann et al., 1984). Initially memory loss and spatial disorientation are evident, followed at a later stage by symptoms of parietal lobe dysfunction (aphasia, apraxia and agnosia) and finally gross dementia. In contrast only 20–40% of Parkinsonian patients present clinically with a rather generalised cognitive decline which is reflected in impairments of verbal and non-verbal memory, localisation of objects in space, complex visual discrimination and abstract reasoning (Pirozzolo et al., 1982; Mortimer et al., 1985).

The accepted neuropathological criteria for

Alzheimer's disease, in both presenile and senile cases, are the presence of senile plaques and neurofibrillary tangles in the cerebral cortex (Tomlinson et al., 1970). Both features should be present as senile plaques frequently occur, albeit at a low density, in the cerebral cortex of mentally normal old people, while neurofibrillary tangles are rarely found in appreciable numbers in the neocortex of non-demented old people (Tomlinson et al., 1968). Other cortical neuropathological features of Alzheimer's disease include cortical atrophy, which is more characteristic of presenile cases (see Perry and Perry, 1983a), and neuronal loss (Terry et al., 1981). The neuropathological changes, as reflected in the density of both senile plaques and neurofibrillary tangles, correlate with the severity of the clinical symptoms (Tomlinson et al., 1970; Wilcock and Esiri, 1982). In contrast, in demented Parkinsonian patients while Alzheimer-type cortical neuropathological changes have been reported in several studies (Hakim and Mathieson, 1979; Boller et al., 1980; see also Mortimer et al., 1985), in a recent study, 11 out of 14 cognitively impaired Parkinsonian patients were found having no significant cortical Alzheimer-type neuropathological changes (Perry et al., 1985). The lack of a clear relationship between cognitive and cortical histological changes in Parkinson's disease confounds the notions that Alzheimer's disease and Parkinson's disease represent two ends of a single disease spectrum (Bowen and Davison, 1975; Drachman and Stahl, 1975; Rossor, 1981), or that the dementia associated with Parkinson's disease necessarily reflects coexisting Alzheimer's disease (Marsden, 1982) — at least in terms of the accepted diagnostic neuropathological markers for Alzheimer's disease.

Neurochemical changes in the cortical cholinergic system in Alzheimer's and Parkinson's diseases

Correlation of choline acetyltransferase activity with clinical and pathological indices of dementia

A landmark for neurochemical research in Alzheimer's disease occurred in 1976–7 with the inde-pendent finding by three groups of a loss of ChAT activity from the cerebral cortex (Davies and Maloney, 1976; Perry et al., 1977a,b; White et al., 1977). More recently it has been shown that ChAT loss is an early feature of the disease (Bowen et al., 1982), and this loss of ChAT activity is reflected in a decreased synthesis of acetylcholine in biopsy samples of cerebral cortex from patients with Alzheimer's disease (Sims et al., 1981). Another enzyme involved in the synthesis of acetylcholine, pyruvate dehydrogenase, has also been shown to have reduced activity in the cerebral cortex in Alzheimer's disease, and the loss of activity of this enzyme appears to be correlated with the level of ChAT activity (Perry et al., 1980a). The decreases in cholinergic synthetic enzyme activities are probably due to the degeneration of cortical cholinergic afferents (see section on histochemical changes in the cortical cholinergic system in Alzheimer's disease and Parkinson's disease). In addition a marked loss of cortical ChAT activity has also been found in cognitively impaired Parkinsonian patients (Perry et al., 1983, 1985).

While changes in several other cortical neurotransmitters, e.g. somatostatinergic (Davies et al., 1980), serotoninergic (Cross et al., 1983) and noradrenergic systems (Perry et al., 1981a), in Alzheimer's disease have subsequently been reported, the loss of ChAT activity still appears to be the most consistent neurochemical change that most strongly correlates with both the dementia rating (Perry et al., 1978, 1981b; Wilcock et al., 1982) and the extent of neuropathological change as defined by the density of senile plaques or neurofibrillary tangles in the cerebral cortex (Perry et al., 1978; Wilcock et al., 1982). In contrast, in demented Parkinsonian patients a loss of cortical ChAT activity, which correlates with the severity of the dementia, has also been reported (Ruberg et al., 1982; Perry et al., 1985), but in this disease there does not appear to be any relation between the extent of cortical ChAT loss and the degree of Alzheimer-type neuropathological change in the cerebral cortex (Perry et al., 1985). These findings suggest that different pathological processes may be responsible for the cholinergic deficit in Parkinson's disease and Alzheimer's disease. The loss of cortical cholinergic activity in Parkinson's disease, which is greatest in demented patients but also occurs to a lesser extent in non-demented patients (Perry et al., 1985), provides a link between the two disease states. In addition, the clear dissociation between the cortical cholinergic and neuropathological changes in Parkinsonian dementia emphasises the importance of the cortical ChAT deficit in relation to cognitive changes that occur in Alzheimer's disease and may provide a neurochemical basis for the impairment in memory processes (Deutsch, 1973; Drachman and Leavitt, 1974) which occur in the two diseases (see section on involvement of cholinergic receptors in cognitive processes).

The neurochemical significance of decreased choline acetyltransferase activity

It is perhaps surprising that the level of ChAT activity should correlate so well with the clinical or neuropathological features of either Alzheimer's or Parkinson's diseases since there is only about a 50% loss of ChAT activity. In addition, the enzyme ChAT is not generally considered to be a rate-limiting factor in acetylcholine synthesis, since the theoretical capacity of ChAT for acetylcholine synthesis greatly exceeds (by at least 20-fold) the in vivo rate of transmitter synthesis — at least at saturating concentrations of the two substrates choline and acetyl-CoA (see Tucek, 1985). However, it has recently been noted, that at the computed cytoplasmic concentrations of these substrates the in vivo activity of ChAT is likely to be up to 30 times less than at maximum substrate concentrations (Tucek, 1984). ChAT activity is therefore likely to be rate limiting in vivo; indeed in cortical biopsies from patients with presenile dementia it has been found that not only is ChAT activity decreased (Bowen et al., 1982) but that there is also a corresponding reduction in the rate of acetylcholine synthesis (Sims et al., 1981). In Alzheimer's disease the activity of pyruvate dehy-

drogenase, the enzyme responsible for the formation of acetyl-CoA, is also decreased (Perry et al., 1980a); this deficit would serve to further limit the rate of acetylcholine synthesis. However, in both biopsy and rapid autopsy studies it has been found that the high affinity uptake of choline is also decreased (Bowen et al., 1982; Rylett et al., 1983), and in the cortical biopsy samples from presenile cases of Alzheimer's disease the decrease in high affinity choline uptake was accompanied by corresponding alterations in ChAT activity (Bowen et al., 1982). This suggests that the reduced level of ChAT and pyruvate dehydrogenase activity may reflect the loss or functional impairment of cortical cholinergic presynaptic terminals.

Choline acetyltransferase and the cerebrovascular system

An additional factor which should be considered when assessing the significance of the loss of ChAT activity in relation to neuronal function in dementing disorders is the presence of ChAT activity in isolated blood vessels in bovine cerebral cortex (Estrada and Kause, 1982; Estrada et al., 1983) and ChAT immunoreactivity in vascular endothelial cells in rat cerebral cortex (Parnavelas et al., 1985). Indeed it has been suggested that up to 35% of the total cortical ChAT activity may be associated with microvessels and capillaries (Estrada et al., 1983). Whether this putative nonneuronal innervation is affected in Alzheimer's and Parkinson's diseases is at present unknown. However, by analogy with the noradrenergic innervation of cortical capillaries, which has the same origin as the cortical neuronal innervation (Hartman et al., 1980), the cortical cholinergic cerebrovascular and neuronal innervation may also have the same origin and be concomitantly reduced in both Alzheimer's and Parkinson's diseases. An interesting area for future research is to determine the functional role of the cholinergic and noradrenergic innervation in regulating cortical blood supply and so — indirectly — the activity of cortical neurons.

Age and choline acetyltransferase activity

During normal ageing (middle to late life), the level of ChAT activity has been reported to be either decreased in certain cortical regions (Davies, 1979; Perry et al., 1981b; Rossor et al., 1981, 1982), or remain unchanged (Bird et al., 1983). However, the rate of acetylcholine synthesis in cortical biopsy samples from mentally normal patients does not appear to vary with age, at least, between 15 and 68 years of age (Sims et al., 1981). In contrast, in presenile cases of Alzheimer's disease the loss of cortical ChAT activity appears to be more severe than in senile cases (Rossor et al., 1982; Bird et al., 1983). Indeed it has been claimed that cases of Alzheimer's disease of over 79 years show no significant loss of ChAT from frontal cortex (Rossor et al., 1981, 1982) — a finding which remains to be confirmed. The influence of age on different cholinergic parameters in the cerebral cortex over a broad post maturation age span, especially the 6th to the 10th decade, clearly needs to be investigated in more detail in both mentally normal and demented patients.

The intralaminar distribution of choline acetyltransferase activity

The intralaminar distribution of ChAT in the temporal cortex (Fig. 1a) has been determined in both mentally normal patients (Amaducci et al., 1981; Perry et al., 1984a) and in senile cases of Alzheimer's disease (Perry et al., 1984a; Sorbi and Amaducci, 1985). The highest levels of ChAT activity were present in the granular layers (II and IV) in normal individuals, while in the senile cases of Alzheimer's disease there was a marked loss of activity from all cortical layers with the greatest loss of activity occurring in layers II and IV (Fig. 1a), which have receptive and associative functions. These cortical ChAT losses are paralleled by a very marked reduction in the activity of this enzyme in the nucleus of Meynert, which supplies the cortical cholinergic afferents (see section on neuropathological and neurochemical changes in

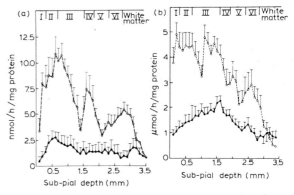

Fig. 1. Laminar distributions of (a) choline acetyltransferase activity and (b) acetylcholinesterase activity in the temporal cortex from normal cases (○- - - -○) and cases of senile dementia of the Alzheimer type (●———●). Points represent mean values (four cases in each of the normal and Alzheimer-type groups, except for AChE with five cases in each group); the bars represent the standard errors. The average positions of the six cortical layers and white matter are indicated. (Perry et al., 1984a)

the nucleus of Meynert in Alzheimer's and Parkinson's diseases).

Acetylcholinesterase activity

In addition to the loss of ChAT activity in Alzheimer's disease, there is also a marked loss of cortical acetylcholinesterase (AChE) activity (Pope et al., 1964; Davies and Maloney, 1976; Perry et al., 1978; Davies, 1979; Bowen et al., 1979). While AChE activity may not always be associated with cholinergic neuronal elements in the cerebral cortex, there does appear to be a close association between its gross distribution in different cortical areas and that of ChAT (Rossor et al., 1982). However, at the microanatomical level the cortical intralaminar distributions of the two enzymes are not identical (Perry et al., 1984a). Thus, a high level of AChE activity was present in layer III (Fig. 1b) in contrast to the distribution of ChAT (Fig. 1a), suggesting that, at least in this particular layer, there may be a dissociation between AChE distribution and the cholinergic input (see section on cortical distribution of choline acetyltransferase and acetylcholinesterase). Nevertheless, in senile cases of Alzheimer's disease there is a marked loss

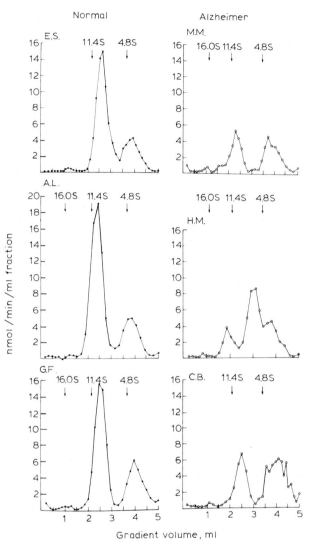

Fig. 2. Distribution of acetylcholinesterase molecular forms in the parietal cortex (Brodman area 40). Figures on the left represent the normal group and figures on the right the senile dementia of Alzheimer-type group. The levels of acetylcholinesterase activity throughout the sucrose density gradient are shown. The internal marker enzymes used were alcohol dehydrogenase (4.8S), catalase (11.4S) and β-galactosidase (16.0S). (Atack et al., 1983)

of AChE activity from all the cortical layers (Fig. 1b) including layer III (Perry et al., 1984a).

AChE exists in the brain, as elsewhere, in several different molecular or polymeric forms (Massoulie and Bon, 1982), and the presence of these various forms have recently been investigated in the cerebral cortex in Alzheimer's disease and Parkinson's disease using sucrose density centrifugation (Atack et al., 1983). In normal human cerebral cortex two major molecular forms of the enzyme are present, which according to the nomenclature of Massoulie and Bon (1982) consist of a G1-monomeric form and a G4-tetrameric form (Atack et al., 1983). In Alzheimer's disease there is a selective loss in the G4 form (sedimentation coefficient of approximately 10 S), while the lighter G1 (3.5 S) form is unchanged (Fig. 2; Atack et al., 1983). A similar selective loss of the 10 S form has also been observed in the cortex of demented Parkinsonian patients (Perry et al., 1985).

Histochemical changes in the cortical cholinergic system in Alzheimer's disease and Parkinson's disease

Methodological approaches

Although sensitive histochemical methods for the detection of AChE activity have been available for several decades (see Silver, 1974), the major difficulty with this approach in mapping cholinergic pathways is that the enzyme is not exclusively localised to the cholinergic system (see Silver, 1974). Although ChAT is the more reliable enzyme marker of the cholinergic system, histochemical methods for its detection (Burt, 1970; Kasa et al., 1970) lack specificity. The recent introduction of a specific inhibitor of ChAT, bromoacetylcholine (Tucek, 1982) may now, however, signal the development of a more satisfactory histochemical method for the enzyme, ChAT. The immunocytochemical localisation of ChAT is probably, at present, the more promising technique, as both polyclonal and monoclonal antibodies against ChAT have recently been produced (see Wainer et al., 1984). There are, nevertheless, certain problems even with this approach; many of the antisera currently produced only demonstrate the presence of ChAT in cell bodies and do not visualise ChAT-containing axonal processes or terminals, also the specificity of the immunostaining staining is difficult to assess routinely since purified ChAT is not yet currently available. Comparison of the distribution of AChE staining with both the immunocytochemical and the neurochemical distribution of ChAT has however, at least partially, validated AChE as a marker enzyme for the cortical cholinergic system.

Cortical distribution of choline acetyltransferase and acetylcholinesterase

Detailed maps of the intralaminar and regional histochemical and immunocytochemical distributions of AChE and ChAT in the cerebral cortex of the human brain are not yet available. However, there appear to be marked variations in the regional and laminar distribution of AChE-stained fibres in the rat (Shute and Lewis, 1967), cat (Krnjevic and Silver, 1965) and primate cerebral cortex (Mesulam et al., 1984). Interestingly, in the primate cerebral cortex the paralimbic areas, which are of prime importance in the modulation of memory and mood, have a much higher density of AChE-containing fibres than the sensory association areas (Mesulam et al., 1984). These findings are consistent with the gross regional distribution of ChAT activity in the primate cerebral cortex (Lehmann et al., 1984) and of AChE and ChAT activities in the human cerebral cortex (Hebb and Silver, 1956; Okinaka et al., 1961; Rossor et al., 1982). A similar widespread cortical distribution of ChAT immunoreactive fibres has also been described in the rat (Houser et al., 1983) and cat (Kimura et al., 1981).

In both the frontal and temporal cortices of the normal elderly human, numerous AChE-stained fibres are present in all cortical layers and, in addition, occasional intensely stained cell bodies are found in layers V and VI (Perry et al., 1985), while many of the pyramidal neurons in layer III of the human cortex show moderate staining (Candy et al., unpublished). A similar distribution of intensely AChE-stained cells in layers V and VI has

also been reported in the cat cerebral cortex (Krnjevic and Silver, 1965). In contrast, in the rat cerebral cortex immunostained cell bodies have been reported to be present in layers II–VI (Houser et al., 1983). However, unlike all other confirmed cholinergic cell bodies in the CNS, the ChAT-positive perikarya in the rat cerebral cortex do not appear to be intensely AChE-positive and the cerebral cortex is devoid of intensely AChE-stained neurons even after pretreatment with diisopropylfluorophosphate (Lehmann et al., 1980). This raises questions concerning their cholinergic status and functional importance, especially since undercutting of the cerebral cortex in animals leads to marked decreases of the cholinergic marker enzymes (Hebb et al., 1963; Krnjevic and Silver, 1965; Green et al., 1970) and decreases in acetylcholine release (Collier and Mitchell, 1967). In addition, intracortical injection of kainic acid fails to decrease cortical ChAT activity (Lehmann et al., 1980). Moreover, a distribution of ChAT immunostained cell bodies, similar to that in the rat, has not been observed in the primate cerebral cortex (Mufson, personal communication). These findings in animals, taken together with the sparse distribution of intensely AChE-stained cell bodies in the human cerebral cortex, suggests that intrinsic cholinergic neurons, if they exist at all, are only a minor component of the cholinergic input (see section on neurochemical and neuroanatomical evidence that the nucleus of Meynert is the source of the cortical cholinergic afferents).

In senile cases of Alzheimer's disease and also in demented cases of Parkinson's disease, where the neuropathological features of Alzheimer's disease are absent, there is a gross loss of AChE-stained fibres from all cortical layers (Candy et al., 1983; Perry et al., 1985). This loss of AChE staining may reflect the loss of the G4 form of AChE in Alzheimer's disease and Parkinson's disease, where dementia is present (Atack et al., 1983; Perry et al., 1985), as it appears that the higher molecular forms of AChE are preferentially demonstrated by histochemical methods (Huther and Luppa, 1979). In addition, the relative solubility of the G4 in non-detergent containing media such as those used in histochemical investigations, is unchanged in Alzheimer's and Parkinson's diseases (Perry et al., unpublished), so eliminating the loss of AChE-histochemical staining in these cases as an artefactual loss of enzyme activity. This finding of a loss of AChE-stained fibres, taken together with the neurochemical loss of ChAT activity and high-affinity choline uptake, strongly suggests that there is a gross degeneration of cholinergic axonal processes projecting to the cerebral cortex in both Alzheimer's disease and Parkinson's disease where dementia is present.

It is of considerable interest that AChE-stained processes have been shown to be present in senile plaques in the cerebral cortex in Alzheimer's disease (Friede, 1965; Perry et al., 1980b), in the mentally normal elderly (Perry et al., 1980b) and in the cerebral cortex of the aged primate (Struble et al., 1982, 1984). Moreover, ChAT immunoreactivity has also been demonstrated in processes in senile plaques of the aged primate (Kitt et al., 1984). Thus, it seems likely that cholinergic processes together with other transmitter processes (Morrison et al., 1984; Armstrong et al., 1985) are associated at some stage in the formation of senile plaques (see section on pathogenic mechanisms).

The nucleus of Meynert in Alzheimer's disease and Parkinson's disease

Neurochemical and neuroanatomical evidence that the nucleus of Meynert is the source of the cortical cholinergic afferents

The most prominent neurons within the substantia innominata of the basal forebrain are the cell bodies of the nucleus of the diagonal band and the nucleus of Meynert. In man, these nuclei are contiguous and often lack a readily identifiable boundary. Lesion studies in animals have demonstrated that the major source of the cortical cholinergic innervation is from the nucleus of Meynert (Johnston et al., 1979, 1981; Wenk et al., 1980; Pedata et al., 1982). Retrograde labelling

experiments have shown that the magnocellular neurons in the nucleus of Meynert (Gorry, 1963) provide an innervation to virtually all areas of the cerebral cortex (Kievet and Kuypers, 1975; Divac, 1975; Jones et al., 1976; Mesulam and Van Hoesen, 1976; Pearson et al., 1983a). In the primate, the nucleus of Meynert can be subdivided into a number of regions on the basis of their cortical connections (Pearson et al., 1983b; Mesulam et al., 1983), suggesting that analogous cortical topographic projections may also exist in the human brain. The importance of this nucleus in man is suggested by phylogenetic studies, which indicate that its size and organisation parallels the development of the neocortex (Gorry, 1963).

The cholinergic nature and development of the nucleus of Meynert in man

The neurons in the nucleus of Meynert stain intensely for AChE activity (Fig. 3A; Candy et al., 1981; Perry et al., 1984b) and the distribution of AChE-stained neurons in the substantia innominata of the basal forebrain has been mapped using a sensitive, specific histochemical method (Fig. 4; Perry et al., 1984b). In addition, high levels of ChAT and AChE activity have been shown to be present in discrete tissue punches from the nucleus of Meynert (Table I; Candy et al., 1981; Perry et al., 1982, Candy et al., 1983; Perry et al., 1984b). These data demonstrate the cholinergic nature of the nucleus of Meynert in man and this has been confirmed by the localisation of ChAT immunoreactivity in neurons in this nucleus (Nagai et al., 1983; Pearson et al., 1983c).

A combined histochemical and biochemical approach has recently demonstrated that the nucleus of Meynert is well defined histochemically and neurochemically within the first 3–4 months of gestation. Thus, at this stage of development intense AChE staining of nucleus of Meynert neurons is observed, while the putamen and caudate nucleus exhibit a much lower level of staining (Fig. 3B; Candy et al., 1985d). Moreover, a relatively high level of ChAT activity

Fig. 3 A

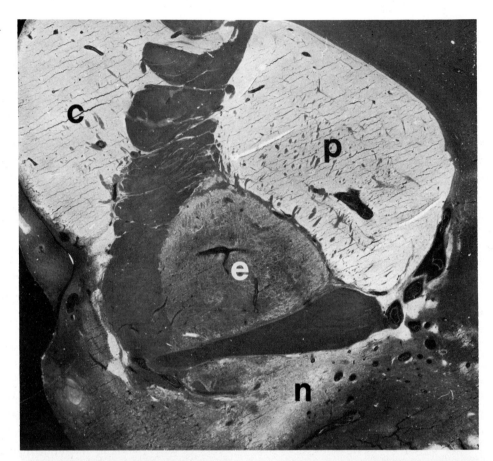

Fig. 3 B

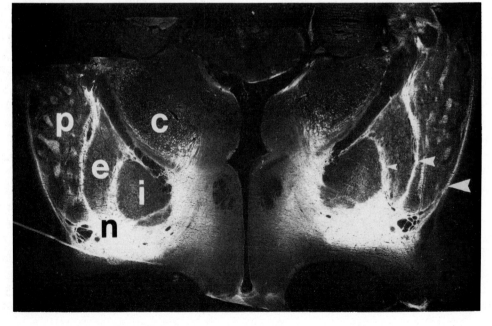

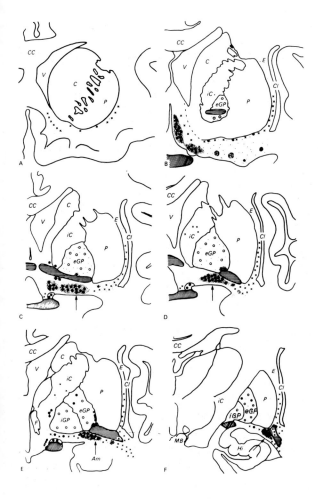

Fig. 4(A–F). Schematic illustrations of the rostrocaudal distribution of AChE staining in the substantia innominata and surrounding areas. Filled and open circles represent intensely and moderately stained cell bodies, respectively. Dots show AChE-stained neuropil and crosses AChE-stained fibres. AChE reactivity in dorsal regions is not shown and for clarity AChE localisation in the caudate nucleus and putamen has been omitted. Horizontally shaded areas represent the anterior commissure and diagonally shaded areas show the position of the optic tract. Arrows indicate the main limits of the nucleus of Meynert. Am, amygdala; c, caudate nucleus; CC, corpus callosum; Cl, claustrum; E, external capsule; eGP, external globus pallidus; F, fornix; Hi, anterior hippocampus; iC, internal capsule; iGP, internal globus pallidus; MB, mammillary body; P, putamen; V, ventricle (Perry et al., 1984b)

Meynert (Krnjevic and Silver, 1965; Perry et al., 1984b). It, therefore, seems likely that the cortical cholinergic system is functional at an early stage of gestation and may consequently play an important role in the development of the cerebral cortex. The demonstration of cholinergic neurons in the nucleus of Meynert during early foetal development presents the possibility of co-culture of these neurons in either dispersed or explant form with foetal cortical neurons and studying their electrophysiological and pharmacological properties (see Gahwiler and Brown, 1985).

Neuropathological and neurochemical changes in the nucleus of Meynert in Alzheimer's and Parkinson's diseases

In presenile cases of Alzheimer's disease a very extensive loss of neurons in the nucleus of Meynert has been reported to occur (Whitehouse et al., 1982; Arendt et al., 1983; Wilcock et al., 1983;

is present in tissue punches from this nucleus at 3–4 months (Candy et al., 1985d), indicating that the neurons possess the adult cholinergic markers at this early stage of development. In addition, almost adult levels of ChAT activity are present in the cortical mantle by 4 months and AChE-stained fibres are present in the external capsule, which has cortical cholinergic afferents from the nucleus of

Fig. 3 (A and B). Shows distribution of AChE staining in coronal sections at the level of the nucleus of Meynert in (A) a 70-year-old mentally normal patient, (B) a foetus at 16 weeks of gestation. These photomicrographs are direct prints from the AChE-stained sections and white therefore represents areas which contain high AChE activity. n, nucleus of Meynert; e, external globus pallidus; i, internal globus pallidus; p, putamen globus pallidus; c, caudate nucleus. Note the high level of AChE activity in both the adult and foetal nucleus of Meynert region, the presence of AChE-stained fibres in the internal (◄) and external medullary laminae (◀) which are absent in the adult, the AChE-stained fibres in the external capsule in both the foetus and adult (◀) and the patches of AChE staining in the foetal putamen.

TABLE I

Choline acetyltransferase and acetylcholinesterase activities in the nucleus of Meynert, adjacent regions, and cerebral cortex in elderly normal patients and in senile cases of Alzheimer's disease

Area	Choline acetyltransferase activity (nmol/h/mg protein)		Acetylcholinesterase activity (μmol/min/mg protein)	
	control $\pm$ SEM	Alzheimer's disease $\pm$ SEM	control $\pm$ SEM	Alzheimer's disease $\pm$ SEM
Brodmann 21	3.7 $\pm$ 1.0	0.7 $\pm$ 0.1**	5.5 $\pm$ 0.5	3.1 $\pm$ 0.4*
Brodmann 10	5.9 $\pm$ 2.6	2.4 $\pm$ 0.4**	6.3 $\pm$ 0.2	4.2 $\pm$ 0.6*
Nucleus of Meynert	196.8 $\pm$ 88.0	13.4 $\pm$ 4.4**	676.7 $\pm$ 101.2	141.9 $\pm$ 33.9**
Putamen	490.1 $\pm$ 98.3	181.8 $\pm$ 34.3*	1479.8 $\pm$ 211.0	676.5 $\pm$ 71.2**
External globus pallidus	26.4 $\pm$ 9.9	14.7 $\pm$ 1.3**	194.8 $\pm$ 37.9	112.5 $\pm$ 26.6
Internal globus pallidus	14.7 $\pm$ 3.8	2.0 $\pm$ 0.5	137.4 $\pm$ 27.3	66.4 $\pm$ 23.5

Asterisked values in the senile dementia of Alzheimer type group show those that are significantly different for the control group. *$p = 0.008$; **$p = 0.004$, Mann-Whitney U test.

Tagliavini and Pilleri, 1983). However, in senile cases of Alzheimer's disease estimates of neuron density or the total number of neurons present in the nucleus of Meynert have indicated a more modest neuron loss (Perry et al., 1982; Candy et al., 1983; Wilcock et al., 1983; Tagliavini and Pilleri, 1983; Perry et al., 1985). A similar modest neuronal loss has also been found in senile cases of Alzheimer's disease using the immunocytochemical localisation of ChAT in the nucleus of Meynert (Pearson et al., 1983c; Nagai et al., 1983). There appears, therefore, to be an inverse relationship between neuronal loss in the nucleus of Meynert and age in Alzheimer's disease (Tagliavini and Pilleri, 1983; Mann et al., 1984a). Indeed the decrease in neuron loss from the nucleus of Meynert with age in Alzheimer's disease, which cannot be explained by tissue atrophy alone (Perry et al., 1985) is such that by 90 years it approaches that found in normal elderly patients (Mann et al., 1984a). Thus between 50 and 90 years of age there is, during normal ageing, about a 35% decrease in the number of nucleus of Meynert neurons (Mann et al., 1984a). The more benign expression of the disease in senile cases, which is reflected both in decreased cortical atrophy and neuron fall-out from the nucleus of Meynert, may result from

some influence of ageing on the disease process or a shorter duration of the disease.

In contrast to the modest neuronal loss in the nucleus of Meynert in senile cases of Alzheimer's disease there is a marked loss of ChAT activity in tissue punches from this nucleus (Table I; Perry et al., 1982, Candy et al., 1983). This suggests that a down-regulation of acetylcholine synthesis occurs, which may be a primary feature of the disease. In agreement with the decreased synthesis of ChAT, reductions in both nucleolar volume and RNA content have been observed in neurons in the nucleus of Meynert in Alzheimer's disease (Mann and Yates, 1982; Mann et al., 1984a,b). In addition, approximately 20% of neurons in this nucleus contain neurofibrillary tangles in senile cases (Candy et al., 1983), the pathological consequences of which may account for a proportion of the loss in ChAT activity.

Fall-out of neurons from the nucleus of Meynert in Parkinson's disease has long been documented (Hassler, 1938; Von Buttlar-Brentano, 1955). A loss of neurons occurs in mentally normal Parkinsonian patients (Candy et al., 1983; Whitehouse et all., 1983; Perry et al., 1985), although in demented Parkinsonian cases the neuronal loss is much greater (Whitehouse et al., 1983; Perry et al., 1985).

Moreover, a decrease in nucleolar volume and RNA content of neurons in the nucleus of Meynert, which is more marked in the mentally impaired cases, has been reported to occur in Parkinson's disease (Mann and Yates, 1983). These findings in Parkinson's disease are in accord with the reported cortical ChAT deficit (see section on correlation of choline acetyltransferase activity with clinical and pathological indices of dementia). In addition, the number of neurons remaining in the nucleus of Meynert has been shown in Parkinson's disease to correlate with the loss of ChAT activity in the cerebral cortex (Perry et al., 1985), which is in contrast to senile cases of Alzheimer's disease where no such correlation exists.

A correlation between the density of cortical senile plaques and the extent of neuron loss has been reported in younger cases of Alzheimer's disease (Arendt et al., 1984; Mann et al., 1985). A similar correlation with cortical neurofibrillary tangles has also been observed (Mann et al., 1985). These findings indicate, at least in presenile cases of Alzheimer's disease, that the neuropathological changes in the cerebral cortex may be of primary importance for neuron loss in the nucleus of Meynert possibly causing retrograde degeneration of the cholinergic afferents with subsequent death of the choline perikarya. In senile cases of Alzheimer's disease, where there is a modest loss of neurons in the nucleus of Meynert, it seems likely that the loss of ChAT activity in the nucleus of Meynert may be a more appropriate marker for the functional status of the Meynert neurons which may reflect the extent of neuropathological change in the cerebral cortex. In contrast, neuron loss in the nucleus of Meynert in demented Parkinsonian patients may reflect primary degenerative changes in the cholinergic perikarya.

Electrophysiological, behavioural and neurochemical studies on cholinergic receptors in the cerebral cortex

Microelectrophysiological evidence for cholinergic receptors in the cerebral cortex

In vivo microiontophoretic studies indicate that acetylcholine has a predominantly excitatory ac-

tion in the deeper layers of the cerebral cortex in the cat (Krnjevic and Phillis, 1963a). The characteristic features of this response are its slow time course and muscarinic nature (Krnjevic and Phillis, 1963a,b). The increased neuronal excitability elicited by acetylcholine is mediated through a decrease in potassium conductance (Krnjevic et al., 1971). Recent evidence suggests that two voltage-dependent potassium conductances are affected by muscarinic agonists: a calcium-dependent conductance, which operates at normal or hyperpolarised membrane potentials and serves to limit the repetitive firing of action potentials (see North and Tokimasa, 1984), and a calcium-independent conductance that is only partly activated at normal resting potentials, but markedly increases with increasing membrane depolarisation and thus serves to stabilise the membrane potential (see Brown, 1983). Both these potassium conductances are decreased by muscarinic agonists (see North and Tokimasa, 1984; Brown, 1983), leading in each case to increased neuronal excitability — a decrease in the calcium-independent potassium conductance leads to an increased firing rate, while a decrease in the calcium-dependent potassium conductance leads to an increased probability of repetitive neuronal firing. Consequently, the excitatory action of the cortical cholinergic input on muscarinic cholinoceptive neurons will be dependent on the level of other excitatory inputs (Krnjevic and Phillis, 1963a; Krnjevic et al., 1971) and will modulate the level of excitability and pattern of neuronal firing. The resultant patterning of responses may be especially important for memory and other cognitive processes.

While purely nicotinic-like effects of acetylcholine in the cerebral cortex have not been observed (Krnjevic and Phillis, 1963b), microiontophoretic studies have revealed the presence of inhibitory effects of acetylcholine, predominantly in the upper layers of the cortex in the cat (Randic et al., 1964; Phillis and York, 1967), that may be mediated through an increased potassium conductance (Hartzell et al., 1977; Dodd and Horne, 1983). This inhibitory action exhibits mixed nicotinic and muscarinic pharmacology (Phillis and York, 1968) suggesting that, in addition to the purely muscarinic excitatory receptor, a receptor with intermediate pharmacological characteristics is present in the cerebral cortex.

Electroencephalographic evidence for a role of cholinergic receptors in cortical arousal

Electroencephalographic studies indicate that the cortical cholinergic system is involved in electrocortical desynchronisation (Bonnet and Bremer, 1937; Bradley and Elkes, 1957) — an action which is dependent on muscarinic receptor activity (Bradley and Elkes, 1957; Monnier and Romanowski, 1962; Rinaldi, 1965; Longo, 1966). The cholinergic nature of cortical arousal is in fact supported by many studies, which have shown that the efflux of acetylcholine from the cortical surface of the cat brain increases during spontaneous or induced periods of alertness or electrocortical desynchronisation (Mitchell, 1963; Belesin et al., 1965; Kanai and Szerb, 1965; Phillis and Chong, 1965; Celesia and Jasper, 1966; Bartolini and Pepeu, 1967; Beani et al., 1968; Phillis, 1968; Jasper and Koyama, 1969).

In view of the cholinergic deficit in both, Alzheimer's and Parkinson's diseases, it is of interest that in both these disease states there are many studies which show that a diffuse slowing of the electrocorticogram occurs, and moreover, that the extent of this change appears to be related to the severity of the disease (Berger, 1932; Weiner and Schuster, 1956; Letemendia and Pampiglione, 1958; England et al., 1959; Gordon and Sim, 1967; Wennberg and Widen, 1974; Muller, 1978; Johannesson et al., 1979; Soininen et al., 1982; Coben et al., 1983; Duffy et al., 1984). A similar diffuse slowing of the electrocortical activity has also been demonstrated after lesioning the major source of the cortical cholinergic afferents, the nucleus of Meynert (Lo Conte et al., 1982; Stewart et al., 1984). This finding of electrocortical changes in Alzheimer's and Parkinson's diseases, where there is a loss of cortical cholinergic afferents, is therefore consistent with the role of the cortical cholinergic system in mediating electrocortical desynchronisation, and suggests that the decrease in fast electroencephalographic activity may be related to cognitive impairment.

Involvement of cholinergic receptors in cognitive processes

Aged primates exhibit marked cognitive changes and, although the status of the cortical cholinergic system in these animals has not been investigated, it is interesting to note that senile plaques frequently occur in the cerebral cortex (Wisniewski et al., 1973). These aged animals have been shown to have a marked deficit in their ability to remember recent sensory stimuli (Bartus et al., 1978, 1980). A very similar change in memory retention can also be elicited in young primates by the specific muscarinic antagonist scopolamine, but not by the peripheral muscarinic antagonist methylscopolamine (Bartus and Johnson, 1976). Moreover, this memory deficit can be at least partially reversed by the acetylcholinesterase inhibitor physostigmine (Bartus, 1978). These data indicate that cholinoceptive neurons are involved in memory processes and they are in accord with the observations in humans that scopolamine in young subjects produces impairments in memory and other cognitive processes, that are similar to those observed in the elderly normal human (Drachman and Leavitt, 1974; Drachman et al., 1980). Further strands of evidence consistent with the involvement of cholinergic mechanisms in human memory, are the facilitation in memory produced by physostigmine in both young (Davis et al., 1978) and elderly subjects (Peters and Levin, 1978; Smith and Swash, 1979; Bartus, 1979; Davis et al., 1979; Christie et al., 1981; Drachman and Sahakian, 1980) and the finding that memory is also facilitated by the muscarinic agonist arecoline in young subjects (Sitaram et al., 1978). While these effects are not necessarily mediated by the cortical cholinergic system, they do provide a link between cholinergic CNS function and memory, and they suggest that memory impairments in old age and Alzheimer's disease, where this is an early, cardinal feature of the disease, may be related to the cholinergic deficit.

Neurochemical investigations on cortical cholinergic binding sites in Alzheimer's disease and Parkinson's disease

Several binding studies have reported that the overall density of muscarinic receptors in the cerebral cortex is unchanged in Alzheimer's disease (White et al., 1977; Davies and Verth, 1977; Perry et al., 1977a, 1978; Reisine et al., 1978; Bowen et al., 1979; Nordberg et al., 1980; Rinne et al., 1984, 1985). In only two studies has a decrease of muscarinic binding sites been observed in the cerebral cortex in Alzheimer's disease (Wood et al., 1983; Mash et al., 1985). In contrast, in demented cases of Parkinson's disease a modest increase in cortical muscarinic binding sites has been reported (Ruberg et al., 1982), which may be related to anticholinergic therapy. However, there seems to be no clear relationship between presynaptic activity and postsynaptic receptor density, as acute lesions of the nucleus of Meynert do not produce a significant change in presumed postsynaptic cortical muscarinic binding sites (McKinney and Coyle, 1982).

The status of muscarinic receptors in pathological conditions such as Alzheimer's disease and Parkinson's disease is complicated by the existence of multiple receptor subtypes. Thus, binding studies in animals have indicated that muscarinic receptors are heterogeneous with two major binding sites with high and low affinities for agonists (Birdsall et al., 1978, 1980). These high- and low-affinity binding sites appear to be interconvertible, thus the high-affinity binding site can be converted to a low-affinity site by guanyl nucleotides (Berrie et al., 1979; Sokolovsky et al., 1980). However, there appears to be a differential distribution of these two binding sites as assessed using carbachol displacement of antagonist binding. Thus in the rat cerebral cortex it appears that only the high-affinity agonist binding site shows regional and laminar variations in its distribution (McKinney and Coyle, 1982; Wamsley et al., 1980), and there is evidence from lesion studies that at least some of the low-affinity binding sites may be presynaptically located (McKinney and Coyle, 1982). Recent investigations using the non-classical muscarinic antagonist pirenzapine have also led to the distinction of more than one antagonist binding site in the cerebral cortex and these sites do not appear to be interconvertible (Hammer et al., 1980; Hammer, 1982; Hammer and Giachetti, 1982; Watson et al., 1982, 1983; Birdsall et al., 1984; Luthin and Wolfe, 1984; Berrie et al., 1985): a high-affinity site (M1 site), which has the highest density of binding sites, and other heterogeneous sites of intermediate and low affinity (M2 sites).

Autoradiographic studies of the cortical laminar distribution of muscarinic antagonist binding sites indicate that the highest densities of binding sites are located in layers II, III and VI (Rotter et al., 1979; Wamsley et al., 1980).

Pirenzapine has been employed to distinguish muscarinic receptor subtypes in the human cerebral cortex (Caulfield et al., 1982; Garvey et al., 1984), and in a preliminary study using pirenzapine to displace *N*-methyl scopolamine from M1 and M2 binding sites, no abnormality was detected in the temporal cortex in senile cases of Alzheimer's disease (Caulfield et al., 1982). It has however, very recently been reported, using either chemical stabilisation or agonist displacement of antagonist binding to differentiate M1 and M2 binding sites, that there is a selective reduction in M2 sites in Alzheimer's disease (Mash et al., 1985; Whitehouse et al., 1985a). In the study employing chemical stabilisation of muscarinic binding sites (Mash et al., 1985), in contrast to most other studies, a reduction of the overall density of muscarinic binding sites was found. Moreover, so-called M2 receptors probably represent a heterogeneous population (Birdsall et al., 1984; Berrie et al., 1985) and further definition of subpopulations of M2 receptors, in normal and pathological human brain, must await a better understanding of the molecular basis of the binding heterogeneity.

It should be noted that most studies of muscarinic binding sites in human brain have used crude tissue homogenates, and a factor which no doubt complicates the interpretation of the results is the presence of muscarinic binding sites on non-neuronal elements. Such sites have been shown to be present not only on astrocytes (Repke and Maderspach, 1982), but also to be associated with intracerebral blood vessels in both the rat and bovine cerebral cortex (Estrada and Krause, 1982; Estrada et al., 1983; Grammas et al., 1983). The reported density of binding sites of these non-neuronal populations of muscarinic binding sites could well mask any alteration in neuronal binding sites in Alzheimer's disease, and further studies to clarify this point are clearly required. The vascular muscarinic receptors appear to be involved in the regulation of vascular permeability (see Rowell and Sastry, 1978) and cerebral blood flow (D'Alecy and Rose, 1977; Heistad et al., 1980). It is of interest, in relation to the cholinergic deficit in Alzheimer's disease, that vascular permeability appears to be impaired (Wisniewski and Kozlowski, 1982) and that a decrease in cerebral blood flow also occurs (Ingvar et al., 1978).

Putative nicotinic cholinergic binding sites have been labelled with α-bungarotoxin, both in the cerebral cortex of animals and humans (McQuarrie et al., 1976; Davies and Feisullin, 1981; Perry and Perry, 1983b). A loss of α-bungarotoxin binding sites has not been consistently found in Alzheimer's disease (Davies and Feisullin, 1981; Perry and Perry, 1983b). However, α-bungarotoxin has no antagonist activity at nicotinic receptors in several neuronal systems (Duggan et al., 1976; Brown and Fumagalli, 1977; Carbonetto et al., 1978) and the relevance of this binding site to nicotinic receptor activity is therefore questionable.

Nicotine (Yoshida and Imura, 1979; Romano and Goldstein, 1980; Martin and Aceto, 1981; Marks and Collins, 1982; Costa and Murphy, 1983; Clarke et al., 1984), acetylcholine (Schwartz et al., 1982) and dihydro-β-erythroidine (Williams and Robinson, 1986) have been used to label

nicotinic-like receptors in animal brain and may be of greater value in investigating these receptors in human brain. Interestingly, two binding sites were identified with dihydro-β-erythroidine and at least one of these sites exhibited muscarinic-like properties (Williams and Robinson, 1985). This nicotinic antagonist may therefore label a receptor with intermediate muscarinic and nicotinic properties with similar characteristics to the one identified electrophysiologically (see section on microelectrophysiological evidence for cholinergic receptors in the cerebral cortex). In the cerebral cortex in Alzheimer's disease a decrease in the density of nicotinic binding has been reported using ^{3}H-acetylcholine as the ligand (Whitehouse et al., 1985b), while a similar reduction has not been found using the ligand ^{3}H-nicotine (Shimohama et al., 1986).

Current evidence, on balance, suggests that in Alzheimer's disease there is no gross change in the putative postsynaptic, cortical muscarinic binding sites. This suggests that, at least in the early stages of the disease, cholinergic agonists may well be effective if the receptors are still functionally coupled. There is good evidence from investigations of animal brains that muscarinic receptors are coupled to either guanylate cyclase (Strange et al., 1977; Hanley and Iversen, 1978) or to the hydrolysis of polyphosphoinositides through activation of phospholipase C (see Mitchell, 1975, 1980; Berridge and Irvine, 1984). Activation of muscarinic receptors consequently leads to the formation of either cyclic GMP or inositol trisphosphate acting as a second messenger for mobilising intracellular calcium and also the formation of diacylglycerol which activates protein kinase C (see Berridge and Irvine, 1984). Low concentrations of potassium have been shown to markedly potentiate the hydrolysis of phosphoinositides elicited by muscarinic agonists (Table II; Candy et al., 1985a; Court et al., in press); this effect may possibly be linked with the potassium conductance changes observed with muscarinic agonists (see section on microelectrophysiological evidence for cholinergic receptors in the cerebral

TABLE II

Effect of K^+ on phosphoinositides hydrolysis in rat and human cerebral cortex and antagonism by pirenzapine

Tissue	[K$^+$] mM	Basal level	Additions	
			carbachol (100 μM)	carbachol (100 μM) + pirenzapine (50 μM)
Fresh rat cortex ($n=9$)	6	0.045 ± 0.009	0.058 ± 0.015*[a]	0.049 ± 0.011
	18	0.049 ± 0.018	0.147 ± 0.052**[a]	0.084 ± 0.028**[b]
Slow frozen human biopsy cortex ($n=3$)	6	0.045 ± 0.007	0.065 ± 0.008*[a]	
	18	0.054 ± 0.003	0.169 ± 0.006***[a]	

Tissue was cross-chopped (350 × 350 μm), labelled with ^{3}H-myo-inositol during a 2-h incubation. Tissue ^{3}H-inositol was reduced by washing slices with excess buffer and phosphatidylinositol hydrolysis measured after a further 1-h incubation in the presence of 10 mM Li$^+$ estimated by the tritium incorporation into the inositol phosphate fraction (Pins). Results are expressed as dpm in Pins/Pins + lipid. [a] Significant difference from basal hydrolysis; [b] significantly different from carbachol alone; *$p < 0.05$, **$p < 0.01$, ***$p < 0.001$, Student's t test.

cortex). Regarding the muscarinic receptor subtype that mediates phosphoinositide hydrolysis, there is recent evidence that the M1 antagonist subtype is linked to this response (Table II; Gonzales and Crews, 1984; Candy et al., 1985b), whereas at least a subpopulation of M2 binding sites is linked to guanylate cyclase.

These muscarinic activated systems present a promising approach for studying muscarinic receptor coupling in the human brain. In cortical biopsy samples it has been possible to elicit carbachol-induced phosphoinositide hydrolysis (Table II; Candy et al., 1984a). However, in post-mortem cortical tissue, incorporation of inositol into polyphosphoinositides, although observed in an initial case (Candy et al., 1984a), has in many subsequent patients been negligible (Court et al., unpublished). Consequently, the only means of monitoring the integrity of this response in the cerebral cortex in Alzheimer's disease or Parkinson's disease is through the use of biopsy tissue.

Therapeutic implications

Based on the electrophysiological and behavioural studies, a potential therapeutic strategy for the cognitive deficit in Alzheimer's disease and Parkinson's disease appears to involve cholinergic replacement therapy. Although trials with precursors of acetylcholine (namely choline and lecithin) or inhibitors of AChE improve cognition in normal patients (see Bartus et al., 1982), in view of the loss of cholinergic afferents in Alzheimer's disease, it is not surprising that these have proved largely ineffective in Alzheimer's disease (see Bartus et al., 1982). A more rational therapeutic approach, and one which has proved at least partially successful for the motor deficit in Parkinson's disease, is the use of receptor agonists. However, any approach involving direct stimulation of cholinergic receptors is obviously dependent not only on a normal complement of functional postsynaptic muscarinic receptors but also on the mode of action of the neurotransmitter. It might at first appear unlikely that cholinergic agonists could mimic the modulatory effect of acetylcholine on neuronal excitability. However, a number of studies, in animals, indicate that acetylcholine is tonically released during electrocortical desynchronisation and behavioural alerting (see section on electroencephalographic evidence for a role of cholinergic receptors in cortical arousal) and it can therefore be inferred that the cortical cholinergic system is tonically active during the waking state. If this is the case, then cholinergic agonists may well be able to effectively replace the normal cholinergic synaptic input, at least during waking periods. In view of the human data on the effect of muscarinic antagonists on memory, it seems likely that muscarinic agonists will be of most value in improving the memory impairment in Alzheimer's disease and Parkinson's disease, if the muscarinic receptors are still functionally coupled to potassium channels and to the phosphatidylinositol response. It is possible that cognitively impaired Parkinsonian patients will benefit most from these drugs, as they frequently appear not to show Alzheimer-type cortical neuropathological changes, implying that the cerebral cortex is more functionally intact. Other potential therapeutic approaches that do not rely on the functional coupling of the muscarinic receptor include the design of drugs, other than cholinomimetics, that can selectively affect the cholinergic potassium conductance changes and directly stimulate or mimic the second messengers produced by activation of the muscarinic receptor.

Pathogenic mechanisms

While cholinergic replacement therapy may ameliorate some of the cognitive deficits in Alzheimer's disease, at least in its early stages, the ultimate aim must be to understand the aberrant neurochemical processes that lead to the neuropathological changes and retrograde degeneration and loss of the cortical cholinergic system.

There is strong evidence that the selective vulnerability to Alzheimer's disease may result from a genetic predisposition. Thus, in many cases, the disease appears to have a familial basis and to be transmitted in an autosomal dominant fashion (Heston et al., 1981; Larsson et al., 1963; Breitner and Folstein, 1984). In addition there is a strong association between Down's syndrome and Alzheimer's disease. Thus, patients with Down's syndrome over the age of 30 almost invariably have

Alzheimer-type neuropathological changes in the cerebral cortex and are frequently demented (see Wisniewski et al., 1985). Cases of Down's syndrome also have a cortical ChAT deficit (Yates et al., 1980) and a loss of neurons in the nucleus of Meynert (Mann et al., 1984a). This clinical, neuropathological and neurochemical link between Down's syndrome and Alzheimer's disease suggests that chromosome 21 may be involved in the disease process. It is clear that genetic linkage analysis combined with recombinant DNA technology may allow localisation and sequencing of the defective gene(s) in Alzheimer's disease by studying familial cases of the disease and also patients with Down's syndrome. Such an approach has been successfully utilised in Huntington's disease where the defective gene has been mapped to chromosome 4 (Gusella et al., 1983). A gene defect in Alzheimer's disease may lead to increased susceptibility to infectious agents (e.g. Scrapie), environmental factors (e.g. aluminium) or altered production of enzymes or neuronotrophic factors.

While there is no convincing evidence for the involvement of an infectious agent, there are a number of lines of evidence that aluminium may be involved in Alzheimer's disease. Thus, increased levels of aluminium have been reported in the brain in Alzheimer's disease (Crapper et al., 1973, 1976) and, in animals, aluminium induces neurofibrillary tangles (Klatzo et al., 1965; Terry and Pena, 1965) and produces cognitive deficits (Crapper, 1976; Petit et al., 1980) in susceptible species. Moreover, aluminium has been implicated in the Parkinsonian-dementia complex of Guam (Garruto et al., 1984), in which there is also a profound loss of neurons from the nucleus of Meynert (Nakano and Hirano, 1983). Recently, electron microprobe energy-dispersive X-ray microanalysis has demonstrated that silicon and aluminium are present in high levels and are focally co-localised in the centre of isolated cortical senile plaque cores and in senile plaque cores in cortical tissue sections in patients with Alzheimer's disease and in elderly normal patients (Fig. 5; Candy et al., 1984b, 1985c). The coincident distribution of silicon and aluminium

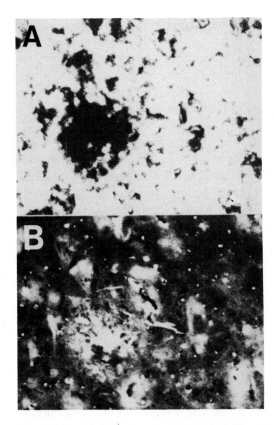

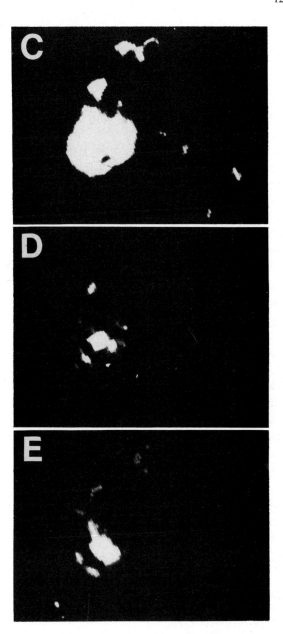

Fig. 5 (A–E). Demonstration of aluminium and silicon in senile plaque cores in situ in the cerebral cortex in Alzheimer's disease. 20-μm) cryostat sections were cut from blocks of formalin-fixed frontal and temporal cortex and silver stained as free floating sections. The stained sections were mounted on melinex (ICI) by drying and then carbon coated. (A) shows the prominent appearance in the frontal cortex of a senile plaque with a silver-stained core light microscopy; (B) shows the scanning electron microscope appearance of the same area shown in (A), the senile plaque cores could be easily discerned by their luminescent appearance; (C) shows the digimap distribution of silver in the area shown in (A), after background subtraction. The silver-stained plaque core is readily seen. (D) and (E) show the digimap distribution of silicon and aluminium, respectively, in the same area, and demonstrate a coincident distribution of silicon and aluminium within the senile plaque core. All the micrographs are at the same magnification.

suggests that these elements may be present as aluminosilicates and this has been confirmed using high-resolution NMR techniques on isolated senile plaque core material (Candy et al., 1986). This raises the possibility that focal formation of an aluminosilicate may be the pathological stimulus that initiates senile plaque formation and affects cholinergic processes with their consequent degen-

eration, (see section of cortical distribution of choline acetyltransferase and acetylcholinesterase).

Neuronal death during neurogenesis is a widespread phenomenon in the CNS and can involve in some nuclei up to 75% of the total neuronal population (see Cowan et al., 1984). A limited supply of specific neuronotrophic factors in the neuronal target tissue provides a possible explanation for this phenomenon (Cowan et al., 1984). It has been observed that lack of a neuronotrophic factor while sparing the neuronal perikarya may selectively eliminate neuronal processes (Campenot, 1977). In the light of these findings it is conceivable that a deficit in specific neuronotrophic factors may be responsible for selective neuronal loss or loss of particular neuronal afferents in neurodegenerative disorders. With respect to the cholinergic system, a number of neuronotrophic factors have been reported that are obligatory for the survival and growth of cholinergic neurons in vitro (Varon and Bunge, 1978; Barde et al., 1982). Moreover, the cortical cholinergic afferents in animals appear to demonstrate a remarkable plasticity after lesions of the nucleus of Meynert (Pedata et al., 1982; Wenk and Olton, 1984), that may be dependent on such factors. An attractive hypothesis based on these findings is that neuronotrophic factors, associated with the cortical cholinergic system, may be selectively reduced or lost in the nucleus of Meynert or cerebral cortex in Alzheimer's disease and Parkinson's disease (Appel, 1981). Such a hypothesis could then explain the differential loss of neurons in the nucleus of Meynert in Alzheimer's and Parkinson's diseases. While preliminary experiments using a neuroblastoma cell line (IMR 32) show that crude cortical extracts have the same ability as those from normal brain to stimulate the activities of both ChAT and AChE (Perry et al., unpublished), it is unlikely that the hypothesis can be adequately tested until brain cholinergic neuronotrophic factors have been identified and their roles defined.

Overview of the current status

An involvement of cholinergic projections to the cerebral cortex in both Alzheimer's and Parkinson's dementia is now widely supported by direct neurochemical and neuropathological investigations of the human brain and indirectly by psychopharmacological and, to a lesser extent, neurophysiological studies. The extent to which the cholinergic deficit may be amenable to some form of therapy — at least in the early stages of dementia — depends on future research aimed at establishing in more detail the status of the cortical cholinergic receptors; at developing novel cholinergic agonists and, more fundamentally, discovering to what extent the cholinergic as opposed to other transmitter systems, also affected in these dementing disorders, is associated with the earlier cognitive symptoms and the pathogenic mechanisms which lead to the neurochemical changes.

Acknowledgement

The authors are grateful to Mrs. D. Hinds for expert secretarial assistance.

References

Amaducci, L., Sorbi, S., Albanese, A. and Gainotti, G. (1981) Choline acetyltransferase (ChAT) activity differs in right and left human temporal lobe. Neurology, 31: 799–805.

Appel, S. H. (1981) A unifying hypothesis for the cause of amyotrophic lateral sclerosis, Parkinsonism and Alzheimer disease. Ann. Neurol., 10: 499–505.

Arendt, T., Bigl, V., Arendt, A. and Tennstedt, A. (1983) Loss of neurons in the nucleus basalis of Meynert in Alzheimer's disease, paralysis agitans and Korsakoff's disease. Acta Neuropathol., 61: 101–108.

Arendt, T., Bigl, V., Tennstedt, A. and Arendt, A. (1984) Correlation between cortical plaque count and neuronal loss in the nucleus basalis in Alzheimer's disease. Neurosci. Lett., 48: 81–85.

Armstrong, D. M., LeRoy, S., Shields, D. and Terry, R. D. (1985) Somatostatin-like immunoreactivity within neuritic plaques. Brain Res., 338: 71–79.

Atack, J. R., Perry, E. K., Bonham, J. R., Perry, R. H., Tomlinson, B. E., Blessed, G. and Fairbairn, A. (1983) Molecular forms of acetylcholinesterase in senile dementia of Alzheimer-type: selective loss of the intermediate (10S) form. Neurosci. Lett., 40: 199–204.

Barde, Y. A., Edgar, D. and Thoenen, H. (1982) New neurotrophic factors. Ann. Rev. Physiol., 45: 601–612.

Bartolini, A. and Pepeu, G. (1967) Investigations into the acetylcholine output from the cerebral cortex of the cat in the presence of hyoscine. Br. J. Pharmacol. Chemother., 31: 66–73.

Bartus, R. T. (1978) Evidence for a direct cholinergic involvement in the scopolamine-induced amnesia in monkeys: effects of concurrent administration of physostigmine and methylphenidate with scopolamine. *Pharmacol. Biochem. Behav.*, 9: 833–836.

Bartus, R. T. (1979) Physostigmine and recent memory: effects in young and aged nonhuman primates. *Science*, 206: 1087–1089.

Bartus, R. T. and Johnson, H. R. (1976) Short-term memory in the rhesus monkey: disruption from the anti-cholinergic scopolamine. *Pharmacol. Biochem. Behav.*, 5: 39–46.

Bartus, R. T., Fleming, D. and Johnson, H. R. (1978) Aging in the rhesus monkey: debilitating effects on short-term memory. *J. Gerontol.*, 33: 858–871.

Bartus, R. T., Dean, R. L. and Beer, B. (1980) Memory deficits in aged Cebus monkeys and facilitation with central cholinomimetics. *Neurobiol. Aging*, 1: 145–152.

Bartus, R. T., Dean, R. L., Beer, B. and Lippa, A. S. (1982) The cholinergic hypothesis of geriatric memory dysfunction. *Science*, 217: 408–417.

Beani, L., Bianchi, C., Santinoceto, L. and Marchetti, P. (1968) The cerebral acetylcholine release in conscious rabbits with semi-permanently implanted epideral cups. *Int. J. Neuropharmacol.*, 7: 469–481.

Belesin, D., Polak, R. L. and Sproull, D. H. (1965) The release of acetylcholine into the cerebral subarachnoid space of anaesthetised cats. *J. Physiol.*, 177: 420–428.

Berger, H. (1932) Uber das Elektroenkephalogramm des Menschen. Fünfte Mitteilung. *Arch. Psychiat. Nervenkr.*, 98: 231–254.

Berridge, M. J. and Irvine, R. F. (1984) Inositol trisphosphate, a novel second messenger in cellular signal transduction. *Nature*, 312: 315–321.

Berrie, C. P., Birdsall, N. J., Burgen, A. S. and Hulme, E. C. (1979) Guanine nucleotide modulate muscarinic receptor binding in the heart. *Biochem. Biophys. Res. Commun.*, 87: 1000–1005.

Berrie, C. P., Birdsall, N. J., Hulme, E. C., Keen, M. and Stockton, J. M. (1985) Solubilisation and characterisation of high and low affinity pirenzapine binding sites from rat cerebral cortex. *Br. J. Pharmacol.*, 85: 697–703.

Bird, T. D., Stanahan, S., Sumi, S. M. and Raskind, M. (1983) Alzheimer's disease: choline acetyltransferase activity in brain tissue from clinical and pathological subgroups. *Ann. Neurol.*, 14: 284–293.

Birdsall, N. J., Burgen, A. S. and Hulme, E. C. (1978) The binding of agonists to brain muscarinic receptors. *Mol. Pharmacol.*, 14: 723–736.

Birdsall, N. J., Hulme, E. C. and Burgen, A. S. (1980) The character of the muscarinic receptors in different regions of the rat brain. *Proc. Roy. Soc. Lond. (Biol.)*, 207: 1–12.

Birdsall, N. J., Hulme, E. C. and Stockton, J. M. (1984) Muscarinic receptor heterogeneity. *Trends Pharmacol. Sci.*, Suppl. 4–8.

Boller, F., Mizutani, T., Roessmann, U. and Gambetti, P. (1980) Parkinson's disease, dementia and Alzheimer's disease — clinicopathological correlations. *Ann. Neurol.*, 7: 329–335.

Bonnet, V. and Bremer, R. (1937) Action du potassium, et de l'acétylcholine sur les activités électriques, spontanées et provoquées, de l'écorce cérébrale. *C. R. Soc. Biol.*, 126: 1271–1275.

Bowen, D. M. and Davison, A. N. (1975) Extrapyramidal diseases and dementia. *Lancet*, 1: 1199–1200.

Bowen, D. M., White, P., Spillane, J. A., Goodhardt, M. J., Curzon, G., Iwangoff, P., Meier-Ruge, W. and Davison, A. N. (1979) Accelerated aging or selective neuron loss as an important cause of dementia? *Lancet*, 1: 11–14.

Bowen, D. M., Benton, J. S., Spillane, J. A., Smith, C. C. and Allen, S. J. (1982) Choline acetyltransferase activity and histopathology of frontal neocortex from biopsies of demented patients. *J. Neurol. Sci.*, 57: 191–202.

Bradley, P. B. and Elkes, J. (1957) The effects of some drugs on the electrical activity of the brain. *Brain*, 80: 77–117.

Breitner, J. C. and Folstein, M. F. (1984) Familial Alzheimer dementia: a prevalent disorder with specific clinical features. *Psychiatry Med.*, 14: 63–80.

Brown, D. A. (1983) Slow cholinergic excitation — a mechanism for increasing neuronal excitability. *Trends Neurosci.*, 6: 302–307.

Brown, D. A. and Fumagalli, L. (1977) Dissociation of bungarotoxin binding and receptor block in the rat superior cervical ganglion. *Brain Res.*, 129: 165–168.

Burt, A. M. (1970) A histochemical procedure for the localisation of choline acetyltransferase activity. *J. Histochem. Cytochem.*, 18: 408–415.

Campenot, R. B. (1977) Local control of neurite development by nerve growth factor. *Proc. Natl. Acad. Sci. USA*, 74: 4516–4519.

Candy, J. M., Perry, R. H., Perry, E. K. and Thompson, J. E. (1981) Distribution of putative cholinergic cell bodies and various neuropeptides in the substantia innominata region of the human brain. *J. Anat.*, 133: 123–124.

Candy, J. M., Perry, R. H., Perry, E. K., Irving, D., Blessed, G., Fairbairn, A. F. and Tomlinson, B. E. (1983) Pathological changes in the nucleus of Meynert in Alzheimer's and Parkinson's diseases. *J. Neurol. Sci.*, 59: 277–289.

Candy, J. M., Court, J. A., Perry, R. H. and Smith, C. J. (1984a) Carbachol-stimulated phosphatidylinositol hydrolysis in the cerebral cortex after freezing and post mortem delay. *Br. J. Pharmacol.*, 83: 356P.

Candy, J. M., Oakley, A. E., Atack, J., Perry, R. H., Perry, E. K. and Edwardson, J. A. (1984b) New observations on the nature of senile plaque cores. In E. S. Vizi and K. Magyar (Eds.), *Regulation of Transmitter Function: Basic and Clinical Aspects, Proceedings of the 5th Meeting European Society of Neurochemistry*, Akademiai Kiado, Budapest, pp. 301–304.

Candy, J. M., Court, J. A. and Smith, C. J. (1985a) Enhancement of the phosphatidylinositol response by raised extracellular potassium in rat cerebral cortex. *Br. J. Pharmacol.*, 84: 61P.

Candy, J. M., Court, J. A. and Hoban, R. P. (1985b) Role of M_1 muscarinic receptors in K^+ facilitation of phosphatidyl-inositol hydrolysis. *Br. J. Pharmacol.*, 86: 607.

Candy, J. M., Edwardson, J. A., Klinowski, J., Oakley, A. E., Perry, E. K. and Perry, R. H. (1985c) Co-localisation of aluminium and silicon in senile plaques: implications for the neurochemical pathology of Alzheimer's disease. In J. Traber and W. H. Gispen (Eds.) *Senile Dementia of the Alzheimer Type. Early Diagnosis, Neuropathology and Animal Models*, Springer–Verlag, Berlin, pp. 183–197.

Candy, J. M., Perry, E. K., Perry, R. H., Bloxham, C. A., Thompson, J., Johnson, M., Oakley, A. E. and Edwardson, J. A. (1985d) Evidence for the early prenatal development of cortical cholinergic afferents from the nucleus of Meynert in the human foetus. *Neurosci. Lett.*, 61: 91–95.

Candy, J. M., Oakley A. E., Kliniowski, T., Carpenter , T. T., Perry, R. H., Atack, R. R., Perry, E. K., Blessed, G., Fairbairn, A. and Edwardson, J. A., (1986) Aluminosilicates and senile plaque formation in Alzheimer's disease, *Lancet*, 1: 354–357.

Carbonetto, S. T., Fambrough, D. M. and Muller, K. J. (1978) Nonequivalence of α-bungarotoxin receptors and acetylcho-line receptors in check sympathetic neurons. *Proc. Natl. Acad. Sci. USA*, 75: 1016–1020.

Caulfield, M. P., Straughan, D. W., Cross, A. J., Crow, T. and Birdsall, N. J. (1982) Cortical muscarinic receptor subtypes and Alzheimer's disease. *Lancet*, 2: 1277.

Celesia, G. G. and Jasper, H. H. (1966) Acetylcholine released from cerebral cortex in relation to state of activation. *Neurology*, 16: 1053–1063.

Christie, J. E., Shering, A., Ferguson, J. and Glen, A. I. (1981) Physostigmine and arecoline: Effect of intravenous infusions in Alzheimer presenile dementia. *Br. J. Psychiat.*, 138: 46–50.

Clarke, P. B., Pert, C. B. and Pert, A. (1984) Autoradiographic distribution of nicotine receptors in rat brain. *Brain Res.*, 323: 390–395.

Coben, L. A., Danziger, W. L. and Berg, L. (1983) Frequency analysis of the resting awake EEG in mild senile dementia of Alzheimer type. *Electroencephalogr. Clin. Neurophysiol.*, 55: 372–380.

Collier, B. and Mitchell, J. F. (1967) The central release of acetylcholine during consciousness and after brain lesion. *J. Physiol.*, 188: 83–98.

Costa, L. G. and Murphy, S. D. (1983) [^{3}H]nicotine binding in rat brain: alteration after chronic acetylcholinesterase inhibi-tion. *J. Pharmacol. Exp. Ther.*, 226: 392–397.

Court, J. A., Fowler, C. T., Candy, J. N., Hoban, P. R. and Smith C. T., (1986) Raising the ambient potassium ion concentration enhances carbachol stimulated phosphoinositide hydrolysis in rat brain hippocampal and cerebral cortical miniprisms. *Naunyn-Schmiedebergs's Arch. Pharmacol.*, in press.

Cowan, W. N., Fawcett, J. W., O'Leary, D. D. and Brent, B. B. (1984) Regressive events in neurogenesis. *Science*, 225: 1258–1265.

Crapper, D. R. (1976) Functional consequences of neurofibril-lary degeneration. In R. D. Terry and S. Gershon (Eds.), *Neurobiology of Aging*, Raven Press, New York, pp. 405–432.

Crapper, D. R., Krishman, S. S. and Dalton, A. J. (1973) Brain aluminium distribution in Alzheimer's disease and experi-mental neurofibrillary degeneration. *Science*, 180: 511–513.

Crapper, D. R., Krishman, S. S. and Quittkat, S. (1976) Aluminium, neurofibrillary degeneration and Alzheimer's disease. *Brain*, 99: 67–80.

Cross, A. J., Crow, T. J., Johnson, J. A., Joseph, M. H., Perry, E. K., Perry, R. H., Blessed, G. and Tomlinson, B. E. (1983) Monoamine metabolism in senile dementia of Alzheimer type. *J. Neurol. Sci.*, 60: 383–392.

D'Alecy, L. G. and Rose, C. J. (1977) Parasympathetic cholinergic control of cerebral blood flow in dogs. *Circ. Res.*, 41: 324–331.

Davies, P. (1979) Neurotransmitter related enzymes in senile dementia of the Alzheimer type. *Brain Res.*, 171: 319–327.

Davies, P. and Maloney, A. J. (1976) Selective loss of cholinergic neurons in Alzheimer's disease. *Lancet*, 2: 1403.

Davies, P. and Verth, A. H. (1977) Regional distribution of muscarinic acetylcholine receptors in normal and Alzheimer's type dementia brains. *Brain Res.*, 138: 385–392.

Davies, P. and Feisullin, S. (1981) Postmortem stability of α-bungarotoxin binding sites in mouse and human brain. *Brain Res.*, 216: 449–454.

Davies, P., Katzman, R. and Terry, R. D. (1980) Reduced somatostatin-like immunoreactivity in cerebral cortex from cases of Alzheimer's disease and Alzheimer senile dementia. *Nature*, 288: 279–280.

Davis, K. L., Mohs, R. C., Tinklenberg, J. R., Pfefferbaum, A., Hollister, L. E. and Kopell, B. S. (1978) Physostigmine improvement of long-term memory processes in normal humans. *Science*, 201: 272–274.

Davis, K. L., Mohs, R. C. and Tinklenberg, J. R. (1979) Enhancement of memory by physostigmine. *New Engl. J. Med.*, 301: 946.

Deutsch, J. A. (1973) The cholinergic synapse and the site of memory. In J. A. Deutsch (Ed.), *The Physiological Basis of Memory*, Academic Press, New York, pp. 59–74.

Divac, I. (1975) Magnocellular nuclei of the basal forebrain project to neocortex, brainstem and olfactory bulb — a review of some functional correlates. *Brain Res.*, 93: 385–398.

Dodd, J. and Horn, J. P. (1983) Muscarinic inhibition of sympathetic neurones in the bullfrog. *J. Physiol.*, 334: 271–291.

Drachman, D. A. and Leavitt, J. (1974) Human memory and the cholinergic system. *Arch. Neurol.*, 30: 113–121.

Drachman, D. A. and Stahl, S. (1975) Extrapyramidal dementia and levodopa. *Lancet*, 1: 809.

Drachman, D. A. and Sahakian, B. J. (1980) Memory and cognitive function in the elderly: a preliminary trial of physostigmine. *Arch. Neurol.*, 37: 674–675.

Drachman, D. A., Noffsinger, D., Sahakian, B. J., Kurzdiel, S.

and Fleming, P. (1980) Aging, memory, and the cholinergic system: a study of dichotic listening. *Neurobiol. Aging*, 1: 39–43.

Duffy, F. H., Albert, M. S. and McAnulty, G. (1984) Brain electrical activity in patients with presenile and senile dementia of the Alzheimer type. *Ann. Neurol.*, 16: 439–448.

Duggan, A. W., Hall, J. G. and Lee, C. Y. (1976) Alpha-bungarotoxin, cobra neurotoxin, and excitation of Renshaw cells by acetylcholine. *Brain Res.*, 107: 166–170.

England, A. C., Schwab, R. S. and Peterson, E. (1959) The electroencephalogram in Parkinson's syndrome. *EEG Clin. Neurophysiol.*, 11: 723–731.

Estrada, C. and Krause, D. N. (1982) Muscarinic cholinergic receptor sites in cerebral blood vessels. *J. Pharmacol. Exp. Ther.*, 221: 85–90.

Estrada, C., Hamel, E. and Krause, D. N. (1983) Biochemical evidence for cholinergic innervation of intracerebral blood vessels. *Brain Res.*, 266: 261–270.

Friede, R. L. (1965) Enzyme histochemical studies of senile plaques. *J. Neuropathol. Exp. Neurol.*, 24: 477–491.

Gahwiler, B. H. and Brown, D. A. (1985) Functional innervation of cultured hippocampal neurons by cholinergic afferents from co-cultured septal explants. *Nature*, 313: 577–579.

Garruto, R. M., Fukatsu, R., Yanagihara, R., Gajdusek, D. C., Hook, G. and Fiori, C. E. (1984) Imaging of calcium and aluminium in neurofibrillary tangle bearing neurones in Parkinsonian-dementia of Guam. *Proc. Natl. Acad. Sci. USA*, 81: 1875–1879.

Garvey, J. M., Rossor, M. and Iversen, L. L. (1984) Evidence for multiple muscarinic receptor subtypes in human brain. *J. Neurochem.*, 43: 299–302.

Gonzales, R. A. and Crews, F. T. (1984) Characterization of the cholinergic stimulation of phosphoinositide hydrolysis in rat brain slices. *J. Neurosci.*, 4: 3120–3127.

Gordon, E. B. and Sim, M. (1967) The EEG in presenile dementia. *J. Neurol. Neurosurg. Psychiat.*, 30: 285–291.

Gorry, J. D. (1963) Studies on the comparative anatomy of the ganglion basale of Meynert. *Acta Anat.*, 55: 51–104.

Grammas, P., Diglio, C. A., Marks, B. H., Giacomelli, F. and Weiner, J. (1983) Identification of muscarinic receptors in rat cerebral cortical microvessels. *J. Neurochem.*, 40: 645–651.

Green, J. R., Halpern, L. M. and Van Niel, S. (1970) Choline acetylase and acetylcholine-esterase changes in chronic isolated cerebral cortex of cat. *Life Sci.*, 9: 481–488.

Gusella, J. F., Wexler, N. S., Conneally, P. M., Naylor, S. L., Anderson, M. A., Tanzi, R. E., Watkins, P. C., Ottina, K., Wallace, M. R., Sakaguchi, A. Y., Young, A. B., Shoulson, I., Bonilla, E. and Martin, J. B. (1983) A polymorphic DNA marker genetically linked to Huntington's disease. *Nature*, 306: 234–238.

Hakim, A. M. and Mathieson, G. (1979) Dementia in Parkinson's disease — A neuropathologic study. *Neurology*, 29: 1209–1214.

Hammer, R. (1982) Subclasses of muscarinic receptors and pirenzapine: further experimental evidence. *Scand. J. Gastroenterol.*, 17, Suppl. 72: 59–67.

Hammer, R. and Giachetti, A. (1982) Muscarinic receptor subtypes M_1 and M_2. Biochemical and functional characterisation. *Life Sci.*, 31: 2991–2998.

Hammer, R., Berrie, C. P., Birdsall, N. J., Burgen, A. S. and Hulme, E. C. (1980) Pirenzapine distinguishes between different subclasses of muscarinic receptors. *Nature*, 283: 90–92.

Hanley, M. R. and Iversen, L. L. (1978) Muscarinic cholinergic receptors in rat corpus striatum and regulation of guanosine 3',5'-cyclic monophosphate. *Mol. Pharmacol.*, 14: 246–255.

Hartman, B. K., Swanson, L. W., Raichle, M. E., Preskorn, S. H. and Clark, H. B. (1980) Central adrenergic regulation of cerebral microvascular permeability and blood flow; anatomic and physiologic evidence. *Adv. Exp. Med. Biol.*, 131: 113–126.

Hartzell, H. C., Kuffler, S. W., Stickgold, R. and Yoshikami, D. (1977) Synaptic excitation and inhibition resulting from direct action of acetylcholine on two types of chemoreceptors on individual amphibian parasympathetic neurones. *J. Physiol.*, 271: 817–846.

Hassler, R. (1938) Zur Pathologie der Paralysis agitans und des postenzephalitischen Parkinsonismus. *J. Psychol. Neurol.*, 48: 387.

Hebb, C. O. and Silver, A. (1956) Choline acetylase in the central nervous system of man and some other mammals. *J. Physiol.*, 134: 718–728.

Hebb, C. O., Krnjevic, K. and Silver, A. (1963) Effect of undercutting on the acetylcholinesterase and choline acetyltransferase activity in the cat's cerebral cortex. *Nature*, 198: 692.

Heistad, D. D., Marcus, M. L., Said, S. I. and Gross, P. M. (1980) Effect of acetylcholine and vasoactive intestinal peptide on cerebral blood flow. *Am. J. Physiol.*, 239: H73–H80.

Heston, L. L., Master, A. R., Anderson, V. E. and White, J. (1981) Dementia of the Alzheimer type: clinical genetics, natural history and associated conditions. *Arch. Gen. Psychiat.*, 38: 1085–1090.

Houser, C. R., Crawford, G. D., Barber, R. P., Salvaterra, P. M. and Vaughn, J. E. (1983) Organisation and morphological characteristics of cholinergic neurons: an immunocytochemical study with a monoclonal antibody to choline acetyltransferase. *Brain Res.*, 266: 97–119.

Huther, G. and Luppa, H. (1979) The multiple forms of brain acetylcholinesterase. *Histochemistry*, 63: 115–121.

Ingvar, D. H., Brun, A., Hagberg, B. and Gustafson, L. (1978) Regional cerebral blood flow in the dominant hemisphere in confirmed cases of Alzheimer's disease, Pick's disease and multi-infarct dementia: relationship to clinical symptomatology and neuropathological findings. In R. Katzman, R. D. Terry and K. L. Bick (Eds.), *Alzheimer's Disease, Senile*

126

Dementia and Related Disorders, Ageing, Vol. 7, Raven Press, New York, pp. 203–211.

Jasper, H. H. and Koyama, I. (1969) Rate of release of amino acids from the cerebral cortex in the cat as affected by brain stem and thalamic stimulation. *Can. J. Physiol. Pharmacol.*, 47: 889–905.

Johannesson, G., Hagberg, B., Gustafson, L. and Ingvar, D. H. (1979) EEG and cognitive impairment in presenile dementia. *Acta Neurol. Scand.*, 59: 225–240.

Johnston, M. V., McKinney, M. and Coyle, J. T. (1979) Evidence for a cholinergic projection to neocortex from neurones in the basal forebrain. *Proc. Natl. Acad. Sci. USA*, 76: 5392–5396.

Johnston, M. V., McKinney, M. and Coyle, J. T. (1981) Neocortical cholinergic innervation: a description of extrinsic and intrinsic components into rat. *Exp. Brain Res.*, 43: 159–172.

Jones, E. G., Burton, H., Saper, C. B. and Swanson, L. W. (1976) Midbrain, diencephalic and cortical relationships of the basal nucleus of Meynert and associated structures in primates. *J. Comp. Neurol.*, 167: 385–420.

Kanai, T. and Szerb, J. C. (1965) Mesencephalic reticular activating system and cortical acetylcholine output. *Nature*, 205: 80–82.

Kasa, P., Mann, S. P. and Hebb, C. (1970) Localisation of choline acetyltransferase. *Nature*, 226: 812–816.

Kievet, J. and Kuypers, H. G. (1975) Basal forebrain and hypothalamic connections to the frontal and parietal cortex in the Rhesus monkey. *Science*, 187: 660–662.

Kimura, H., McGeer, P. L., Peng, J. H. and McGeer, E. G. (1981) The central cholinergic system studied by choline acetyltransferase immunocytochemistry in the cat. *J. Comp. Neurol.*, 200: 151–201.

Kitt, C. A., Price, D. L., Struble, R. G., Cork, L. C., Wainer, B. H., Becher, M. W. and Mobley, W. C. (1984) Evidence for cholinergic neurites in senile plaques. *Science*, 226: 1443–1444.

Klatzo, I., Wisniewski, H. and Streicher, E. (1965) Experimental production of neurofibrillary degeneration. *J. Neuropathol. Exp. Neurol.*, 24: 187–199.

Krnjevic, K. and Phillis, J. W. (1963a) Acetylcholine-sensitive cells in the cerebral cortex. *J. Physiol.*, 166: 296–327.

Krnjevic, K. and Phillis, J. W. (1963b) Pharmacological properties of acetylcholine-sensitive cells in the cerebral cortex. *J. Physiol.*, 166: 328–350.

Krnjevic, K. and Silver, A. (1965) A histochemical study of cholinergic fibres in the cerebral cortex. *J. Anat.*, 99: 711–759.

Krnjevic, K., Pumain, R. and Renaud, L. (1971) The mechanism of excitation by acetylcholine in the cerebral cortex. *J. Physiol.*, 215: 247–268.

Larsson, T., Sjögren, T. and Jacobson, G. (1963) A clinical, sociomedical and genetic study. *Acta Psychiat. Scand.*, Suppl. 167: 1–259.

Lehmann, J., Nagy, J. T., Atmadja, S. and Fibiger, H. C. (1980) The nucleus basalis magnocellularis: the origin of a cholinergic project to the neocortex of the rat. *Neuroscience*, 5: 1161–1174.

Lehmann, J., Struble, R. G., Antuono, P. G., Coyle, J. T., Cork, L. C. and Price, D. L. (1984) Regional heterogeneity of choline acetyltransferase activity in primate neocortex. *Brain Res.*, 322: 361–364.

Letemendia, F. and Pampiglione, G. (1958) Clinical and electroencephalographic observations in Alzheimer's disease. *J. Neurol. Neurosurg. Psychiat.*, 21: 167–172.

Lo Conte, G., Casamenti, F., Bigl, V., Milaneschi, E. and Pepeu, G. (1982) Effect of magnocellular forebrain nuclei lesions on acetylcholine output from the cerebral cortex, electrocorticogram and behaviour. *Arch. Ital. Biol.*, 120: 176–188.

Longo, V. G. (1966) Behavioural and electroencephalographic effects of atropine and related compounds. *Pharmacol. Rev.*, 18, 965–996.

Luthin, G. R. and Wolfe, B. B. (1984) Comparison of ^{3}H-pirenzapine and ^{3}H-quinuclidinyl-benzilate binding to muscarinic cholinergic receptors in rat brains. *J. Pharmacol. Exp. Ther.*, 228: 648–655.

Mann, D. M. and Yates, P. O. (1982) Is the loss of cerebral choline acetyltransferase activity in Alzheimer's disease due to degeneration of ascending cholinergic nerve cells? *J. Neurol. Neurosurg. Psychiat.*, 45: 936.

Mann, D. M. and Yates, P. O. (1983) Pathological basis for neurotransmitter changes in Parkinson's disease. *Neuropathol. Appl. Neurobiol.*, 9: 3–19.

Mann, D. M., Yates, P. O. and Marcyniuk, B. (1984a) Alzheimer's presenile dementia, senile dementia of Alzheimer type and Down's syndrome form an age-related continuum of pathological changes. *Neuropathol. Appl. Neurobiol.*, 10: 185–207.

Mann, D. M., Yates, P. O. and Marcyniuk, B. (1984b) A comparison of changes in the nucleus basalis and locus coeruleus in Alzheimer's disease. *J. Neurol. Neurosurg. Psychiat.*, 47: 201–203.

Mann, D. M., Yates, P. O. and Marcyniuk, B. (1985) Correlation between senile plaque and neurofibrillary tangle counts in cerebral cortex and neuronal counts in cortex and subcortical structures in Alzheimer's disease. *Neurosci. Lett.*, 56: 51–55.

Marks, M. J. and Collins, A. C. (1982) Characterization of nicotine binding in mouse brain and comparison with the binding of α-bungarotoxin and quinuclidinyl benzilate. *Mol. Pharmacol.*, 22: 554–564.

Marsden, C. D. (1982) Basal ganglia disease. *Lancet*, 2: 1141–1147.

Martin, B. R. and Aceto, M. D. (1981) Nicotine binding sites and their localization in the central nervous system. *Neurosci. Behav. Rev.*, 5: 473–478.

Mash, D. C., Flynn, D. D. and Potter, L. T. (1985) Loss of M_2 muscarinic receptors in the cerebral cortex in Alzheimer's disease and experimental cholinergic denervation. *Science*, 228: 1115–1117.

Massoulie, J. and Bon, S. (1982) The molecular forms of cholinesterase and acetylcholinesterase in vertebrates. *Ann. Rev. Neurosci.*, 5: 57–106.

McKhann, G., Drachman, D., Folstein, M., Katzman, R., Price, D. and Stadlan, E. (1984) Clinical diagnosis of Alzheimer's disease: report of the NINCDS-ADRDA work group under the auspices of Department of Health and Human Services Task Force on Alzheimer's disease. *Neurology*, 34: 939–944.

McKinney, M. and Coyle, J. T. (1982) Regulation of neocortical muscarinic receptors: effects of drug treatment and lesions. *J. Neurosci.*, 2: 97–105.

McQuarrie, C., Salvaterra, P. M., De Blas, A., Routes, J. and Mahler, H. R. (1976) Studies on nicotinic acetylcholine receptors in mammalian: preliminary characterization of membrane bound α-bungarotoxin receptors in rat cerebral cortex. *J. Biol. Chem.*, 251: 6335–6339.

Mesulam, M.-M., and Van Hoesen (1976) Acetylcholinesterase-rich projections from the basal forebrain of the Rhesus monkey to neocortex. *Brain Res.*, 109: 152–157.

Mesulam, M.-M., Mufson, C. J., Levey, A. I. and Wainer, B. H. (1983) Cholinergic innervation of cortex by the basal forebrain: cytochemistry and cortical connections of the septal area, diagonal bound nuclei, nucleus basalis (substantia innominata) and hypothalamus in the Rhesus monkey. *J. Comp. Neurol.*, 214: 170–197.

Mesulam, M.-M., Rosen, A. D. and Mufson, E. J. (1984) Regional variations in cortical cholinergic innervation: chemoarchitectonics of acetylcholinesterase-containing fibres in the Macaque brain. *Brain Res.*, 311: 245–258.

Mitchell, J. F. (1963) The spontaneous and evoked release of acetylcholine from the cerebral cortex. *J. Physiol.*, 165: 98–116.

Mitchell, R. H. (1975) Inositol phospholipids and cell surface receptor function. *Biochem. Biophys. Acta*, 415: 81–147.

Mitchell, R. H. (1980) Muscarinic acetylcholine receptors. In D. Schulster and A. Levitzki (Eds.), *Cellular Receptors for Hormones and Neurotransmitters*, John Wiley and Sons Ltd, London, pp. 353–368.

Monnier, M. and Romanowski, W. (1962) Les systèmes cholinoceptifs cérébraux — actions de l'acétylcholine, de la physostigmine, pilocarpine et de GABA. *Electroencephalogr. Clin. Neurophysiol.*, 14: 486–500.

Morrison, J. H., Roger, J., Scherr, S., Benoit, R. and Bloom, F. E. (1984) Somatostatin immunoreactivity in neuritic plaques of Alzheimer patients. *Nature*, 314: 90–92.

Mortimer, J. A., Christensen, K. J. and Webster, D. D. (1985) Parkinsonian dementia. In P. J. Vinken, G. W. Bruyn and H. L. Klawans (Eds.), *Neurobehavioural Disorders, Handbook of Clinical Neurology, Vol. 46*, Elsevier, Amsterdam, pp. 371–384.

Muller, H. F. (1978) The electroencephalogram in senile dementia. In K. Nandy (Ed.), *Senile Dementia: a Biomedical Approach*, Elsevier/North Holland Biomedical Press, New York, pp. 237–250.

Nagai, T., McGeer, P. L., Peng, J. H., McGeer, E. G. and Dolman, C. E. (1983) Choline acetyltransferase immunohistochemistry in brains of Alzheimer's disease patients and controls. *Neurosci. Lett.*, 36: 195–199.

Nakano, I. and Hirano, A. (1983) Neuron loss in the nucleus basalis of Meynert in Parkinsonism dementia complex of *Guam. Ann. Neurol.*, 13: 87–91.

Nordberg, A., Adolfson, R., Aquilonius, S. -M., Marklund, S., Oreland, L. and Winblad, B. (1980) Brain enzymes and acetylcholine receptors in dementia of Alzheimer type and chronic alcohol abuse. In L. Amaducci, A. N. Davison and P. Anatuono (Eds.), *Aging of the Brain and Dementia, Aging, Vol. 13*, Raven Press, New York, pp. 169–171.

North, R. A. and Tokimasa, T. (1984) Muscarinic suppression of calcium-activated potassium conductance. *Trends Pharmacol. Sci.*, Suppl: 35–38.

Okinaka, S., Toshikawa, M., Uono, M., Muro, T., Mozai, T., Iqata, A., Tanabe, H., Ueda, S. and Tomonaga, M. (1961) Distribution of cholinesterase activity in the human cerebral cortex. *Am. J. Physiol. Med.*, 40: 135–146.

Parnavelas, J. G., Kelly, W. and Burnstock, G. (1985) Ultrastructural localization of choline acetyltransferase in vascular endothelial cells in rat brain. *Nature*, 316: 724–725.

Pearson, R. C., Gatter, K. C. and Powell, T. P. (1983a) The cortical relationships of certain basal ganglia and the cholinergic basal forebrain nuclei. *Brain Res.*, 261: 327–330.

Pearson, R. C., Gatter, K. C., Brodal, P. and Powell, T. P. (1983b) The projection of the basal nucleus of Meynert upon the neocortex in the monkey. *Brain Res.*, 259: 132–136.

Pearson, R. C., Sofroniew, M. V., Cuello, A. C., Powell, T. P., Eckenstein, F., Esiri, M. M. and Wilcock, G. K. (1983c) Persistence of cholinergic neurons in the basal nucleus in a brain with senile dementia of the Alzheimer type demonstrated by immunohistochemical staining for choline acetyltransferase. *Brain Res.*, 289: 375–379.

Pedata, F., Lo Conte, G., Sorbi, S., Marconcini-Pepeu, I. and Pepeu, G. (1982) Changes in high affinity choline uptake in rat cortex following lesions of the magnocellular forebrain nuclei. *Brain Res.*, 233: 359–367.

Perry, R. and Perry, E. (1983a) The ageing brain and its pathology. In R. Levy and F. Post (Eds.), *The Psychiatry of Late Life*, Blackwell Sci. Publ., Oxford, pp. 1–67.

Perry, E. K. and Perry, R. H. (1983b) Acetylcholinesterase in Alzheimer's disease. In B. Reisberg (Ed.), *Alzheimer's Disease the Standard Reference*, Free Press, New York, pp. 93–99.

Perry, E. K., Gibson, P. H., Blessed, G., Perry, R. H. and Tomlinson, B. E. (1977a) Neurotransmitter enzyme abnormalities in senile dementia. *J. Neurol. Sci.*, 34: 247–265.

Perry, E. K., Perry, R. H., Blessed, G. and Tomlinson, B. E. (1977b) Necropsy evidence of central cholinergic deficits in senile dementia. *Lancet*, 1: 189.

Perry, E. K., Tomlinson, B. E., Blessed, G., Bergmann, K., Gibson, P. H. and Perry, R. H. (1978) Correlations of cholinergic abnormalities with senile plaques and mental test scores in senile dementia. *Br. Med. J.*, 2: 1427–1429.

Perry, E. K., Perry, R. H., Tomlinson, B. E., Blessed, G. and Gibson, P. H. (1980a) Coenzyme A-acetylating enzymes in Alzheimer's disease: possible cholinergic 'compartment' of pyruvate dehydrogenase. *Neurosci. Lett.*, 18: 105–110.

Perry, R. H., Blessed, G., Perry, E. K. and Tomlinson, B. E. (1980b) Histochemical observations on the cholinesterase activities in the brains of elderly normal and demented (Alzheimer-type) patients. *Age Ageing*, 9: 9–16.

Perry, E. K., Tomlinson, B. E., Blessed, G., Perry, R. H., Cross, A. J. and Crow, T. J. (1981a) Neuropathological and biochemical observations on to noradrenergic system in Alzheimer's disease. *J. Neurol. Sci.*, 51: 279–287.

Perry, E. K., Blessed, G., Tomlinson, B. E., Perry, R. H., Crow, T. J., Cross, A. J., Dockray, G. J., Dimaline, R. and Arregui, A. (1981b) Neurochemical activities in human temporal lobe related to aging and Alzheimer-type changes. *Neurobiol. Aging*, 2: 251–256.

Perry, R. H., Candy, J. M., Perry, E. K., Irving, D., Blessed, G., Fairbairn, A. F. and Tomlinson, B. E. (1982) Extensive loss of choline acetyltransferase activity is not reflected by neuronal loss in the nucleus of Meynert in Alzheimer's disease. *Neurosci. Lett.*, 33: 311–315.

Perry, R. H., Tomlinson, B. E., Candy, J. M., Blessed, G., Foster, J. F., Bloxham, C. A. and Perry, E. K. (1983) Cortical cholinergic deficit in mentally impaired Parkinsonian patients. *Lancet*, 2: 789–790.

Perry, E. K., Atack, J. R., Perry, R. H., Hardy, J. A., Dodd, P. R., Edwardson, J. A., Blessed, G., Tomlinson, B. E. and Fairbairn, A. F. (1984a) Intralaminar neurochemical distributions in human midtemporal cortex: comparisons between Alzheimer's disease and the normal. *J. Neurochem.*, 42: 1402–1410.

Perry, R. H., Candy, J. M., Perry, E. K., Thompson, J. and Oakley, A. E. (1984b) The substantia innominata and adjacent regions in the human brain: histochemical and biochemical observations. *J. Anat.*, 138: 713–732.

Perry, E. K., Curtis, M., Dick, D. J., Candy, J. M., Atack, J. R., Bloxham, C. A., Blessed, G., Fairbairn, A., Tomlinson, B. E. and Perry, R. H. (1985) Cholinergic correlates of cognitive impairment in Parkinson's disease: comparisons with Alzheimer's disease. *J. Neurol. Neurosurg. Psychiat.*, 48: 413–421.

Peters, B. H. and Levin, H. S. (1978) Effects of physostigmine and lecithin on memory in Alzheimer's disease. *Ann. Neurol.*, 6: 219–221.

Petit, T. L., Biederman, G. B. and McMullen, P. A. (1980) Neurofibrillary degeneration, dendritic dying back and learning memory deficits after aluminium administration: implications for brain aging. *Exp. Neurol.*, 67: 152–162.

Phillis, J. W. (1968) Acetylcholine release from the cerebral cortex: its role in cortical arousal. *Brain Res.*, 7: 378–389.

Phillis, J. W. and Chong, G. C. (1965) Acetylcholine release from the cerebral and cerebellar cortices: its role in cortical arousal. *Nature*, 207: 1253–1255.

Phillis, J. W. and York, D. H. (1967) Cholinergic inhibition in the cerebral cortex. *Brain Res.*, 5: 517–520.

Phillis, J. W. and York, D. H. (1968) Pharmacological studies on a cholinergic inhibition in the cerebral cortex. *Brain Res.*, 10: 297–306.

Pirozzolo, F. J., Hansch, E. C., Mortimer, J. A., Webster, D. D. and Kuskowski, M. A. (1982) Dementia in Parkinson's disease: a neuropsychological analysis. *Brain Cognition*, 1: 71–83.

Pope, A., Hess, H. H. and Lewin, E. (1964) Studies on the microchemical pathology of human cerebral cortex. In M. M. Cohen and R. S. Snider (Eds.), *Morphological Correlates of Neural Activity*, Hoeber-Harper, New York, pp. 98–111.

Randic, M., Siminoff, R. and Straughan, D. W. (1964) Acetylcholine depression of cortical neurons. *Exp. Neurol.*, 9: 236–242.

Reisine, T. D., Yamamura, H. I., Bird, E. D., Spokes, E. and Enna, S. J. (1978) Pre- and postsynaptic neurochemical alterations in Alzheimer's disease. *Brain Res.*, 159: 477–481.

Repke, H. and Maderspach, K. (1982) Muscarinic acetylcholine receptors on cultured glia cells. *Brain Res.*, 232: 206–211.

Rinaldi, F. (1965) Direct action of atropine on the cerebral cortex of the rabbit. In W. A. Himwich and J. P. Schadé (Eds.), *Horizons in Neuropsychopharmacology*, *Progress in Brain Research*, *Vol. 16*, Elsevier, Amsterdam, pp. 229–244.

Rinne, J. O., Rinne, J. K., Laakso, K., Paljarvi, L. and Rinne, U. K. (1984) Reduction in muscarinic receptor binding in limbic areas of Alzheimer brain. *J. Neurol. Neurosurg. Psychiat.*, 47: 651–653.

Rinne, J. O., Laakso, K., Lonnberg, P., Molsa, P., Paljarvi, L., Rinne, J. K., Sako, E. and Rinne, U. K. (1985) Brain muscarinic receptors in senile dementia. *Brain Res.*, 336: 19–25.

Romano, C. and Goldstein, A. (1980) Stereo-specific nicotine receptors on rat brain membranes. *Science*, 210: 647–650.

Rossor, M. N. (1981) Parkinson's disease and Alzheimer's disease as disorders of the isodendritic core. *Br. Med. J.*, 283: 1588–1590.

Rossor, M. N., Iversen, L. L., Johnson, A. J., Mountjoy, C. Q. and Roth, M. (1981) Cholinergic deficit in frontal cerebral cortex in Alzheimer's disease is age dependent. *Lancet*, 2: 1422.

Rossor, M. N., Garrett, N. J., Johnson, A. J., Mountjoy, C. Q., Roth, M. and Iversen, L. L. (1982) A post mortem study of the cholinergic and GABA systems in senile dementia. *Brain*, 105: 313–330.

Rotter, A., Birdsall, N. J., Field, P. M. and Raisman, G. (1979) Muscarinic receptors in the central nervous system of the rat. II. Distribution of binding of [^{3}H]propylbenzilylcholine mustard in the midbrain and hindbrain. *Brain Res. Rev.*, 1: 167–183.

Rowell, P. P. and Sastry, B. V. (1978) The influence of cholinergic blockade on the uptake of β-aminoisobutyric acid by isolated human placenta villi. *Toxicol. Appl. Pharmacol.*, 45: 79–93.

Ruberg, M., Ploska, A., Javoy-Agid, F. and Agid, Y. (1982) Muscarinic binding and choline acetyltransferase activity in Parkinsonian subjects with reference to dementia. *Brain Res.*, 232: 129–139.

Rylett, R. J., Ball, M. J. and Colhoun, E. H. (1983) Evidence for high affinity choline transport in synaptosomes prepared from hippocampus and neocortex of patients with Alzheimer's disease. *Brain Res.*, 289: 169–175.

Schwartz, R. D., McGee, R. and Kellar, K. J. (1982) Nicotinic cholinergic receptors labelled by [^{3}H]acetylcholine in rat brain. *Mol. Pharmacol.*, 22: 56–62.

Shimohama, S., Taniguchi, T., Fujiwara, M. and Kameyama, M. (1986) Changes in nicotinic and muscarinic cholinergic receptors in senile dementia of the Alzheimer-type. *J. Neurochem.*, 46: 288–293.

Shute, C. C. and Lewis, P. R. (1967) The ascending cholinergic reticular system: neocortical olfactory and subcortical projections. *Brain*, 90: 497–520.

Silver, A. (1974) *Biology of Cholinesterases*. North-Holland, Amsterdam.

Sims, N. R., Bowen, D. M. and Davison, A. N. (1981) [^{14}C]acetylcholine synthesis and [^{14}C]carbon dioxide production from [U-^{14}C]glucose by tissue prisms from human neocortex. *Biochem. J.*, 196: 867–876.

Sitaram, N., Weingartner, H. and Gillin, J. C. (1978) Human serial learning: Enhancement with arecoline and choline and impairment with scopolamine. *Science*, 201: 274–276.

Smith, A. M. and Swash, M. (1979) Physostigmine in Alzheimer's disease. *Lancet*, 1: 42.

Soininen, H., Partanen, V. J., Helkala, E.-L. and Reikkinen, P. J. (1982) EEG findings in senile dementia and normal aging. *Acta Neurol. Scand.*, 65: 59–70.

Sokolovsky, M., Gurwitz, D. and Galeon, R. (1980) Muscarinic receptor binding in mouse brain: regulation by guanine nucleotides. *Biochem. Biophys. Res. Commun.*, 94: 487–492.

Sorbi, S. and Amaducci, L. (1985) Intracortical microchemistry in Alzheimer's disease. *J. Neurochem.*, 44, Suppl.: S192.

Stewart, D. J., Macfabe, D. F. and Vanderwolf, C. H. (1984) Cholinergic activation of the electrocorticogram: role of the substantia innominata and effects of atropine and quinuclidinyl benzilate. *Brain Res.*, 322: 219–232.

Strange, P. G., Birdsall, N. J. and Burgen, A. S. (1977) Occupancy of muscarinic acetylcholine receptors stimulates a guanylate cyclase in neuroblastoma cells. *Biochem. Soc. Trans.*, 5: 189–191.

Struble, R. G., Cork, L. C., Whitehouse, P. J. and Price, D. L. (1982) Cholinergic innervation in neuritic plaques. *Science*, 216: 413–415.

Struble, R. G., Hedreen, J. C., Cork, L. C. and Price, D. L. (1984) Acetylcholinesterase activity in senile plaques of aged Macaques. *Neurobiol. Aging*, 5: 191–198.

Tagliavini, F. and Pilleri, G. (1983) Neuronal counts in basal nucleus of Meynert in Alzheimer disease and in simple senile dementia. *Lancet*, 1: 469–670.

Terry, R. D. and Pena, C. (1965) Experimental production of neurofibrillary degeneration. 2. Electron microscopy, phosphatase histochemistry and electron probe analysis. *Exp. Neurol.*, 24: 200–210.

Terry, R. D., Peck, A., De Teresa, R., Schechter, R. and Horoupian, D. S. (1981) Some morphometric aspects of the brain in senile dementia of the Alzheimer type. *Ann. Neurol.*, 10: 184–192.

Tomlinson, B. E., Blessed, G. and Roth, M. (1968) Observations on the brains of non demented old people. *J. Neurol. Sci.*, 7: 331–356.

Tomlinson, B. E., Blessed, G. and Roth, M. (1970) Observations on the brains of demented old people. *J. Neurol. Sci.*, 11: 205–242.

Tucek, S. (1982) The synthesis of acetylcholine in skeletal muscles of the rat. *J. Physiol.*, 322: 53–60.

Tucek, S. (1984) Problems in the organisation and control of acetylcholine synthesis in brain neurons. *Prog. Biophys. Mol. Biol.*, 44: 1–46.

Tucek, S. (1985) Regulation of acetylcholine synthesis in the brain. *J. Neurochem.*, 44: 11–24.

Varon, S. S. and Bunge, R. P. (1978) Trophic mechanisms in the peripheral nervous system. *Ann. Rev. Neurosci.*, 1: 326–361.

Von Buttlar-Brentano, K. (1955) Das Parkinson Syndrom im Lichte der lebensgeschichtlichen Veränderungen des Nucleus basali. *J. Hirnforsch.*, 2: 55–76.

Wainer, B. H., Levey, A. I., Mufson, E. J. and Mesulam, M.-M. (1984) Cholinergic systems in mammalian brain identified with antibodies against choline acetyltransferase. *Neurochem. Int.*, 6: 163–182.

Wamsley, J. K., Zarbin, N. A., Birdsall, N. J. and Kuhar, M. J. (1980) Muscarinic cholinergic receptors: Autoradiographic localisation of high and low affinity agonist binding sites. *Brain Res.*, 200: 1–12.

Watson, M., Roeske, W. R. and Yamamura, H. I. (1982) [^{3}H]pirenzapine selectively identifies a high affinity population of muscarinic cholinergic receptors in the rat cerebral cortex. *Life Sci.*, 31: 2019–2123.

Watson, M., Yamamura, H. I. and Roeske, W. R. (1983) A unique regulatory profile and regional distribution of [^{3}H]pirenzapine binding in the rat provide evidence for distinct, M_1 and M_2 muscarinic receptor subtypes. *Life Sci.*, 32: 3001–3011.

Weiner, H. and Schuster, D. B. (1956) The electroencephalogram in dementia — some preliminary observations and correlations. *EEG Clin. Neurophysiol.*, 8: 479–488.

Wenk, G. L. and Olton, D. S. (1984) Recovery of neocortical choline acetyltransferase activity following ibotenic acid injection into the nucleus basalis of Meynert in rats. *Brain Res.*, 293: 184–186.

Wenk, H., Bigl, V. and Meyer, U. (1980) Cholinergic projections from magnocellular nuclei of the basal forebrain to cortical areas in the rat. *Brain Res. Rev.*, 2: 295–316.

Wennberg, A. and Widen, L. (1974) EEG och electroneurografi vid organisk demens. *Lakartidningen*, 71: 1282–1284.

White, P., Hiley, C. R., Goodhardt, M. J., Carrasco, L. H., Keet, J. P., Williams, I. E. and Bowen, D. M. (1977) Neocortical cholinergic neurons in elderly people. *Lancet*, 1: 668–670.

Whitehouse, P. J., Price, D. L., Struble, R. G., Clark, A. W., Coyle, J. T. and De Long, M. R. (1982) Alzheimer's disease and senile dementia; loss of neurons in the basal forebrain. *Science*, 215: 1237–1239.

Whitehouse, P. J., Hedreen, J. C., White, C. L. and Price, D. L. (1983) Basal forebrain neurons in the dementia of Parkinson disease. *Ann. Neurol.*, 13: 243–248.

Whitehouse, P. J., Kopajtic, T., Jones, B. E., Kuhar, M. J. and Price, D. L. (1985a) An in vitro receptor autoradiographic study of muscarinic cholinergic receptor subtypes in the amygdala and neocortex of patients with Alzheimer's disease. *Neurology*, 35, Suppl. 1: 217.

Whitehouse, P. J., Martino, A. M., Antuono, P. G., Coyle, J. T., Price, D. L. and Kellart, K. J. (1985b) Reductions in nicotinic cholinergic receptors measured using [³H]acetylcholine in Alzheimer's disease. *Soc. Neurosci.*, Abstracts, 11: 134.

Wilcock, G. K. and Esiri, M. M. (1982) Plaques, tangles and dementia. *J. Neurol. Sci.*, 56: 343–356.

Wilcock, G. K., Esiri, M. M., Bowen, D. M. and Smith, C. C. (1982) Alzheimer's disease: Correlation of cortical choline acetyltransferase activity with the severity of dementia and histological abnormalities. *J. Neurol. Sci.*, 57: 407–417.

Wilcock, G. K., Esiri, M. M., Bowen, D. M. and Smith, C. C. (1983) The nucleus basalis in Alzheimer's disease: cell counts and cortical biochemistry. *Neuropath. Appl. Neurobiol.*, 9: 175–179.

Williams, M. and Robinson, J. L. (1986) Binding of the nicotinic cholinergic antagonist, dihydro-β-erythroidine (DBE) to rat brain tissue. *J. Neurosci.*, in press.

Wisniewski, H. M. and Kozlowski, P. B. (1982) Evidence for blood–brain barrier changes in senile dementia of the Alzheimer type (SDAT). *Ann. NY Acad. Sci.*, 396: 119–129.

Wisniewski, H. M., Ghetti, B. and Terry, R. D. (1973) Neuritic (senile) plaques and filamentous changes in aged Rhesus monkey. *J. Neuropathol. Exp. Neurol.*, 32: 566–584.

Wisniewski, K. E., Wisniewski, H. M. and Wen, G. Y. (1985) Occurrence of neuropathological changes and dementia of Alzheimer's disease in Down's syndrome. *Ann. Neurol.*, 17: 278–282.

Wood, P. L., Etienne, P., Nair, N. P., Finlayson, M. H., Gauthier, S., Palo, J., Haltia, M., Paeptau, A. and Bird, E. D. (1983) A post-mortem comparison of the cortical cholinergic system in Alzheimer's disease and Pick's disease. *J. Neurol. Sci.*, 62: 211–217.

Yates, C. M., Simpson, J., Maloney, A. F., Gordon, A. and Reid, A. H. (1980) Alzheimer-like cholinergic deficiency in Down's syndrome. *Lancet*, 2: 979.

Yoshida, K. and Imura, H. (1979) Nicotinic cholinergic receptors in brain synaptosomes. *Brain Res.*, 172: 453–459.

Discussion

D. F. SWAAB: The loss of nucleus basalis of Meynert neurons you mentioned is based upon density measurements. There is of course a possibility that, e.g. by a change in glial cell number, the total volume of the nucleus is changing. This might give changes in neuron density without changes in neuron number. Do you know how the volume of the nucleus basalis is changing in normal aging, Alzheimer and Parkinson?

ANSWER: That is a pertinent point, which unfortunately we have not as yet been able to resolve, due to the fact that the spatial configuration of the nucleus of Meynert makes volume measurements extremely difficult. However, atrophy is generally more marked in presenile cases of Alzheimer's disease and it is in these cases that a marked loss of nucleus of Meynert neurons occurs. This seems to make it unlikely that changes in the volume of the nucleus of Meynert per se can account for the dissimilar neuronal loss in this nucleus in presenile and senile cases of Alzheimer's disease.

J. M. RABEY: (1) Do you think the patients you described as Parkinsonian with dementia with choline acetyltransferase (ChAT) loss and without senile plaques will later on develop senile plaques? Is that for these the end of the process?

(2) Do you know of patients with a lot of senile plaques and neurofibrillary tangles and without loss of ChAT?

ANSWER: (1) The cognitively impaired Parkinsonian patients (average age 72 years) did have senile plaques in the cerebral cortex with a density at the upper end of the normal range (Perry et al., 1985). The fact that the loss of cortical ChAT was as great as that seen in Alzheimer's disease makes it unlikely that abnormalities in the cortical cholinergic system are responsible for the formation of senile plaques.

(2) We have data on a moderately severe case of senile dementia of Alzheimer-type. In this patient, the ChAT level in both the cerebral cortex and nucleus of Meynert was within the normal range, however, there was a marked loss of the 10 S form of acetylcholinesterase in the cerebral cortex.

H. VAN RIEZEN: Parkinson patients were previously treated with anticholinergics. If about half of the Parkinsonian patients have a deficient cholinergic system, why did nobody notice that this therapy provoked dementia while it was clear in depressed patients treated with antidepressants which are (less) anticholinergic?

ANSWER: Estimates of the prevalence of dementia in Parkinson's disease have varied widely (see Mortimer et al., 1985) and it is possible that some of the higher estimates may have been due to anticholinergic therapy. However, Dr. Van Riezen has raised a crucial question regarding the relationship between dysfunction of the cortical cholinergic system and the severity of the dementing process. While the loss of cortical ChAT in cognitively impaired Parkinsonian patients is of a similar magnitude to that found in Alzheimer's disease, the dementia in Alzheimer's disease is generally more severe than that seen in Parkinson's disease. This apparent dissociation is reinforced by the finding that a much lower correlation exists between loss of ChAT and mental test performance below a score of about 20 (Perry et al., 1985).

A. J. CROSS: Have you looked at the composition of plaques in other disease states, e.g. scrapie and Creutzfeldt-Jacob disease?

ANSWER: As you know senile plaques occur in only 10–15% of patients with Creutzfeldt-Jacob disease which presents a difficulty. We are planning to examine the distribution of aluminium and silicon in scrapie plaques.

P. W. M. RAAYMAKERS: (1) What is the nature of the cognitive impairment in your studies?
(2) Do you know whether there is a relation between cognitive impairment and decrease in cortical ChAT activity in aged Down's syndrome patients? This would be of importance for the 'cholinergic hypothesis of geriatric memory dysfunction'.

ANSWER: (1) A mental test was used which measures short-term memory, personal memory and concentration (Blessed et al., 1968). The scores of the cognitively impaired Parkinsonian patients ranged from 0 to 27 out of a possible score of 37. A study is in progress in Newcastle to determine more precisely the nature of the cognitive impairment in Parkinson's disease. Previous studies have reported a generalised cognitive deficit which includes impairment in both verbal and non-verbal memory, complex visual discrimination and abstract reasoning (see Mortimer et al., in press).
(2) A decrease in cortical ChAT (Yates et al., 1980) and loss of nucleus of Meynert neurons (Mann et al., 1984; Casanova et al., 1985) has been reported in Down's syndrome. There is a controversy regarding the prevalence of dementia in older cases of Down's syndrome who have Alzheimer-type neuropathological changes in the cerebral cortex, which may be at least partly due to the difficulty of assessing cognitive performance in these patients. I am not aware of any studies which have attempted to relate loss of cortical ChAT with cognitive impairment in Down's syndrome.

R. D. TERRY: What is the ultrastructural appearance of the neocortex in Parkinson's disease with dementia without plaques?

ANSWER: That is an interesting question which we have not, as yet, addressed.

F. MIZOBE: I am impressed that marked and selective reduction of 10 S form acetylcholinesterase occurs in Alzheimer's brain. I would like to know whether or not a similar selective reduction of 10 S form occurs in pseudo-cholinesterase from Alzheimer's brain. Have you looked at that?

ANSWER: There is no significant loss of either the G1 or G4 forms of pseudo-cholinesterase in senile cases of Alzheimer's disease (Perry et al., unpublished).

J. M. PALACIOS: The results in impaired Parkinsonian patients suggest (1) that there is no correlation between the presence of senile plaques and neurochemical cholinergic deficits. This is a central question and these results indicate that both processes are independent. What is your opinion?
(2) Do the impaired Parkinsonian patients present the other neurochemical deficits seen in SDAT (somatostatin, S2 receptors).

ANSWER: (1) Our findings suggest that the cortical cholinergic abnormalities in cognitively impaired patients with Parkinson's disease may be a consequence of primary degenerative changes in the nucleus of Meynert — analogous to the loss of neurons in the substantia nigra, whereas the cortical cholinergic deficits in Alzheimer's disease may result from the cortical pathological changes.
(2) The density of serotoninergic S2-binding sites is unchanged in cognitively impaired Parkinsonian patients, in contrast to the decrease observed in senile dementia of Alzheimer-type (Perry et al., 1984). We do not yet have data on possible changes in the cortical somatostatinergic system in mentally impaired cases of Parkinson's disease where Alzheimer-type neuropathological changes were absent. Decreased levels of somatostatin immunoreactivity in the cerebral cortex have been reported in demented cases of Parkinson's disease (Epelbaum et al., 1983), however, the patients in this study also had the neuropathological features of Alzheimer's disease.

R. T. BARTUS: Some of your data suggest that there may indeed be at least two forms of AD, which you define as early (less than 71 years) and late (+71 years). However, your age-

132

differentiation contrasts with both the classic distinction of presenile and senile dementia (age cut off at 60–65 years) and more recent classifications by Rossor (age cut off at 81 years). How did you decide the age which should be used to classify the two forms you define, and how different would your conclusions be if your cut-off age was either 60 or 81?

ANSWER: Unfortunately it is usually extremely difficult to determine retrospectively the precise age of onset of Alzheimer's disease. Since in presenile cases of Alzheimer's disease the onset is generally considered to occur before 65 years of age, it seems reasonable to consider senile cases as those aged over 70 at death. The more benign expression of the disease in senile cases, which is reflected in both cortical atrophy and neuronal loss from the nucleus of Meynert, may result from some influence of ageing on the disease process or a shorter duration of the disease. Before definite conclusions can be drawn it will be necessary to determine the influence of both age and disease duration on cholinergic parameters in longitudinal studies.

K. IQBAL: Dr. Bowen from London has shown that there are some Alzheimer cases which show no cholinergic deficit in the neocortex. What were the controls used for measuring aluminum silicate in plaque cores and was aluminium silicate seen in any other structures?

ANSWER: Aluminosilicates are a constant, central feature of only senile plaque cores and do not show the peripheral or homogeneous distribution pattern seen for other elements such as iron, calcium and magnesium. Aluminium and silicon have not been detected, for example, in Pick bodies (Oakley et al., unpublished).

References

Blessed, G., Tomlinson, B. E. and Roth, M. (1968) The association between quantitative measures of dementia and of senile changes in the cerebral grey matter of aged subjects. *Br. J. Psychiat.*, 114: 797–811.

Casanova, M. F., Walker, L. C., Whitehouse, P. J. and Price, D. L. (1985) Abnormalities of the nucleus basalis in Down's syndrome. *Ann. Neurol.*, 18: 310–313.

Epelbaum, J., Ruberg, M., Moyse, E., Javoy-Agid, F., Dubois, B. and Agid, Y. (1983) Somatostatin and dementia in Parkinson's disease. *Brain Res.*, 278: 376–379.

Mann, D. M., Yates, P. O. and Marcyniuk, B. (1980) Alzheimer's presenile dementia, senile dementia of Alzheimer type and Down's syndrome from an age-related continuum of pathological changes. *Neuropathol. Appl. Neurobiol.*, 10: 185–207.

Mortimer, J. H., Christensen, K. J. and Webster, D. D. (1985) Parkinsonian dementia. In P. J. Vinken, G. W. Bruyn and H. L. Klawans (Eds.), *Neuro-behavioural Disorders, Handbook of Clinical Neurology, Vol. 46*, Elsevier, Amsterdam, pp. 371–384.

Perry, E. K., Perry, R. H., Candy, J. M., Fairbairn, A. F., Blessed, G., Dick, D. J. and Tomlinson, B. E. (1984) Cortical serotonin-S2 receptor binding abnormalities in patients with Alzheimer's disease: comparisons with Parkinson's disease. *Neurosci. Lett.*, 51: 353–357.

Perry, E. K., Curtis, M., Dick, D. J., Candy, J. M., Atack, J. R., Bloxham, C. A., Blessed, G., Fairbairn, A., Tomlinson, B. E. and Perry, R. H. (1985) Cholinergic correlates of cognitive impairment in Parkinson's disease: Comparisons with Alzheimer's disease. *J. Neurol. Neurosurg. Psychol.*, 48: 413–421.

Yates, C. M., Simpson, J., Maloney, A. F., Gordon, A. and Reid, A. H. (1980) Alzheimer-like cholinergic deficiency in Down's syndrome. *Lancet*, 2: 979.

D. F. Swaab, E. Fliers, M. Mirmiran, W. A. Van Gool and F. Van Haaren (Eds.)
Progress in Brain Research, Vol. 70.
© 1986 Elsevier Science Publishers B.V. (Biomedical Division)

CHAPTER 8

Monoamines and myelin components in aging and dementia disorders

C. G. Gottfries

Department of Psychiatry and Neurochemistry, St. Jörgens Hospital, S-422 03 Hisings Backa, Sweden

Introduction

In advanced age mental impairment is seen and assumed to be due to a normal aging process and/or dementia disorders.

Before trying to classify different dementias, the question of distinguishing normal aging from dementia disorders must be raised. From a theoretical point of view it is possible to differentiate normal aging from age-related diseases. The normal aging process has an insidious onset, is slowly progressive, and is assumed to take place on a subcellular level without immediately giving rise to signs or symptoms. However, when the reserve capacity of the brain is finally destroyed, the cumulated effect will give rise to symptoms of insufficiency.

In cerebrovascular disorders (CVD) the dementia is assumed to be caused by infarctions of the brain and therefore this form is called multiinfarction dementia (MID). Dementia due to primary degenerative disorders are senile dementia (SD), Alzheimer's presenile dementia, Pick's disease and Huntington's chorea.

Alzheimer's presenile dementia was described in 1907 and this disorder is characterized by an onset in middle life with senile plaques and fibrillary tangles in the brain. SD is a clinically similar disorder but the onset is over 65 years of age. Since the 'Alzheimer lesions' are also found in the brains of patients with SD the name senile dementia of Alzheimer type (SDAT) is used for the latter group. The two forms will here be classified together under the name of Alzheimer's disease.

Since long, neuropathologists have carefully described structural changes in brains from patients with dementia disorders and the current classification is based on these findings. During the last two decades there has been biochemical research in this field. Post-mortem investigations of human brains have revealed interesting changes in normal aging as well as in dementia disorders. In this paper, biochemical findings made in post-mortem material will be discussed. The data presented are derived from a still ongoing investigation (Gottfries et al., 1986), which in more detail will be published later. Also biochemical post-mortem findings from other groups will be discussed.

Material and methods

In our ongoing investigation 21 brains from controls were collected at autopsy. The patients forming the control group had not suffered from psychiatric or neurologic disorders before death. Death was due to bronchopneumonias, circulatory disorders or cancer. At autopsy, which was performed within 72 h after death, the brain was carefully dissected. By geographical landmarks several nuclei or regions of the brain were dissected and within 2 h the tissue was deep-frozen to minus 80°C. Before chemical analysis, the samples were homogenized in deep frozen condition to a powdery homogenate. Subsamples of the homogenate were then transported to the various laboratories that performed the chemical analyses. In this way several analyses could be made from one and the same tissue sample. The brains from 22 patients with Alzheimer's disease and nine patients with MID were dissected in the same way. The diagnoses were made clinically, by macroscopic inspection of the brain at autopsy and by histopathological examination of the hippocampus and the frontal cortex.

Lipids were determined in white matter (centrum semiovale) and in frontal cortex (c.f. Gottfries et al., 1985). Choline acetyltransferase (CAT), monoamine oxidase (MAO), biogenic amines and their metabolites were determined in gray matter (c.f. Gottfries et al., 1983).

Results

The mean age and standard deviation (SD) in the control group was 73.6 ± 7.5, in the Alzheimer group 79.6 ± 8.9 and in the MID group 82.2 ± 6.0 years. In white matter there was a significant negative correlation between neutral phospholipids and cholesterol on one side and age on the other. In gray matter, cholesterol was negatively correlated with age on a significant level (Table I).

TABLE I

Correlations (Pearson's r) between lipids and sialoglycoproteins on one side and age on the other in white matter (centrum semiovale) and gray matter (cortex of frontal lobe)

	White matter		Gray matter	
	n	r	n	r
Phospholipids				
neutral	17	-0.49^a	17	-0.43
acidic	17	-0.16	17	-0.26
Cholesterol	17	-0.66^b	17	-0.63^b
Cerebrosides	17	-0.10	–	–
Sulfatides	14	-0.22	–	–

$^a p < 0.05$; $^b p < 0.01$.

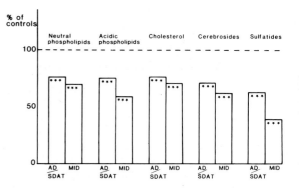

Fig. 1. White matter (centrum semiovale) changes expressed as percentage of controls ($n=21$), in a group of AD patients ($n=22$) and a group of MID patients ($n=9$). ***, $p < 0.05$; group differences according to Student's t test.

TABLE II

Levels of myelin components in white matter in a group of controls and a group of patients with Alzheimer dementia

	Controls			Alzheimer dementia		
	n	mean	SD	n	mean	SD
Phospholipids						
neutral (μmol/g)	17	75.9	9.2	13	57.1^a	11.3
acidic (μmol/g)	17	21.1	2.6	13	15.9^a	3.6
Cholesterol (μmol/g)	17	112.0	16.2	13	84.3^a	20.2
Cerebrosides (μmol/g)	17	39.5	6.4	13	28.2^a	5.4
Sulfatides (μmol/g)	14	15.9	4.0	13	10.0^a	2.6

Group differences according to Student's t test $^a p < 0.005$. n, number of cases; SD, standard deviation.

As is evident from Fig. 1 and Table II, neutral and acidic phospholipids, cholesterol, cerebrosides and sulfatides were all significantly reduced in white matter in the Alzheimer group as well as in the MID group as compared with controls.

In post-mortem analyses of brains from normally aged individuals a decrease in some neurotransmitter levels, as compared to younger individuals has been reported (Carlsson and Winblad, 1976; Carlsson, 1981; Gottfries et al., 1983). The old individuals were considered 'normally aged'

TABLE III

Correlations between age on one side and amines and their metabolites on the other

	Age/5-HT		Age/5-HIAA		Age/NA		Age/HMPG		Age/DA		Age/HVA		Age/CAT	
	n	r	n	r	n	r	n	r	n	r	n	r	n	r
Hypothalamus	21	0.34	22	0.30	22	−0.38[a]			22	0.03	22	−0.28		
Caudate nucleus	22	−0.60[c]	22	−0.02	22	0.34	22	0.23	22	−0.24	22	−0.29	10	0.59[a]
Putamen left	22	−0.73[c]	22	0.24	22	−0.47[b]			22	−0.43[b]	22	−0.34	10	0.31
Putamen right	22	−0.60[c]	22	0.17	22	−0.21			22	−0.32	22	−0.25	11	0.53[a]
Mesencephalon	22	−0.05	22	0.32	22	−0.41[a]	22	0.35	22	−0.13	22	−0.04		
Hippocampus	22	−0.09	22	0.15	22	−0.45[b]	22	0.23	22	−0.65[c]	22	−0.05	11	0.22
Cortex gyrus hippocampus	22	−0.29	22	0.20	22	−0.47[b]			22	0.08	22	0.12	10	−0.25
Cortex lobus temporalis	21	−0.17	21	0.05	20	−0.54[b]	22	0.30	22	−0.04	22	−0.05	9	0.33

5-HT, 5-hydroxytryptamine; 5-HIAA, 5-hydroxyindoleacetic acid; NA, noradrenaline; HMPG, 3-methoxy-4-hydroxyphenylglycol; DA, dopamine; HVA, homovanillic acid; CAT, choline acetyltransferase. Group differences according to Student's t test [a]$p < 0.10$; [b]$p < 0.05$; [c]$p < 0.005$.

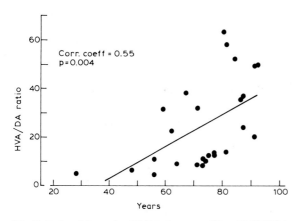

Fig. 2. Ratio of dopamine (DA) to homovanillic acid (HVA) in the hippocampus of controls plotted versus age.

and consequently the transmitter reduction did not go together with any detectable functional loss. In our ongoing investigation, we can confirm an age-dependent decrease in dopamine (DA), noradrenaline (NA) and 5-hydroxytryptamine (5-HT) (Table III). Of interest is that any concomitant decrease in the metabolites, 3-methoxytyramine (MT), 3,4-dihydroxyphenylacetic acid (DOPAC), homovanillic acid (HVA), 3-methoxy-4-hydroxyphenylglycol (HMPG) or 5-hydroxyindoleacetic acid (5-HIAA) is

not seen. Consequently there is a significant increase in the ratio of the metabolites to transmitters as seen in Fig. 2 (after Carlsson, 1985). CAT, a marker of the cholinergic system, seems to be less age-dependent than, e.g., tyrosine hydroxylase (McGeer, 1978). In this investigation as well as in a previous one (Gottfries et al., 1983) we failed to detect any age-dependent decrease in CAT (Table III).

As can be seen from Fig. 3 and Table IV there

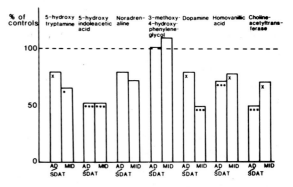

Fig. 3. Changes in the caudate nucleus expressed as percentage of controls ($n = 21$), in a group of AD patients ($n = 22$) and a group of MID patients ($n = 9$). ×, p < 0.10; *, $p < 0.05$; ***, $p < 0.005$; group differences according to Student's t test.

TABLE IV

Mean values and standard deviations (SD) of biochemical variables in the nucleus caudatus from a group of controls, a group of patients with Alzheimer dementia and a group with multiinfarction dementia (MID)

	Controls			Alzheimer dementia			MID		
	n	mean	SD	n	mean	SD	n	mean	SD
5-Hydroxytryptamine (ng)	22	250	96	20	200[a]	74	9	163[b]	95
5-Hydroxyindoleacetic acid (nmol/g)	22	590	329	20	3.19[c]	113	9	319[c]	137
Noradrenaline (ng)	22	28	15	20	22	19	9	20	21
3-Methoxy-4-hydroxy-phenylglycol (nmol/g)	22	0.35	0.21	20	0.36	0.11	9	0.38	0.16
Dopamine (ng)	22	1878	774	20	1454[a]	699	9	937[c]	492
3,4-Dihydroxyphenyl-acetic acid (ng)	22	655	265	20	524[b]	261	9	403[b]	229
3-Methoxytyramine (ng)	22	1141	370	20	777[b]	299	9	696[b]	365
Homovanillic acid (nmol/g)	22	17.96	5.64	20	12.76[c]	5.01	9	13.77[a]	5.58
Choline acetyltransferase (μkat/kg protein)	10	4087	1359	18	2027[c]	740	8	2896[a]	1454
Monoamineoxidase-A (μkat/kg protein)	17	8.28	1.6	17	8.38	1.27	9	7.73	1.74
Monoamineoxidase-B (μkat/kg protein)	17	15.56	3.57	17	19.53[c]	4.64	9	18.71[b]	3.6

Group differences according to Student's t test [a]$p < 0.10$; [b]$p < 0.05$; [c]$p < 0.01$. The dementia groups are compared to the controls.

are severe disturbances in the biochemical variables in the caudate nucleus. 5-HT is significantly reduced in the MID group and borders significance in the Alzheimer group. 5-HIAA is significantly reduced in the two groups. NA is slightly but not significantly reduced, while HMPG is unchanged. DA is significantly reduced in the MID group and the reduction in the Alzheimer group borders significance. HVA is significantly reduced in the Alzheimer group and the reduction in the MID group borders significance. There are also significant reductions in the metabolites DOPAC and MT in the two dementia groups. In the caudate nucleus a reduced activity of CAT was found, which is significant in the Alzheimer group and borders significance in the MID group (Table IV and Fig. 3). MAO-A is unchanged while MAO-B is significantly increased in the two dementia groups.

The pattern of damage is about the same in the hippocampus (Fig. 4, Table V). 5-HT as well as 5-

HIAA are significantly decreased, NA is reduced in the Alzheimer group on a level that borders significance, while there is no reduction in the MID group. HMPG is unchanged. DA is significantly reduced while HVA is unchanged in the two dementia groups. DOPAC and MT are also

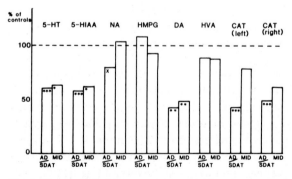

Fig. 4. Changes in the hippocampus expressed as percentage of controls ($n = 21$), in a group of AD patients ($n = 22$) and a group of MID patients ($n = 9$). $\times$, $p < 0.10$; *, $p < 0.05$; **, $p < 0.01$; ***, $p < 0.005$; group differences according to Student's t test.

TABLE V

Mean values and standard deviations (SD) of biochemical variables in the hippocampus from a group of controls, a group of patients with Alzheimer dementia and a group with multiinfarction dementia (MID)

	Controls			Alzheimer dementia			MID		
	n	mean	SD	n	mean	SD	n	mean	SD
5-Hydroxytryptamine (ng)	22	51.7	24.8	19	31[d]	15	8	32[b]	18
5-Hydroxyindoleacetic acid (nmol/g)	22	284.7	112.9	19	164[d]	69	8	178.4[b]	84.3
Noradrenaline (ng)	22	19.0	6.3	19	15[a]	6	8	20	12
3-Methoxy-4-hydroxy-phenylglycol (nmol/g)	22	0.36	0.16	20	0.39	0.17	9	0.33	0.16
Dopamine (ng)	22	21.0	15.8	19	9.1[c]	10.8	8	10[c]	6
3,4-Dihydroxyphenyl-acetic acid (ng)	22	22	8	19	17[b]	7	8	15[b]	5
3-Methoxytyramine (ng)	10	46	22	13	27[b]	22	3	32[b]	18
Homovanillic acid (nmol/g)	22	1.80	0.70	20	1.60	1.34	9	1.59	1.26
Choline acetyltransferase (left) (μkat/kg protein)	11	363	166	16	157[d]	107	6	284	184
Choline acetyltransferase (right) (μkat/kg protein)	10	363	133	16	180[d]	161	6	224	191

Group differences according to Student's t test [a] $p < 0.10$; [b] $p < 0.05$; [c] $p < 0.01$; [d] $p < 0.005$. The dementia groups are compared to the controls.

reduced. As is evident from Fig. 4 and Table IV the most severe reduction of CAT activity is seen in the Alzheimer group.

Discussion

The concentrations of DA, NA and 5-HT are significantly reduced with age, which may indicate a neuron loss in these systems. The metabolites are, however, not reduced and the ratio between the metabolites and the amines are significantly increased with age. This may indicate an increased speed of turnover in the remaining neurons, which may be a compensation for the neuron loss. This means that in normal aging the remaining neurons are in a healthy state, they can respond to feedback mechanisms. In brains from patients with Alzheimer's disease DA and 5-HT as well as their metabolites are reduced, indicating that at least in these two systems there is not only a cell loss but also a neurochemical defect in the remaining

neurons, at least as reflected by reduced concentrations of metabolites. The NA system is to some extent an exception. NA is decreased but HMPG is not, it may even be increased (Gottfries et al., 1983).

Structural changes of white matter are reported by Brun and Gustafson (1978). These findings are described as incomplete infarctions of white matter (Brun, 1983) and they are seen more often in patients with a late onset of the dementia. The changes are found both in patients with Alzheimer's disease and in patients with MID. As reported by DeLeon et al. (1985), investigations by nuclear magnetic resonance (NMR) also have revealed white matter changes in patients with dementia disorders. Again the changes were seen both in patients with Alzheimer's disease and in patients with MID. Chia et al. (1984) have reported evidence for myelin disorders in brains from patients with Alzheimer's disease. Higher levels of malondialdehyde and conjugated dienes in white matter from diseased brain suggested that free radical mediated lipid peroxidation might be the source of the increased myelin disorder.

Our present findings of reduced myelin components in Alzheimer's disease and in MID are in agreement with the neuropathological and NMR findings. There seems to be a rather severe disturbance of white matter in these dementia conditions. The white matter changes may of course be secondary to neuron death followed by an axon/myelin degeneration. According to Brun the changes were suggestive of incomplete infarctions, which may mean that there has been hypoxia in the brain. In fact, investigations of cerebrospinal fluid (CSF) have also indicated hypoxia in patients with Alzheimer dementia (Gottfries et al., 1974). Of interest is that Sourander et al. (1985) have reported an increased frequency of sleep apnea and hypoxia in patients with dementia. It can of course be assumed that the demented brain cannot control its own blood supply sufficiently and therefore hypoxia attacks may take place causing white matter changes. One may, however, also make the speculative hypothesis that healthy elderly people can have difficulties in controlling the supply of blood to the brain. Blood pressure falls in the elderly may cause hypoxia and white matter changes, which may have pathogenetic importance for the dementia process.

In several reports, neurotransmitter disturbances of the brain from patients with Alzheimer's disease are shown. Some authors (c.f. Reisberg, 1983) have emphasized the importance of the reduced activity of the acetylcholine system for Alzheimer's disease. There are, however, several reports indicating disturbances of other neurotransmitters (c.f. Hardy et al., 1985). Our present findings are in agreement with a more general damage of neurotransmitter systems in the brains of patients with Alzheimer's disease. Of interest is that also in patients with MID there are reduced concentrations of neurotransmitters. Rather general disturbances are found. Perhaps the reduced activity of CAT is somewhat more severe in patients with Alzheimer's disease than in patients with MID.

It seems logical to assume that the infarctions in MID would cause selective reductions of neurotransmitter functioning. This seems, however, not to be the case. In our material of MID patients the amount and the localization of infarction could hardly explain the extended biochemical defects recorded.

In patients with MID, the neuropathological investigations revealed changes also in the small vessels. It may be assumed that MID is a disorder with rather general cerebrovascular disturbances in the brain. This explanation would indeed also be in agreement with the clinical picture. Some of the patients were severely demented although there were few and small macroinfarctions of the brain.

Summary and conclusions

In a material of 21 normally aged individuals, 22 patients with Alzheimer's disease and nine patients with multiinfarction dementia, biochemical investigations were made on post-mortem brain samples. As was already shown in previous investigations, an age-dependent decrease was found in the concentrations of DA, NA and 5-HT while a concomitant reduction in the metabolites of these transmitters was not seen. In normally aged individuals changes were found in white matter as some myelin components were reduced with age.

In brains from patients with Alzheimer dementia reduced concentrations of DA and 5-HT and of the main metabolites of these transmitters were observed. A slight reduction of NA was seen while the end-metabolite of this transmitter was not reduced. The activity of MAO-A was unchanged while the MAO-B was significantly increased. CAT is often used as a marker for the cholinergic system of the human brain. The activity of this enzyme was decreased in brains from patients with Alzheimer dementia. Of interest is that in material from MID patients rather general biochemical changes were found. The relationship between the amount of infarcted brain tissue or the location of brain infarctions and the biochemical changes was unclear. In some brains, small and few infarctions of the brain existed although general neurotransmitter disturbances were found. A microscopic investigation of the brain revealed changes in small vessels, which were rather general in brains with multiinfarction dementia.

Significant reductions of myelin components in the dementia groups were observed. The white matter changes may indicate attacks of hypoxia in the white matter. Among the dementias with late onset there may be a subgroup of 'white matter dementias', where changes of white matter have pathogenetic importance for the dementia syndrome.

References

Alzheimer, A. (1907) Ueber eine eigenartige Erkrankung der Hirnrinde. *Cbl. Nervenheilk. Psychiat.*, 18: 177–179. Cited in: Torack, R. (1971) In C. Wells (Ed.), *Dementia*, F. A. Davis & Co., Philadelphia.

Brun, A. (1983) An overview of light and electron microscopic changes. In B. Reisberg (Ed.), *Alzheimer's Disease, the Standard Reference*. The Free Press, McMillan, New York, pp. 37–47.

Brun, A. and Gustafson, L. (1978) Limbic lobe involvement in presenile dementia. *Arch. Psychiatr. Nervenkr.*, 226: 76–93.

Carlsson, A. (1981) Aging and brain neurotransmitters. In Th. Crook and S. Gershon (Eds.), *Strategies for the Development of an Effective Treatment for Senile Dementia*, Mark Powley Ass. Inc., New Canaan, pp. 93–104.

Carlsson, A. (1985) Neurotransmitters in old age and dementia. In H. Hafner, N. Sartorius and G. Moschel (Eds.), *Mental Health in the Elderly: A Review of the Present State of Research*, Springer Verlag, Heidelberg, in press.

Carlsson, A. and Winblad, B. (1976) Influence of age and time interval between death and autopsy on dopamine and 3-methoxytyramine levels in human basal ganglia. *J. Neurol. Transm.*, 38: 271–276.

Chia, L. S., Thompson, J. E. and Moscarello, M. A. (1984) X-ray diffraction evidence for myelin disorder in brain from humans with Alzheimer's disease. *Biochim. Biophys. Acta*, 775: 308–312.

DeLeon, M. J., George, A. E., Ferris, S. H., Christman, D., Gentes, C. I., Miller, J. D., Fowler, J., Reisberg, B. and Wolf, A. P. (1985) CT, PET and NMR brain imaging in aging and Alzheimer's disease. In C. G. Gottfries (Ed.), *Normal Aging, Alzheimer's Disease and Senile Dementia. Aspects on Etiology, Pathogenesis, Diagnosis and Treatment*, Proceedings of two symposia held at the C.I.N.P. 14th Congress, June 22 and 23, 1984, Florence, Italy. L'Université de Bruxelles, pp. 199–202.

Gottfries, C. G., Kjällquist, Å., Ponten, U., Roos, B. E. and Sundbärg, G. (1974) Cerebrospinal fluid pH and monoamine and glucolytic metabolites in Alzheimer's disease. *Br. J. Psychiat.*, 124, 280–287.

Gottfries, C. G., Adolfsson, R., Aquilonius, S. M., Carlsson, A., Eckernäs, S. Å., Nordberg, A., Oreland, L., Svennerholm, L., Wiberg, Å. and Winblad, B. (1983) Biochemical changes in dementia disorders of Alzheimer type (AD/S-DAT). *Neurobiol. Aging*, 4: 261–271.

Gottfries, C. G., Karlsson, I. and Svennerholm, L. (1985) Senile dementia — A 'white matter' disease? In C. G. Gottfries (Ed.), *Normal Aging, Alzheimer's Disease and Senile Dementia. Aspects on Etiology, Pathogenesis, Diagnosis and Treatment*, Proceedings of two symposia held at the C.I.N.P. 14th Congress, June 22 and 23, 1984, Florence, Italy. L'Université de Bruxelles, Bruxelles, pp. 111–118.

Gottfries, C. G., Alafuzoff, I., Carlsson, A., Eckernäs, S. Å., Karlsson, I., Oreland, L., Svennerholm, L. and Winblad, B. (1986), in preparation.

Hardy, J., Adolfsson, R., Alafuzoff, I., Bucht, G., Marcusson, J., Nyberg, P., Perdahl, E., Wester, P. and Winblad, B. (1985) Review. Transmitter deficits in Alzheimer's disease. *Neurochem. Int.*, 7: No. 4, 545–563.

McGeer, E. G. (1978) Aging and neurotransmitter metabolism in the human brain. In R. Katzman, R. D. Terry and K. L. Bick (Eds.), *Aging*, Raven Press, New York, pp. 427–440.

Reisberg, B. (Ed.) (1983) *Alzheimer's Disease. The Standard Reference*. The Free Press, New York.

Sourander, L., Polo, O. and Alihanka, J. (1985) Sleep apnea and hypoxia in patients with senile dementia. Paper presented at the Nordic Psychiatric Congress in Odense, May 29 – June 1, 1985, in press.

Discussion

P. D. COLEMAN: Comment: Recent data from our laboratories show that indeed the cholinergic system may decline without neuronal loss. Others have shown age-related declines in selected aspects of the cholinergic system in rodents. We have found in C57B1/6 mice no loss of basal forebrain cholinergic neurons with an oldest group of 53 months. Since cholinergic declines are evident well before 53 months in C57B1/6 mice the decline in some aspects of transmitter function is not an immediate precursor of neuronal death.

I would also like to point out that in considering changes in the dopaminergic system we must not focus only on the substantia nigra since other brain regions — e.g. ventral tegmental nucleus — are also important sources of dopamine.

M. C. JORI: Do you think there is any possible correlation between therapeutic effects of drugs acting on monoaminergic systems and CSF level changes of their metabolites in vivo?

ANSWER: There are CSF changes as reduced concentrations of HVA and 5-HIAA in AD patients (Gottfries, 1983). There are, however, no data from treatment studies in which the CSF finding has determined the way of treatment. In a study of our own we gave AD patients L-DOPA. We did not see any improvement. Also the patients with low HVA in the CSF did not improve.

J. E. PISETSKY: Are there changes in the blood vessels in AD patients? Are there blood–brain barrier and permeability changes? Dr. Terry says that no such changes occur; others say that there may be alterations.

ANSWER: In our MID material the neuropathologist found changes in small vessels in all the cases. In the AD material there was also pathology of small blood vessels in around 25% of the patients examined.

G. S. ROTH: I have a question related to both of this morning's presentations concerning the possible distinctions between neurochemical deficits and cell loss. Since therapeutically it may be easier to deal with the former, I wonder whether the two processes can be dissociated, and in fact whether they are causally related.

ANSWER: I think some data in our studies may answer your question. We have found reduced concentrations of the active amines. This reduction may indicate cell loss. In the normally aged individuals, we found no reduced concentrations of the metabolites. However, in the AD group we found reduced concentrations of the amines as well as of the metabolites. This may indicate that the neurons in the AD brains cannot increase the speed of turnover and, therefore, it can be assumed that in the AD brains there is a neurochemical defect.

R. D. TERRY: Comment: The differences between early and late onset Alzheimer's disease are not adequate at this time to separate these two groups on the basis of age alone.

ANSWER: I don't agree with Dr. Terry's point of view that early and late onset AD should be sampled into one group. According to an investigation in Sweden (Larsson et al., 1963), the hereditary patterns of the two disorders are different. There are also biochemical differences between early and late onset AD (Rossor et al., 1984; Gottfries et al., 1983). Our present findings of white matter changes seem to be most pronounced in the dementia form with late onset. From a scientific point of view it seems wiser to keep these two forms apart.

D. R. CRAPPER McLACHLAN: In your data and also in Dr. Candy's data on cortical CAT activity, decreases in the absence of concomitant cell loss may reflect an alteration in gene expression rather than axonal loss. Have you considered this alternative explanation?

ANSWER: This possibility exists.

References

Gottfries, C. G. (1983) Biochemical changes in blood and cerebrospinal fluid. In B. Reisberg (Ed.), *Alzheimer's Disease. The Standard Reference.* The Free Press, Collier McMillan Publ., London, pp. 122–130.

Gottfries, C. G., Adolfsson, R. Aquilonius, S. M., Carlsson, A., Eckernäs, S. A., Nordberg, A., Oreland, L., Svennerholm, L., Wiberg, A. and Winblad, B. (1983) Biochemical changes in dementia disorders of Alzheimer type (AD/SDAT). *Neurobiol. Aging*, 4: 261–271.

Larsson, T., Sjögren, T. and Jacobson, G. (1963) Senile dementia. A clinical, sociomedical and genetic study. *Acta Psychiat. Scand.*, Suppl. 167.

Rossor, M. N., Iversen, L. L., Reynolds, G. P., Mountjoy, C. Q. and Roth, M. (1984) Neurochemical characteristics of early and late onset types of Alzheimer's disease. *Br. Med. J.*, 288: 961–964.

D. F. Swaab, E. Fliers, M. Mirmiran, W. A. Van Gool and F. Van Haaren (Eds.)
Progress in Brain Research, Vol. 70.
© 1986 Elsevier Science Publishers B.V. (Biomedical Division)

CHAPTER 9

Neuropeptide changes in aging and Alzheimer's disease

E. Fliers and D.F. Swaab

Netherlands Institute for Brain Research, Meibergdreef 33, 1105 AZ Amsterdam ZO, The Netherlands

Introduction

Neuropeptides are an ever growing group of putative neurotransmitters. Although the exact function of any of these peptides is not known at present, they are capable of eliciting a variety of effects upon central or peripheral administration (for a review see Swaab, 1982). Neuropeptide effects have also been demonstrated on functions, which are known to change in aging and Alzheimer's disease, such as cognitive functions. This is one of the reasons why interest in changes in neuropeptide systems in senescence and Alzheimer's disease has increased over the past decade. In addition, research on peptidergic changes in brain areas which are known to exhibit changes in other neurotransmitter systems such as acetylcholine (Candy et al., 1986) or monoamines (Gottfries, 1986), may yield information with respect to the specificity of alterations in neurotransmitter systems with aging or in Alzheimer's disease. Any selectivity in neurotransmitter changes in Alzheimer's disease may contribute to a better understanding of its pathogenesis, which is a prerequisite for the development of a rational therapeutic approach (Swaab and Fliers, 1986).

In various earlier studies, changes were demonstrated in neuropeptide systems which in general seemed to be indicative of degeneration. For instance, the level of somatostatin (SOM) was found to be reduced in a number of cortical areas in patients with Alzheimer's disease (Davies et al., 1980; Rossor et al., 1980a). These findings were

confirmed in later studies (Davies and Terry, 1981; Arai et al., 1984). Ferrier et al. (1983) reported decreased SOM levels in several cortical areas in Alzheimer's disease, without significant reductions in neurotensin (NT) or substance P (SP) levels. However, the decrease in SOM did not simply reflect the pattern of neuropathological changes, since in the hippocampus no difference was observed between patients with Alzheimer's disease and controls. Furthermore, there was no close correlation between changes in the cholinergic system and SOM changes in the cortical areas studied, suggesting a rather indirect relationship between these two systems. This was also illustrated by the fact that in the substantia innominata, where a 50% reduction in choline acetyltransferase (CAT) activity was found, concentrations of SOM were increased, which points towards selective neuropeptide changes in Alzheimer's disease, that are probably not directly related to changes in e.g. the cholinergic system.

Spatial selectivity of changes in neuropeptide systems also appeared from a study of Sanders et al. (1982), showing increased concentrations of glucagon in the grey matter of the temporal cortex in Alzheimer's disease, without differences in the occipital cortex. Other examples of reduced peptide concentrations in Alzheimer's disease are vasoactive intestinal polypeptide (VIP) in insular and angulate cortex (Arai et al., 1984) and, in contrast to the study of Ferrier et al. (1983), cortical substance P (Crystal and Davies, 1982).

Neuropeptide concentrations in brain areas

reflect, however, only a balance between the rates of production, transport, release and degradation. Consequently, changes in neuropeptide concentrations do not give any indication with respect to the direction in which the activity of peptidergic neurons has changed. Conversely, the absence of a decreased concentration does not rule out a marked reduction in the total number of afferent fibers, for example in the case of cortical atrophy. Consequently, it seems impossible to interpret changes in concentrations in terms of functional integrity of a particular peptidergic system. In that respect it might, however, be of interest that also in the cerebrospinal fluid (CSF), decreased neuropeptide concentrations have been reported in Alzheimer's disease e.g. for oxytocin (OXT) (Unger et al., 1971), ACTH (Facchinetti et al., 1984) and SOM (Oram et al., 1981; Soininen et al., 1984).

Vasopressin, aging and Alzheimer's disease

One peptide which has received much attention in relation to aging and Alzheimer's disease is vasopressin (VP), in view of its effects on certain aspects of memory as originally demonstrated by the group of De Wied (for review see De Wied, 1983). VP cells are present in the supraoptic and paraventricular nuclei (SON and PVN), from which they project to the neurohypophysis, where the peptide is released into the blood. These are the 'classical' neurosecretory cells of the hypothalamo-neurohypophyseal system (HNS), involved in the maintenance of water and salt homeostasis. VP cells are also present in the suprachiasmatic nucleus (SCN), both in the rat (Swaab et al., 1975; Vandesande et al., 1975) and in man (Dierickx and Vandesande, 1977; Swaab et al., 1985). VP fibers are present in many extrahypothalamic brain areas both in the rat and in man (Buijs et al., 1978; Fliers et al., 1986), where they most probably act as neurotransmitters (Buijs, 1982). Recent work in the rat showed that in many of these extrahypothalamic areas of termination, VP fibers are dependent upon the levels of circulating androgens (De Vries et al., 1985). Many of the areas of termination

contain VP fibers that are derived from the bed nucleus of the stria terminalis (BST), which, along with the dorsomedial hypothalamus, medial amygdaloid nucleus and locus ceruleus, was found to contain VP-immunoreactive cells in colchicine-pretreated rats (Van Leeuwen and Caffé, 1983; Caffé and Van Leeuwen, 1983). The human BST was also found to contain VP neurons, but the pattern of extrahypothalamic VP fiber distribution was found to be different from that in the rat (Fliers et al., 1986).

With respect to the neurosecretory pathway, degenerative changes with aging were proposed by Legros (1975), who showed decreased blood levels of neurophysins in a group of healthy men aged 50–60, as compared with younger age groups. In aged rodents, neurohypophyseal failure was proposed already in the 1950's (Friedman and Friedman, 1957). Effects of aging on the regulation of VP secretion were also observed. An increased VP response to hypertonic saline infusion has been reported (Helderman et al., 1978; Robertson and Rowe, 1980), while VP secretion in response to hemodynamic stimuli was found to decrease with aging (Rowe et al., 1982). However, these observations may give information regarding receptor sensitivity rather than the integrity of the HNS as such.

Because of the importance of salt and water homeostasis for the organism, the effects of treatment of aged rats with suspensions of posterior pituitary extracts on lifespan were tested. A significant prolongation of the mean lifespan was indeed observed after long-term treatment of old rats (Friedman and Friedman, 1963). However, in later experiments, this effect turned out to be due to OXT rather than to VP (Bodanszky and Engel, 1966). This surprising observation has not had any recent follow-up.

Legros' observations (1975), together with results of experiments indicating effects of VP on memory functions (see De Wied, 1983) have led to a number of clinical trials, in which VP or its analogs were administered to patients with Alzheimer's disease (for review see Jolles, 1983; Jolles,

1986). Moderate improvement of certain aspects of cognition was found in some studies, involving mildly impaired AD patients. However, major improvement of memory functions was not found (Jolles, 1986).

With respect to the integrity of centrally projecting VP cells in senescence and Alzheimer's disease, only very few data were available until recently. Rossor et al. (1980b) reported a non-significant decrease in VP concentrations in a number of extrahypothalamic brain areas in Alzheimer's disease, while a significant decrease was found in globus pallidus. In the aged rat brain, Dorsa and Bottemiller (1982) reported decreased VP concentrations in a number of extrahypothalamic areas. However, again these data were hard to interpret in terms of activity changes (see before). In human CSF, lower (Sundquist et al., 1983; Sørensen et al., 1983) as well as higher (Tsuji et al., 1981) VP levels in Alzheimer's disease have been reported, making unequivocal conclusions impossible.

In our studies on VP and OXT in the human brain, we have tried to circumvent the methodological pitfalls mentioned before by studying both cells of origin and areas of innervation, and by applying morphometric techniques that would indicate the direction of functional changes to immunocytochemically identified neurons. VP cells were studied from early infancy into senescence, while also brain material from patients with neuropathologically verified Alzheimer's disease was studied.

Hypothalamic VP cells in aging and Alzheimer's disease

In the SON and PVN, the size of immunocytochemically identified VP and OXT neurons and their nucleoli was measured as a parameter of neurosecretory activity (cf. Zambrano and De Robertis, 1968; Russel, 1983). No significant changes were observed in cellular profile areas of OXT cells from early infancy into senescence. However, VP cellular profile area was significantly increased both in the PVN and in the SON from 80–100 years of age,

pointing to activation of VP neurons. The Alzheimer's disease patients showed similar values as controls (Fliers et al., 1985a). A similar differential pattern of changes was found for the size of nucleoli of VP and OXT cells, viz., a significant increase in nucleolar size of VP cells after 80 years of age without changes in nucleolar size of OXT cells. The values of the Alzheimer's disease patients were commensurate with their age-matched controls (Hoogendijk et al., 1985). A highly significant correlation was found between mean nucleolar diameter and mean cellular profile area per patient of VP cells in the SON and PVN ($p < 0.001$). These results were indicative of increased neurosecretory activity of VP cells in senescence, as opposed to earlier reports in the literature (cf. Legros, 1975; Rowe et al., 1982). Two arguments plead against the possibility that the observed activation of neurosecretory VP cells has to be considered as a compensatory mechanism for cell loss from the PVN or SON: (a) recent studies reported elevated plasma levels of VP, both in the aged rat and in man (Frolkis et al., 1982; Fliers and Swaab, 1983; Miller, 1985; Kirkland et al., 1984), (b) determination of total cell numbers in the SON and PVN in the same material revealed no cell loss during normal aging. Cell numbers in the SON of Alzheimer's disease patients were somewhat lower than in age-matched controls, but this difference was not statistically significant. In the PVN, similar cell numbers were found in Alzheimer's disease patients and controls (Goudsmit et al., 1986; Swaab et al., 1986).

In aged rats, a strongly diminished VP binding in renal distal convolutes and collecting ducts was found (Ravid et al., 1986a). This opens the possibility of the activation of neurosecretory VP cells being a consequence of decreased renal sensitivity for VP in senescence. Another factor of possible causal importance is changes in gonadal function in senescence. Blood levels of testosterone decrease during aging, both in man (Deslypere and Vermeulen, 1984) and in the rat (Kaler and Neaves, 1981; Ravid et al., 1986b). Since castration of male rats has been shown to result in increased neurosecretory activity in the SON and PVN (Swaab and Jongkind, 1970) and in increased VP blood levels (Skowsky et al., 1979), the decreased levels of testosterone in senescence may contribute to the activation of neurosecretory VP cells in senescence. In addition, changes in the afferent innervation of the SON and PVN may play a role in the observed age-related changes. Sladek et al. (1983) observed a decrease in the catecholaminergic innervation of the SON in aged rats. No data are available on the human SON and PVN in this respect.

A completely different pattern of age-related changes was found in another VP cell containing hypothalamic nucleus, viz., the suprachiasmatic nucleus (SCN). This nucleus is considered to be the major circadian pacemaker of the mammalian brain, coordinating hormonal and behavioral circadian rhythms (e.g. Rusak and Zucker, 1979). Age-related changes in circadian rhythms have been reported in man as well as in other species (for review see Van Gool and Mirmiran, 1986). Among the most prominent changes is a fragmentation of sleep-wake patterns which occurs in senescence (Van Gool and Mirmiran, 1983), a phenomenon that is even more obvious in Alzheimer's disease patients (Prinz et al., 1982). Since the human SCN is hardly recognizable in conventionally stained material (Lydic et al., 1980), immunocytochemical staining of VP cells was used in order to visualize the nucleus, making it accessible to morphometric investigation.

A marked decrease in SCN volume, VP cell number and total cell number was found in subjects aged 80–100, while in Alzheimer's disease patients these changes were more pronounced than in age-matched controls (Swaab et al., 1985). Since the size of the SCN has been shown to be directly related to the expression of its pacemaker properties (Pickard and Turek, 1983), the observed decrease in SCN volume and cell number in senescence and Alzheimer's disease suggests a causal relationship between degenerative changes in the SCN and disturbances of circadian rhythmicity in these conditions.

The observations of increased activity of neurosecretory VP cells in senescence and Alzheimer's disease without concomitant cell loss in the SON and PVN, and of decreased SCN volume and cell number point towards differential changes with aging within one brain area, viz., the anterior hypothalamus, even among neurons of one peptidergic type, viz., VP neurons. The fact that all morphometric analyses were performed in one series of brain material gives extra support to this point. Since in the SCN, neither VP-cell density nor total cell density showed any significant changes with aging or in Alzheimer's disease, it can be concluded that determination of cell density does not necessarily give information with respect to cell loss. Apparently, marked cell loss may go together with unaltered cell density in case the volume of a particular structure decreases.

The pronounced changes observed in the SCN in senescence and Alzheimer's disease at first glance suggest that neurotransmitter changes in these conditions are not restricted to the cholinergic system. However, data concerning a possible cholinergic innervation of the human SCN are lacking. Therefore, our observations at present do not rule out cholinergic involvement in the disrupted circadian organization in Alzheimer's disease.

Changes in extrahypothalamic VP fibers in the aging brain

In order to investigate what the consequences of the differential changes with aging in VP cells are for the vasopressinergic innervation of extrahypothalamic brain areas, young and old Brown-Norway rats were compared with respect to the density of VP fibers in a number of brain areas. A marked decrease of VP fiber density was found in 34-months-old rats as compared with the 5-months-old control animals in the vertical limb of the diagonal band, the basal nucleus of Meynert (Fig. 1), the lateral habenular nucleus, the medial amygdaloid nucleus, the substantia nigra, the ventral hippocampus, the central grey, the locus

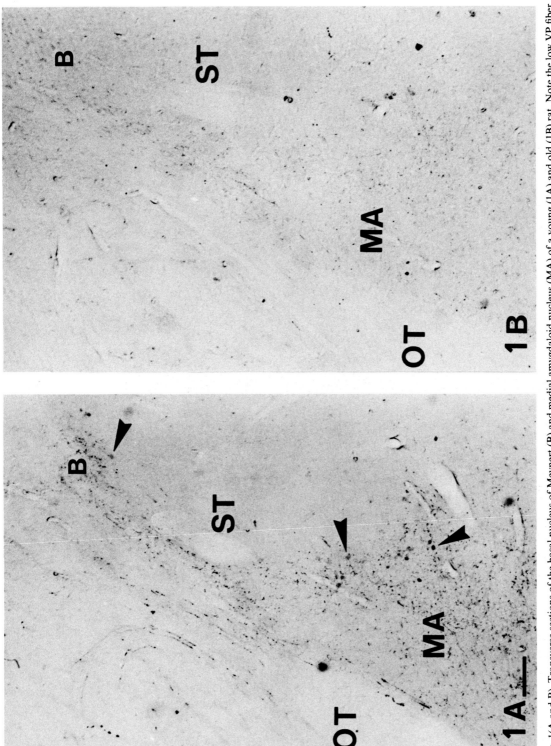

Fig. 1(A and B). Transverse sections of the basal nucleus of Meynert (B) and medial amygdaloid nucleus (MA) of a young (1A) and old (1B) rat. Note the low VP fiber density in both areas in 1B. Arrows point towards weakly staining VP immunoreactive cells that were found in both MA and B of young animals only. OT, optic tract; ST, stria terminalis. Bar represents 100 μm.

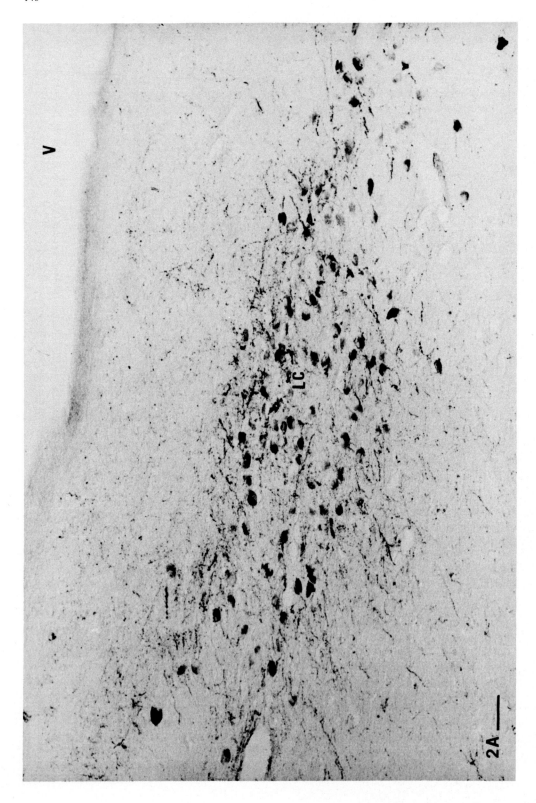

147

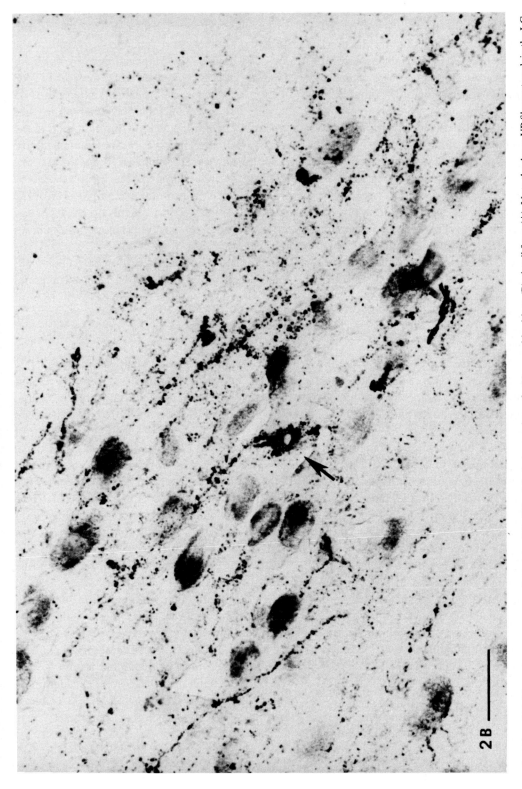

2 B

Fig. 2(A and B). Transverse cryostate section, stained for VP, of the locus ceruleus of a 74-year-old subject. (B), detail from (A). Note the dense VP fiber network in the LC between the neuromelanin-containing cell bodies. Arrow points towards structure, suggestive of perineuronal innervation. LC, locus ceruleus; V, fourth ventricle. Bars represent 100 μm (A) and 50 μm (B), respectively.

ceruleus and the ambiguus nucleus. The VP innervation of the lateral septum and the dorsomedial hypothalamic nucleus was moderately, although not significantly reduced. No age difference was found in the VP innervation of the paraventricular thalamic nucleus or in the nucleus of the solitary tract. OXT fiber density did not differ in any of the brain areas studied. Thus, the aging process appeared to affect centrally projecting VP cells in a differential way as well (Fliers et al., 1985b).

There is a remarkable similarity between the pattern of decrease in VP fiber density with aging and that observed following castration (cf. De Vries et al., 1985). In view of this parallel and since testosterone levels decrease during aging in rats of various strains (Kaler and Neaves, 1981; Chambers and Phoenix, 1984; Ravid et al., 1986b), the observed decrease in VP fiber density might be explained in part by age-related decline in testosterone levels. Therefore, long-term testosterone treatment of aged rats may yield interesting information with respect to the possible reversibility of these innervation changes and its potential behavioral consequences.

Also in the human brain a start was made with the investigation of the VP innervation of extrahypothalamic brain areas. Until recently, only little information was available on the morphologic distribution of VP fibers in the human brain, since most of the studies so far were performed by radioimmunoassay (RIA) (Rossor et al., 1981; Jenkins et al., 1984). However, also by means of immunocytochemistry as applied to post-mortem brain tissue, VP fibers could be demonstrated in the brain stem and spinal cord (Sofroniew et al., 1981), while the presence of VP fibers in the septum and spinal cord was found already by 17 weeks of gestation (Swaab and Ter Borg, 1981).

In a recent study, the VP and OXT innervation in brain material of human subjects aged 18–90 was investigated by means of immunocytochemistry (Fliers et al., 1986). In contrast to the rat brain, VP fibers were found only in low numbers in the septum, where, in contrast to the situation in rat,

no sex difference in VP fiber density was found. Very few VP fibers were found to be present in the amygdala and in the hippocampus. By contrast, the locus ceruleus contained dense networks of VP fibers over its entire rostro-caudal extension (Fig. 2). The extrahypothalamic VP innervation thus appears to be quite different from that seen in the rat, in that the innervation of human limbic structures is less pronounced than in the rat, whereas the innervation of the locus ceruleus is denser in the human brain as compared with the rat brain. As opposed to the rat, no effects of age on VP fiber density was found in any of the brain areas studied.

In future studies, the extrahypothalamic VP innervation will be investigated in brain material from Alzheimer's disease patients as well.

Summary and conclusions

In the present chapter, the pattern of peptidergic changes in Alzheimer's disease is reviewed and compared with changes during normal aging. Many peptides have been measured in Alzheimer's disease brain tissue and age-matched control material. Reduced cortical levels of SOM have been reported consistently, while reports of reductions in other neuropeptide systems (e.g. substance P) were not consistent. VP was reported to be reduced in a number of extrahypothalamic brain regions, although statistical significance was reached only in the globus pallidus. In the CSF, ACTH, SOM and OXT have been reported to be reduced in Alzheimer's disease. It is argued, however, that the mere determination of peptide concentrations in brain areas is not sufficient to investigate age-related or disease-related changes in peptidergic systems, since the observed changes cannot be interpreted in functional terms.

A different approach towards the elucidation of peptidergic changes during aging and Alzheimer's disease is the assessment of parameters that indicate changes in cell function, i.e. cell size or nucleolar size, in immunocytochemically identified peptidergic neurons. Application of such procedures to VP and OXT neurons in the human SON and PVN revealed increased neurosecretory activity of VP, but not of OXT cells in senescence and Alzheimer's disease. By contrast, extensive cell loss was found in the SCN, a VP cell containing hypothalamic area which is essential for the coordination of hormonal and behavioral circadian rhythms. Therefore, changes in VP cells during aging and Alzheimer's disease were found to be specific for the hypothalamic area studied. A topographic selectivity of age-related changes was also found in the VP innervation of the rat brain. The VP innervation of the human brain was found to differ from the rat brain, without any apparent age differences being found so far.

From these data it can be concluded that:

(a) changes in neurotransmitter systems in senescence and Alzheimer's disease are not restricted to cholinergic or monoaminergic neurons, but also include neuropeptides;

(b) changes in peptidergic neurons show a strong topographic selectivity, even among neurons of one peptidergic type;

(c) marked species differences may exist with respect to the neuroanatomy of peptidergic systems.

For these reasons, and in particular because there is no animal experimental model for Alzheimer's disease so far, it is essential to investigate such neurotransmitter changes in the human brain in order to obtain an insight into the neurotransmitter changes occurring in this disease.

Acknowledgements

The authors are indebted to the Foundation for Medical Research (FUNGO) and the Stichting Onderzoek op het gebied van de Ouder wordende Mens (SOOM) for financial support, to Dr. F. Van Haaren for checking the English and to Ms. T. Eikelboom for typing the manuscript.

References

Arai, H., Moroji, T. and Kosaka, K. (1984) Somatostatin and vasoactive intestinal polypeptide in postmortem brains from patients with Alzheimer-type dementia. *Neurosci. Lett.*, 52: 73–78.

Bodanszky, M. and Engel, S. L. (1966) Oxytocin and the lifespan of male rats. *Nature*, 210: 751.

Buijs, R. M. (1982) The ultrastructural localization of amines, amino acids and peptides in the brain. In R. M. Buijs, P. Pévet and D. F. Swaab (Eds.), *Chemical Transmission in the Brain. The Role of Amines, Amino Acids and Peptides, Progress in Brain Research, Vol. 55*, Elsevier, Amsterdam, pp. 167–183.

Buijs, R. M., Swaab, D. F., Dogterom, J. and Van Leeuwen, F. W. (1978) Intra- and extrahypothalamic vasopressin and oxytocin pathways in the rat. *Cell Tiss. Res.*, 186: 423–433.

Caffé, A. R. and Van Leeuwen, F. W. (1983) Vasopressin-immunoreactive cells in the dorsomedial hypothalamic region, medial amygdaloid nucleus and locus coeruleus of the rat. *Cell Tiss. Res.*, 233: 23–33.

Candy, J. M., Perry, E. K., Perry, R. H., Court, J. A., Oakley, A. E. and Edwardson, J. A. (1986) The current status of the cortical cholinergic system in Alzheimer's disease and Parkinson's disease. In D. F. Swaab, E. Fliers, M. Mirmiran, W. A. Van Gool and F. Van Haaren (Eds.), *Aging of the Brain and Alzheimer's Disease, Progress in Brain Research, this volume*, pp. 105–132.

Chambers, K. C. and Phoenix, C. H. (1984) Testosterone and the decline of sexual behavior in aging male rats. *Behav. Neural Biol.*, 40: 87–97.

Crystal, H. A. and Davies, P. (1982) Cortical substance P like immunoreactivity in senile dementia of the Alzheimer type. *J. Neurochem.*, 38: 1781–1784.

Davies, P. and Terry, R. D. (1981) Cortical somatostatin-like immunoreactivity in cases of Alzheimer's disease and senile dementia of the Alzheimer type. *Neurobiol. Aging*, 2: 9–14.

Davies, P., Katzman, R. and Terry, R. D. (1980) Reduced somatostatin-like immunoreactivity in cerebral cortex from cases of Alzheimer disease and Alzheimer senile dementia. *Nature*, 288: 279–280.

Deslypere, J. P. and Vermeulen, A. (1984) Leydig cell function in normal men: effect of age, lifestyle, residence, diet and activity. *J. Clin. Endocrinol. Metabol.*, 59: 955–962.

De Vries, G. J., Buijs, R. M., Van Leeuwen, F. W., Caffé, A. R. and Swaab, D. F. (1985) The vasopressinergic innervation of the brain in normal and castrated rats. *J. Comp. Neurol.*, 233: 236–254.

De Wied, D. (1983) Central actions of neurohypophysial hormones. In B. A. Cross and G. Leng (Eds.), *The Neurohypophysis: Structure, Function and Control, Progress in Brain Research, Vol. 60*, Elsevier, Amsterdam, pp. 155–168.

Dierickx, K. and Vandesande, F. (1977) Immunocytochemical localization of the vasopressinergic and oxytocinergic neurons in the human hypothalamus. *Cell Tiss. Res.*, 184: 15–27.

150

Dorsa, D. M. and Bottemiller, L. (1982) Age-related changes of vasopressin content of microdissected areas of the rat brain. *Brain Res.*, 242: 151–156.

Facchinetti, F., Nappi, G., Petraglia, F., Martignoni, E., Sinforiani, E. and Genazzani, A. R. (1984) Central ACTH deficit in degenerative and vascular dementia. *Life Sci.*, 35: 1691–1697.

Ferrier, I. N., Cross, A. J., Johnson, J. A., Roberts, G. W., Crow, T. J., Corsellis, J. A. N., Lee, Y. C., O'Shaughnessy, D., Adrian, T. E., McGregor, G. P., Baracese-Hamilton, A. J. and Bloom, S. R. (1983) Neuropeptides in Alzheimer type dementia. *J. Neurol. Sci.*, 62: 159–170.

Fliers, E. and Swaab, D. F. (1983) Activation of vasopressinergic and oxytocinergic neurons during aging in the Wistar rat. *Peptides*, 4: 165–170.

Fliers, E., Swaab, D. F., Pool, C. W. and Verwer, R. W. H. (1985a) The vasopressin and oxytocin neurons in the human supraoptic and paraventricular nucleus; changes with aging and in senile dementia. *Brain Res.*, 342: 45–53.

Fliers, E., De Vries, G. J. and Swaab, D. F. (1985b) Changes with aging in the vasopressin and oxytocin innervation of the rat brain. *Brain Res.*, 348: 1–8.

Fliers, E., Guldenaar, S. E. F., Van der Wal, N. and Swaab, D. F. (1986) Extrahypothalamic vasopressin and oxytocin in the human brain; presence of vasopressin cells in the bed nucleus of the stria terminalis. *Brain Res.*, 375: 363–367.

Friedman, S. M. and Friedman, C. L. (1957) Salt and water balance in ageing rats. *Gerontologia*, 1: 107–121.

Friedman, S. M. and Friedman, C. L. (1963) Effects of posterior pituitary extracts on the life-span of old rats. *Nature*, 200: 237–238.

Frolkis, V. V., Golovchenko, S. F., Medved, V. I. and Frolkis, R. A. (1982) Vasopressin and cardiovascular system in aging. *Gerontology*, 28: 290–302.

Gottfries, C. G. (1986) Monoamines and myelin components in aging and dementia disorders. In D. F. Swaab, E. Fliers, M. Mirmiran, W. A. Van Gool and F. Van Haaren (Eds.), *Aging of the Brain and Alzheimer's Disease, Progress in Brain Research, this volume*, pp. 133–140.

Goudsmit, E., Fliers, E. and Swaab, D. F. (1986) Unaltered cell numbers in the human supraoptic and paraventricular nucleus with aging and senile dementia, in preparation.

Helderman, J. H., Vestal, R. E., Rowe, J. W., Tobin, J. D., Andres, R. and Robertson, G. L. (1978) The response of arginine vasopressin to intravenous ethanol and hypertonic saline in man: the impact of aging. *J. Gerontol.*, 33: 39–47.

Hoogendijk, J. E., Fliers, E., Swaab, D. F. and Verwer, R. W. H. (1985) Activation of vasopressin neurons in the human supraoptic and paraventricular nucleus in senescence and senile dementia. *J. Neurol. Sci.*, 69: 291–299.

Jenkins, J. S., Ang, V. T. Y., Hawthorn, J., Rossor, M. N. and Iversen, L. L. (1984) Vasopressin, oxytocin and neurophysins in the human brain and spinal cord. *Brain Res.*, 291: 111–117.

Jolles, J. (1983) Vasopressin-like peptides and the treatment of memory disorders in man. In B. A. Cross and G. Leng (Eds.), *The Neurohypophysis: Structure, Function and Control, Progress in Brain Research, Vol. 60*, Elsevier, Amsterdam, pp. 169–182.

Jolles, J. (1986) Neuropeptides and the treatment of cognitive deficits in aging and dementia. In D. F. Swaab, E. Fliers, M. Mirmiran, W. A. Van Gool and F. Van Haaren (Eds.), *Aging of the Brain and Alzheimer's Disease, Progress in Brain Research, this volume*, pp. 429–441.

Kaler, L. W. and Neaves, W. B. (1981) The androgen status of aging male rats. Endocrinology, 108: 712–719.

Kirkland, J., Ley, M., Goddard, C., Vargas, E. and Davies, J. (1984) Plasma arginine vasopressin in dehydrated elderly. *Clin. Endocrinol.*, 20: 451–456.

Legros, J. J. (1975) The radioimmunoassay of human neurophysins: contribution to the understanding of the physiopathology of neurohypophyseal function. *Ann. NY Acad. Sci.*, 248: 281–303.

Lydic, R., Schoene, W. C., Czeisler, C. A. and Moore-Ede, M. C. (1980) Suprachiasmatic region of the human hypothalamus: homolog to the primate circadian pacemaker? *Sleep*, 2: 355–361.

Miller, M. (1985) Influence of aging on vasopressin secretion and water regulation. In R. W. Schrier (Ed.), *Vasopressin*, Raven Press, New York, pp. 249–258.

Oram, J. J., Edwardson, J. and Millard, P. H. (1981) Investigation of cerebrospinal fluid neuropeptides in idiopathic senile dementia. *Gerontology*, 27: 216–223.

Pickard, G. E. and Turek, F. W. (1983) The suprachiasmatic nuclei: two circadian clocks? *Brain Res.*, 268: 201–210.

Prinz, P. N., Vitaliano, P. P., Vitiello, M. V., Bokan, J., Raskind, M., Perskind, E. and Gerber, C. (1982) Sleep EEG and mental function changes in senile dementia of the Alzheimer's type. *Neurobiol. Aging*, 3: 361–370.

Ravid, R., Swaab, D. F., Fliers, E. and Hoogendijk, J. J. (1986a) Increased vasopressin production in senescence and dementia due to kidney changes. In A. Fisher, I. Hanin and C. Lachman (Eds.), *Alzheimer's and Parkinson's Disease: Strategies in Research and Development*, Plenum Press, New York, pp. 121–128.

Ravid, R., Fliers, E. and Swaab, D. F. (1986b) Changes in renal vasopressin (VP) binding sites, urinary VP excretion and plasma testosterone in aging male Brown-Norway rats, submitted for publication.

Robertson, G. L. and Rowe, J. (1980) The effect of aging on neurohypophyseal function. *Peptides*, 1: Suppl. 1, 159–162.

Rossor, M. N., Emson, P. C., Mountjoy, C. Q., Roth, M. and Iversen, L. L. (1980a) Reduced amounts of immunoreactive somatostatin in the temporal cortex in senile dementia of Alzheimer type. *Neurosci. Lett.*, 20: 373–377.

Rossor, M. N., Iversen, L. L., Mountjoy, C. Q., Roth, M., Hawthorn, J., Ang, V. T. Y. and Jenkins, J. S. (1980b) Arginine vasopressin and choline acetyltransferase in brains of patients with Alzheimer type senile dementia. *Lancet*, 2: 1367–1368.

Rossor, M. N., Iversen, L. L., Hawthorn, J., Ang, V. T. Y. and Jenkins, J. S. (1981) Extrahypothalamic vasopressin in human brain. *Brain Res.*, 214: 349–355.

Rowe, J. W., Minaker, K. L., Sparrow, D. and Robertson, G. L. (1982) Age-related failure of volume-pressure-mediated vasopressin release. *J. Clin. Endocrinol. Metabol.*, 54: 661–664.

Rusak, B. and Zucker, I. (1979) Neural regulation of circadian rhythms. *Physiol. Rev.*, 59: 449–526.

Russel, J. A. (1983) Combined morphometric and immunocyto-chemical evidence that in the paraventricular nucleus of the rat oxytocin — but not vasopressin — neurons respond to the suckling stimulus. In B. A. Cross and G. Leng (Eds.), *The Neurohypophysis: Structure, Function and Control, Progress in Brain Research, Vol. 60*, Elsevier, Amsterdam, pp. 31–38.

Sanders, D. J., Zahedi-Asl, S. and Marr, A. P. (1982) Glucagon and CCK in human brain: controls and patients with senile dementia of Alzheimer type. In R. M. Buijs, P. Pévet and D. F. Swaab (Eds.), *Chemical Transmission of the Brain. The Role of Amines, Amino Acids and Peptides, Progress in Brain Research, Vol. 55*, Elsevier, Amsterdam, pp. 465–471.

Skowsky, W. R., Swan, L. and Smith, P. (1979) Effects of sex steroid hormones on arginine vasopressin in intact and castrated male and female rats. *Endrocrinology*, 104: 105–108.

Sladek, J. R., Schöler, J. and Armstrong, W. E. (1983) Norepinephrine-vasopressin interactions during aging. In Y. Sano et al. (Eds.), *Structure and Function of Peptidergic and Aminergic Neurons*, Japan Scientific Society Press, Tokyo, pp. 289–298.

Sofroniew, M.V., Weindl, A., Schrell, U. and Wetzstein, R. (1981) Immunohistochemistry of vasopressin, oxytocin and neurophysin in the hypothalamus and extrahypothalamic region of the human and primate brain. *Acta Histochem.*, Suppl. 24: 79–95.

Soininen, H., Jolkkonen, J. T., Reinikainen, K. J., Halonen, T. O. and Riekkinen, P. J. (1984) Reduced cholinesterase activity and somatostatin like immunoreactivity in the cerebrospinal fluid of patients with dementia of the Alzheimer type. *J. Neurol. Sci.*, 63: 167–172.

Sørensen, P. S., Hammer, M., Vorstrup, S. and Gjerris, F. (1983) CSF and plasma vasopressin concentrations in dementia. *J. Neurol. Neurosurg. Psychiat.* 46: 911–916.

Sundquist, J., Forsling, M. L., Olsson, J. E. and Akerlund, M. (1983) Cerebrospinal fluid arginine vasopressin in degenerative disorders and other neurological diseases. *J. Neurol. Neurosurg. Psychiat.*, 46: 14–17.

Swaab, D. F. (1982) Neuropeptides. Their distribution and function in the brain. In R. M. Buijs, P. Pévet and D. F. Swaab (Eds.), *Chemical Transmission in the Brain. The Role of Amines, Amino Acids and Peptides, Progress in Brain Research, Vol. 55*, Elsevier, Amsterdam, pp. 97–122.

Swaab, D. F. and Fliers, E. (1986) Clinical strategies in the treatment of Alzheimer's disease. In D. F. Swaab, E. Fliers, M. Mirmiran, W. A. Van Gool and F. Van Haaren (Eds.), *Aging of the Brain and Alzheimer's Disease, Progress in Brain Research, this volume*, pp. 413–427.

Swaab, D. F. and Jongkind, J. F. (1970) The hypothalamic neurosecretory activity during the oestrous cycle, pregnancy, parturition, lactation, and persistent oestrous, and after gonadectomy in the rat. *Neuroendocrinology*, 6: 133–145.

Swaab, D. F. and Ter Borg, J. P. (1981) Development of peptidergic systems in the rat brain. In K. Elliot and J. Whelan (Eds.), *The Fetus and Independent Life*, Pittman Medical, London, pp. 271–294.

Swaab, D. F., Pool, C. W. and Nijveldt, F. (1975) Immunofluo-rescence of vasopressin and oxytocin in the rat hypothalamo-neurohypophyseal system. *J. Neural Transm.*, 36: 195–215.

Swaab, D. F., Fliers, E. and Partiman, T. S. (1985) The suprachiasmatic nucleus of the human brain in relation to sex, age and senile dementia. *Brain Res.*, 342: 37–44.

Swaab, D. F., Fliers, E. and Goudsmit, E. (1986) Differential cell loss in (peptide) neurons in the hypothalamus anterior with aging and in Alzheimer's disease. Lack of changes in cell density. In K. Poeck (Ed.), *Proceedings of the 13th World Congress of Neurology, Hamburg, Sept. 1–6*, Springer Verlag, Berlin, in press.

Tsuji, M., Takahashi, S. and Akazawa, S. (1981) CSF vasopressin and cyclic nucleotide concentrations in senile dementia. *Psychoneuroendocrinology*, 6: 171–176.

Unger, H., Pommrich, G. and Beck, R. (1971) Der Oxytocinge-halt im menschlichen pathologischen Liquor. *Experientia*, 27: 1486.

Vandesande, F., Dierickx, K. and De Mey, J. (1975) Identifi-cation of the vasopressin-neurophysin producing neurons of the rat suprachiasmatic nuclei. *Cell Tiss. Res.*, 156: 377–380.

Van Gool, W. A. and Mirmiran, M. (1983) Age-related changes in the sleep pattern of male adult rats. *Brain Res.*, 279: 394–398.

Van Gool, W. A. and Mirmiran, M. (1986) Aging and circadian rhythms. In D. F. Swaab, E. Fliers, M. Mirmiran, W. A. Van Gool and F. Van Haaren (Eds.), *Aging of the Brain and Alzheimer's Disease. Progress in Brain Research, this volume*, pp. 255–277.

Van Leeuwen, F. W. and Caffé, A. R. (1983) Vasopressin-immunoreactive cell bodies in the bed nucleus of the stria terminalis of the rat. *Cell Tiss. Res.*, 228: 525–534.

Zambrano, D. and De Robertis, E. (1968) The effect of castration upon the ultrastructure of the rat hypothalamus. Part I. Supraoptic and paraventricular nuclei. *Z. Zellforsch.*, 86: 487–498.

Discussion

R. S. J. FRACKOWIAK: Do you think your observation of differential sensitivity of neurons in one neurotransmitter system (which though anatomically distinct are spatially closely related) has any pathogenic implication or gives us any insight into pathogenic mechanisms in Alzheimer's disease?

ANSWER: Indeed, we are currently trying to elucidate the mechanisms underlying these differential changes. In the SCN a change in ACh innervation belongs to the possibilities. However, recent immunocytochemical staining with CAT antibodies failed to reveal a cholinergic innervation of the human SCN. Studies in rat have shown a reduction in both amplitude and period of circadian rhythm in senescence (Van Gool and Mirmiran, 1986), which may be related to a reduction in cell numbers in the SCN. Current experiments in aged rats are directed towards environmental manipulation of the age related changes in circadian rhythms. For the changes which we observed in the extrahypothalamic VP innervation of the rat brain, decreased blood levels of testosterone may be responsible, since the VP innervation of a number of brain areas has been shown to be dependent upon the levels of circulating androgens, both during development and in adulthood (De Vries et al., 1985). Recent experiments involving immunocytochemical staining of VP binding sites in the kidney suggest a role for the kidney in the increased neurosecretory activity of VP cells in senescence. All of these possibilities will be tested in future research.

D. M. GASH: What was the range in the number of vasopressin neurons in the SCN of AD patients? Was there an overlap between cell numbers found in AD patients and in the normal aged population?

ANSWER: There was an overlap. However, a comparison of AD patients with age- and sex-matched controls revealed a statistically significant difference in the number of SCN neurons between AD patients and controls.

R. D. TERRY: I do not believe that replacement of one or several neurotransmitters will provide effective improvement in Alzheimer's disease. Only finding and preventing the etiologic agent would seem to offer major help. L-DOPA's success in Parkinson's disease seems actually to have delayed research on the cause of that disease.

ANSWER: I fully agree with your point regarding replacement therapy in Alzheimer's disease, but I do think that our immunocytochemical approach towards the elucidation of changes in certain neurotransmitter systems may help us in obtaining a better insight into parts of the pathogenesis of AD.

A.J. CROSS: Two points about Dr. Terry's comments: (1) In Parkinson's disease there are many transmitter disturbances present in the brain at autopsy, yet L-DOPA still proves to be a useful therapeutic agent.

(2) I do not think that the relationship between plaques and the presence of dementia has been proved. In scrapie in animals, in some models one can get a proliferation of plaques without any obvious behavioral changes.

D.F. SWAAB: There are also theoretical reservations with respect to the proposed substitution therapies with neurotransmitters. It may be somewhat naive to think that we can replace the integrating capacity of the lost neurons by administrating their neurotransmitters. The brain is more than a solution of 1.5 litres of neurotransmitter!

P.W.M. RAAIJMAKERS: Do you know of any changes in afferents to the VP cells in SON and PVN that might be causing the age-dependent increase in VP that you find?

ANSWER: In aged rats, a decrease in the catecholaminergic innervation of the SON has been demonstrated (Sladek et al., 1983). However, we do not have data on age-related changes in other afferents to the PVN and SON in the rat. No data are available on the human brain in this respect. However, endocrine factors may be of importance as well. Recent results showed that VP binding to renal collecting ducts and distal convolutes is strongly diminished in aged rats. Hence, the activation of neurosecretory VP cells in the senescent brain might be secondary to decreased renal sensitivity for VP. A third factor of possible importance for the observed activation of VP cells is decreased levels of testosterone in senescence, since castration of adult rats has been shown to induce elevated VP blood levels (Skowsky et al., 1979) and increased neurosecretory activity of VP cells in the SON and PVN (Swaab and Jongkind, 1970). These possibilities will be investigated in future research.

References

De Vries, G. J., Buijs, R. M., Van Leeuwen, F. W., Caffé, A. R. and Swaab, D. F. (1985) The vasopressin innervation of the brain in normal and castrated rats. *J. Comp. Anat.*, 233: 236–254.

Skowsky, W. R., Swan, L. and Smith, P. (1979) Effects of sex steroid hormones on arginine vasopressin in intact and castrated male and female rats. *Endocrinology*, 104: 105–108.

Sladek, J. R., Schöler, J. and Armstrong, W. E. (1983) Norepinephrine-vasopressin interactions during aging. In Y. Sano et al. (Eds.), *Structure and Function of Peptidergic and Aminergic Neurons*, Japan Scientific Society Press, Tokyo, pp. 289–298.

Swaab, D. F. and Jongkind, J. (1970) The hypothalamic neurosecretory activity during the oestrous cycle, pregnancy, parturition, lactation, and persistent oestrus, and after gonadectomy, in the rat. *Neuroendocrinology*, 6: 133–145.

Van Gool, W. A. and Mirmiran, M. (1986) Aging and circadian rhythms. In D. F. Swaab, E. Fliers, M. Mirmiran, W. A. Van Gool and F. Van Haaren (Eds.), *Aging of the Brain and Alzheimer's Disease. Progress in Brain Research, this volume*, pp. 255–277.

D. F. Swaab, E. Fliers, M. Mirmiran, W. A. Van Gool and F. Van Haaren (Eds.)
Progress in Brain Research, Vol. 70.
© 1986 Elsevier Science Publishers B.V. (Biomedical Division)

CHAPTER 10

Cortical neurochemistry in Alzheimer-type dementia

A. J. Cross, T. J. Crow and T. J. Peters

Department of Physiology, University of Manchester, Manchester M13 9PT, and Divisions of Psychiatry and Clinical Cell Biology, Clinical Research Centre, Harrow HA1 3UJ, UK

Introduction

The occurrence of numerous senile plaques and neurofibrillary tangles in cerebral cortex and some limbic structures are considered to be the predominant pathological features of Alzheimer-type dementia (e.g. Tomlinson et al., 1970). In addition, it has become evident that neuronal loss and atrophy may also occur in some areas of the cerebral cortex and limbic system (Terry et al., 1981; Mountjoy et al., 1983; Mann et al., 1985), and degeneration of several subcortical structures which project to the cerebral cortex has been implicated in the disease process. These areas include the nucleus basalis of Meynert (Whitehouse et al., 1981), the locus coeruleus (Tomlinson et al., 1981) and some raphe nuclei (Mann et al., 1984).

Post-mortem neurochemical studies have demonstrated a severe loss of cortical neurochemical markers contained within the terminals of ascending neurons, particularly cholinergic (Bowen et al., 1976; Davies and Maloney, 1976; Perry et al., 1977) and to a lesser extent, noradrenergic (Adolfsson et al., 1979; Cross et al., 1981) and serotonergic (Bowen et al., 1983; Cross et al., 1983b). It has become clear that the loss of these markers in cortex do not correlate with the loss of their respective cell bodies in brain stem and basal forebrain (Candy et al., 1983; Perry et al., 1982; Pearson et al., 1983), although this may occur in Parkinsonian patients with dementia (Perry et al., 1985).

It would seem likely, therefore, that in Alzheimer-type dementia, changes in ascending neurons are secondary to pathological changes in cerebral cortex and some limbic structures. The degenerative changes observed in the brain-stem nuclei and the basal forebrain may consequently be the result of retrograde degeneration, a process which has been shown to occur in cholinergic and adrenergic neurons following cortical lesion (Pearson et al., 1983).

Neuropathological studies have suggested that the temporal lobe may be an early focus of the disease (summarised by Wilcock, 1983), and limbic structures within the temporal lobe such as the hippocampus and amygdala (Hooper and Vogel, 1976) are particularly affected. Neurochemical studies of markers of intrinsic cortical neurons have demonstrated a selective loss of somatostatin (Davies and Terry, 1981; Rossor et al., 1982; Ferrier et al., 1983), and in the most severely affected, GABA (Rossor et al., 1982). These changes may be limited to the temporal lobe in the less severely demented subjects (Rossor et al., 1984).

It would seem likely, therefore, that the temporal lobe is of central importance in the pathogenesis of Alzheimer-type dementia, and we have concentrated our neurochemical studies on this region. In the present report, we describe studies on the neurochemistry of the temporal cortex using two quite different approaches. Firstly, we have examined a series of neurotransmitter receptors using ligand-binding techniques. The neurochemical markers of intrinsic cortical neurons previously studied have been either neuropeptides or GABA. As neurotransmitter receptors in cortex are predominantly post-synaptic, these are also considered as markers of the integrity of cortical cell bodies and dendrites. Whilst demonstrating the selectivity of the degenerative process, studies of neurotransmitters and receptors have provided little information on the sequence of metabolic changes which lead to the selective cell loss. An alternative to measuring markers of particular cells is to study markers of subcellular organelles, and this forms the basis of the second part of this study. The technique involves quantifying components specific to membranes or organelles as markers of the integrity and functional activity of the organelle (Peters and Seymour, 1978).

In addition, we have compared the activities of the various neurochemical markers in Alzheimer-type dementia patients with a group of Huntington's disease patients. Both of these groups of patients suffer under broadly similar conditions of terminal illness, which are extremely difficult to control (Spokes, 1980). By comparison of these groups, we hope to eliminate any non-specific changes due to agonal status and terminal anoxia.

Post-mortem brains

Two series of post-mortem brains were studied:

(1) A series of 14 brains from subjects with Alzheimer-type dementia (ATD) collected by Professor J. A. N. Corsellis, Runwell Hospital, Middlesex, and a series of matched controls. Brains were obtained at autopsy, halved sagitally and one half was frozen for subsequent dissection and neurochemical analysis, the other half being fixed in formalin for neuropathological assessment. Brains were stored and dissected as previously described (Ferrier et al., 1983), temporal cortex consisted of Brodmann areas 21 and 22 combined. Whilst the control group contained no cases with a history of neuropsychiatric disease, no histological examination of the brain was made. The clinical diagnosis of Alzheimer-type dementia was confirmed neuropathologically by the presence of numerous senile plaques and neurofibrillary tangles in cerebral cortex and hippocampus. Cases with evidence of moderate to severe vascular changes were not included. The groups were matched for age, sex and post-mortem delay, details of which are given in Table I. All the patients in the ATD group suffered from protracted terminal illnesses associated with hypoxia, the majority with bronchopneumonia.

(2) A series of 16 brains from subjects with Huntington's chorea, collected by Dr. Gavin Reynolds, at the MRC Neurochemical Pharmacology Unit, Cambridge, and 17 matched controls. Details of the methods of collection, storage and dissection of these samples have been described previously (Spokes, 1980). Frontal cortex tissue was taken from Brodmann area 4. The clinical diagnosis of Huntington's disease was confirmed neuropathologically. The post-mortem details of the control and Huntington's disease patients are shown in Table I, in this case the majority of the Huntington's disease patients died with bronchopneumonia. Most of the patients had been treated with phenothiazine or butyrophenone neuroleptics, whereas none of the control patients had received neuroleptics.

TABLE I

Post-mortem details

	Age (y)	Sex (M/F)	Post-mortem delay (h)
Controls	77.6 ± 14.8	5/5	52.5 ± 20.6
Alzheimer-type dementia	81.3 ± 11.7	5/5	45.0 ± 20.3
Controls	63.2 ± 11.7	14/3	52.4 ± 25.4
Huntington's disease	64.9 ± 10.2	12/4	49.4 ± 23.1

Values are mean $\pm$ SD. Post-mortem delay is the time from death to autopsy in hours.

Ligand-binding studies

Serotonin receptors in Alzheimer-type dementia

Our initial studies using ^{3}H-LSD as ligand (Cross et al., 1984a) demonstrated a marked loss of serotonin receptors in cortex and hippocampus in ATD. However, it is apparent that ^{3}H-LSD labels at least two types of serotonin receptor in rat and human brain (Peroutka and Snyder, 1979; Cross, 1982), and we have therefore used ligands selective for these subtypes in the present study. Thus, ^{3}H-serotonin was used to label S1 receptors and ^{3}H-ketanserin to label S2 receptors (Peroutka and Snyder, 1979; Leysen et al., 1982).

The binding of ^{3}H-serotonin to membrane preparations of control and ATD brains is shown in Table II. In controls, highest binding values

TABLE II

^{3}H-Serotonin binding to S1 receptors in controls and ATD patients

	Control	ATD	% Control
Temporal cortex	51.4 ± 5.2 (11)	27.2 ± 3.6[b] (10)	54
Frontal cortex	136 ± 9.3 (12)	116 ± 13.2 (11)	85
Cingulate cortex	103 ± 14.4 (12)	75.3 ± 15.0 (10)	73
Hippocampus	53.6 ± 7.6 (10)	31.9 ± 6.4[a] (12)	60
Amygdala	23.9 ± 2.2 (12)	11.4 ± 2.9[b] (12)	48
Olfactory tubercle	36.3 ± 4.2 (12)	28.7 ± 4.1 (12)	79
Substantia nigra	39.2 ± 4.3 (12)	22.6 ± 7.1 (6)	58
Substantia innominata	39.6 ± 3.0 (5)	22.2 ± 5.7 (5)	56
Septum	27.0 ± 3.6 (5)	15.5 ± 4.7 (6)	57
Caudate nucleus	77.8 ± 8.6	80.6 ± 9.6	103

Values are expressed as fmol ligand bound/mg protein, mean ± SEM. Numbers of samples are given in parentheses. [a]$p < 0.05$, [b]$p < 0.01$. Comparisons were made using Students t test (2-tailed).

TABLE III

^{3}H-Ketanserin binding to S2 receptors in controls and ATD patients

	Control	ATD	% Control
Temporal cortex	56.3 ± 6.44 (11)	20.0 ± 3.0[a] (10)	36
Frontal cortex	90.4 ± 9.8 (12)	48.6 ± 6.4[a] (12)	54
Cingulate cortex	57.6 ± 5.9 (12)	30.4 ± 3.1[a] (9)	53
Hippocampus	17.4 ± 2.2 (12)	11.6 ± 1.8 (12)	67
Amygdala	20.6 ± 2.4 (12)	12.4 ± 2.0[a] (12)	60
Olfactory tubercle	22.2 ± 3.2 (12)	17.6 ± 2.8 (12)	79
Substantia nigra	14.4 ± 1.3 (12)	14.2 ± 2.8 (6)	99
Substantia innominata	30.2 ± 8.0 (5)	17.4 ± 1.6 (5)	58
Septum	22.6 ± 4.0 (7)	12.4 ± 2.8 (6)	55

Values are expressed as fmol ligand bound/mg protein, mean ± SEM. Numbers of samples are given in parentheses. [a]$p < 0.01$ (Students t test, 2-tailed).

were observed in frontal and cingulate cortex and caudate nucleus. ^{3}H-serotonin binding was lowest in basal forebrain regions such as septum and amygdala. Significant reductions in ^{3}H-serotonin binding were observed in temporal cortex, hippocampus and amygdala in the ATD group. The distribution of ^{3}H-ketanserin binding to control brain membranes (Table III) differed from ^{3}H-serotonin binding. Highest binding values were observed in frontal cortex, temporal cortex and cingulate cortex, with considerably lower values in the other brain regions studied. Whereas hippocampus contained moderate levels of ^{3}H-serotonin binding, this was one of the lowest areas for ^{3}H-ketanserin binding. Significant differences between controls and ATD patients were observed in neocortex and amygdala. Again, whilst mean binding values were considerably reduced in

TABLE IV

Saturation analysis of ^{3}H-serotonin and ^{3}H-ketanserin binding to control and ATD temporal cortex

Ligand	Binding constant	Control	ATD
^{3}H-Serotonin	K_D	1.77 ± 0.21	1.72 ± 0.35
	B_{max}	53.5 ± 8.2	33.9 ± 6.5^a
^{3}H-Ketanserin	K_D	1.52 ± 0.19	1.53 ± 0.16
	B_{max}	104 ± 12	43.2 ± 7.7^a

Binding values were derived from Scatchard plots of saturation data using ^{3}H-serotonin concentrations of 0.5–8.0 nM and ^{3}H-ketanserin concentrations of 0.2–4.0 nM. K_D values are given as nM and B_{max} values as fmol ligand bound/mg. All values are mean $\pm$ SEM of 3 samples. $^a p < 0.05$ (Students t test, 2-tailed).

septum and substantia innominata, these reductions were not statistically significant.

Binding parameters derived from saturation analysis of ^{3}H-serotonin and ^{3}H-ketanserin binding to temporal cortex membranes of three controls and three ATD patients are given in Table IV. The reduction in binding of both ^{3}H-serotonin and ^{3}H-ketanserin in ATD samples was characterised by a loss of binding sites (B_{max}) with no change in affinity (K_D).

The selectivity of the reduction in serotonin receptors

In view of the marked reduction in serotonin S2 receptors in temporal cortex (to 36% of control), this area was chosen for further study. The specificity of the reduction was examined by studying a range of other receptors using ligand binding assays. The binding of the various ligands tested to membrane preparations of control and ATD temporal cortex is given in Table V. Of the 13 ligand binding sites studied, only two were significantly reduced in the ATD group. Of these, the serotonin S2 receptor was the only monoamine receptor found to be reduced, to 57% of control values, with no change in serotonin S1 receptors or adrenergic receptors. Among the other binding

TABLE V

Ligand binding in temporal cortex of controls and ATD patients

Receptor	Control ($n = 13$)	ATD ($n = 13$)	% Control
β-adrenergic	49.6 ± 1.8	50.0 ± 2.9	101
α_1-adrenergic	99.1 ± 4.2	87.3 ± 8.0	88
α_2-adrenergic	33.6 ± 2.0	32.0 ± 2.1	95
Serotonin S1	47.0 ± 2.8	41.0 ± 4.4	87
Serotonin S2	116.0 ± 5.0	66.9 ± 4.4^a	57
Adenosine A1	57.8 ± 5.4	56.0 ± 5.3	106
Histamine H1	69.3 ± 4.6	58.5 ± 4.2	85
Benzodiazepine	458 ± 16	587 ± 12^a	84
Opiate μ	81.9 ± 6.9	82.1 ± 7.2	100
Opiate K$^+$	32.3 ± 2.7	36.0 ± 3.2	111
GABA	258 ± 13	244 ± 20	95
Muscarinic	290 ± 11	272 ± 12	
Kainic acid	130 ± 12	132 ± 11	102

Values are expressed as fmol ligand bound/mg protein, mean $\pm$ SEM. $^a p < 0.01$ (Students t test, 2-tailed).

sites, only benzodiazepine receptors were reduced, to 84% of controls; although a reduction of similar magnitude in histamine H1 receptors was observed, this was not statistically significant. The reduction in serotonin S2 receptors in the ATD group was significantly greater than the loss of benzodiazepine receptors (paired t test $p < 0.01$).

Relationship between ligand binding and pre- and post-mortem variables

No differences between males and females were observed for any of the parameters studied. In the control group, no significant relationships were observed between age and ligand binding in any brain region. It should be noted that the age range of the control group was restricted (69–92 years). Similarly, in the ATD group, no significant relationship between ^{3}H-ketanserin binding and age was apparent. In contrast, a significant age effect on ^{3}H-serotonin binding in the ATD group was noted (Fig. 1). When the ATD group was divided on the basis of younger or older than 75

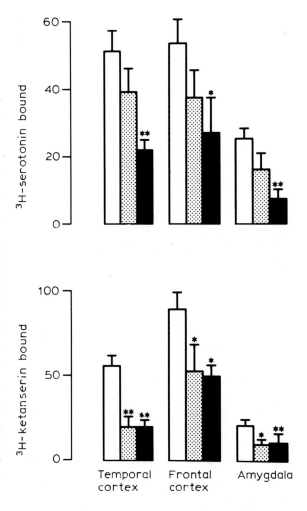

Fig. 1. Relationships between serotonin receptors and age in ATD brains. Control values are given as open columns; ▨, ATD patients older than 75 years; ■, ATD patients younger than 75 years. Binding values are as fmol ligand bound/mg protein, bars represent SEM; $_*p < 0.05$, $_{**}p < 0.01$ vs. controls.

(see discussion by Rossor et al., 1982), the significant decreases in ³H-serotonin binding in the ATD group were only observed in the younger subjects. Both younger and older ATD patients demonstrated significantly reduced ³H-ketanserin binding compared to controls.

None of the neurochemical parameters studied correlated significantly with post-mortem delay or agonal status in either the control or ATD groups.

Relationship between serotonin receptors and other neurochemical parameters

In the combined control and ATD groups, significant correlations were observed between ³H-ketanserin binding and choline acetyltransferase activity in temporal cortex ($r = 0.543$, $p < 0.05$) and hippocampus ($r = 0.517$, $p < 0.05$), and between ³H-serotonin binding and choline acetyltransferase

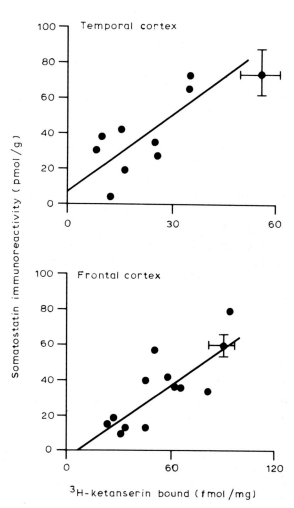

Fig. 2. Relationships between ³H-ketanserin binding and somatostatin-like immunoreactivity in temporal cortex (upper) and frontal cortex (lower) of ATD patients. Mean control values are included with bars representing SEMs. Somatostatin immunoreactivity values are those previously published (Ferrier et al., 1984). For frontal cortex $r = 0.666$, $p < 0.05$, and for temporal cortex, $r = 0.678$, $p < 0.05$.

activity in temporal cortex ($r = 0.523$, $p < 0.05$) and hippocampus ($r = 0.702$, $p < 0.01$). None of these relationships were significant in the ATD group alone. None of the other ligand binding sites studied correlated with choline acetyltransferase activity in either the combined group or the ATD group alone. In contrast to S2 receptors, none of these binding sites was related to age within the ATD group.

[3]H-Ketanserin binding in the ATD group was significantly correlated with somatostatin-like immunoreactivity (SRIF) (assayed in the same samples and reported by Ferrier et al., 1983) in temporal cortex ($r = 0.678$, $p < 0.05$) and frontal cortex ($r = 0.666$, $p < 0.05$) but not in other areas where ^{3}H-ketanserin binding was reduced (cingulate cortex $r = 0.633$ NS, amygdala $r = 0.077$ NS). These relationships are shown in Fig. 2. The binding of ^{3}H-ketanserin in cingulate cortex of the ATD group was highly significantly correlated with GABA concentrations in this region ($r = 0.924$, $p < 0.01$) (Fig. 3). In contrast, ^{3}H-ketanserin binding in temporal and frontal cortex was not significantly correlated with GABA concentrations ($r = 0.072$ and $r = 0.216$, respectively).

Significant correlations were observed between

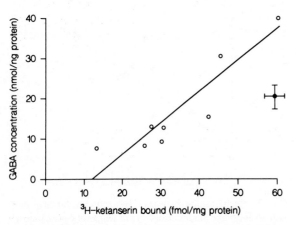

Fig. 3. Relationship between ^{3}H-ketanserin binding and GABA concentration in cingulate cortex of ATD patients (○). The mean control value is included (●), bars represent SEM; $r = 0.924$, $p < 0.01$. GABA concentrations were determined using a radioreceptor assay (Enna and Snyder, 1976).

[3]H-serotonin binding and ^{3}H-ketanserin binding in frontal cortex ($r = 0.542$, $p < 0.01$), temporal cortex ($r = 0.744$, $p < 0.01$) and cingulate cortex ($r = 0.709$, $p < 0.01$) of the control and ATD groups combined. Only the relationship in temporal cortex remained significant in the ATD group alone ($r = 0.661$, $p < 0.05$).

Relationship between serotonin receptors and cholinergic neurons

Although the reductions in serotonin receptors in Alzheimer-type dementia did not correlate with the cholinergic marker enzyme choline acetyltransferase, the possibility exists that serotonin receptors may be present on some cholinergic terminals. The loss of cortical serotonin receptors in Alzheimer-type dementia would then merely reflect the cholinergic deficit. We have examined this possibility by studying cortical serotonin receptor subtypes in rats after excitotoxin lesions of the basal forebrain. Ten days after unilateral ibotenic acid injections into the nucleus basalis, a 50–60% loss of cortical choline acetyltransferase activity was observed on the lesioned side, whereas the activity of glutamic acid decarboxylase, a marker of intrinsic cortical neurons, was unaffected by the lesion, as were dopamine and serotonin metabolism.

Serotonin receptors were assessed in two groups of animals after unilateral ibotenic acid injections. In both groups of animals, serotonin S1 receptors, as labelled by ^{3}H-serotonin, were significantly reduced on the lesioned side. The magnitude of the change was small but reproducible. In contrast, ^{3}H-ketanserin binding to S2 receptors was unaffected by the lesion procedure (Table VI).

The present results are therefore consistent with a loss of some cortical serotonin S1 but not S2 receptors after lesion of cortical afferents. The observation that cortical serotonin S2 receptors are independent of cortical cholinergic afferents complements the findings of Leysen et al. (1983). In these studies, serotonin S2 receptors were unaffected by lesions of the ascending serotonergic

TABLE VI

Effects of nucleus basalis lesions on serotonin S1 and S2 receptors in rat cortex

	Receptor	Control	Lesion	% Control
Expt 1. ($n = 8$)	Serotonin S1	41.8 ± 6.4	33.4 ± 8.7	80[a]
	Serotonin S2	49.2 ± 7.6	48.0 ± 7.3	98
Expt 2. ($n = 6$)	Serotonin S1	42.1 ± 2.9	32.3 ± 3.8	77[a]
	Serotonin S2	45.6 ± 9.2	41.5 ± 6.5	91

All values as fmol ligand bound/mg protein, mean $\pm$ SD.
[a]$p < 0.05$ (paired t test, 2-tailed).

system, but reduced by almost 80% by kainic acid lesions of intrinsic neurons. Thus, the majority of cortical serotonin S2 receptors may be present on intrinsic neurons (or on other extrinsic systems).

Serotonin receptors in Huntington's disease

To control for the non-specific effects of the protracted terminal illnesses associated with chronic neuropsychiatric diseases, serotonin receptors were studied in a group of Huntington's disease patients, and a group of controls (Table VII). In contrast to Alzheimer-type dementia, serotonin S2 receptors were not significantly reduced in the cortex in Huntington's disease

patients. This suggests that the reduction in S2 receptors in ATD is not related to the non-specific factors associated with chronic hospitalisation but may relate specifically to the disease process. Interestingly, serotonin S1 receptors were reduced in both cortex and hippocampus in Huntington's disease.

Markers of subcellular organelles

Markers of subcellular organelles in temporal cortex

The distribution of subcellular markers in temporal cortex of control and Alzheimer-type dementia patients is shown in Table VIII. No differences were observed between the groups for the plasma membrane marker enzymes, γ-glutamyltransferase and 5'-nucleotidase. Of the lysosomal enzymes, β-glucuronidase activity was significantly increased in the ATD group (to 145% of control $p < 0.02$), whereas acid phosphatase activity was unchanged. DNA concentrations were used as an index of the nucleus, and RNA concentrations as a marker of ribosomes and neither were altered in the ATD group. Catalase activity was used as a marker of peroxisomes, and was found to be highly variable in the samples studied, enzyme activity in the ATD group was not significantly different from controls. The activity of 2'3'cyclic nucleotide phosphohydrolase was used as a myelin marker and again no

TABLE VII

Serotonin receptors in Huntington's disease

Receptor	Brain region		Huntington's	% Control
S1 Receptor (^{3}H-serotonin binding)	Frontal cortex	121 ± 12	81 ± 12	67[a]
	Hippocampus	229 ± 18	146 ± 16	64[b]
S2 Receptor (^{3}H-ketanserin binding)	Frontal cortex	76 ± 7	59 ± 7	79
	Hippocampus	N.D.	N.D.	

Values are fmol ligand bound/mg protein, mean $\pm$ SEM.
N.D., no significant binding.
[a]$p < 0.05$, [b]$p < 0.01$ (Students t test, 2-tailed).

TABLE VIII

Subcellular organelle marker activities in ATD temporal cortex

Organelle	Marker	Activity in control (n = 10)		ATD (n = 10)	
Plasma membrane	5'nucleotidase	109	± 34	125	± 56
	γ-glutamyltransferase	1.19 ±	0.15	1.31 ±	0.26
Lysosome	acid phosphatase	7.62 ±	2.81	7.29 ±	1.71
	β-glucuronidase	0.055±	0.012	0.080±	0.070[b]
Mitochondria	total MAO	3.15 ±	0.69	3.74 ±	0.35[a]
	MAO-A	1.31 ±	0.42	1.00 ±	0.19
	MAO-B	1.80 ±	0.53	2.59 ±	0.74[a]
Peroxisome	catalase	32.2 ±	15.0	54.1 ±	33.9
Myelin	2'3'CNPase	3250	±940	3794	±430
Endoplasmic reticulum	neutral α-glucosidase	0.182±	0.105	0.088±	0.060[b]
Ribosome	RNA	3.97 ±	0.68	4.68 ±	0.75
Nucleus	DNA	5.88 ±	1.05	5.15 ±	1.77

Enzyme activities are expressed as nmol product formed/mg protein/min and nucleic acid concentrations as μg/mg protein, mean ± SD. [a]$p < 0.05$ [b]$p < 0.02$ (Students t test, 2-tailed).

difference was found between controls and ATD patients.

Total monoamine oxidase activity, assessed using tyramine as substrate, was used initially as a marker of mitochondria. Enzyme activity was marginally but significantly increased to 119% of control values ($p < 0.05$). Further analysis using benzylamine as a substrate for monoamineoxidase-B demonstrated that the increase in monoamine oxidase activity resided solely in the B isoenzyme which was increased to 143% of control values ($p < 0.05$).

Neutral α-glucosidase was used as a marker of endoplasmic reticulum and was found to be markedly reduced in temporal cortex (to 48% of control values $p < 0.02$).

Glycoside hydrolase activities in temporal cortex

In view of the increase in lysosomal β-glucuronidase activity with no change in acid phosphatase, the activities of a range of glycoside hydrolases with acidic pH optima were studied in temporal cortex of controls and ATD patients (Table IX).

Whilst the majority of the glycoside hydrolases studied were unchanged in Alzheimer-type dementia, a significant increase was observed in β-xylosidase activity, to 123% of control ($p < 0.05$). In contrast, the activity of α-fucosidase was significantly decreased to 72% of control ($p < 0.05$).

Golgi-endoplasmic reticulum-associated enzymes in temporal cortex

Subsequent to the demonstration of reduced activity of the endoplasmic reticulum marker, neutral α-glucosidase (Table VIII), a number of other enzymes associated with this fraction were studied. NADPH-cytochrome c reductase may be taken as a marker of smooth endoplasmic reticulum, whereas inosine diphosphatase may be associated with both smooth and rough endoplasmic reticulum. None of the enzyme activities were changed in Alzheimer-type dementia temporal cortex (Table X). In addition, the Golgi-associated enzymes, galactosyltransferase and fucosyltransferase were also unchanged in Alzheimer-type dementia (Table X).

elements (see Peroutka et al., 1980; Henn et al., 1980). However, in experimental animals, ^{3}H-ketanserin binding to S2 receptors is considered to be present on intrinsic cortical neurons (Leysen et al., 1983; Cross and Deakin, 1985). Similarly, SRIF and GABA are thought to be present in intrinsic cortical neurons in animals (Emson and Lindvall, 1979) and man (Sorensen, 1982; Vincent et al., 1982). The present results are therefore consistent with a loss of neuronal cell bodies or dendrites in temporal cortex. Whilst a loss of cortical neurons has been reported in some cases of ATD (Brun and Eglund, 1981; Terry et al., 1981) this may be less consistent than hippocampal changes (Tomlinson and Henderson, 1976). A loss of dendritic morphology and volume has also been demonstrated in ATD (Schiebel and Tomiyasu, 1978; Buell and Coleman, 1979). The reduction in serotonin S2 receptors in ATD, coupled with the absence of changes in other ligand binding sites suggests that such processes may be selective to certain subpopulations of cortical neurons.

The binding of ^{3}H-serotonin to S1 receptors did not correlate with measures of choline acetyltransferase activity, GABA concentrations or somatostatin immunoreactivity, SRIF (Ferrier et al., 1983) in the ATD group. In temporal and frontal cortex, the binding of ^{3}H-ketanserin to S2 receptors was significantly correlated with SRIF; however, this relationship was not significant in other regions where S2 receptors were reduced in ATD. S2 receptors did, however, correlate with GABA concentrations in cingulate cortex of the ATD group. Two interpretations of the present data are possible. Firstly, that distinct sets of cortical neurons carrying S2 receptors in temporal, frontal and cingulate cortex, and separate sets of neurons containing SRIF in frontal and temporal cortex and perhaps GABA in cingulate cortex, may degenerate in ATD. Alternatively, intrinsic cortical neurons which carry S2 receptors may degenerate in ATD, and these cells could contain SRIF in temporal and frontal cortex, and GABA in cingulate cortex. The present data do not differentiate between these interpretations. However, it is

noteworthy that the intralaminar distribution of S2 receptors in human temporal cortex (Luaboya et al., 1984) differs from the distribution of both somatostatin immunoreactivity (Perry et al., 1983) and choline acetyltransferase activity (Perry et al., 1984a). Moreover, cortical layers III and IV, which are the layers most abundant in S2 receptors in normal brain (Luaboya et al., 1984), also show the greatest degree of abnormal dendritic morphology in ATD (Paula-Barbosa et al., 1980).

It is unlikely that the progression of pathological changes in the serotonergic system occurs primarily in the raphe nucleus and spreads to terminal fields, as changes in serotonin and 5-HIAA concentrations (Adolfsson et al., 1979; Cross et al., 1984b) are not evenly distributed throughout terminal areas such as cortex and basal ganglia. It would seem probable that changes in serotonergic cell bodies in raphe nucleus are secondary to pathological changes in areas where 5-HIAA concentrations are reduced (i.e. neocortex and hippocampus). In the present study, serotonin receptors and particularly S2 receptors were selectively reduced in these areas. Our results suggest also that changes in S2 receptors occur relatively early, as has been proposed for SRIF (Rossor et al., 1984). It is possible, therefore, to envisage that changes in neurons expressing S2 receptors in neocortex and hippocampus might lead to degeneration of serotonergic terminals and, hence, to changes in dorsal raphe nucleus.

It is difficult to determine how these changes in serotonin receptors relate to the cholinergic abnormalities in ATD. It is clear that a similar process does not occur in the cholinergic system in ATD, as muscarinic receptors are within the normal range in ATD (Perry et al., 1977; Davies and Verth, 1978; Caulfield et al., 1982; present results). In the present study, serotonergic receptors were assessed in septum and substantia innominata, the areas of basal forebrain containing cholinergic cell bodies which project to hippocampus and cortex, respectively (see Fibiger, 1983). In these regions, serotonin receptors were markedly reduced in ATD. The levels of serotonin receptors were low and the sample size was small, consequently with the large variability in the results, none of the differences were statistically significant. The substantia innominata as dissected in the present study (Ferrier et al., 1983), whilst containing some of the areas rich in intensely cholinesterase-positive neurons (Whitehouse et al., 1981; Candy et al., 1983), may also contain other structures. Thus, the present results provide no conclusive evidence that serotonin receptors are reduced in septum and substantia innominata in ATD. The use of quantitative autoradiographic techniques or tissue punches of specific regions may resolve this problem.

The cholinergic deficits in ATD that have been extensively studied (see Rossor et al., 1982) appear to be an early neurochemical change, and in some cases, may precede neuropathological change (Rossor et al., 1982). At present there is no obvious neuroanatomic connection between actylcholine- and somatostatin-containing structures in cortex and hippocampus. Our studies in animals with neurotoxin-induced lesions suggest that S2 receptors are not detectable on cholinergic terminals in rat cortex and also that muscarinic cholinergic receptors are not present on serotonergic terminals (Cross and Deakin, unpublished data). An alternative explanation is that somatostatin-containing neurons carry S2 receptors and that somatostatin receptors are on cholinergic terminals. It is interesting that in Parkinson's disease patients with dementia, who have cortical cholinergic and SRIF deficits, a reduction in somatostatin receptors has recently been reported (Agid, 1983). It should also be noted that Parkinsonian patients with dementia do not have low cortical serotonin S2 receptors, although S1 receptors may be reduced (Perry et al., 1984b). This change is very similar to the loss of S1 receptors we have observed in cortex and hippocampus of Huntington's disease patients, with no change in S2 receptors. Thus, the reduction of S2 receptors seems to be specifically associated with Alzheimer-type dementia.

The studies of subcellular markers in ATD demonstrated a number of significant differences from controls. The activity of MAO-B was significantly increased, as has also been observed by Gottfries and co-workers (Adolfsson et al., 1980). It would seem this does not reflect an increase in the density or activity of mitochondria, as MAO-A activity was unchanged. Other studies of mitochondrial markers have not shown increases in activity in ATD (Bowen et al., 1977; Pope et al., 1964). In experimental animals, a high proportion of MAO-B immunoreactivity may be present in astrocytes (Levitt et al., 1982), and therefore the increase in MAO-B may reflect the reactive gliosis which occurs in ATD (Duffy et al., 1980).

A number of changes were observed in acid glycoside hydrolases, the most prominent of which was an increase in β-glucuronidase activity. The activity of β-xylosidase was also increased. These increases in enzyme activities are unlikely to be due to tissue shrinkage as other lysosomal enzymes were unchanged. Studies in experimental animals have shown that brain lysosomal glycoside hydrolase activities increase after infection with some conventional viruses (Bowen et al., 1974) and also the slow virus diseases, scrapie (Millson and Boutiff, 1973) and Creutzfeldt-Jakob disease (Annunziata and Federico, 1981). In Creutzfeldt-Jakob disease in man, an increase has been observed in the activity of β-glucuronidase and also β-galactosidase (Annunziata and Federico, 1981) which was unchanged in the present study. Histochemical studies in ATD have revealed areas of high activity of lysosomal hydrolases in the regions of neuritic plaques (Robinson, 1969), again, suggestive of reactive gliosis. Taken together, these studies would suggest that the increases in glycoside hydrolases might also reflect either reactive gliosis or an active degenerative process.

A large and significant decrease in neutral α-glucosidase activity was observed in ATD temporal cortex, and to a lesser extent, in hippocampus. Whilst neutral α-glucosidase is mainly associated with the endoplasmic reticulum (Peters and Seymour, 1978), it seems there is not a generalised deficiency of endoplasmic reticulum in ATD as the other marker enzymes were unchanged in temporal cortex (Table X). This agrees with an earlier histochemical study in which nucleoside phosphatase activity (also associated with endoplasmic reticulum) was unchanged in ATD (Johnson, 1968). The neutral α-glucosidase activity assessed with 4-methylumbelliferyl-α-glucoside as substrate probably reflects the combined activity of both glucosidases I and II (Hettkamp et al., 1984). Both of these enzymes are involved in the processing of precursor glycoconjugates in the synthesis of the complex oligosaccharides of N-linked glycoproteins and glycolipids (Grinna and Robbins, 1979). Amongst other enzymes studied, both galactosyltransferase and fucosyltransferase are involved in glycoconjugate processing. The lack of change in the enzymes suggests that a generalised deficit in glycoconjugate synthesis is unlikely to occur in ATD. Several other studies have suggested that abnormalities in glycoconjugate processing occur in ATD. A number of studies have found decreases in glycolipid concentrations, including gangliosides and cerebrosides (Pope et al., 1964; Dekosky and Bass, 1982). More recently, abnormalities in dolichol metabolism have been described, which may also be consistent with defective glycoprotein processing (Wolfe et al., 1982).

The reduction in α-glucosidase activity in Huntington's disease (HD) suggests that the enzyme is concentrated in certain neurons (small intrinsic cells) which are known to degenerate in the striatum. Similarly, in Alzheimer-type dementia, the reduction of α-glucosidase activity may reflect loss of neurons in temporal cortex. Histochemical studies suggest that α-glucosidase is localised to specific neuronal populations in cortex of the rat (unpublished data). As previously reported, the neurotransmitter profile of neurons lost in Alzheimer-type dementia cortex and Huntington's disease putamen differs in that somatostatin is the only transmitter intrinsic to cortex so far known to be reduced in Alzheimer-type dementia (Davies and Terry, 1981; Rossor et al., 1980; Ferrier et al., 1983), and yet is one of the few intrinsic transmitters which is retained in Huntington's disease putamen (Aronin et al., 1983). If α-glucosidase is localised to particular groups of neurons in human brain, these apparently are unrelated in terms of neurotransmitter content. Neuronal cell loss in ATD cortex has been demonstrated in several studies, however, the relationship between this and the reduction in neutral α-glucosidase activity awaits further examination.

Neutral α-glucosidase is involved in glycoconjugate processing, and in HD a deficit in fucosyltransferase activity which is also involved in glycoconjugate processing, was also observed. Glycoconjugates and glycoproteins in particular are present in significant amounts on the cell surface, and may be concentrated in synaptic regions (Gurd, 1980). Neuronal glycoproteins may function as neurotransmitter and hormone receptors (Cross et al., 1983a), as binding sites for immunoglobulins, viruses and lectins and may also be involved in cell-cell recognition and the development and stabilisation of synapses (Olden et al., 1982). It is clear, therefore, that deficits in neuronal glycoconjugate processing may lead to the disruption of many functions which are essential for the viability of neurons. Whilst the present results are not consistent with the deficits of glycoconjugate-processing enzymes being the primary event in neuronal degeneration, it remains possible that it may be related to the susceptibility of particular groups of neurons to the degenerative process of ATD.

Summary

Two separate approaches have been used to study the neurochemistry of the temporal cerebral cortex in post-mortem brain samples from controls and patients with Alzheimer-type dementia (ATD) or Huntington's disease (HD).

Of a range of neurotransmitter receptors studied, only serotonin receptors were significantly reduced in ATD, the reduction being greatest in S2 receptors. This reduction appeared to be a relatively early change, and correlated significantly with the loss of somatostatin immunoreactivity in ATD. Cortical serotonin S2 receptors were unchanged in HD. These changes may reflect a loss of a specific subset of cortical neurons in ATD.

In the second study, the activities of a range of enzymic markers of subcellular fractions were studied in cerebral cortex. Whilst most markers were unchanged in ATD, a significant increase in lysosomal enzymes was observed, possibly relating to an active degenerative process. In addition, a significant reduction in α-glucosidase activity (a marker of endoplasmic reticulum) was also observed in ATD cortex. As this enzyme appears to be localised to specific groups of neurons in cortex, this loss may again reflect a degeneration of some cortical neurons.

References

Adolfsson, R., Gottfries, C. G., Roos, B. E. and Winblad, B. (1979) Changes in brain catecholamines in patients with dementia of Alzheimer-type. *Br. J. Psychiat.*, 135: 216–223.

Adolfsson, R., Gottfries, C. G., Oreland, L., Wiberg, A. and Winblad, B. (1980) Increased activity of brain and platelet monoamine oxidase in dementia of Alzheimer-type. *Life Sci.*, 27: 1029–1034.

Agid, Y. (1983) *Neuropeptides in Parkinson's Disease*, presented at 'Peptides and Neurological Disease'. Robinson College, Cambridge.

Annunziata, F. and Federico, A. (1981) Brain glycosidases in Creutzfeldt-Jakob disease. *J. Neurol. Sci.*, 49: 325–328.

Aronin, N., Cooper, P. E., Lorenz, L. J., Bird, E. D., Sagar, S. M., Leeman, S. E. and Martin, J. B. (1983) Somatostatin is increased in the basal ganglia in Huntington's disease. *Ann. Neurol.*, 13: 519–526.

Bowen, D. M., Flack, R. H. A., Martin, R. O., Smith, C. B., White, P. and Davison, A. N. (1974) Biochemical studies on degenerative neurological disorders. 1. Acute experimental encephalitis. *J. Neurochem.*, 22: 1099–1107.

Bowen, D. M., Smith, C. B., White, P. and Davison, A. N. (1976) Neurotransmitter-related enzymes and indices of hypoxia in senile dementia and other abiotrophies. *Brain*, 99: 459–496.

Bowen, D. M., Smith, C. B., White, P., Goodhardt, M. J., Spilane, J. A., Flack, R. H. A. and Davison, A. N. (1977) Chemical pathology of the organic dementias. *Brain*, 100: 397–426.

Bowen, D. M., White, P., Spillane, J. A., Goodhardt, M. J., Curzon, G., Iwangoff, P., Meier-Rouge, W. and Davison, A. N. (1979) Accelerated ageing or selective neuronal loss as an important cause of dementia? *Lancet*, i: 11–14.

Bowen, D. M., Allen, S. J., Benton, J. S., Goodhardt, M. J., Haan, E. A., Palmer, A. M., Sims, N. R., Smith, C. C. T., Spilane, J. A., Esiri, M. H., Neary, D., Snowdon, J. S., Wilcock, G. K. and Davison, A. N. (1983) Biochemical assessment of serotonergic and cholinergic dysfunction and cerebral atrophy in Alzheimer's disease. *J. Neurochem.*, 41: 266–272.

Brun, A. and Englund, E. (1981) Regional pattern of degeneration in Alzheimer's disease: neuronal loss and histopathological grading. *Histopathology*, 5: 549–564.

Buell, S. J. and Coleman, P. D. (1979) Dendritic growth in the aged human brain and failure of growth in senile dementia. *Science*, 206: 854–856.

Candy, J. M., Perry, R. H., Perry, E. K., Irving, D., Blessed, G., Fairbairn, A. F. and Tomlinson, B. E. (1983) Pathological changes in the nucleus of Meynert in Alzheimer's and Parkinson's diseases. *J. Neurol. Sci.*, 59: 277–289.

Caulfield, M. P., Straughan, D. W., Cross, A. J., Crow, T. J. and Birdsall, N. J. M. (1982) Cortical muscarinic receptor subtypes and Alzheimer's disease. *Lancet*, ii: 1277.

Cross, A. J. (1982) Interactions of ^{3}H-LSD with serotonin receptors in human brain. *Eur. J. Pharmacol.*, 82: 77–80.

Cross, A. J. and Deakin, J. F. W. (1985) Cortical serotonin receptor subtypes after lesion of ascending cholinergic neurones. *Neurosci. Lett.*, in press.

Cross, A. J., Crow, T. J., Perry, E. K., Perry, R. H., Blessed, G. and Tomlinson, B. E. (1981) Reduced dopamine-Ω-hydroxylase activity in Alzheimer's disease. *Br. Med. J.*, 282: 93–94.

Cross, A. J., Crow, T. J. and Johnson, J. A. (1983a) Neurotransmitter receptors as glycoproteins. *Experientia*, 39: 1168–1171.

Cross, A. J., Crow, T. J., Johnson, J. A., Joseph, M. H., Perry, E. K., Perry, R. H., Blessed, G. and Tomlinson, B. E. (1983b) Monoamine metabolism in senile dementia of Alzheimer type. *J. Neurol. Sci.*, 60: 383–392.

Cross, A. J., Crow, T. J., Johnson, J. A., Perry, E. K., Perry, R. H., Blessed, G. and Tomlinson, B. E. (1984a) Studies on neurotransmitter receptor systems in cortex and hippocampus in senile dementia of the Alzheimer-type. *J. Neurol. Sci.*, 64: 109–111.

Cross, A. J., Crow, T. J., Ferrier, I. N., Johnson, J. A., Bloom, S. R. and Corsellis, J. A. N. (1984b) Serotonin receptor changes in dementia of the Alzheimer type. *J. Neurochem.*, 43: 1574–1581.

Davies, P. and Maloney, A. J. (1976) Selective loss of central cholinergic neurones in Alzheimer's disease. *Lancet*, ii: 1403.

Davies, P. and Terry, R. D. (1981) Cortical somatostatin-like immunoreactivity in cases of Alzheimer's disease and senile dementia of the Alzheimer-type. *Neurobiol. Ageing*, 2: 9–14.

Davies, P. and Verth, A. H. (1978) Regional distribution of

muscarinic acetylcholine receptor in normal and Alzheimer-type dementia brains. *Brain Res.*, 138: 383–392.

Dekosky, S. T. and Bass, N. H. (1982) Ageing, senile dementia, and the intralaminar microchemistry of cerebral cortex. *Neurology*, 32: 1227–1233.

Duffy, P. E., Rapport, M. and Graf, L. (1980) Glial fibrillary acidic protein and Alzheimer-type senile dementia. *Neurology*, 30: 778–782.

Emson, P. C. and Lindvall, O. (1979) Distribution of putative neurotransmitters in the neocortex. *Neuroscience*, 4: 1–30.

Enna, S. J. and Snyder, S. H. (1976) A simple sensitive and specific radio receptor assay for endogenous GABA in brain tissue. *J. Neurochem.*, 26: 221–224.

Farmery, S., Owen, F., Poulter, M. and Crow, T. J. (1985) Iodinated somatostatin binding in human brain membranes: a comparison of controls and ATD patients. *Br. J. Pharmacol.*, 85: 8P.

Ferrier, I. N., Cross, A. J., Johnson, J. A., Roberts, G. W., Crow, T. J., Corsellis, J. A. N., Lee, Y. C., O'Shaughnessy, D., Adrian, T. E., McGregor, G. P., Bacarese-Hamilton, A. J. and Bloom, S. R. (1983) Neuropeptides in Alzheimer-type dementia. *J. Neurol. Sci.*, 62: 159–170.

Fibiger, H. C. (1983) The organisation and some projections of cholinergic neurons of the mammalian forebrain. *Brain Res. Rev.*, 4: 327–388.

Grinna, L. S. and Robinson, P. W. (1979) Glycoprotein biosynthesis. Rat liver microsomal glucosidases which process oligosaccharides. *J. Biol. Chem.*, 254: 8814–8818.

Gurd, J. W. (1980) Subcellular distribution and partial characterisation of the three major classes of concanavalin A receptors associated with rat brain synaptic junctions. *Can. J. Biochem.*, 58: 941–951.

Hays, S. E. and Paul, S. M. (1982) CCK receptors and human neurological disease. *Life Sci.*, 31: 319–322.

Henn, F. A., Deering, J. and Anderson, P. (1980) Receptor studies on isolated astroglial cell fractions prepared with and without trypsin. *Neurochem. Res.*, 5: 459–464.

Hettkamp, H., Legler, G. and Bause, E. (1984) Purification by affinity chromatography of glucosidase I, an endoplasmic reticulum hydrolase involved in the processing of asparagine-like oligosaccharides. *Eur. J. Biochem.*, 142: 85–90.

Hooper, M. W. and Vogel, F. S. (1976) The limbic system in Alzheimer's disease. *Am. J. Pathol.*, 85: 1–13.

Hubbard, B. M. and Anderson, J. M. (1981) A quantitative study of cerebral atrophy in old age and senile dementia. *J. Neurol. Sci.*, 50: 135–145.

Johnson, A. B. (1968) Apparent nucleoside phosphatase activity in the neurofibrillary tangles of Alzheimer's disease. *J. Neuropathol. Exp. Neurol.*, 27: 155–156.

Levitt, P., Pintar, J. E. and Breakfield, Y. O. (1982) Immunocytochemical demonstration of monoamine oxidase B in brain astrocytes and serotonergic neurons. *Proc. Natl. Acad. Sci. USA*, 79: 6385–6389.

Leysen, J. E., Niemegeers, C. J. E., Van Neuten, J. M. and Laduron, P. M. (1982) ^{3}H-Ketanserin (R 41468), a selective ^{3}H-ligand for serotonin$_2$ receptor binding sites. *Mol. Pharmacol.*, 21: 301–314.

Leysen, J. E., Van Gompel, P., Verwimp, M. and Niemegeers, C. J. E. (1983) Role and localisation of serotonin S2 receptor-binding sites: effects of neuronal lesions. In P. Mandel and F. V. De Feudis (Eds.), *CNS Receptors — from Molecular Pharmacology to Behaviour*, Raven Press, New York, pp. 373–383.

Luaboya, M. K., Maloteaux, J. M. and Laduron, P. M. (1984) Regional and cortical laminar distributions of serotonin S2 benzodiazepine, muscarine and dopamine D2 receptors in human brain. *J. Neurochem.*, 43: 1068–1071.

Mann, D. M. A., Yates, P. O. and Marcynick, B. (1984) Monoaminergic neurotransmitter systems in presenile Alzheimer's disease and in senile dementia of Alzheimer type. *Clin. Neuropathol.*, 3: 199–205.

Mann, D. M. A., Yates, P. O. and Marcynick, B. (1985) Correlation between senile plaque and neurofibrillary tangle counts in cerebral cortex and neuronal counts in cortex and subcortical structures in Alzheimer's disease. *Neurosci. Lett.*, 56: 51–55.

Millson, G. C. and Bountiff, L. (1973) Glycosidases in normal and scrapie mouse brain. *J. Neurochem.*, 20: 541–546.

Mountjoy, C. Q., Roth, M., Evans, N. J. R. and Evans, H. M. (1983) Cortical neurone counts in normal and elderly controls and demented patients. *Neurobiol. Ageing*, 4: 1–12.

Olden, K., Parent, J. B. and White, S. L. (1982) Carbohydrate moieties of glycoproteins. A re-evaluation of their function. *Biochem. Biophys. Acta*, 650: 209–232.

Paula-Barbosa, M. M., Cardoso, R. M., Guimaraes, H. L. and Cruz, C. (1980) Dendritic degeneration and regrowth in the cerebral cortex of patients with Alzheimer's disease. *J. Neurol. Sci.*, 45: 129–134.

Pearson, R. C. A., Gatter, K. C. and Powell, T. P. S. (1983) Retrograde cell degeneration in the basal nucleus in monkey and man. *Brain Res.*, 261: 321–326.

Peroutka, S. J. and Snyder, S. H. (1979) Multiple serotonin receptors: differential binding of ^{3}H-5-hydroxytryptamine, ^{3}H-lysergic acid diethylamide and ^{3}H-spiroperidol. *Mol. Pharmacol.*, 16: 687–699.

Peroutka, S. J., Moskowitz, M. A., Reinhard, J. F. and Snyder, S. H. (1980) Neurotransmitter receptor binding in bovine cerebral microvessels. *Science*, 208: 610–612.

Perry, E. K. and Perry, R. H. (1983) Human brain neurochemistry — some post-mortem problems. *Life Sci.*, 33: 1733–1743.

Perry, E. K., Gibson, P. H., Blessed, G., Perry, R. H. and Tomlinson, B. E. (1977) Neurotransmitter enzyme abnormalities in senile dementia. *J. Neurol. Sci.*, 34: 247–265.

Perry, E. K., Atack, J. R., Perry, R. H., Hardy, J. A., Dodd, P. R., Edwardson, J. A., Blessed, G., Tomlinson, B. E. and Fairbairn, A. F. (1984a) Intralaminar neurochemical distributions in human midtemporal cortex: comparison between

Alzheimer's disease and the normal. *J. Neurochem.*, 42: 1402–1410.

Perry, E. K., Perry, R. H., Candy, J. M., Fairbairn, A. F., Blessed, G., Dick, D. J. and Tomlinson, B. E. (1984b) Cortical serotonin S2 receptor binding abnormalities in patients with Alzheimer's disease: comparisons with Parkinson's disease. *Neurosci. Lett.*, 51: 353–357.

Perry, E. K., Curtis, M., Dick, D. J., Candy, J. M., Atack, J. R., Bloxham, C. A., Blessed, G., Fairbairn, A., Tomlinson, B. E. and Perry, R. M. (1985) Cholinergic correlates of cognitive impairment in Parkinson's disease: comparisons with Alzheimer's disease. *J. Neurol. Neurosurg. Psychiat.*, 48: 413–421.

Perry, R. H., Candy, J. M., Perry, E. K., Irvine, D., Blessed, G., Fairbairn, A. F. C. and Tomlinson, B. E. (1982) Extensive loss of cholineacetyltransferase activity is not reflected by neuronal loss in the nucleus of Maynert in Alzheimer's disease. *Neurosci. Lett.*, 33: 311–315.

Perry, R. H., Candy, J. M. and Perry, E. K. (1983) Some observations and speculations concerning the cholinergic system and neuropeptides in Alzheimer's disease. In R. Katzman (Ed.), *Biological Aspects of Alzheimer's Disease, Barbury Report 15*, Cold Spring Harbor Laboratory, pp. 351–360.

Peters, T. J. and Seymour, C. A. (1978) Analytical subcellular fractionation of needle-biopsy specimens from human liver. *Biochem. J.*, 174: 435–446.

Pope, A., Hess, H. H. and Lewin, E. (1964) Studies on the microchemical pathology of human cerebral cortex. In M. M. Cohen and R. S. Snider (Eds.), *Morphological and Biochemical Correlates of Neural Activity*, Hoeber-Harper, New York, pp. 98–111.

Robinson, N. (1969) Creutzfeldt-Jakob's disease: a histochemical study. *Brain*, 92: 581–588.

Rossor, M. N., Emson, P. C., Mountjoy, C. Q., Roth, M. and Iversen, L. L. (1980) Reduced amounts of immunoreactive somatostatin in the temporal cortex in senile dementia of Alzheimer type. *Neurosci. Lett.*, 20: 373–377.

Rossor, M. N., Garrett, N. J., Johnson, A. L., Mountjoy, C. Q., Roth, M. and Iversen, L. L. (1982) A post-mortem study of the cholinergic and GABA systems in senile dementia. *Brain*, 105: 313–330.

Rossor, M. N., Iversen, L. L., Reynolds, O. P., Mountjoy, C. Q. and Roth, M. (1984) Neurochemical characteristics of early and late onset types of Alzheimer's disease. *Br. Med. J.*, 288: 961–964.

Schiebel, A. B. and Tomiyasu, U. (1978) Dendritic sprouting in Alzheimer's presenile dementia. *Exp. Neurol.*, 60: 1–8.

Sorensen, K. V. (1982) Somatostatin: localisation and distribution in the cortex and the subcortical white matter of the human brain. *Neuroscience*, 7: 1227–1232.

Spokes, E. G. S. (1980) Neurochemical alterations in Huntington's chorea. *Brain*, 103: 179–210.

Terry, R. D., Peck, A., De Teresa, R., Schecter, R. and Horoupian, D. S. (1981) Some morphometric aspects of the brain in senile dementia of the Alzheimer type. *Ann. Neurol.*, 10: 184–192.

Tomlinson, B. E., Blessed, G. and Roth, M. (1970) Observations on the brains of demented old people. *J. Neurol. Sci.*, 11: 205–242.

Tomlinson, B. E. and Henderson, G. (1976) Some quantitative cerebral findings in normal and demented old people. In R. D. Terry and S. Gershan (Eds.), *Neurobiology of Ageing*, Raven Press, New York, pp. 183–204.

Tomlinson, B. E., Irving, D. and Blessed, G. (1981) Cell loss in the locus coeruleus in senile dementia of the Alzheimer type. *J. Neurol. Sci.*, 49: 419–428.

Vincent, S. R., Johansson, O., Hokfelt, T., Heyerson, B., Sachs, C., Elde, R. P., Terenius, L. and Kinmel, J. (1982) Neuropeptide coexistence in human cortical neurones. *Nature*, 298: 65–67.

Whitehouse, P. J., Price, D. L., Clark, A. W., Coyle, T. T. and Delong, M. (1981) Alzheimer's disease: evidence for a selective loss of cholinergic neurones in the nucleus basalis. *Ann. Neurol.*, 10: 122–126.

Wilcock, G. K. (1983) The temporal lobe in dementia of Alzheimer's type. *Gerontology*, 29: 320–324.

Wolfe, L. S., Ng Ying Kin, N. M. K., Palo, J. and Halita, M. (1982) Raised levels of cerebral cortex dolichols in Alzheimer's disease. *Lancet*, ii: 99.

Discussion

J. M. PALACIOS: Most peptidergic neurons contain a co-transmitter, for example somatostatin neurons contain GABA as a co-transmitter and yet there is no report of decreased GABA in AD. Do you have an explanation for that?

ANSWER: The number of GABA neurons in some layers of rat cortex can represent a very high percentage of the total neurons, however somatostatin is co-localised in only a very low percentage of these cells (Schmechel et al., 1984). We would therefore be looking for a very small change in GABA, which is probably not within the resolution of these types of study.

D. F. SWAAB: You mentioned the problem of controlling for the way the subjects died. Is it not possible to use brain pH matched controls in order to correct for the agonal state?

ANSWER: This would be a useful control group, however I think it would be difficult to obtain a large series of normal controls which would match the AD patients for pH changes. Nonetheless pH measurement would be a useful measure of some agonal changes in these groups of patients.

R. N. KALARIA: Since there is high capacity binding of some neurotransmitter receptors on microvessels or capillaries, how did you account for these effects in your receptor studies? Were the binding studies done on membranes from whole homogenates?

ANSWER: All our binding assays were performed on homogenates. Recent work from Prof. Agid's group in Paris has studied the density of binding sites on microvessels and found them to be a very low proportion of the total number of sites in homogenates (personal communication). It would be most interesting to look at receptors on isolated microvessels in AD.

J. M. RABEY: During the last years there have been publications showing a relationship between depression and serotonin availability (pre- and post-synaptic). Did you compare your results in the AD group with depressed patients or did you use a depression scale in the AD patients?

ANSWER: We have no data on the incidence of depression in the AD patients we studied. However, in two separate groups (Crow et al., 1985) of depressed patients we have found no change in serotonin receptors in cortex and hippocampus.

K. IQBAL: You have shown a loss of α-glucosidase activity in hippocampus in AD/SDAT and in putamen in HD. Since these two brain areas are known to show a very marked neuron loss in these conditions, is it possible that what you have observed is just reflecting the loss of neurons.

ANSWER: This is indeed the most appropriate interpretation of the data. However, one has to ask why these neurons degenerate. In this respect it is interesting that neurons containing α-glucosidase also degenerate in Huntington's disease, although the neurotransmitters associated with these neurons are different. Therefore, I think it is possible that this may reflect a particular susceptibility of α-glucosidase-containing neurons. It could be speculated that this may relate to the synthesis of cell-surface markers by α-glucosidase, which might be recognised by toxins, viruses or the immune system.

R. RAVID: (1) Are there any changes in plasma membranes with ageing which are similar to those in binding?

(2) Do you have any data on differences in affinity of S1 and S2 serotonin receptors as reflected in the difference between Huntington disease and SDAT?

ANSWER: The changes we have observed in ligand binding to crude membrane preparations in ATD appear to be highly selective to the serotonin S2 receptor. On this basis it would seem unlikely that this reflects a generalised alteration in plasma membranes. However, in Huntington's disease, there is evidence supporting a change in GABA receptors which may relate to membrane alterations (Lloyd and Davidson, 1979). In both diseases the losses of receptors are associated with reductions in the number of binding sites with no change in affinity.

References

Crow, T. J., Cross, A. J. and Cooper, S. J. (1984) Neurotransmitter receptors and monoamine metabolites in the brains of patients with Alzheimer-type dementia and depression and suicide. *Neuropharmacology*, 23: 1561–1569.

Lloyd, K. G. and Davidson, L. (1979) ^{3}H-GABA binding to brains from Huntington's chorea patients: altered regulation by phospholipids? *Science*, 205: 1147–1149.

Schmechel, D. E., Vickrey, B. G., Fitzpatrick, D. and Elde, R. P. (1984) GABAergic neurons of mammalian cerebral cortex: widespread subclass defined by somatostatin content. *Neurosci. Lett.*, 47: 227–232.

D. F. Swaab, E. Fliers, M. Mirmiran, W. A. Van Gool and F. Van Haaren (Eds.)
Progress in Brain Research, Vol. 70.
© 1986 Elsevier Science Publishers B.V. (Biomedical Division)

CHAPTER 11

Lipofuscin: characteristics and significance

R. S. Sohal[a] and L. S. Wolfe[b]

[a]*Department of Biology, Southern Methodist University, Dallas, Tx 75275, USA and* [b]*Donner Laboratory of Experimental Neurochemistry, Montreal Neurological Institute, McGill University, Montreal, Canada*

Introduction

Most of the cell types in the body of multicellular organisms exhibit an age-associated increase in the content of a specific organelle, which has been given a variety of different names including, age pigment, chromolipid, lipopigment and lipofuscin (Fig. 1). Indeed, accretion of lipofuscin is the only consistent age-related morphological alteration detected thus far. A related structure, usually termed ceroid, is formed in some cell types under certain experimental and pathological conditions (Hartroft and Porta, 1965; Porta and Hartroft, 1969; Siakotos and Koppang, 1973), however, it is as yet uncertain if lipofuscin and ceroid are products of similar qualitative events. During the last century, considerable information has been gathered on lipofuscin and an increasing amount of evidence suggests that an understanding of the mechanisms of lipofuscin formation may provide useful clues to the underlying causes of cellular senescence. The objective of this paper is to provide a brief, synthetic overview of the current status of this organelle in relation to the aging process. Readers can gain detailed background information from other recent reviews on this topic by Strehler (1964), Toth (1968), Bourne (1973), Wolman (1975, 1980), Glees and Hasan (1976), Miquel et al. (1977), Dolman and MacLeod (1981), Donato and Sohal (1981) and the compendium 'Age Pigments' (Sohal, 1981a).

Characteristics of lipofuscin

The key to the understanding of the nature and potential significance of lipofuscin is the realization that mature lipofuscin is formed by a dynamic process during which morphology and chemical composition of the organelle undergo progressive modifications. Furthermore, the composition of lipofuscin may vary in different cell types and under different dietary and physiological conditions.

According to the classification proposed by DeDuve and Wattiaux (1966), lipofuscin is a secondary lysosome of the residual body variety. On the basis of the information, gathered from different lines of investigation, it can be generalized that lipofuscin, as an organelle, serves the function of a depot or storehouse of indigestable, unexcreted cellular wastes primarily consisting of intracellular membranes. It follows, then, that the nature of the contained material should reflect the composition and activity of the specific cell type. Hence, the highly variable morphology and chemical composition of lipofuscin, within different cell types, and even in the same cell, can be rationalized. Nevertheless, mature lipofuscin, from various tissues and organisms, shares certain common features which lend to its recognition. On the basis of current information, lipofuscin can be defined as a "membrane-bound lysosomal organelle, which contains lipoidal moieties, exhibits yellow to brown coloration, emits yellow to greenish autofluorescence under UV, and accumulates in the cytoplasm progressively with age under normal physiological conditions". Ceroid can be contrasted with lipofuscin as an organelle which shares some of the above characteristics, but is formed under pathological conditions traceable to a certain, albeit presently unknown, biochemical inadequacy whereby the quantity of indigestable residues is abnormally enhanced. Since the underlying mechanisms of lipofuscin and ceroid formation are not as yet clearly understood, it is advisable not to use a single conjoined designation, e.g., ceroid-lipofuscin, for these organelles.

Mode of lipofuscinogenesis

The structure and composition of lipofuscin is best understood in context of the processes involved in the formation of lipofuscin. The most widely accepted view, based on electron microscopic, cytochemical and biochemical studies is that the initial step in the formation of lipofuscin is the autophagocytosis of cytoplasmic components (Koenig, 1963; DeDuve and Wattiaux, 1966; Frank and Christensen, 1968). Focal areas of the cytoplasm are isolated within a limiting membrane, usually contributed by the cisternae of endoplasmic reticulum, forming an autophagic vacuole. Primary lysosomes fuse with these vacuoles to form autolysosomes or secondary lysosomes. Enclosed cytoplasmic components undergo hydrolysis by the lytic activity of lysosomal enzymes and most of the monomeric molecules diffuse into the extralysosomal cytoplasm for reuse by the cell. Focal degeneration of mitochondria, presumably following fusion with primary lysosomes, also seems to contribute to the formation of autolysosomes (Hasan and Glees, 1972a; Gopinath and Glees, 1974; Glees and Hasan, 1976; Miquel et al., 1977). Conceptually, the newly formed autolysosome represents the first stage in the genesis of lipofuscin. Lipid droplets in the cytoplasm can also fuse with autolysosomes thus increasing their relative lipoidal content (Wolman, 1975, 1980). In addition, autolysosomes of various ages, representing different stages of development, can fuse with each other.

In the next step, apparently, there is considerable chemical interaction between various residues in the autolysosomes. Although the nature of such interactions would be determined by the actual residues present, one consistent outcome is the formation of fluorescent material. There is some lack of agreement concerning the chemical nature of fluorophores, but it is widely believed that oxidative molecular damage, involving oxygen-derived free radicals, plays a role in the formation of fluorescent materials (for references, see Tappel, 1975; Miquel et al., 1977; Wolman, 1980; Donato, 1981). According to a currently popular scheme, originally developed by Tappel and co-workers (for references, see Tappel, 1975, 1980), malondialdehyde or a similar substance formed as a result of free radical induced lipid peroxidation reactions as well as free radical damage to other biological molecules, such as proteins and nucleic acids (Gutteridge, 1982) plays a key role in the polymerization of amine-containing molecules. Conjugated Schiff bases, formed as a result of such malondialdehyde-mediated polymerization of amine-containing molecules, are believed to contribute a ubiquitous category of fluorophores. This view is strengthened by the presence of blue-emitting fluorescent material in chloroform extracts of purified lipofuscin granules (Tappel, 1975) as well as in tissue homogenates of a variety of species (for references, see Donato and Sohal, 1981).

Recently, increasing doubts have been expressed about lipid peroxidation as the sole or dominant mechanism for the formation of fluorophores or lipofuscin. Some of the reasons for this shift of opinion are the following. The blue-emitting fluorescent material in chloroform extracts of isolated lipofuscin and tissues has not been definitely identified as a conjugated Schiff base. In vitro lipofuscin granules emit yellow to green rather than blue fluorescence (Pearse, 1972; Oliver, 1981; Eldred et al., 1982). It is unclear how yellow-emitting fluorophores can arise as a result of lipid peroxidation. In organisms such as the housefly, which is incapable of synthesizing polyunsaturated fatty acids, the lipid composition of the animals can be manipulated. A 200-fold difference in the level of polyunsaturated fatty acids did not result in a detectable difference in the morphometrically-determined volume of lipofuscin (Sohal et al., 1984a). Only a 15% difference was observed in the concentration of chloroform-soluble blue-emitting fluorescent material between the flies containing high and low levels of polyunsaturated fatty acids (Bridges and Sohal, 1980). It seems that the Schiff-base-like blue-emitting fluorescent material can arise from sources other than polyunsaturated fatty acids. Such findings have prompted a search for other mechanisms of fluorophore formation. Experimental studies dealing with the induction of ceroid suggest that inhibition of lysosomal enzymes in general and thiol proteases in particular accelerate the formation of ceroid (Ivy et al., 1985; Jolly et al., 1985). The resultant structures are initially non-fluorescent. Since the fatty acid and the protein composition of ceroid do not seem to be significantly different from that of the normally-occurring lipofuscin granules (Siakotos et al., 1970; Siakotos and Koppang, 1973; Jolly et al., 1985), it suggests that defects in lipid metabolism may not be the sole factor in the formation of ceroid or lipofuscin. Wolfe et al. (1981) are of the opinion that inadequate disposal and build-up of dolichol lipids, within lysosomes, is the main factor responsible for ceroid and lipofuscin formation.

Chemical composition

The chemical composition of lipofuscin and ceroid is very heterogeneous (Hendley et al., 1963a,b; Bjorkerud, 1964; Siakotos and Koppang, 1973; Wolfe et al., 1981; Elleder, 1981; Palmer et al., 1986a,b). As also stated above, the basis of this heterogeneity appears to be the dynamic nature of the organelle's maturational process as well as the differences in the chemical constituents of different tissues and organisms. On the basis of histochemical and biochemical studies, proteins and lipids have been identified as the main constituents of ceroid and lipofuscin (Elleder, 1981; Siakotos and Munkres, 1981; Ng Ying Kin et al., 1983; Jolly et al., 1985; Palmer et al., 1986a,b). Dominant lipids are the lysosomal marker bis(monoacylglycero)phosphate, dolichols, dolichyl esters and ubiquinone. In addition, cholesterol, phosphatidylcholine, phosphatidylinositol, phosphatidylserine, phosphatidylethanolamine and free fatty acids are also present (Elleder, 1981; Wolfe, 1981; Ng Ying Kin et al., 1983; Palmer et al., 1986a,b). Proteins, which constitute more than half of the weight of ceroid or lipofuscin granules, have not as yet been well characterized. Metals such as copper and iron are also detectable in relatively high concentrations (Sohal et al., 1977; Armstrong, 1984). Chromatographic analyses of materials extractable in organic solvents have indicated the presence of up to 14 fluorophores (Palmer et al., 1986a). In addition, in tissues such as liver and retinal pigment epithelium, lipofuscin granules may also contain compounds with properties of a retinoid-protein complex (Wolfe et al., 1977).

Presently, the chemical basis of autofluorescence of lipofuscin and ceroid is unclear. It has been suggested that autofluorescence is due to degradation of lipids (Strehler, 1964) or 1-amino-3-iminopropenes (Tappel, 1975) or retinoid complexes (Wolfe et al., 1977) or modified proteins (Jolly et al., 1985; Palmer et al, 1986a,b).

That the composition of lipofuscin is dependent on cellular constituents, present in a particular cell type, is clearly demonstrable in the autonomic ganglia and substantia nigra. These neurons contain dopa and dopamine, which apparently become incorporated into lipofuscin granules (Barden, 1978, 1979), abolishing the autofluorescence of lipofuscin in these cells. Such melanized lipofuscin regains its fluorescence upon oxidation by hydrogen peroxide. Similarly, ceroid and lipofuscin granules tend to be more lipoidal in tissues rich in lipids (Wolman, 1975, 1980). Thus, on the basis of the dynamic changes occurring during lipofuscinogenesis, together with intercellular variations in the composition of lipofuscin granules, the diversity of structure and composition, reported in this organelle, can be appreciated.

At present, it is difficult to draw a definitive distinction between the chemical composition of ceroid and lipofuscin because of the variations encountered in different tissues and species as well as lack of detailed knowledge about their composition. Although some differences between ceroid and lipofuscin have been noted (Siakotos and Koppang, 1973), they do not appear to be so fundamental or consistent as to be of diagnostic value. Nevertheless, from the causal point of view, ceroid is induced by specific biochemical lesions resulting in the enhancement of autophagocytosis and/or oxidative polymerizations and the general buildup of undigested residual material. Lipofus-

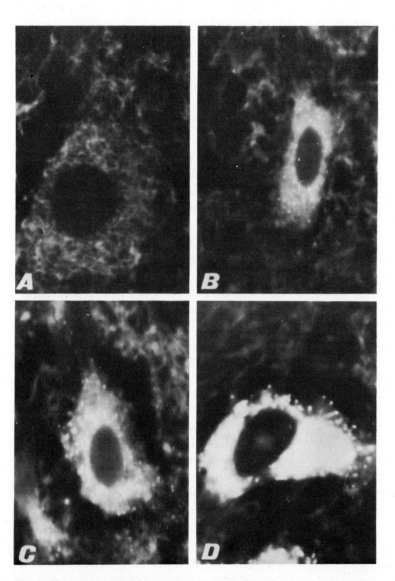

Fig. 1. Fluorescence microscope preparations showing progressive age-associated accumulation of lipofuscin in the neurons of oculomotor nucleus of rhesus monkey. The ages of the animals were: A, 1 day; B, 4 years; C, 10 years; D, 19.5 years. × 1 950. (From Brizzee et al., 1974, reproduced with permission)

cin, on the other hand, is considered to be a product of 'normal' cellular activity. It is possible, but as yet unsubstantiated, that lipofuscin formation may, like ceroid, be ultimately caused by the inefficiency of certain biochemical mechanisms which manifests gradually during the aging process.

Structure of lipofuscin granules

As would be expected, the morphology of lipofuscin varies at different stages of its development and in different cell types (Braak and Goebel, 1978; Brizzee and Ordy, 1981). Newly formed autolysosomes consist of a limiting membrane enclosing identifiable cytoplasmic organelles, which undergo progressive degeneration (Brandes, 1966). At this early stage, the autolysosomes are non-fluorescent under UV light. The next phase, which gives rise to the formation of mature lipofuscin, is marked by polymerization of residues, which also results in the formation of characteristic fluorescent material. Fine structure of lipofuscin in the neurons of an old rat is presented in Fig. 2.

Ultrastructurally, mature lipofuscin granules exhibit up to four different components: a finely granular electron dense material, coarse dense granules, osmiophilic lamellae and lipid-like vacuoles (Samorajski et al., 1965; Hasan and Glees, 1972b; Bourne, 1973; Sekhon and Maxwell, 1974). There do not appear to be any fundamental or characteristic differences in the ultrastructure of ceroid and lipofuscin. It should be noted that the relative development of the different structural components varies in different lipofuscin granules depending upon age and cell type. Lipofuscin granules vary between 0.5–3 μm in diameter. They are smaller and sparser in young cells and tend to increase in size with age (Fig. 1), probably due to fusion (Nandy, 1971; Brizzee et al., 1974; Miquel et al., 1977).

Factors influencing lipofuscinogenesis

Rates of formation of lipofuscin granules as well as chloroform-soluble fluorescent material (SFM),

presumably derived from lipofuscin, have been shown to respond to certain physiological and pathological conditions (Wolman, 1975, 1980, 1981). Three different factors seem to affect the rate of lipofuscin and ceroid formation: (1) an increase in functional activity, (2) oxidative stress, and (3) a disturbance or inadequacy of lysosomal function.

Functional activity and oxidative stress

There is considerable evidence to indicate that functionally active cells accumulate relatively more lipofuscin, but this generalization must be modified in light of certain exceptions. For example, flight muscles of dipteran insects such as flies, which have an extremely high metabolic rate, do not contain any lipofuscin granules. Extensive ultrastructural examination of flight muscles of the housefly, *Musca domestica*, in this laboratory, has rarely detected any lipofuscin-like structures (Sohal, 1976).

Dolman and MacLeod (1981) have cited several examples of a correlation between functional activity of cells and their lipofuscin levels. Postural muscles of humans have lesser amounts of lipofuscin than muscles involved in movement (Kny, 1937). Paralyzed muscles of stroke victims have paucity of lipofuscin (Kny, 1937). Friede (1962) found a strong correlation between lipofuscin content of neurons in human brain and activities of two oxidative enzymes, viz., DPN diaphorase and succinic dehydrogenase. In one-eyed persons, neurons of the lateral geniculate body, which received terminals from the blind eye, contained a lesser amount of lipofuscin than neurons in the layers connected to the seeing eye (Friede, 1962; Scholtz and Brown, 1978). Rate of lipofuscin accumulation in cardiac myocytes of dogs is about 5.5 times faster than in humans (Munnell and Getty, 1968), whereas metabolic rate of dogs is higher and life span shorter than that of humans by about the same 5.5 times ratio.

A direct experimental relationship between metabolic rate and rates of lipofuscin and fluores-

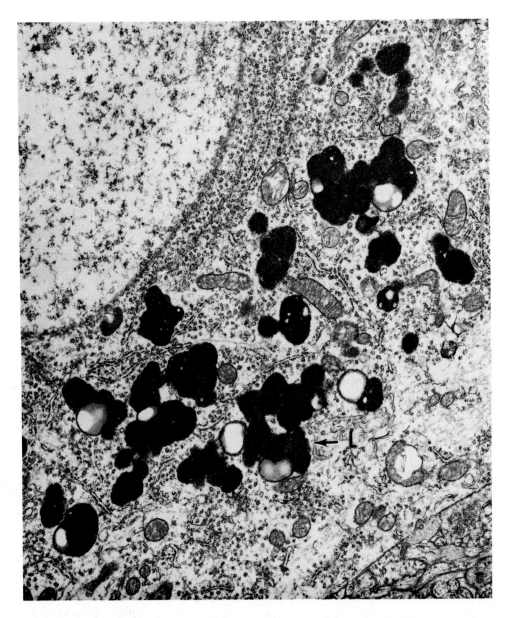

Fig. 2. Electron micrograph of cortical neurons of a 25-months-old rat showing lipofuscin granules (L). × 17 000. (Courtesy of Dr. T. Samorajski).

cent age pigment (FAP) accumulation was established in this laboratory in the adult housefly and by Miquel's group in *Drosophila* (Miquel et al., 1977). Physical activity and, consequently, the metabolic rate of houseflies was experimentally manipulated by varying their flying activity. Rate of oxygen consumption of flies increases around 60 to 100-fold during flight as compared to the resting state (Davis and Fraenkel, 1940). Flying activity of flies was altered by housing the flies in 0.027-m³ cages, where they could fly, or in urine-specimen bottles (about 150 ml), partitioned with cardboard, where flies could walk but were unable to fly. The average and the maximum life span of flies kept under conditions of high physical activity (cages) were more than 2.5-fold shorter than those kept under conditions of low physical activity (Sohal and Donato, 1978, 1979; Sohal, 1981b,c). The rate of FAP accumulation was 3.6 times faster in short-lived high activity flies; however, the maximal levels reached were similar in the two groups (Sohal and Donato, 1978).

To determine whether a direct relationship existed between the rate of FAP accumulation and the rate of aging, FAP values were plotted against the physiological age of the population (Sohal and Donato, 1978). Physiological age was defined as 'relative nearness to the end point or death'. It was assumed that death represented, in both populations, an identical level of vulnerability and physiological age. The physiological age was estimated in relation to the time of 20% mortality of the population and was obtained by dividing the chronological age by the age when 20% mortality had been reached. When FAP concentration was plotted in relation to the physiological age, there were no statistically significant differences in the slopes of the lines between the two groups which indicated that FAP was associated with the physiological rather than the chronological age of the flies. Rate of FAP accumulation has also been shown to be faster in tissues of rats undergoing chronic treadmill exercise (Basson et al., 1982).

In other studies, rates of lipofuscin accumulation in three different cell types of the housefly were found to be faster in flies kept under conditions of high physical activity as compared to those kept under conditions at low physical activity (Sohal and Donato, 1978; Sohal, 1981b). The maximal levels reached were similar in the two groups, but were reached later in the low activity flies. Similar results have been reported in hibernating mammals. Life-spans of Turkish hamsters are prolonged in proportion to the period spent under hibernation (Lyman et al., 1981). Rates of lipofuscin accumulation in the heart and the brain were slower in hibernators as compared to non-hibernators (Papafrangos and Lyman, 1982).

The mechanism by which changes in metabolic rate affect life span and lipofuscin accumulation probably involves oxygen free radicals generated during univalent reduction of oxygen. There is a large body of irrefutable evidence indicating that steady-state concentrations of oxygen free radicals are present under normal physiological conditions in aerobic cells. It has been shown that following exhaustive physical exercise in rats, concentrations of a free radical species and lipid peroxidation products increase while mitochondrial respiratory efficiency decreases (Davies et al., 1982). Increase in the metabolic rate of houseflies has been shown to greatly increase the rate of lipid peroxidation in vivo as indicated by n-pentane exhalation (Sohal et al., 1985).

Comprehensive studies on houseflies have indicated that antioxidant defenses tend to decline with age, whereas products of oxygen free radical reactions tend to increase with age (Sohal et al., 1984b; Sohal and Allen, 1985). Levels of superoxide, oxidised glutathione (GSH) and vitamin E declined in the old flies (Sohal et al., 1984b). Concentrations of hydrogen peroxide, oxidised glutathione and exhalation of n-pentane increased in old flies (Sohal et al., 1984b; Sohal et al., 1985). Tissues of old flies were also more vulnerable to lipid peroxidative damage than tissues of younger flies (Sohal et al., 1981).

The relationship between oxygen metabolites and lipofuscin accumulation has been elegantly demonstrated by Thaw et al. (1984) in cultured human glial cells. Rate of lipofuscin accumulation in cells, grown in an atmosphere containing 5%, 10%, 20% and 40% oxygen, was higher at higher concentrations of ambient oxygen. The presence of prooxidant (vitamin C/iron) increased while that of antioxidants (vitamin E/selenium, GSH, DMSO) decreased the rate of lipofuscin accumulation. Iron, a catalyst for the interaction of superoxide radical, also accelerates the formation of FAP in houseflies (Sohal et al., 1985).

Free radical-induced reactions, involving peroxidation of polyunsaturated fatty acids, play a causal role in the formation of ceroid granules as well as FAP material as has been amply demonstrated, experimentally. Animals fed on vitamin-E-deficient diets invariably exhibit increased levels of ceroid and FAP in different tissues (Tappel, 1980; Wolman, 1981).

Lysosomal activity

The involvement of lysosomal enzymes in the formation of ceroid was recently examined by Ivy et al. (1984a,b, 1985). They found that inhibitors of lysosomal enzymes and of thiol proteases, in particular, cause the accumulation of structures which in some morphological and histochemical respects resemble ceroid. Specifically, rats receiving continuous intraventricular infusions of the thiol protease inhibitor leupeptin, or of the general lysosomal enzyme inhibitor chloroquine, exhibited accumulation of ceroid bodies in the cytoplasm of neurons and glial cells in various regions of the brain. Leupeptin treatment caused the build-up of numerous dense bodies of heterogeneous nature (Fig. 3), whereas chloroquine infusion caused a similar build-up of dense bodies in hippocampal neurons. The dense bodies, induced by leupeptin and chloroquine, were stained positively by periodic acid-Schiff, toluidine blue, Schmorl's ferric-ferricyanide method, carbol fuchsin, Sudan black B, oil red O, and Nile blue sulfate in approximate descending order of affinity, indicating that these bodies contained polysaccharides or compounds with groups capable of oxidation to aldehydes, carbonyl groups and some lipids. However, unlike mature lipofuscin, these dense bodies exhibited faint autofluorescence under UV exposure.

The accumulation of the dense bodies was noticeable by electron microscopic techniques as soon as 8 h after an intraventricular injection of leupeptin. Upon termination of leupeptin adminis-tration, the ceroid gradually disappeared until, after 10 weeks, the amount of the dense substance in the cytoplasm of dentate gyrus granule cells was similar to that present in untreated age-matched rats. Dolichol content was significantly higher in the brains of rats treated with leupeptin and chloroquine than in brains of rats treated with saline or aprotonin, a serine protease inhibitor (Ivy et al., 1984b). Results of these studies raise the possibility that decrease in specific proteases may play a role in ceroid formation. Altogether, it seems reasonable to conclude that ceroidosis occurs if there is an overproduction of undegradable material or if the lytic capacity of the cell is exceeded by the production of materials requiring degradation.

Relationship of lipofuscin to aging

Although lipofuscin is the most ubiquitous age-related cytological alteration known thus far, its relationship to the aging process has remained rather ambiguous. There is no evidence that presence of lipofuscin in the cytoplasm hampers cellular function. It is conceivable that congestion of the cytoplasm by lipofuscin, which is a component of the lysosomal system, may reduce the degradative efficiency of this system, resulting in a slowdown of organelle membrane turnover and/or receptor-mediated endocytosis and/or exocytotic mechanisms. It is reasonable to view lipofuscin as a depot of unexcreted waste products. There is suggestive evidence that some lipofuscin granules may be exocytosed and after further breakdown may be voided from the body (Braunmuhl, 1957; Spoerri et al., 1974). The accumulation of lipofuscin is in itself an indication that the rate of exocytosis is exceeded by the rate of formation.

Although lipofuscin formation is influenced by dietary and pathological conditions, under specified and highly controlled conditions, lipofuscin

---

Fig. 3(A and B). Electron micrographs of granule cells in the dentate gyrus of rats which received an infusion of saline (A) and leupeptin (B) (a thiol protease inhibitor) for 2 weeks before death. Note the accumulation of lipofuscin-like dense bodies in the leupeptin-injected rat. (Courtesy of Dr. G. O. Ivy)

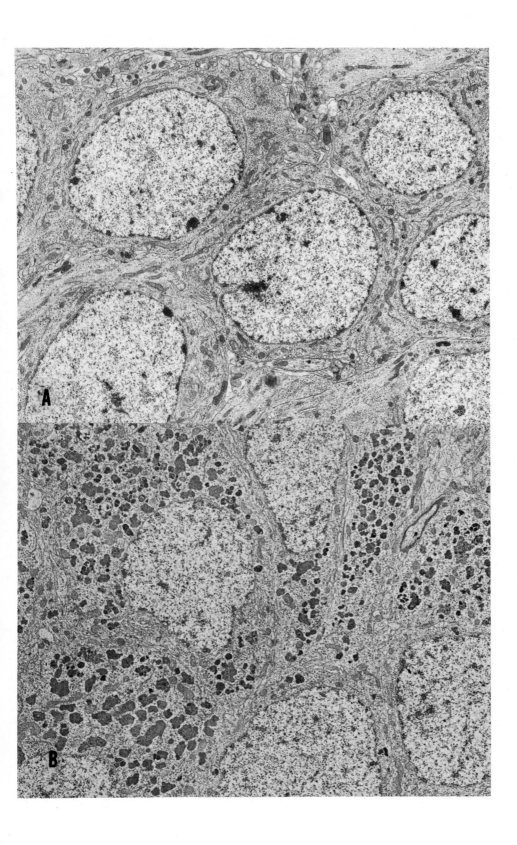

Fig. 3(A, B)

can be used as a marker of aging as indicated by studies on the Turkish hamster (Papafrangos and Lyman, 1982) and the housefly (Sohal, 1981c).

Preponderance of current knowledge is consistent with the view that metabolic rate, lipofuscin formation and aging are linked together, probably by oxygen free radicals. Lipofuscin is not believed to be a causal factor in aging but is regarded as a by-product of cellular reactions which may play a role in the aging process. The relationship of lipofuscin to aging has been poignantly stated by Wolman (1980) as follows: "Lipid pigments should be regarded somewhat like monuments erected on the sites of old battles. Their biological meaning is that at that site a destructive oxidative process took place. This autocatalytic process went on until it was stopped by free radical trapping and polymerization in which oxidants and antioxidants participated. The presence of numerous lipid pigment granules, like the presence of numerous war monuments, indicates that the organism is not very young, and that it has been the scene of many (victorious) battles". Another view, championed by Wolfe et al. (1981, 1983), on the basis of studies on lysosomal storage diseases, is that the storage material in ceroid and lipofuscin granules arises due to defects in enzyme(s) involved in the normal degradation and disposal of lysosomal membranes. It is possible that materials in ceroid and lipofuscin may well arise by a combination of independent or interrelated processes. The relative importance of any process would depend on the particular intracellular physiological situation. For example, under conditions of antioxidant deficiency, oxidative damage to membranes may be the main contibutory factor, whereas, in a lysosomal storage disease such as ceroid-lipofuscinosis, a defect in lysosomal enzymes may play a major part in the formation of undigested residues in ceroid bodies.

Concluding remarks

Although much knowledge concerning the morphology, origin and chemical composition of lipofuscin has been gathered, the precise relationship between lipofuscin and aging process still remains obscure. This is clearly due to the current ignorance about the nature of the underlying biochemical mechanisms of aging. It is possible that lipofuscin may contribute to the study of the underlying causes of aging since it is currently the most reliable marker of aging. However, to fully exploit this potential, a complete chemical characterization of lipofuscin would be a necessary step. Current knowledge in this area leaves much to be desired.

Acknowledgements

Valuable comments of Dr. G. Ivy on the manuscript are gratefully acknowledged. Research of R.S.S. has been financially supported by grants from the American Heart Association, NASA, N.I.H., and The Glenn Foundation for Medical Research. Research of L.S.W. has been supported by the grant MT1345 from the Medical Research Council of Canada.

References

Armstrong, D. (1984) Free radical involvement in the formation of lipopigments. In D. Armstrong, R. S. Sohal, R. G. Cutler and T. F. Slater (Eds.), *Free Radicals in Molecular Biology, Aging, and Disease*, Raven Press, New York, pp. 129–141.

Barden, H. (1978) Further histochemical studies characterizing the lipofuscin component of human neuromelanin. *J. Neuropathol. Exp. Neurol.*, 37: 437–451.

Barden, H. (1979) Acid-fast staining of oxidized neuromelanin and lipofuscin in the human brain. *J. Neuropathol. Exp. Neurol.*, 38: 453–462.

Basson, A. B. K., Terblanche, S. E. and Oelofsen, W. (1982) A comparative study on the effects of aging and training on the levels of lipofuscin in various tissues of the rat. *Comp. Biochem. Physiol.*, 71A: 369–374.

Bjorkerud, S. (1964) Isolated lipofuscin granules — a survey of new field. *Adv. Gerontol. Res.*, 1: 257–288.

Bourne, G. H. (1973) Lipofuscin. In D. H. Ford (Ed.), *Neurological Aspects of Maturation and Aging, Progress in Brain Research, Vol. 40*, Elsevier, Amsterdam, pp. 187–201.

Braak, H. and Goebel, H. H. (1978) Loss of pigment-laden stellate cells: a severe alteration of the isocortex in juvenile neuronal ceroid lipofuscinosis. *Acta Neuropathol.*, 42: 53–58.

Brandes, D. (1966) Lysosomes and aging pigment. In P. L. Krohn (Ed.), *Topics in the Biology of Aging*, Interscience, New York, pp. 149–158.

Braunmuhl, A. V. (1957) Alterserkrankungen des Zentralnervensystems. In O. Lubarsch, F. Henke and R. Rosle (Eds.), *Handbuch der Soziellen Pathologie, Anatomie und Histologie, Vol. 14* (I) A, Springer-Verlag, Berlin, pp. 337–359.

Bridges, R. G. and Sohal, R. S. (1980) Relationship between age-associated fluorescence and polyunsaturated fatty acids in the adult housefly, *Musca domestica. Insect Biochem.*, 10: 557–562.

Brizzee, K. R. and Ordy, J. M. (1981) Cellular features, regional accumulation and prospects of modification of age pigments in mammals. In R. S. Sohal (Ed.), *Age Pigments*, Elsevier/North-Holland, Amsterdam, pp. 101–154.

Brizzee, K. R., Ordy, J. M. and Kaack, B. (1974) Early appearance and regional differences in intraneuronal and extraneuronal lipofuscin accumulation with age in the brain of a nonhuman primate (*Macaca mulatta*). *J. Gerontol.*, 29: 366–381.

Davies, K. J. A., Quintanilha, A. T., Brooks, G. A. and Packer, L. (1982) Free radicals and tissue damage during exercise. *Biochem. Biophys. Res. Commun.*, 107: 1198–1205.

Davis, R. A. and Fraenkel, G. F. (1940) The oxygen consumption of flies during flight. *J. Exp. Biol.*, 17: 402–407.

DeDuve, C. and Wattiaux, R. (1966) Functions of lysosomes. *Ann. Rev. Physiol.*, 28: 435–492.

Dolman, C. L. and MacLeod, P. M. (1981) Lipofuscin and its relation to aging. In S. Fedoroff and L. Hertz (Eds.), *Advances in Cellular Neurobiology, Vol. 2*, Academic Press, New York, pp. 205–247.

Donato, H. (1981) Lipid peroxidation, cross-linking reactions and aging. In R. S. Sohal (Ed.), *Age Pigments*, Elsevier/North-Holland, Amsterdam, pp. 63–82.

Donato, H. and Sohal, R. S. (1981) Lipofuscin. In J. Florini (Ed.), *Handbook of Biochemistry in Aging*, CRC Press, Cleveland, pp. 221–227.

Eldred, G., Miller, G. V., Stark, W. and Feeney-Burns, L. (1982) Lipofuscin: resolution of discrepant fluorescence data. *Science*, 216: 757–759.

Elleder, M. (1981) Chemical characterization of age pigments. In R. S. Sohal (Ed.), *Age Pigments*, Elsevier/North-Holland, Amsterdam, pp. 204–241.

Frank, A. L. and Christensen, A. K. (1968) Localization of acid phosphatase in lipofuscin granules and possible autophagic vacuoles in interstitial cells of the guinea pig testis. *J. Cell Biol.*, 36: 1–13.

Friede, R. L. (1962) The relation of the formation of lipofuscin to the distribution of oxidative enzymes in the human brain. *Acta Neuropathol.*, 2: 113–125.

Glees, P. and Hasan, M. (1976) Lipofuscin in neuronal aging and disease. *Norm. Pathol. Anat.*, 32: 1–68.

Gopinath, G. and Glees, P. (1974) Mitochondrial genesis of lipofuscin in the mesencephalic nucleus of the V nerve of aged rats. *Acta Anat.*, 89: 14–20.

Gutteridge, J. M. C. (1982) Free radical damage to lipids, amino acids, carbohydrates and nucleic acids determined by thiobarbituric acid reactivity. *Int. J. Biochem.*, 14: 649–654.

Hartroft, W. S. and Porta, E. A. (1965) Ceroid. *Am. J. Med. Sci.*, 134: 324–345.

Hasan, M. and Glees, P. (1972a) Genesis and possible dissolution of neuronal lipofuscin. *Gerontologia* (Basel), 18: 217–236.

Hasan, M. and Glees, P. (1972b) Electron microscopical appearance of neuronal lipofuscin using different preparative techniques including freeze etching. *Exp. Gerontol.*, 7: 345–351.

Hendley, D. D., Mildvan, A. S., Reporter, M. C. and Strehler, B. L. (1963a) The properties of isolated human cardiac age pigment. I. Preparation and physical properties. *J. Gerontol.*, 18: 144–150.

Hendley, D. D., Mildvan, A. S., Reporter, M. C. and Strehler, B. L. (1963b) The properties of isolated human cardiac age pigment. II. Chemical and enzymatic properties. *J. Gerontol.*, 18: 250–259.

Ivy, G. O., Schottler, F., Wenzel, J., Baudry, M. and Lynch, G. (1984a) Inhibition of lysosomal enzymes: accumulation of lipofuscin-like dense bodies in the brain. *Science*, 226: 985–987.

Ivy, G. O., Wolfe, L. S., Huston, K., Baudry, M. and Lynch, G. (1984b) Lysosomal enzyme inhibitors cause the accumulation of ceroid-lipofuscin and dolichols in rat brain. *Neurosci. Abstr.*, 10: 885.

Ivy, G. O., Baudry, M. and Lynch, G. S. (1985) Experimental production of lipofuscin-like dense bodies in the brain. *Proceedings of the International Workshop on Age Pigments: Biological Markers in Aging and Environmental Stress*, Naples, Italy, p. 28.

Jolly, R. D., Bube, A., Hobman, B. L., Barnes, G. E. and Palmer, D. N. (1985) Ovine ceroid-lipofuscinosis: chemical constituents of the lipopigment, their pathogenic significance and similarities to other lipopigments. *Proceedings of the International Workshop on Age Pigments: Biological Markers in Aging and Environmental Stress*, Naples, Italy, p. 29.

Kny, W. (1937) Uber die Verteilung des Lipofuschsins in der Skelettmuskulatur in ihrer Beziehung zur Funktion. *Virch. Arch. Pathol. Anat. Physiol.*, 229: 468–478.

Koenig, H. (1963) The autofluorescence of lysosomes. Its value for the identification of lysosomal constituents. *J. Histochem. Cytochem.*, 11: 556–557.

Lyman, C. P., O'Brien, R. C., Green, G. C. and Papafrangos, E. D. (1981) Hibernation and longevity in the Turkish hamster *Mesocricetus brandti. Science*, 221: 668–670.

Miquel, J., Oro, J., Bensch, I. and Johnson, J. (1977) Lipofuscin: fine structural and biochemical studies, In W. A. Pryor (Ed.), *Free Radicals in Biology, Vol. 3*, Academic Press, New York, pp. 133–182.

Munnel, J. and Getty, R. (1968) Rate of accumulation of cardiac lipofuscin in the aging canine. *J. Gerontol.*, 23: 154–158.

Nandy, K. (1971) Properties of neuronal lipofuscin pigment in mice. *Acta Neuropathol.*, 19: 25–32.

Ng Ying Kin, N. M. K., Palo, J., Haltia, M. and Wolfe, L. S. (1983) High levels of brain dolichols in neuronal ceroid-lipofuscinosis and senescence. *J. Neurochem.*, 40: 1465–1473.

Oliver, C. (1981) Lipofuscin and ceroid accumulation in experimental animals. In R. S. Sohal (Ed.), *Age Pigments*, Elsevier/North-Holland, Amsterdam, pp. 335–353.

Palmer, D. N., Husbands, D. R., Winter, P. J., Blunt, J. W. and Jolly, R. D. (1986a) Ceroid-lipofuscinosis in sheep. I. Bis(monoacylglycero)phosphate, dolichol, ubiquinone, phospholipids, fatty acids and fluorescence in liver lipopigment lipids. *J. Biol. Chem.*, 261: 1766–1772.

Palmer, D. N., Barns, G., Husbands, D. R. and Jolly, R. D. (1986b) Ceroid-lipofuscinosis in sheep. II. The major component of the lipopigment in liver, kidney, pancreas and brain is low molecular weight protein. *J. Biol. Chem.*, 261: 1773–1777.

Papafrangos, E. D. and Lyman, C. P. (1982) Lipofuscin accumulation and hibernation in Turkish hamster, *Mesocricetus brandti. J. Gerontol.*, 37: 417–421.

Pearse, A. G. E. (1972) *Histochemistry, Vol. 2*, 3rd Ed., Williams and Wilkins, Baltimore.

Porta, E. and Hartroft, W. S. (1969) Lipid pigments in relation to aging and dietary factors (lipofuscins). In W. Wolman (Ed.), *Pigments in Pathology*, Academic Press, New York, pp. 191–235.

Samorajski, T., Ordy, J. M. and O'Keefe, J. R. (1965) The fine structure of lipofuscin age pigment in the nervous system of aged mice. *J. Cell Biol.*, 26: 779–795.

Scholtz, C. L. and Brown, A. (1978) Lipofuscin and transsynaptic degeneration. *Virch. Arch., A.*: 35–40.

Sekhon, S. S. and Maxwell, D. S. (1974) Ultrastructural changes in neurons of the spinal anterior horn of aging mice with particular reference to the accumulation of lipofuscin pigment. *J. Neurocytol.*, 3: 59–72.

Siakotos, A. M. and Koppang, N. (1973) Procedures for the isolation of lipopigments from brain, heart and liver, and their properties: a review. *Mech. Ageing Develop.*, 2: 177–200.

Siakotos, A. M. and Munkres, K. D. (1981) Purification and properties of age pigments. In R. S. Sohal (Ed.), *Age Pigments*, Elsevier/North-Holland, Amsterdam, pp. 181–202.

Siakotos, A. M., Watanabe, I., Saito, A. and Fleischer, S. (1970) Procedures for the isolation of two distinct lipopigments from human brain. Lipofuscin and ceroid. *Biochem. Med.*, 4: 361–375.

Sohal, R. S. (1976) Aging changes in insect flight muscle. *Gerontology*, 22: 317–333.

Sohal, R. S. (Ed.), (1981a) *Age Pigments*, Elsevier/North-Holland, Amsterdam.

Sohal, R. S. (1981b) Relationship between metabolic rate, lipofuscin accumulation and lysosomal enzyme activity during aging in the adult housefly, *Musca domestica. Exp. Gerontol.*, 16: 347–355.

Sohal, R. S. (1981c) Metabolic rate, aging and lipofuscin accumulation. In R. S. Sohal (Ed.), *Age Pigments*, Elsevier/North-Holland, Amsterdam, pp. 303–316.

Sohal, R. S. and Allen, R. G. (1985) Relationship between metabolic rate, free radicals, differentiation and aging: a unified theory. In Woodhead, A. D., Blackett, A. D. and Hollaender, A. (Eds.), *The Molecular Basis of Aging*, Plenum, New York, pp. 75–104.

Sohal, R. S. and Donato, H. (1978) Effects of experimentally altered life spans on the accumulation of fluorescent age pigment in the housefly, *Musca domestica. Exp. Gerontol.*, 13: 335–341.

Sohal, R. S. and Donato, J. (1979) Effect of experimental prolongation of life span on lipofuscin content and lysosomal enzyme activity in the brain of the housefly, *Musca domestica. J. Gerontol.*, 34: 489–496.

Sohal, R. S., Peters, P. D. and Hall, T. A. (1977) Structure, origin, composition and age-dependence of mineralized dense bodies (concretions) in the midgut of the adult housefly, *Musca domestica. Tissue Cell*, 9: 87–102.

Sohal, R. S., Donato, H. and Biehl, E. R. (1981) Effect of age and metabolic rate on lipid peroxidation in the housefly, *Musca domestica. Mech. Ageing Develop.*, 16: 159–167.

Sohal, R. S., Bridges, R. G. and Howes, E. A. (1984a) Relationship between lipofuscin granules and polyunsaturated fatty acids in the housefly, *Musca domestica. Mech. Ageing Develop.*, 25: 355–363.

Sohal, R. S., Farmer, K. J., Allen, R. G. and Cohen, N. R. (1984b) Effect of age on oxygen consumption, superoxide dismutase, catalase, glutathione, inorganic peroxides and chloroform-soluble antioxidants in the adult housefly, *Musca domestica. Mech. Ageing Develop.*, 24: 185–195.

Sohal, R. S., Muller, A., Koletzko, B. and Sies, H. (1985) Effect of age and ambient temperature on *n*-pentane production in adult housefly, *Musca domestica. Mech. Ageing Develop.*, 29: 317–326.

Sohal, R. S., Allen, R. G., Farmer, K. J. and Newton, R. K. (1985) Iron induces oxidative stress and may alter the rate of aging in the housefly, *Musca domestica. Mech. Ageing Dev.*, 32: 33–38.

Spoerri, P. E., Glees, P. and El Ghazzawi, E. (1974) Accumulation of lipofuscin in the myocardium of senile guinea pigs. Dissolution and removal of lipofuscin following dimethylaminoethyl-*p*-chloro-phenoxyacetate administration. An electron microscopic study. *Mech. Ageing Develop.*, 3: 311–321.

Strehler, B. L. (1964) On the histochemistry and ultrastructure of age pigments. *Adv. Gerontol. Res.*, 1: 343–384.

Tappel, A. L. (1975) Lipid peroxidation and fluorescent molecular damage to membranes. In B. F. Trump and A. V. Arstila (Eds.), *Pathobiology of Cell Membranes, Vol. 1*, Academic Press, New York, pp. 145–170.

Tappel, A. L. (1980) Measurement and protection from in vivo lipid peroxidation. In W. A. Pryor (Ed.), *Free Radicals in Biology, Vol. 4*, Academic Press, New York, pp. 1–47.

Thaw, H. H., Brunk, U. T. and Collins, P. V. (1984) Influence of oxygen tension, pro-oxidants and antioxidants on the formation of lipid peroxidation products (lipofuscin) in individual cultivated human glial cells. *Mech. Ageing Develop.*, 24: 211–223.

Toth, S. E. (1968) The origin of age pigment. *Exp. Gerontol.*, 3, 19–20.

Wolfe, L. S., Ng Ying Kin, N. M. K., Baker, R. R., Carpenter, S. and Andermann, F. (1977) Identification of retinoyl complexes as the autofluorescent component of the neuronal storage material in Batten's disease. *Science*, 195: 1360–1362.

Wolfe, L. S., Ng Ying Kin, N. M. K. and Baker, R. R. (1981)

Batten disease and related disorders: new findings on the chemistry of the storage material. In J. W. Callahan and J. A. Lowden (Eds.), *Lysosomes and Lysosomal Storage Diseases*, Raven Press, New York, pp. 315–330.

Wolfe, L. S., Ng Ying Kin, N. M. K., Palo, J. and Haltia, M. (1983) Dolichols in brain and urinary sediment in neuronal ceroid lipofuscinosis. *Neurology*, 33: 103–103.

Wolman, M. (1975) Biological peroxidation of lipids and membranes. *Israel J. Med. Sci.*, Suppl. 10, 11: 1–248.

Wolman, M. (1980) Lipid pigments (chromolipids): their origin, nature and significance. In H. L. Ioachim (Ed.), *Pathobiology Annual, Vol. 10*, Raven Press, New York, pp. 253–267.

Wolman, M. (1981) Factors affecting lipid pigment formation. In R. S. Sohal (Ed.), *Age Pigments*, Elsevier/North-Holland, Amsterdam, pp. 265–281.

Discussion

D. F. SWAAB: Shouldn't we make a differentiation between body and brain metabolism, in that increased body metabolism seems to lead to a shorter life-span, while increased brain metabolism may lead to a longer life-span? (Hofman, 1983).

ANSWER: To do so, one has to assume that brain cells somehow fundamentally differ from non-neuronal cells. I do not know any evidence which would prompt this assumption (See Hofman, 1983).

D. M. GASH: Is your data complementary with the suggestions of Dr. C. Finch and others of the hormonal theory of aging? That is, can hormonal increase of metabolism in a cell lead to the aging of the cell and associated tissue?

ANSWER: Yes! the main point of my hypothesis is that rate of metabolism and rate of aging are linked together.

K. IQBAL: You have shown very interesting data supporting increase in life-span with decrease in metabolic activity in houseflies. What are your thoughts on metabolic activity and life-span in humans?

ANSWER: A minimal amount of physical activity is essential in mammals to prevent atrophy of muscles. Beyond this minimal level, there is no evidence that exercise is beneficial. On the contrary, it may in fact be harmful as suggested by the data of Davies et al. (1982) on rats.

E. FLIERS: Could you please speculate on possible effects of lipofuscin accumulation on cell function?

ANSWER: I do not believe that the mere presence of lipofuscin

is deleterious. Instead, lipofuscin should be considered as an indicator or marker of the rate of aging. It is not possible to establish, unambiguously, a direct relationship between the functional capacity of the cells and the volume of lipofuscin. A correlation will, of course, be insufficient to demonstrate a structural-functional relationship because the possibility that some other intracellular age-related alteration may be playing a contributory role cannot be ruled out.

A. J. CROSS: How do changes in oxidative free radicals during aging produce specific cellular changes within the brain?

ANSWER: There is a very large body of evidence documenting specific deleterious effects of oxygen free radicals on biological molecules and cellular functions.

H. R. LIEBERMAN: I wish to suggest that your earlier comment concerning exercise may be true. However, humans in their natural environment are much more active than we are. We may be like the animals who had no exercise opportunity.

ANSWER: Humans get considerably more exercise than the laboratory animals confined to a small cage throughout their life. I can assure you that our life cannot be compared to that of a rat in a cage.

References

Davies, K. J. A., Quintanilha, A. T., Brooks, G. A. and Packer, L. (1982) Free radicals and tissue damage during exercise. *Biochem. Biophys. Res. Commun.*, 107: 1198–1205.

Hofman, M. A. (1983) Energy metabolism, brain size and longevity in mammals. *Quart. Rev. Biol.*, 58: 495–512.

D. F. Swaab, E. Fliers, M. Mirmiran, W. A. Van Gool and F. Van Haaren (Eds.)
Progress in Brain Research, Vol. 70.
© 1986 Elsevier Science Publishers B.V. (Biomedical Division)

CHAPTER 12

Ratio of pyramidal cells versus non-pyramidal cells in the human frontal isocortex and changes in ratio with ageing and Alzheimer's disease

H. Braak and E. Braak

Department of Anatomy, Theodor Stern Kai 7, 6000 Frankfurt/Main 70, FRG

Introduction

The neuronal constituents of the mammalian telencephalic cortex can generally be classified as either pyramidal neurons or non-pyramidal neurons. In general, pyramidal cells and the modified forms of pyramidal cells can be considered projection neurons while most non-pyramidal cells can be referred to as local circuit neurons (H. Braak, 1980, 1984).

Evaluation of the ratio of the non-pyramidal neurons versus the pyramidal neurons and knowledge of their pattern of laminar distribution is essential for a better understanding of cortical circuitry and function. Unfortunately, most types of non-pyramidal cells cannot reliably be distinguished from pyramidal neurons by light microscopic examination of Nissl preparations alone. Particular difficulties arise if cells of small soma size are to be classified. Using autopsy material, differentiation of nerve cells in Nissl preparations is additionally impeded by issues of suboptimal and delayed fixation. The Golgi techniques, in contrast, show details of the cellular processes often necessary for a reliable classification of the neuronal type but, unfortunately, they demonstrate, in a non-representative manner, only a small percentage of the nerve cells present in the tissue (Scheibel and Scheibel, 1978). It is on this account that quantitative studies cannot be based upon analyses of Golgi impregnated material.

Lipofuscin pigment granules can frequently be encountered in nerve cells of the human adult. The size, shape, stainability and pattern of distribution of these granules can serve as characteristics for differentiation of the various neuronal types forming the human brain. Pigmented nerve cells show a slight increase in the number of lipofuscin granules with age (Mann and Yates, 1974; Mann et al., 1978; West, 1979; Brizzee and Ordy, 1981a,b; Rösler and Kemnitz, 1983), but this does not change the typical pattern of pigmentation. The lipofuscin characteristics have been analyzed using a transparent Golgi technique (H. Braak, 1983) that allows examination of the pigment deposits of individual nerve cells through a translucent impregnation of the soma and the cellular processes (E. Braak and H. Braak, 1983; H. Braak and E. Braak, 1982a,b, 1983a,b, 1984a,b). The pigmentation of pyramidal cells and modified pyramidal cells differs considerably from that seen in the non-pyramidal neurons. After demonstration of the correspondence of the pigment characteristics and the nerve cell type as seen in the Golgi preparation, a combined pigment Nissl preparation will allow one to quantitatively analyze the proportions of the various types of cortical constituents at light microscopical level and enables one to study their pattern of distribution throughout the various cortical layers.

The present study is aimed at assessing the

percentages of both the pyramidal neurons and the non-pyramidal cells in the various layers of a defined prefrontal isocortical area of the human adult and it has the ultimate goal of examining whether changes of these percentages occur with ageing and in Alzheimer's disease.

Material and methods

Brains from 24 cadavers obtained at autopsy were used for this study (Table I). The brains Nrs. 1–18 were from patients without known neurological disorder. Apart from an age-related widening of both ventricles and frontal and temporal sulci in brains Nrs. 7–12, no significant pathological changes were found. The brains Nrs. 19–24 were from patients afflicted with presenile dementia

TABLE I

Material used for the study

Nr.	Sex	Age	Brain weight	Cause of death
1	♂	28	1430	M. Hodgkin
2	♂	35	1490	pancreatitis
3	♂	41	1443	myocardial infarction
4	♂	41	1510	cancer of pancreas
5	♂	41	1400	colitis ulcerosa
6	♀	48	1317	pneumonia
7	♂	88	1430	lung cancer
8	♀	89	1329	bronchopneumonia
9	♂	91	1291	bronchopneumonia
10	♀	92	1193	coma hepaticum
11	♀	93	1297	cancer of the stomach
12	♀	96	993	cardiac infarction
13	♀	56	1421	pyelonephritis
14	♂	59	1636	pulmonary embolism
15	♂	61	1564	myocardial infarction
16	♂	62	1271	myocardial infarction
17	♂	62	1480	myocardial infarction
18	♀	65	1376	myocardial infarction
19	♀	57	1165	bronchopneumonia, M. Alzh.
20	♀	57	1000	bronchopneumonia, M. Alzh.
21	♀	58	1000	bronchopneumonia, M. Alzh.
22	♂	61	1280	bronchopneumonia, M. Alzh.
23	♂	62	1240	bronchopneumonia, M. Alzh.
24	♀	66	1000	bronchopneumonia, M. Alzh.

of the Alzheimer type (neuropathologically confirmed). The time from death to removal of the brain varied from 12 to 30 h. The post-mortem delay is in this study not a crucial point since intraneuronally deposited lipofuscin granules are inert structures insensitive to suboptimal fixation. Brains were fixed by immersion in an aqueous solution of formaldehyde (4%).

Coronal slices of frontobasal isocortex of the left hemisphere were cut 3 mm anterior to the entrance of the olfactory tract and three blocks, each comprising portions of the gyrus rectus and the adjacent orbitofrontal gyri, were cut out of these slices. Since the olfactory sulcus runs sagittally, most of the brain tissue along its walls is cut perpendicular to the surface. Only these portions were analyzed to facilitate differentiation between the various types of nerve cells. The area investigated corresponds to area 11 of Brodmann (1909).

For thick sections, the first block was cut with the aid of a freezing microtome at 800 μm and 100 μm. The sections were oxidized with performic acid, stained with aldehydefuchsin (800 μm), and used for pigmentoarchitectonic studies, or they were stained with lithium hematoxylin (100 μm) for myeloarchitectonic examination (Schroeder, 1939; H. Braak, 1980).

The second block was cut with the aid of a vibrating-blade microtome. These sections were cut for quantitative analysis at 40 μm to minimize counting errors and to facilitate cell classification (Haug, 1967). Possible changes in brain volume due to effects of fixation were not corrected for, since the material had been kept in formaldehyde for more than a year. After this time period, the initial swelling and subsequent shrinkage has come to an end and a stable volume is achieved (Haug et al., 1983). The sections were stained with a combination of aldehydefuchsin and gallocyanin chrome alum referred to as combined 'pigment-Nissl' preparation (H. Braak, 1980). Preliminary studies showed that paraffin embedding causes severe distortion and partial destruction of nerve cells in autopsy material, thus mainly accounting for a large number of unclassifiable neurons.

Vibratome sections, in contrast, display in addition to the pattern of pigmentation the typical shapes of neuronal cell bodies and are, therefore, better suited for quantitative analyses. The vibratome sections were fixed on gelatinized slides, oxidized with dilute performic acid (Wall, 1975) for 5 h, thoroughly washed under running tap water, and stained for 12 h with aldehydefuchsin (H. Braak, 1980). After washing with 70% ethanol, the sections were transferred into distilled water and counterstained with gallocyanin chrome alum (Einarson, 1932; Berube et al., 1966; Marshall and Horobin, 1972) for 6 h, rapidly dehydrated in ethanol, cleared with xylene, and mounted in a synthetic resin (Permount, Fisher). It should be emphasized that using autopsy material the preservation of the tissue is far from being optimal and by the relatively high thickness of the sections in addition, the brilliancy of the photographs is considerably reduced. Photographs of various neuronal types from the vibratome sections used for quantitative analyses are nevertheless shown intentionally, so as to allow the reader to form his own opinion concerning the suitability of pigment characteristics for differentiation of cortical neuronal types (Figs. 1–3).

For quantitative evaluation, stripes of area 11 running through the entire depth of the cortex between the pia mater and white matter were drawn with the aid of a drawing tube using a $\times 6.7$ eye piece and a $\times 63$ oil immersion objective lens (Zeiss). The width of the field was 230 μm. Only cells displaying a nucleolus were taken into consideration (Haug, 1967). Approximately 450 projection areas of nerve cells were outlined within each stripe. The thickness of each preparation was verified (Haug, 1979) and the counting results were corrected to compensate for differences in section thickness. Using a MOP, the surface area of the vibratome sections was measured prior to and after the staining and embedding procedures and corrections were made for changes in size. In general, the shrinkage found was less than 1%.

Nerve cells were distinguished on account of characteristics seen in the combined pigment Nissl preparation. These will be described in detail in the first part of the observations. The preparations were sufficiently thick to delineate the cortical laminae and, therefore, layers were counted separately.

Some of the vibratome sections were processed with a reduced silver technique proposed by Gallyas (1971) for demonstration of neurofibrillary changes of the Alzheimer type. Patients ranging in age from 28 to 48 did not show tangles in frontal isocortex, those in the age group of 56 to 65 showed no more than a few occasional tangles; older patients of up to 96 years had some tangles but none of them in a density comparable to that found in the cases of Alzheimer's disease. Between 10 and 20% of well-preserved old people have occasional isocortical tangles (Tomlinson and Henderson, 1976). All of our Alzheimer cases had massive isocortical tangles.

The third block was embedded in paraffin and cut at 12, 15, and 30 μm. Paraffin sections were stained with cresylviolet (Nissl preparations).

Results

Cytoarchitecture of prefrontal area 11

Area 11 mainly spreads over the inferior facies of the frontal lobe, almost totally constituting the cortex which covers the gyrus rectus and the medial orbital gyrus. The olfactory sulcus passes through the field, dividing it into two portions of roughly the same extent. The field corresponds approximately to area F_G of Von Economo and Koskinas (1925), the fields 4–6 of Vogt (1910), and the fields 4–6 of Sanides (1962).

In Nissl preparations, the prefrontal area displays features of a homotypic frontal isocortex with neither a predominance of small or large nerve cells. The boundaries between the layers can easily be identified in this area. Layer I contains only a few non-pigmented nerve cells. Layer II is a little less broad than the first one and harbors closely packed tiny nerve cells. Layer III averages approximately one third of the total thickness of the cortex and contains well-formed pyramidal cells. A more or less abrupt increase in the average cell size marks the border between sublayer IIIab and sublayer IIIc. Layer IV contains tiny nerve cells, not as closely packed as in layer II. Layer V is divisible into an upper cell rich sublayer Va harboring small to medium-sized nerve cells and a lower cell-sparse sublayer Vb with large nerve cells. Layer VI is prevalently composed of nerve cells with spindle-shaped or triangular cell bodies. In Nissl preparations, the exact border between layers V and VI is difficult to define but it can easily be determined in combined pigment Nissl preparations on account of characteristic features of the lipofuscin deposits in nerve cells of layer VI. The profound portions of layer VI thin out gradually towards the white matter. A fair number of nerve cells can be found scattered throughout the white substance underlying the prefrontal cortex.

Normal morphology of prefrontal isocortex

Pyramidal neurons and modified pyramidal neurons
Golgi preparations display mature prefrontal isocortical pyramidal cells in layers III and V as endowed with a stout apical dendrite and several less conspicuous and shorter basal dendrites. The long axis of the cell body and the shaft of the main dendrite are oriented perpendicular to the cortical surface. The dendrites are covered with numerous spines. The axon is generated from the cell body or a proximal dendrite by way of a cone-shaped initial segment. It heads towards the white matter giving off on its way a number of recurrent collaterals.

Cells deviating more or less substantially from the stereotypical pyramidal cells are also present and referred to as 'modified pyramidal cells'. The location and normal appearance of modified pyramidal cells should be noted, to avoid misinterpretation as pathological constituents of the cortex (H. Braak, 1980, 1984; Feldman, 1984). In some forms of pyramidal cells, the apical dendrite is reduced to only a short and very thin process. In superficial portions of layer II many modified pyramidal cells are found generating fork-like two

or three short dendrites into the molecular layer (O'Leary, 1941; Kirsche et al., 1973). One of the main constituents of layer VI, the 'pair of compass cells' (De Crinis, 1933) emits, apart from a regularly oriented apical dendrite, a second main dendrite that runs in various directions, ranging from a horizontal course to a vertical one (H. Braak, 1980).

In combined pigment Nissl preparations, the rounded nucleus of pyramidal cells and modified pyramidal cells is generally found in a slightly eccentric position. It is pale, of uniform density and contains a conspicuous nucleolus. The soma is endowed with a variable amount of Nissl material that generally extends into the proximal portions of the major dendrites. The cone shaped dendritic roots can therefore be recognized and can serve as a criterion for differentiating pyramidal cells and modified pyramidal cells from non-pyramidal neurons. Small lipofuscin granules are randomly dispersed throughout wide portions of the cell body but do not occur within dendrites. The axon hillock is devoid of both Nissl material and lipofuscin granules (H. Braak and E. Braak, 1976). The small lipofuscin granules of pyramidal cells have only a weak capacity to be stained by aldehydefuchsin. The amount of pigment depends on the type of the pyramidal cells and the location of the pyramidal cell within the isocortical layers. The pigmentation of modified pyramidal cells does not differ from that seen in typical pyramidal cells.

Layer I contains a few, probably dislocated, small pyramidal cells.

The tightly packed pyramidal cells of layer II are weakly stained. The pale nucleus is surrounded by only a small rim of cytoplasm with a few small lipofuscin granules.

Layer IIIab is mainly formed of slender pyramidal cells endowed with a small amount of basophilic material. Cells of this type gradually increase in size from the upper border of the layer to the lower one and can be found scattered throughout layer IIIc as well (Fig. 1, a–c).

Layer IIIc is dominated by large pyramidal cells with well-formed flocks of Nissl substance often concentrated in peripheral portions of the soma and extending into the roots of the dendrites. The stout and radially oriented stem of the apical dendrite is easily distinguished from the thinner basal dendrites. Lipofuscin is frequently concentrated in one pole of the cell body (Fig. 1, d,e).

In layer IV, tiny pyramidal cells prevail. The small cell body contains a pale nucleus and a few intensely stained pigment granules with light lipid droplets. Despite their small number, the characteristic pigment granules facilitate the differentiation of layer IV pyramidal cells from other types of small neurons belonging to the class of non-pyramidal cells (Fig. 1, f–i). Small pyramidal cells similar to those of layer IV can be found scattered throughout layers IIIc and V.

Layer V pyramidal cells show a wide range in their soma size, running from small to large, with the larger cells preferentially located within the lower half of the layer (Fig. 1, k–m).

Layer VI is formed of two basic neuronal types. The 'pair of compass cells' mentioned above are modified pyramidal cells generating two main dendrites, both of approximately the same length and caliber. The first and apical one is regularly oriented while the second one runs in various directions. The soma shape, therefore, varies and is often triangular or rhombic. Cells of this type are sparsely pigmented and the fine granules are spaced widely apart (Fig. 1, n–p). The second type of layer VI neurons is more easily classified with the group of pyramidal cells displaying a club-shaped pallid soma that gradually tapers into a thick apical dendrite. The 'club-shaped' neurons accumulate vast amounts of intensely stained lipofuscin granules that assemble to form tightly packed agglomerations close to the nucleus in one side of the cell body (Fig. 1, q–t). The distinguishing pattern of pigmentation allows clear differentiation between the two basic types of layer VI neurons.

Non-pyramidal neurons

Non-pyramidal cells comprise a variety of neuronal types distinguishable in Golgi impregnations but ill-defined in Nissl preparations.

The non-pyramidal neurons lack a typical apical dendrite. In Golgi preparations, the dendrites appear to emerge more or less abruptly from various points of the soma. They are smoothly contoured or bear only a few spines. The dendrites branch infrequently and often display a slightly varicose or beaded outline. The axon is given off from any point of the soma, frequently from the upper surface, and runs in various directions to ramify profusely in the vicinity of the parent soma.

In the combined pigment Nissl preparation, the cell bodies of the non-pyramidal cells appear polygonal, rounded or spindle-shaped in outline. Some types of non-pyramidal cells are richly endowed with basophilic material while others are marked by their pallid appearance. In general, the basophilic material does not extend into the proximal portions of the dendrites, a characteristic that helps to differentiate non-pyramidal cells from the class of pyramidal cells and modified pyramidal cells. Non-pyramidal cells are either filled with coarse and intensely stained lipofuscin granules or they are devoid of pigment or contain only a few faintly stained granules.

Pigment-laden non-pyramidal cells are mainly located in layer II and subjacent portions of layer III. They have a small spindle-shaped cell body with its longer axis oriented perpendicular to the cortical surface (Fig. 1, 1–4). Larger ones occur in small numbers within profound portions of the cortex (H. Braak, 1974a, 1978a,b,c; E. Braak, 1976; Schlegelberger and Braak, 1982).

Non-pyramidal cells, devoid or almost devoid of pigment, prevail in the isocortex and can be encountered in all layers (Fig. 1, 5–17). Forms with small polygonal somata can be found in layers I and II. The majority of the supragranular non-pyramidal cells shows a small, vertically aligned spindle-shaped cell body (Fig. 1, 5–9). The elongated nucleus is frequently relatively dark and shows infoldings of the nuclear membrane, often in form of a deep cleft oriented parallel to the long axis of the nucleus (Fig. 1, 7). Layer IIIc and the deep layers accomodate, in addition, a small number of large non-pyramidal cells with rounded

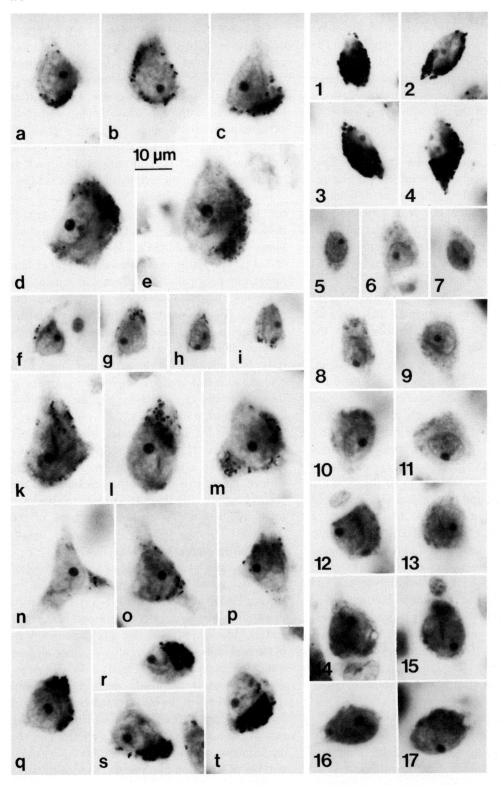

10 μm

Fig. 1

or irregularly polygonal cell bodies. These show often some concentrations of basophilic material in peripheral portions of the soma. The eccentrically located large and pallid nucleus contains patchy clumps of chromatin and shows several deep indentations of the nuclear membrane (Fig. 1, 10–13). Similarly large basophilic cells can be found in layer VI (Fig. 1, 14–17).

Distribution pattern of different nerve cell classes in prefrontal isocortex

Combined pigment Nissl preparations are used for quantitative evaluation of different classes of cortical nerve cells and their pattern of distribution. Stripes of cortex passing through the entire depth of the prefrontal area 11 were analyzed, and each of the nucleolated nerve cells found within these stripes was grouped into either the class of pyramidal cells including the modified forms or into the class of non-pyramidal cells, the latter being further classified into pigment-laden and non-pigmented forms.

Stripes of the prefrontal cortex of 12 different patients are displayed in Figs. 4 and 5. The cortex of young to middle-aged patients is shown in the left half of Fig. 4, as opposed to that of old-aged patients in the right half. Fig. 5, in addition, shows the cortex of cases of Alzheimer's disease and their age-matched controls. The contours of pyramidal neurons and modified pyramidal cells are lightly outlined throughout, whereas the non-pyramidal cells are black regardless of whether they are of the pigment-laden or of the non-pigmented type.

Changes in the size and packing density of the pyramidal cells mainly account for the typical lamination pattern of the prefrontal isocortical area.

The non-pyramidal cells are scattered throughout all cortical layers. The majority of these cells, nevertheless, is concentrated within the supragranular layers II and III with maximum packing density in layer IIIab. It appears worthwhile to point out that layer IV contains comparably few non-pyramidal cells. The deep layers V and VI are likewise sparsely endowed with non-pyramidal cells.

For demonstration of their distribution pattern, Figs. 6 and 7 display — besides the lightly outlined pyramidal cells and modified pyramidal cells — only the pigment-laden non-pyramidal cells as dark spots. These cells are not confined to a certain isocortical layer but, in large numbers, they occur only in the supragranular layers II and III.

Figs. 8 and 9 display, in the same manner, the distribution pattern of only the non-pyramidal cells that are devoid of lipofuscin deposits. Comparison with Figs. 6 and 7 shows that cells of this class outnumber considerably the pigment-laden neurons. On closer examination, it becomes apparent that the non-pigmented neurons are mainly found in lower portions of layer III whence they can be found with gradually decreasing packing density scattered throughout all the other isocortical laminae as well.

Proportions of the different nerve cell classes as evaluated in pigment Nissl preparations

The number of pyramidal neurons and modified pyramidal neurons within the supragranular layers (I–III) is roughly the same as within the deep layers IV to VI in the six stripes of the normative cases. As regards the non-pyramidal cells, in contrast, the bulk of these neurons is found within the supra-

Fig. 1. Pyramidal and non-pyramidal neurons of area 11 as seen in combined pigment-Nissl preparations of patients ranging in age from 28 to 48 (Vibratome section, 40 μm). (a,b,c) The medium-sized pyramidal neurons of layer IIIab contain only a few lipofuscin granules. (d,e) In layer IIIc pyramidal neurons the lipofuscin granules tend to accumulate in one cell pole. (f–i) Layer IV is mainly composed of small pyramidal neurons showing a few intensely stained lipofuscin granules. (k–m) Layer V pyramidal neurons. (n–p) The 'pair of compass cells' in layer VI are characterized by two main dendrites and a sparse number of lipofuscin granules. (q–t) The 'club-shaped neurons' of layer VI accumulate vast amounts of intensely stained lipofuscin granules. (1–4) Pigment-laden non-pyramidal cells of layers II and III. (5–17) Non-pyramidal cells devoid of pigment. (5–9) Small and mostly spindle-shaped neurons in layer IIIab. (10–13) Basket cells of layer IIIc. (14–17) Polygonal cells of layer VI.

TABLE II

Median of the percentage of pyramidal neurons and non-pyramidal cells in prefrontal area 11 (Brodmann) of the human brain

Groups	Age range (years)	Number of subjects	Pyramidal neurons (layers I–VI)		Non-pyramidal neurons (layers I–VI)	
			number per stripe (range)	% of total ±SD	number per stripe (range)	% of total ±SD
1. Young non-dem.	28–48	6	295–436	85.1±1.7	52–81	14.9±1.7
2. Aged non-dem.	88–96	6	326–484	91.6±1.2	22–52	8.4±1.2[a]
3. Controls	56–65	6	353–484	86.0±0.8	55–84	14.0±0.8
4. M. Alzheimer	57–66	6	313–493	90.1±1.4	24–55	9.9±1.4[a]

[a]Group 2 significantly different from group 1 and group 4 significantly different from group 3, $p < 0.005$, Mann-Whitney U test.

granular layers. There is relatively little interindividual difference in the ratio of pyramidal cells versus non-pyramidal neurons. 2 761 nerve cells were classified. The cortex is formed of about 85% pyramidal cells which are intermixed with about 15% non-pyramidal neurons. Following the cortex from the pial surface downwards, an abrupt decrease in the packing density of non-pyramidal cells occurs at the boundary between layer IIIc and layer IV. Approximately 20% of the nerve cells of the supragranular layers belong to the class of non-pyramidal cells as opposed to the deep layers IV to VI containing only about 10% of these cells (Table II).

Changes of prefrontal isocortex in old age

Pyramidal neurons and modified pyramidal neurons

The extent and the severity of the morphological changes seen in pyramidal neurons and their modified forms depends on the type of the pyramidal cell and its location within the various layers. In general, the basis of the pyramidal cell somata in the supragranular layers (I–III) narrows down considerably and gives the cells a slender appearance.

Layer II pyramidal neurons appear relatively well preserved. A very large number of the layer IIIab pyramidal cells, in contrast, shows a conspicuous age-related change in that they develop fusiform pigment-laden expansions interposed between the base of the cell body and the initial segment of the axon filled with lipofuscin granules (Fig. 2, a–c). These swellings are referred to as meganeurites. During the first stage of their formation, the axon hillock is filled with pigment. In the next step, perpendicularly arranged rows of a few lipofuscin granules can be seen within the slender expansion (H. Braak, 1979; E. Braak, 1980; E. Braak et al., 1980). Some of the meganeurites may become quite voluminous, and occasionally the volume of the spindle exceeds that of the parent

Fig. 2. Pyramidal and non-pyramidal neurons of area 11 of patients ranging in age from 88 to 96 (Vibratome sections, 40 μm, combined pigment Nissl preparation). (a–c) A large number of layer IIIab pyramidal cells develop pigment filled expansions of the proximal axonal segment ('meganeurites') with age. (d–f) The density of the cytoplasm is increased in layer IIIc pyramidal cells. The pyramidal neurons of layers IV (g–k), and V (l–n), as well as the 'pair of compass cells' (o–q), and the 'club-shaped neurons' of layer VI (r–t) remain almost unchanged. (1,2) Pigment-laden non-pyramidal cells of layer II. (3–5) Extraneuronally located pigment deposits. (6–17) These non-pyramidal neurons remain devoid of lipofuscin granules even in old age. There is a general decrease in basophilic material in the cytoplasm of non-pyramidal cells with age. (6–8) Spindle-shaped cells with foamy cytoplasm in layer IIIab. (9–12) Basket cells of layer IIIc. (13–17) Polygonal cells of layer VI.

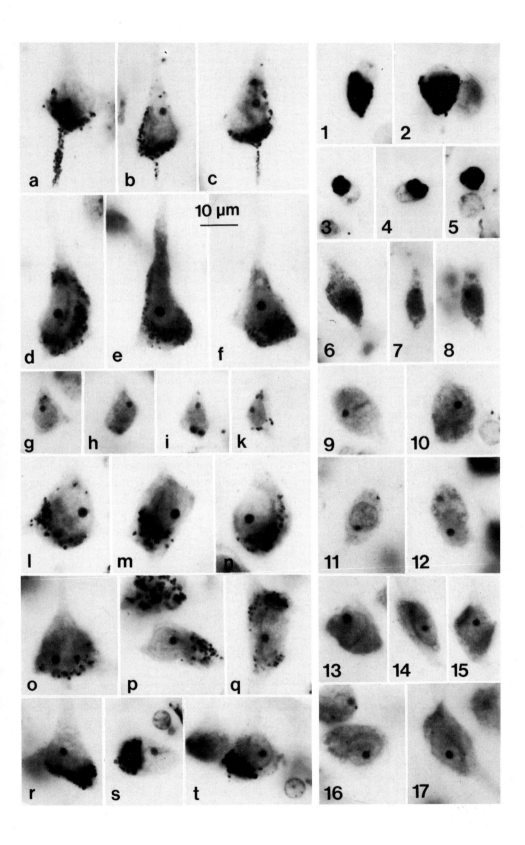

10 µm

Fig. 2

soma. Pyramidal cells with giant meganeurites frequently show only a few lipofuscin granules within their cell bodies. The large layer IIIc pyramidal cells generally do not show meganeurite formation. Besides being changed into slender elements they show a remarkable increase in the density of their cytoplasm (Fig. 2, d–f).

The tiny pyramidal cells of layer IV appear well preserved (Fig. 2, g–k). In general, the deep layers do not show age-related changes that are immediately obvious in pigment Nissl preparations. Layer V pyramidal cells (Fig. 2, l–n), the 'pair of compass cells' (Fig. 2, o–q), and 'club-shaped neurons' of layer VI (Fig. 2, r–t) remain almost unchanged.

Non-pyramidal neurons

Pigment-laden non-pyramidal neurons are rarely encountered within the supragranular layers of the senescent isocortex (Fig. 2, 1–2). With age, there is a severe loss of these nerve cells (H. Braak, 1984). Conjointly, a fair number of extraneuronally located pigment deposits can be found with lipofuscin granules showing the same tinctorial characteristics as those found in the small pigment-laden non-pyramidal neurons (Fig. 2, 3–5). Normally, the astrocytes of layers II and IIIab do not contain pigment that can intensely be stained by aldehydefuchsin and, therefore, the appearance of extraneuronally deposited lipofuscin pigment within the supragranular layers is a further feature of an age-changed human isocortex.

Non-pyramidal neurons devoid of pigment occur in all isocortical layers. They remain to be non-pigmented even in old age. The spindle-shaped forms in layer IIIab show a dark nucleus and a foamy cytoplasm with numerous vacuoles in peripheral portions (Fig. 2, 6–8). The large neurons found at midcortical level (Fig. 2, 9–12) and in layer VI (Fig. 2, 13–17) show a considerable decrease in their content of basophilic material.

Distribution pattern and proportions of different nerve cell classes in aged prefrontal isocortex

The right halves of Figs. 4, 6, and 8 show stripes of the prefrontal cortex of three old-aged patients. The number and laminar distribution of pyramidal neurons appears almost unchanged. In particular, layer IV is well preserved. The non-pyramidal cells, in contrast, are severely reduced in number.

Even in old age, the supragranular layers (I–III) harbor approximately the same number of pyramidal neurons as are found in the deep laminae (IV–VI). And again, the bulk of non-pyramidal cells is located within the supragranular layers. The ratio of pyramidal neurons including their modified forms versus non-pyramidal neurons does not show much variation from one individual to another. 2 569 nerve cells were classified. The pyramidal cells account for about 92% of all cortical neurons in this age group and there are only about 8% non-pyramidal cells. The ratio of pyramidal cells versus non-pyramidal cells, therefore, is changed with age from 85:15 to about 92:8. Provided that the number of pyramidal cells has not changed much, there is a loss of approximately 47% of the non-pyramidal cells (Table II).

Changes of prefrontal isocortex in Alzheimer's disease

Qualitative examination of cortical nerve cells

The qualitative changes of cortical neuronal constituents as seen in pigment Nissl preparations

Fig. 3. Pyramidal and non-pyramidal neurons of area 11 of patients suffering from Alzheimer's disease (Vibratome section, 40 μm, combined pigment-Nissl preparation). (a–c) Layer IIIab pyramidal neurons rarely develop 'meganeurites' in Alzheimer's disease. Pyramidal cells of layers IIIc (d–f), and IV (g–k), appear almost unchanged as well as the 'pair of compass cells' (o–q) and the 'club-shaped neurons' (r–t) of layer VI. Many layer V pyramidal neurons (l–n) develop tangles, concomitantly the lipofuscin shows an unusual clustering (l). (1–4) Pigment-laden non-pyramidal neurons of layer II. Pigment granules occur within proximal portions of the cellular processes. (5) Extraneuronally located pigment accumulation. (6–16) The non-pigmented non-pyramidal cells (6–16) have lost much of their basophilic cytoplasmic material. (6–8) Spindle-shaped neurons of layer IIIab. (9–12) Basket cells of layer IIIc. (13–16) Polygonal cells of layer VI.

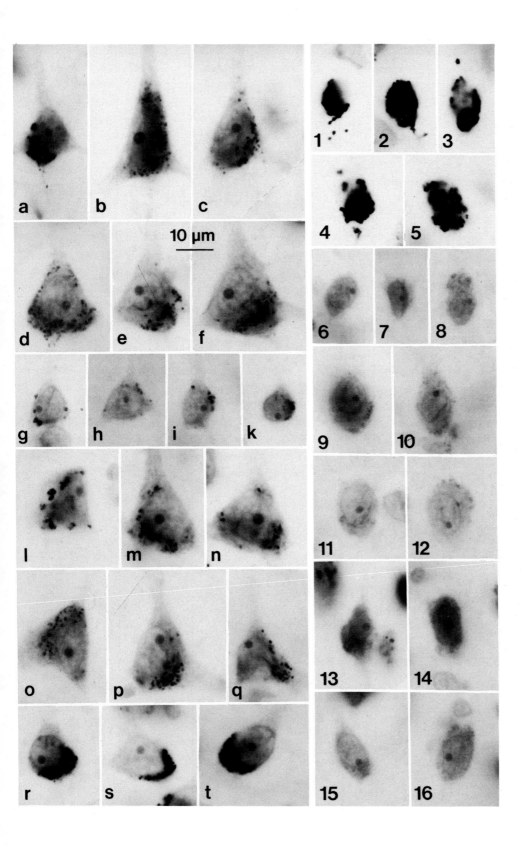

10 µm

Fig. 3

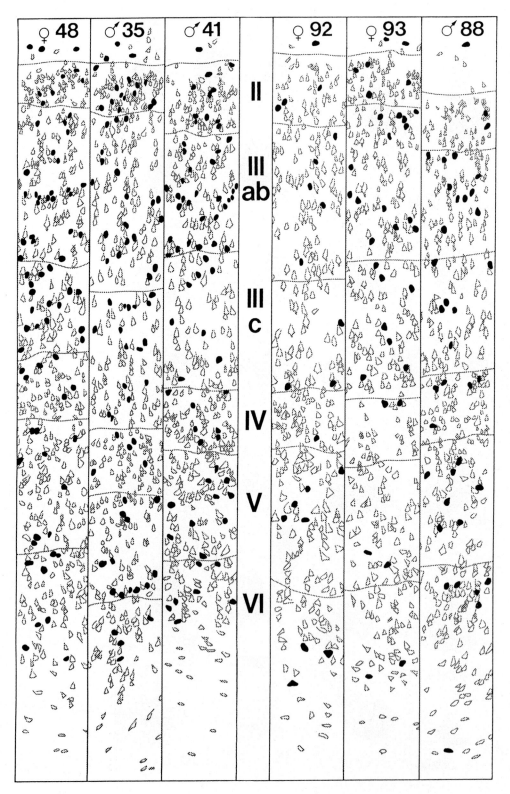

♀ 48 ♂ 35 ♂ 41 ♀ 92 ♀ 93 ♂ 88

II

III
ab

III
c

IV

V

VI

Fig. 4
(legend on p. 198)

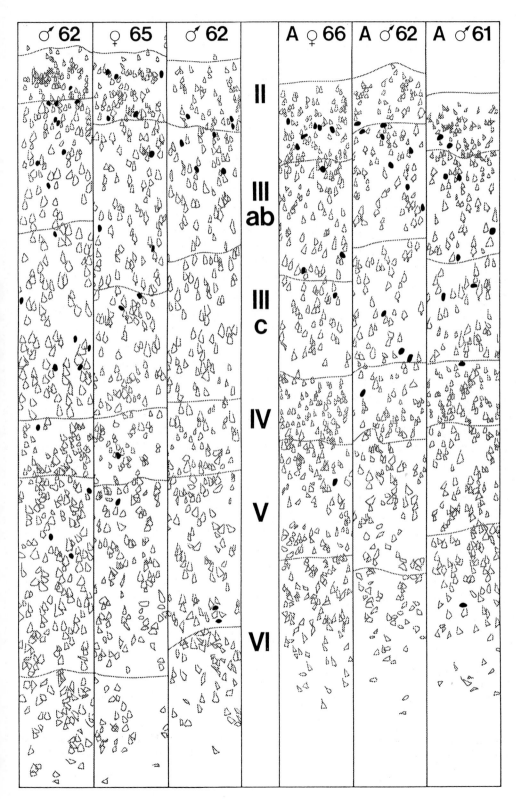

Fig. 5
(legend on p. 198)

partially resemble those described above for the senile brain and, therefore, need not be repeated here. Pigment-filled meganeurites are rarely encountered in layer IIIab pyramidal cells (Fig. 3, a–c). Layer IIIc pyramidal neurons show a normal size and shape of the cell body (Fig. 3, d–f). Layer IV pyramidal cells are well preserved (Fig. 3, g–k). Many of the layer V pyramidal cells show pigment granules in clusters (Fig. 3, l–n), while layer VI cells appear almost unchanged (Fig. 3, o–t). Pigment-laden non-pyramidal cells are reduced in number and often some of the lipofuscin granules can be found in proximal portions of their cellular processes (Fig. 3, 1–4). Occasionally, coarse flocks of extraneuronally located pigment can be seen with a size and shape closely resembling those of the pigment-laden non-pyramidal cells (Fig. 3, 5). In general, the non-pyramidal cells devoid of pigment have lost much of their basophilic cytoplasmic material (Fig. 3, 6–16).

Gallyas preparations show abundant, particularly tightly packed plaques in the supragranular layers and numerous pyramidal cells filled with flame-shaped tangles. These are mainly found in layer V and with decreasing density in layers IIIc and VI as well. The tangles are never encountered in isocortical non-pyramidal cells. In the pigment Nissl preparation, some of the larger plaques can be identified due to their content of pigment-laden glial cells. Frequently, these are tightly packed together and form one of the components of the plaque. It should be emphasized that glial cells tightly filled with pigment that can be stained by aldehydefuchsin are not a normal constituent of the isocortex and can be considered unusual and pathologically changed elements. The presence of

tangles can occasionally be recognized in pigment Nissl preparations as well due to a characteristic clustering of the pigment granules. A probably tangle-bearing layer V pyramidal neuron is displayed in Fig. 3, l.

Distribution pattern and proportions of different nerve cell classes in Alzheimer's disease and in age-matched controls

The right halves of Figs. 5, 7, and 9 display stripes of prefrontal isocortex of three demented patients afflicted with Alzheimer's disease, opposed to three stripes of age-matched controls in the left halves of the same Figs. The total thickness of the cortex is considerably reduced in Alzheimer's disease and each of the various layers contributes to this change. The laminar distribution pattern of the pyramidal cells is well preserved but the number of non-pyramidal neurons per stripe is considerably reduced.

The counting results of the six demented patients can be compared with the values found in non-demented age-matched controls both shown in Table II. Despite the marked overall decrease in cortical thickness in Alzheimer's disease, there is no obvious reduction in the total number of pyramidal cells per stripe in comparison to controls.

The bulk of non-pyramidal neurons is found in layers II and III. 2 663 nerve cells were identified in the six cases of Alzheimer's disease. The pyramidal cells account for approximately 90%, and the non-pyramidal neurons for about 10% of all cortical nerve cells. In the non-demented controls, 2 803 nerve cells have been differentiated. The cortical neurons are formed of about 86% pyramidal neurons intermixed with 14% non-pyramidal cells.

Fig. 4 (see p. 196). Camera lucida drawings of three stripes of prefrontal area 11 of patients ranging in age from 28 to 48 in comparison to three similar stripes of patients ranging in age from 88 to 96. Pyramidal cells and modified pyramidal cells are lightly outlined. Both the pigment-laden and the non-pigmented non-pyramidal cells are filled in with black. The size of the non-pyramidal cells is considerably exaggerated to permit recognition of their laminar distribution pattern. Note the severe loss of non-pyramidal neurons in the old age group.

Fig. 5 (see p. 197). Camera lucida drawings of three stripes of prefrontal area 11 of patients afflicted with Alzheimer's disease (right half) in comparison to similar stripes of age-matched controls (left half). Technical details as in Fig. 4. In Alzheimer's disease, there is a considerable loss of non-pyramidal cells.

The 86:14 ratio of the controls corresponds closely to the 85:15 ratio found in the group of non-demented young individuals. In Alzheimer's disease, in contrast, the 90:10 ratio is already close to the 92:8 ratio found in the non-demented aged patients. There are no signs of a remarkable loss of pyramidal cells in Alzheimer's disease. Accordingly, in comparison to the age-matched controls, there is a neuronal loss of about 29% of the non-pyramidal cells (Table II).

Discussion

Qualitative analysis

Pyramidal neurons and modified pyramidal neurons

Pyramidal and modified pyramidal cells are, in number, the predominant neuronal constituents of the isocortex (Braitenberg, 1978; Sloper et al., 1979; Winfield et al., 1980). The equivalence of pyramidal cells as seen in Golgi impregnated material and in Nissl preparations is generally accepted (Feldman, 1984). Studies using transparent Golgi impregnations counterstained for lipofuscin pigment, in addition, show that isocortical pyramidal cells generally contain fine lipofuscin granules that are only weakly stained by aldehyde-fuchsin (H. Braak, 1980, 1984). In this context it should be mentioned that some rare forms of pyramidal neurons such as the Betz pyramidal cells contain densely packed masses of pigment (H. Braak and E. Braak, 1976); however, these special types of pyramidal cells do not occur in the prefrontal area under consideration.

In Nissl preparations, cut exactly perpendicular to the cortical surface, medium-sized to large pyramidal cells can be recognized on account of their characteristic soma-shape. Small pyramidal cells, in contrast, are hardly distinguishable from non-pyramidal cells of similar soma-size, in particular in layers II and IV, where these cells often appear as polygonal 'granule' cells without the typical gradual blending of the cell body into the apical dendrite. The sparse but characteristic pigmentation of the small layer II and layer IV pyramidal cells, therefore, facilitates their recognition and distinction from non-pyramidal cells. The prevalence of small 'granule' cells in layers II and IV has often led to the assumption that both layers are predominantly formed of stellate cells (Tömböl, 1974; Brody and Vijayashankar, 1977). The results of the present study however indicate a clear predominance of pyramidal cells in layer IV comparable to that found in all the other cellular layers of the isocortex. Using electron microscopic criteria for differentiation of pyramidal cells from non-pyramidal neurons, Peters and Kara (1985a) arrive at the same conclusion for the rat visual cortex.

A large number of reports exists dealing with modified forms of pyramidal cells in various areas and laminae of the mammalian brain (Ngowyang, 1932; De Crinis, 1933; Juba, 1934; O'Leary, 1941; Sanides and Sanides, 1972; Kirsche et al., 1973; H. Braak, 1980; Feldman, 1984). Transparent Golgi impregnations counterstained for pigment reveal that modified pyramidal cells show the same pigmentation characteristics as the pyramidal cells; they are, therefore, included into the class of pyramidal cells in Table II.

Relatively little effort has been made to differentiate the nerve cells forming the sixth isocortical layer. Using the Golgi technique, Tömböl (1984) distinguishes a large number of neuronal types displaying only subtle differences. It remains to be seen whether these cells cannot be considered merely individual expressions of a wide range of forms of only a few basic types. Our findings point to the latter possibility. Due to the characteristic differences in pigmentation, two main neuronal types can be distinguished in layer VI of the human brain, and these are 'the pair of compass cells' and the 'club-shaped neurons' (H. Braak, 1974b, 1980). Unfortunately, these neuronal types cannot be differentiated in Nissl preparations with certainty and were thus not recognized. Existence of these two main forms in the subhuman mammalian brain has not been demonstrated as yet.

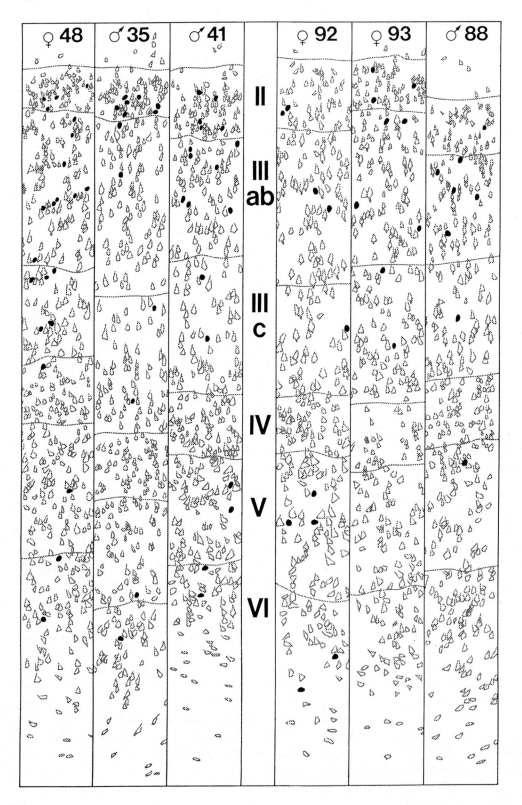

Fig. 6.

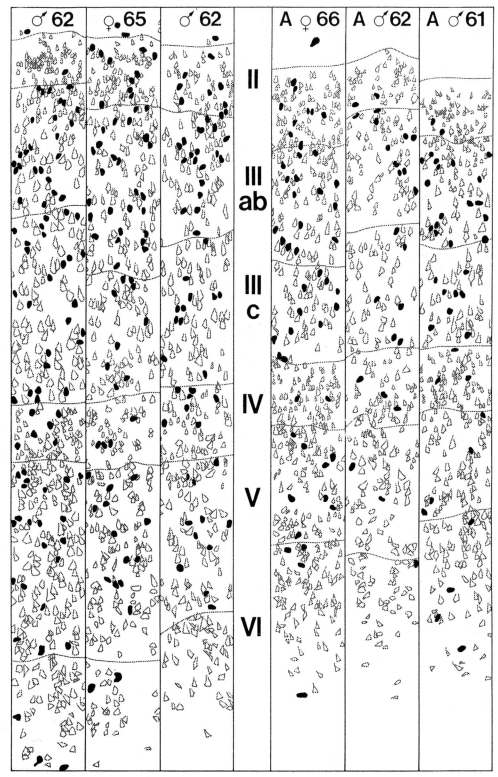

Fig. 7

Figs. 6 and 7. The same stripes as seen in Figs. 4 and 5. These drawings show only the pigment-laden non-pyramidal neurons. They are preferentially localized in layers II and IIIab.

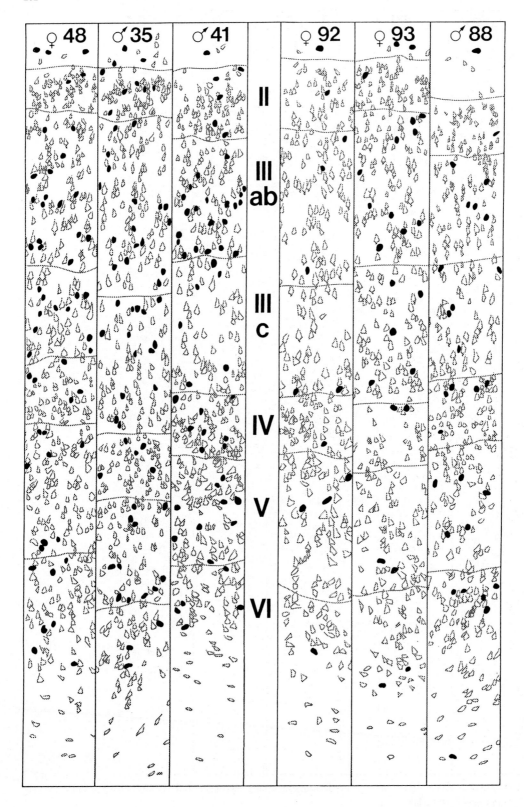

♀48 ♂35 ♂41 ♀92 ♀93 ♂88

II

III
ab

III
c

IV

V

VI

Fig. 8

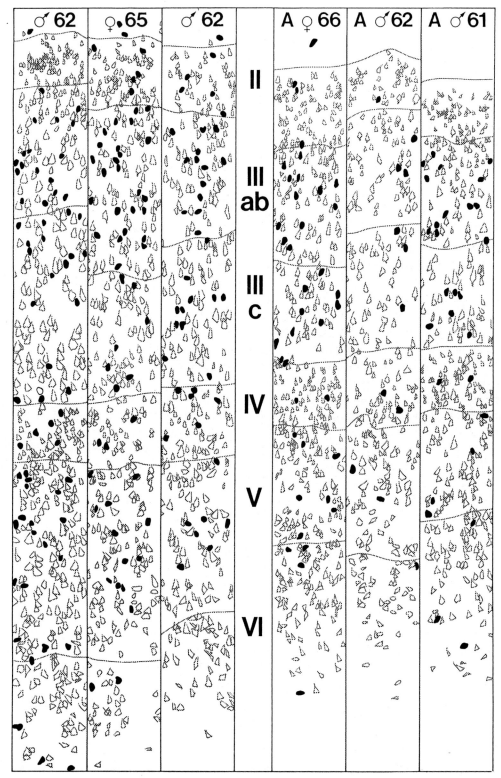

Fig. 9

Figs. 8 and 9. The same stripes as seen in Figs. 4 and 5. These drawings show only the non-pyramidal cells devoid of pigment. They are preferentially located at midcortical level.

Non-pyramidal neurons

Combined pigment-Nissl preparations reveal the existence of two basic types of non-pyramidal cells: the pigment-laden cells and neurons devoid of lipofuscin granules.

The pigment-laden non-pyramidal cells are mainly encountered in the outer cortical layers. They occur in large numbers in phylogenetically late appearing portions of the isocortex, such as in the opercula of the lateral cerebral sulcus. They are, correspondingly, sparsely distributed in older portions such as the proisocortical areas of the cingulate gyrus (E. Braak, 1976; H. Braak, 1974a, 1978a,b,c; Schlegelberger and Braak, 1982). At present, there are no data which allow the pigment-laden stellate cells to be compared with an equivalent, specific neuronal type known from Golgi studies; even their existence in the subhuman mammalian brain has not been demonstrated yet.

Non-pyramidal cells devoid of pigment comprise a variety of forms. Most conspicuous are large cells that are relatively rich in basophilic material. They are mainly located at midcortical level and form apparently a homogeneous population. Transparent Golgi impregnations counterstained for lipofuscin pigment reveal that large non-pigmented neurons of layers IIIc–Va correspond to basket cells known from Golgi studies. The basket cells are ubiquitous constituents of the isocortex (Jones and Hendry, 1984). In man and in the non-human primate, basket cells can mainly be encountered in a horizontal strip extending from the lower portions of layer III to the upper portions of layer V. This pattern of laminar distribution corresponds exactly to that of the large basophilic non-pyramidal cells devoid of pigment.

It has been shown that basket cells receive a dense thalamic input. The dendrites of neighboring cells are interconnected by gap junctions (Sloper and Powell, 1978, 1979). The thick axon gives rise to several terminal branches forming symmetrical synapses on the somata of pyramidal cells in the neighborhood. Basket cells contain glutamic acid decarboxylase. It can, therefore, be assumed that the putative GABAergic cells are inhibitory neurons involved in the control of the activity of the pyramidal cells at midcortical level (Hendry et al., 1983, Houser et al., 1983, Jones and Hendry, 1984).

Difficulties arise if further classification of the small non-pyramidal cells, which are meager in Nissl material, is attempted. These cells are mainly found in the supragranular layers and frequently have spindle-shaped and radially oriented cell bodies. Although detailed correlations have to be worked out, it seems likely that a large number of these cells corresponds to the bipolar and double bouquet cells with dendritic arborizations preferentially oriented in narrow and radially aligned columns (Peters, 1984; Somogyi and Cowey, 1984). The best that can be presently achieved is a distinction between the small spindle-shaped neurons of layers II and III and the relatively large polygonal neurons of layer VI.

Martinotti cells are among the first non-pyramidal cells to appear during ontogenesis. A large number of these cells persist into adulthood forming a ubiquitous constituent of the mature isocortex. They have a relatively large soma size and are mainly encountered within the sixth layer but can, in smaller numbers, also be found in layers III to V. Unfortunately, the distinguishing feature of Martinotti cells is the axon that vertically ascends, splitting off into its terminal branches within the molecular layer (Fairén et al., 1984). Cells of this type do not display cytoplasmic characteristics that would allow them to be distinguished from other types of non-pyramidal cells. Transparent Golgi impregnations counterstained for pigment show medium-sized multipolar layer VI neurons with smoothly contoured dendrites and ascending axon that are devoid of lipofuscin granules. Martinotti cells therefore probably belong to the group of non-pigmented non-pyramidal cells.

Quantitative evaluation

In the brain of the human adult, pyramidal neurons and modified pyramidal cells can be distinguished from non-pyramidal neurons in combined pigment Nissl preparations. These permit examination of the distribution pattern of the various neuronal types in different laminae and areae and allow evaluation of their ratio to each other by light microscopical investigation. The use of pigment deposits as a criterion for differentiating neuronal types permits to examine a large amount of material and to study the neuropathology of non-pyramidal cells (H. Braak and Goebel, 1978; H. Braak et al., 1983; H. Braak, 1984). The fact that the pigment is a stable cytoplasmic component, practically unchanged by suboptimal and delayed fixation, is a prerequisite for the examination of age-related and disease-related changes of the neuronal composition of the human cortex.

Proportion of cortical nerve cell types

Unfortunately, only a few studies are devoted to the evaluation of the percentages of cortical neuronal types and, therefore, comparison of the findings presented with those given by other authors is difficult. As regards the human brain, data are only available on the neuronal composition of sector CA1 of the ammonshorn (Olbrich and Braak, 1985). In experimental animals, the neuronal composition of the cortex has been analyzed on basis of the appearance of the different cell types in Nissl preparations (Werner et al., 1979, 1981, 1982; Werner and Voss, 1981). As already indicated, Nissl interpretation is rendered difficult by issues of post-mortem delay and autolytic changes, and even in experimental animals there is an increasing ambiguity in the interpretation of Nissl preparations with a decrease in the size of the neurons that have to be classified. Percentages of isocortical nerve cell classes are therefore at present mainly studied by electron microscopy (Sloper, 1973; Tömböl, 1974; Sloper et al., 1979; Powell, 1981; Peters and Kara, 1985a,b) with somatic features as distinguishing criteria (Colonnier, 1968, 1981).

By studying narrow stripes of cortex passing through the entire depth of the monkey motor and somato-sensory cortex, Sloper (1973) and Sloper et al. (1979) have found that 72% of the nerve cells belong to the class of pyramidal neurons. The remainder is considered to be comprised of 7% large and 22% small stellate cells in the motor cortex and of 5% large and 23% small stellate cells in the somato-sensory cortex, respectively. Only cells with a centrally cut nucleus have been taken into consideration, and the stripes examined resulted in a final sample of about 100 classified nerve cells.

In her study of the monkey visual cortex, Tömböl (1974) has reported similar percentages of approximately 60%, 7%, and 33%, respectively, for the three categories of cortical constituents mentioned above. Only nucleolated nerve cells have been taken into account in this study.

Winfield et al. (1980), extending this type of cortical analysis on primary motor and visual areas of the cat and rat, have found similar values of 62–72% pyramidal neurons and they as well consider the remaining nerve cells as local circuit neurons being comprised of 3–8% large and 23–33% small stellate cells. Again, only a limited number of about 100 neuronal profiles has been identified for each area of each species.

Peters and Kara (1985a,b), studying in a similar manner area 17 in the rat, in contrast, have found a far larger proportion of pyramidal cells that accounted for about 85% of all cortical nerve cells.

One possible reason for this discrepancy is probably the fact that cell bodies of small pyramidal cells — in particular those of layer IV — are easily misinterpreted as non-pyramidal neurons. Numerous, so-called 'spiny stellate cells', typical layer IV neurons in the visual cortex of many mammalian species (Lund, 1984), are easily classified with the non-pyramidal cells. Spiny stellate cells have several traits in common with pyramidal cells and should be considered as belonging to the group of modified pyramidal neurons (H. Braak, 1976, 1980; E. Braak, 1978, 1982; Sloper et al., 1979; Lund, 1984). Such a classification will of course considerably change the overall proportion of the pyramidal neurons. It is fortuitous that in the human brain, the small pyramidal cells of layer IV are marked by pigment granules that allow their differentiation from non-pyramidal cells. We agree with the statement of Peters and Kara (1985a) emphasizing that most of the small neurons in layer IV are pyramidal cells. Precariousness in the classification of small nerve cells and the small total number of profiles identified go a long way in explaining the discrepancies between the results reviewed above and the data presented in this text.

Age changes

Several authors report a considerable overall loss of cortical nerve cells with ageing and this is often considered a major factor accounting for the age-related decline in intellectual capabilities (Brody, 1955, 1976; Hanley, 1974). With regard to the isocortex, recent investigations have raised serious doubts as to the existence of a marked neuronal loss with ageing in experimental animals (Brizzee et al., 1968; Curcio and Coleman, 1982; Diamond and Connor, 1982) as well as in man (Haug, 1975; Haug et al., 1981, 1983, 1984).

Our results do not point to a severe reduction of pyramidal cells with age; in contrast, the absolute number of pyramidal neurons per cortical stripe of the young individuals corresponds closely to that found in the old-aged group. Although our data are corrected for shrinkage and other factors influencing the counting results we would not like to put emphasis on the absolute numbers. Influences of secular acceleration (Haug, 1984), age-related differences in the extent of tissue shrinkage (Sass, 1982; Eggers et al., 1984), and changes in the volume of the neuropil caused by dendritic distortion, and increase in the number of glial cells are not taken into account, and the number of cases studied appears to be too low to provide a solid basis for such a statement. Our results, nevertheless, buttress the assumption that there is little or no loss of pyramidal neurons with age.

From Golgi studies it is known that the cellular processes of pyramidal cells undergo severe destruction with age and occasionally somata can be found that have virtually lost all of their processes (Scheibel, 1981; Schierhorn, 1981). Unfortunately, the ultimate fate of the surviving pyramidal cell somata has not clearly been demonstrated as yet. It should be stressed, however, that a mere preservation of cell bodies into old age does not imply that pyramidal cell function is preserved as well.

Even a mild neuronal loss may affect the cortex in remarkably different manners. It appears questionable, in the least, as to whether a weak and random loss of nerve cells will really hamper cortical functions. A loss of nerve cells confined to specific neuronal types, in contrast, which like most types of non-pyramidal cells are scattered only in small numbers throughout the cortex, will probably severely impair normal function. There is growing evidence that non-pyramidal cells are unusually vulnerable in various pathological conditions and that they are, in particular, sensitive to disconnection of their afferents. In storage diseases, a marked loss of isocortical local circuit neurons has been reported (H. Braak and Goebel, 1978; H. Braak et al., 1983) and, following hypoxia, selective degeneration of inhibitory interneurons has been found in the monkey motor cortex (Sloper et al., 1980). The large number of mitochondria found in isocortical basket cells and some other types of non-pyramidal cells suggests a high metabolic activity of these cells and — as the other side of the coin — a particular sensitivity to a variety of noxious influences (Ribak and Anderson, 1980; Sloper et al., 1980; Schwartzkroin and Kunkel, 1985).

Again, we would not like to put too much emphasis on the absolute numbers of the non-pyramidal cells. The ratio of pyramidal neurons versus non-pyramidal neurons appears far better suited to demonstrate an age-related decline of non-pyramidal cells since it is independent of all the potentially important variables mentioned above.

General loss of cortical nerve cells linked with a reduction of all neuronal types present in the tissue to roughly the same extent, will yield no change in the ratio of pyramidal neurons versus non-pyramidal cells, but if differences in the vulnerability of these two classes of cortical constituents exist, these will clearly show up. Our results reveal a conspicuous change of this ratio with age pointing to a severe loss of non-pyramidal cells. Both types of non-pyramidal cells, the pigment-laden forms and the neurons devoid of pigment, suffer from a numerical decrease of about the same extent.

Changes in Alzheimer's disease

Presenile and senile dementia of the Alzheimer type are associated with a number of complex structural changes of not only allocortical and isocortical areas but also of many subcortical nuclei (Von Braunmühl, 1957; Jamada and Mehraein, 1968, 1977; Hooper and Vogel, 1976; Kemper, 1978). Many of the isocortical changes observed in Alzheimer's disease such as the development of senile plaques, the dendritic degeneration, and appearance of neurofibrillary changes in certain types of pyramidal cells — mimic, in a sense, the destructions seen to occur inevitably as age advances (Tomlinson et al., 1970; Mehraein et al., 1975; Wisniewski and Soifer, 1979; Scheibel, 1981; Iqbal et al., 1982).

The present results show that the isocortical pathology seen in Alzheimer's disease is incompletely described if only the development of senile plaques and the appearance of neurofibrillary tangles are taken into consideration. The marked loss of isocortical non-pyramidal cells is a further feature that has to be added to the already large number of structural changes recognized in Alzheimer's disease.

The large pyramidal cells of the deep layers V and VI and of layer IIIc are particularly prone to develop tangles in Alzheimer's disease and often the cell body is found almost completely filled with changed fibrils. The cells show a reduced protein synthetic capability and a significant reduction of their nuclear and nucleolar volume (Mann and Sinclair, 1978; Uemura and Hartmann, 1978; Mann and Yates, 1981; Mann et al., 1981a,b; Mann, 1982). Extraneuronally located tangles can

occasionally be found within the neuropil engulfed by glial cells. Tangles have not been shown to develop outside of nerve cells and, therefore, extraneuronal tangles are probably remnants of destroyed neurons with neurofibrillary change (Probst et al., 1982). Hence, there must be some loss of pyramidal cells, though it may be too little to be detectable in quantitative evaluations.

Until now, neurofibrillary changes of the Alzheimer type have not been described to occur in cortical non-pyramidal cells. Neurons of this class do not show other conspicuous changes or impairments of their cellular processes and somata. For all that, it is mainly the class of non-pyramidal cells that is severely reduced in number. A convincing explanation for this specific neuronal loss cannot be offered at present and, on this account, it appears worthwhile to carry out systematic investigations of the conditions responsible for the pronounced vulnerability of the non-pyramidal cells.

Summary and conclusions

Most of the nerve cells constituting the cerebral cortex of the human adult contain large amounts of lipofuscin pigment. Transparent Golgi impregnations counterstained for pigment reveal that the amount, shape, stainability, and pattern of distribution of the pigment granules characterize the neuronal type. In isocortical pyramidal cells and modified pyramidal cells, the pigment is generally finely granulated and randomly dispersed. Isocortical non-pyramidal cells, in contrast, are either filled with coarse lipofuscin granules or are devoid of pigment. Nissl preparations counterstained for pigment, therefore, allow recognition of the main neuronal types of the human cortex and can be used to evaluate the ratio between pyramidal neurons and non-pyramidal cells. This ratio was determined in stripes passing through the full depth of the cortex in a defined frontal field (area 11, Brodmann). All nucleolated nerve cells present within these stripes were classified, drawn, and counted. Twenty four brains of subjects ranging in age from 28 to 96 years were used for this study. A total number of 10 796 neurons was classified. There was only a slight overall loss of cortical nerve cells with age or in Alzheimer's disease.

Pyramidal neurons and modified pyramidal cells together formed about 85% of all cortical nerve cells in non-demented patients up to an age of 65; non-pyramidal cells accounted for about 15% of the nerve cells in these samples.

Approximately two thirds of the non-pyramidal cells were located within the supragranular layers I–III. The packing density of non-pyramidal cells decreased abruptly at the border between layer IIIa and layer IV. The supragranular layers, accordingly, were made up of about 20% non-pyramidal cells while layers IV to VI contained only about 10% of these neurons.

Pigment-laden non-pyramidal cells were mainly encountered within the lower portions of layer II and subjacent portions of layer IIIab. They formed about one fourth of the isocortical non-pyramidal cells. The non-pyramidal cells devoid of pigment were found in all cortical layers and were particularly densely packed at midcortical level.

In brains of non-demented patients ranging in age from 88 to 96 years, a far smaller percentage of non-pyramidal cells was found. In this age group, non-pyramidal cells accounted for only about 8%

of all cortical nerve cells. A similar reduction to about 10% of all cortical neurons was recognized in brains of patients suffering from Alzheimer's disease, and ranging in age from 57 to 66 years.

The data point to a fairly constant number of pyramidal cells even in old age and in Alzheimer's disease. The non-pyramidal cells, in contrast, show a considerable loss of about 47% with age and of about 30% in Alzheimer's disease.

Acknowledgements

The authors are indebted to Prof. Dr. Hübner and Prof. Dr. Stutte (Department of Pathology, Frankfurt) for providing the autopsy material. They would also like to express their appreciation to Prof. Dr. Schlote (Department of Neuropathology, Edinger Institute, Frankfurt), to Prof. Dr. Goebel (Department of Neuropathology, Mainz), Prof. Dr. Mehraein and Dr. Rothemund (Department of Neuropathology, Munich) for supplying material from Alzheimer patients, and they wish to thank Dr. Schleicher (Department of Anatomy, Cologne) for his help with the statistical evaluation. Funding for the research was kindly supplied by the Deutsche Forschungsgemeinschaft.

References

Berube, G. R., Powers, M. M., Kerkay, J. and Clark, G. (1966) The gallocyanin-chrome alum stain; influence of methods of preparation on its activity and separation of active staining compound. *Stain Technol.*, 41: 73–81.

Braak, E. (1976) On the fine structure of the small, heavily pigmented non-pyramidal cells in lamina II and upper lamina III of the human isocortex. *Cell Tissue Res.*, 169: 233–245.

Braak, E. (1978) On the structure of the human striate area. Lamina IV cβ. *Cell Tissue Res.*, 188: 217–234.

Braak, E. (1980) On the structure of lamina IIIab-pyramidal cells in the human isocortex. A Golgi and electron microscopical study with special emphasis on the proximal axon segment. *J. Hirnforsch.*, 21: 439–444.

Braak, E. (1982) On the structure of the human striate area. In: F. Beck, W. Hild, J. Van Limborgh, R. Ortmann, J. E. Pauly and T. H. Schiebler (Eds.), *Advances in Anatomy, Embryology*

and Cell Biology, Vol. 77, Springer, Berlin, New York, Heidelberg, pp. 1–87.

Braak, E. and Braak, H. (1983) On three types of large nerve cells in the granular layer of the human cerebellar cortex. *Anat. Embryol.*, 166: 67–86.

Braak, E., Braak, H., Strenge, H. and Muhtaroglu, U. (1980) Age-related alterations of the proximal axon segment in lamina IIIab-pyramidal cells of the human isocortex. A Golgi and fine structural study. *J. Hirnforsch.*, 21: 531–535.

Braak, H. (1974a) On pigment-loaded stellate cells within layer II and III of the human isocortex. A Golgi and pigmentarchitectonic study. *Cell Tissue Res.*, 155: 91–104.

Braak, H. (1974b) On club-shaped neurons establishing part of the deep moiety of layer VI in the human isocortex. A Golgi and pigmentarchitectonic study. *Cell Tissue Res.*, 156: 113–125.

Braak, H. (1976) On the striate area of the human isocortex. A Golgi and pigment-architectonic study. *J. Comp. Neurol.*, 166: 341–364.

Braak, H. (1978a) On the pigmentarchitectonics of the human telencephalic cortex. In: M. A. B. Brazier and H. Petsche (Eds.), *Architectonics of the Cerebral Cortex*, Raven Press, New York, pp. 137–157.

Braak, H. (1978b) On magnopyramidal temporal fields in the human brain — probable morphological counterparts of Wernicke's sensory speech region. *Anat. Embryol.*, 152: 141–169.

Braak, H. (1978c) The pigment architecture of the human temporal lobe. *Anat. Embryol.*, 154: 213–240.

Braak, H. (1979) Spindle-shaped appendages of the IIIab-pyramids filled with lipofuscin: a striking pathological change of the senescent human isocortex. *Acta Neuropathol.*, 46: 197–202.

Braak, H. (1980) Architectonics of the human telencephalic cortex. In: V. Braitenberg, H. B. Barlow, E. Bizzi, E. Florey, O. J. Grüsser and H. van der Loos (Eds.), *Studies of Brain Function, Vol. 4*, Springer, Berlin, Heidelberg, New York, pp. 1–147.

Braak, H. (1983) Transparent Golgi impregnations: a way to examine both details of cellular processes and components of the nerve cell body. *Stain Technol.*, 58: 91–95.

Braak, H. (1984) Architectonics as seen by lipofuscin stains. In: A. Peters and E. G. Jones (Eds.) *Cerebral Cortex, Vol. 1, Cellular Organization of the Cerebral Cortex*, Plenum Press, New York, pp. 59–104.

Braak, H. and Braak, E. (1976) The pyramidal cells of Betz within the cingulate and precentral gigantopyramidal field in the human brain. A Golgi and pigmentarchitectonic study. *Cell Tissue Res.*, 172: 103–119.

Braak, H. and Braak, E. (1982a) Neuronal types in the claustrum of man. *Anat. Embryol.*, 163: 447–460.

Braak, H. and Braak, E. (1982b) Neuronal types in the striatum of man. *Cell Tissue Res.*, 227: 319–342.

Braak, H. and Braak, E. (1983a) Morphological studies of local circuit neurons in the cerebellar dentate nucleus of man. *Human Neurobiol.*, 2: 49–57.

Braak, H. and Braak, E. (1983b) Neuronal types in the basolateral amygdaloid nuclei of man. *Brain Res. Bull.*, 11: 349–365.

Braak, H. and Braak, E. (1984a) Neuronal types in the lateral geniculate nucleus of man. A Golgi-pigment study. *Cell Tissue Res.*, 237: 509–520.

Braak, H. and Braak, E. (1984b) Neuronal types in the neocortex-dependent thalamic nuclei of man. A Golgi-pigment study. *Anat. Embryol.*, 169: 61–72.

Braak, H. and Goebel, H. H. (1978) Loss of pigment-laden stellate cells: a severe alteration of the isocortex in juvenile neuronal ceroid-lipofuscinosis. *Acta Neuropathol.*, 42: 53–57.

Braak, H., Braak, E. and Goebel, H. H. (1983) Isocortical pathology in type C Niemann-Pick disease. *J. Neuropathol. Exp. Neurol.*, 42: 671–687.

Braitenberg, V. (1978) Cortical architectonics: general and areal. In: M. A. B. Brazier and H. Petsche (Eds.), *Architectonics of the Cerebral Cortex*, Raven Press, New York, pp. 443–465.

Brizzee, K. R. and Ordy, J. M. (1981a) Cellular features, regional accumulation, and prospects of modification of age pigments in mammals. In: R. S. Sohal (Ed.), *Age Pigments*, Elsevier, Amsterdam, New York, Oxford, pp. 101–154.

Brizzee, K. R. and Ordy, J. M. (1981b) Age pigments, cell loss and functional implications in the brain. In: R. S. Sohal (Ed.), *Age Pigments*, Elsevier, Amsterdam, New York, Oxford, pp. 317–334.

Brizzee, K. R., Sherwood, N. and Timiras, P. S. (1968) A comparison of various depth levels in cerebral cortex of young and aged Long-Evans rats. *J. Gerontol.*, 23: 289–297.

Brodmann, K. (1909) *Vergleichende Lokalisationslehre der Großhirnrinde*, J. A. Barth, Leipzig.

Brody, H. (1955) Organization of the cerebral cortex. III. A study of aging in the human cerebral cortex. *J. Comp. Neurol.*, 102: 511–556.

Brody, H. (1976) An examination of cerebral cortex and brainstem aging. In: R. D. Terry and S. Gershon (Eds.), *Neurobiology of Aging, Vol. 3*, Raven Press, New York, pp. 177–181.

Brody, H. and Vijayashankar, N. (1977) Cell loss with aging. In: K. Nandy and J. Sherwin (Eds.), *The Aging Brain and Senile Dementia*, Plenum Press, New York, pp. 15–21.

Colonnier, M. (1968) Synaptic patterns on different cell types in the different laminae of the cat visual cortex. An electron microscope study. *Brain Res.*, 9: 268–287.

Colonnier, M. (1981) The electron-microscopic analysis of the neuronal organization of the cerebral cortex. In: F. O. Schmitt, F. G. Worden, G. Adelman and S. G. Dennis (Eds.), *The Organization of the Cerebral Cortex*, MIT Press, Cambridge, Mass., pp. 125–152.

Curcio, C. A. and Coleman, P. D. (1982) Stability of neuron number in cortical barrels of aging mice. *J. Comp. Neurol.*, 212: 158–171.

De Crinis, M. (1933) Über die Spezialzellen in der menschlichen Großhirnrinde. *J. Psychol. Neurol.*, 45: 439–449.

Diamond, M. C. and Connor, J. R. (1982) Plasticity of the aging cerebral cortex. In: S. Hoyer (Ed.), *The Aging Brain, Suppl. 5, Exp. Brain Res.*, Springer, Berlin, Heidelberg, New York, pp. 36–44.

Eggers, R., Haug, H. and Fischer, D. (1984) Preliminary report on macroscopic age changes in the human prosencephalon. A stereologic investigation. *J. Hirnforsch.*, 25: 129–139.

Einarson, L. (1932) A method for progressive selective staining of Nissl and nuclear substance in nerve cells. *Am. J. Pathol.*, 8: 295–307.

Fairén, A., DeFelipe, J. and Regidor, J. (1984) Nonpyramidal neurons: General account. In: A. Peters and E. G. Jones (Eds.), *Cerebral Cortex, Vol. 1, Cellular Organization of the Cerebral Cortex*, Plenum Press, New York, pp. 201–253.

Feldman, M. L. (1984) Morphology of the neocortical pyramidal neuron. In: A. Peters and E. G. Jones (Eds.),

Cerebral Cortex, Vol. 1, Cellular Organization of the Cerebral Cortex, Plenum Press, New York, pp. 123–200.

Gallyas, F. (1971) Silver staining of Alzheimer's neurofibrillary changes by means of physical development. *Acta Morph. Acad. Sci. Hung.*, 19: 1–8.

Hanley, T. (1974) 'Neuronal fall-out' in the ageing brain: a critical review of the quantitative data. *Age Ageing*, 3: 133–151.

Haug, H. (1967) Über die exakte Feststellung der Anzahl der Nervenzellen pro Volumeneinheit des Cortex cerebri, zugleich ein Beispiel für die Durchführung genauer Zählungen. *Acta Anat.*, 67: 53–73.

Haug, H. (1975) Neuere Aspekte über den biologischen Altersvorgang im menschlichen Gehirn. *Verh. Anat. Ges.*, 67: 389–395.

Haug, H. (1979) The evaluation of cell densities and of nerve-cell size distribution by stereological procedures in a layered tissue (cortex cerebri). *Microsc. Acta*, 82: 147–161.

Haug, H. (1984) Der Einfluß der säkularen Acceleration auf das Hirngewicht des Menschen und dessen Änderung während der Alterung. *Gegenbaurs Morphol. Jahrb.*, 130: 481–500.

Haug, H., Knebel, G., Mecke, E., Orun, C. and Sass, N. L. (1981) The aging of cortical cytoarchitectonics in the light of stereological investigations. In: E. A. Vidrio and M. A. Galina (Eds.), *Eleventh International Congress of Anatomy*, Liss, New York, pp. 193–197.

Haug, H., Barmwater, U., Eggers, R., Fischer, D., Kühl, S. and Sass, N. L. (1983) Anatomical changes in aging brain. *Aging*, 21: 1–12.

Haug, H., Kühl, S., Mecke, E., Sass, N. L. and Wasner, K. (1984) The significance of morphometric procedures in the investigation of age changes in cytoarchitectonic structures of human brain. *J. Hirnforsch.*, 25: 353–374.

Hendry, S. H. C., Houser, C. R., Jones, E. G. and Vaughn, J. E. (1983) Synaptic organization of immunocytochemically identified GABA neurons in the monkey sensory-motor cortex. *J. Neurocytol.*, 12: 639–660.

Hooper, W. M. and Vogel, F. S. (1976) The limbic system in Alzheimer's disease. A neuropathologic investigation. *Am. J. Pathol.*, 25: 1–20.

Houser, C. R., Hendry, S. H. C., Jones, E. G. and Vaughn, J. E. (1983) Morphological diversity of immunocytochemically identified GABA neurons in the monkey sensory-motor cortex. *J. Neurocytol.*, 12: 617–638.

Iqbal, K., Grundke-Iqbal, I., Merz, P. A. and Wisniewski, H. M. (1982) Alzheimer neurofibrillary tangle: Morphology and biochemistry. In: S. Hoyer (Ed.), *The Aging Brain, Suppl. 5, Exp. Brain Res.*, Springer, Berlin, Heidelberg, New York, pp. 10–14.

Jamada, M. and Mehraein, P. (1968) Verteilungsmuster der senilen Veränderungen im Gehirn. Die Beteiligung des limbischen Systems bei hirnatrophischen Prozessen des Seniums und bei Morbus Alzheimer. *Z. Ges. Neurol.*, 211: 308–324.

Jamada, M. and Mehraein, P. (1977) Verteilungsmuster der senilen Veränderungen in den Hirnstammkernen. *Folia Psychiat. Neurol. Jpn.*, 31: 219–224.

Jones, E. G. and Hendry, S. H. C. (1984) Basket cells. In: A. Peters and E. G. Jones (Eds.), *Cerebral Cortex, Vol. 1, Cellular Organization of the Cerebral Cortex*, Plenum Press, New York, London, pp. 309–336.

Juba, A. (1934) Über seltenere Ganglienzellformen der Großhirnrinde. *Z. Zellforsch.*, 21: 441–447.

Kemper, T. L. (1978) Senile dementia: a focal disease in the temporal lobe. In: K. Nandy (Ed.), *Senile Dementia: a Biomedical Approach.* Elsevier, Amsterdam, pp. 105–113.

Kirsche, W., Kunz, G., Wenzel, J., Wenzel, M., Winkelmann, A. and Winkelmann, E. (1973) Neurohistologische Untersuchungen zur Variabilität der Pyramidenzellen des sensorischen Cortex der Ratte. *J. Hirnforsch.*, 14: 117–135.

Lund, J. S. (1984) Spiny stellate neurons. In: A. Peters and E. G. Jones (Eds.), *Cerebral Cortex, Vol. 1, Cellular Organization of the Cerebral Cortex*, Plenum Press, New York, pp. 255–308.

Mann, D. M. A. (1982) Nerve cell protein metabolism and degenerative disease. *Neuropathol. Appl. Neurobiol.*, 8: 161–176.

Mann, D. M. A. and Sinclair, K. G. A. (1978) The quantitative assessment of lipofuscin pigment, cytoplasmic RNA and nucleolar volume in senile dementia. *Neuropathol. Appl. Neurobiol.*, 4: 129–135.

Mann, D. M. A. and Yates, P. O. (1974) Lipoprotein pigments — their relationship to ageing in the human nervous system. I. The lipofuscin content of nerve cells. *Brain*, 97: 481–488.

Mann, D. M. A. and Yates, P. O. (1981) The relationship between formation of senile plaques and neurofibrillary tangles and changes in nerve cell metabolism in Alzheimer type dementia. *Mech. Ageing Dev.*, 17: 395–401.

Mann, D. M. A., Yates, P. O. and Stamp, J. E. (1978) The relationship between lipofuscin pigment and ageing in the human nervous system. *J. Neurol. Sci.*, 37: 83–93.

Mann, D. M. A., Neary, D., Yates, P. O., Lincoln, J., Snowden, J. S. and Stanworth, P. (1981a) Neurofibrillary pathology and protein synthetic capability in nerve cells in Alzheimer's disease. *Neuropathol. Appl. Neurobiol.*, 7: 37–47.

Mann, D. M. A., Neary, D., Yates, P. O., Lincoln, J., Snowden, J. S. and Stanworth, P. (1981b) Alterations in protein synthetic capability of nerve cells in Alzheimer's disease. *J. Neurol. Neurosurg. Psychiat.*, 44: 97–102.

Marshall, P. N. and Horobin, R. W. (1972) The chemical nature of gallocyanin-chrome alum staining complex. *Stain Technol.*, 47: 155–161.

Mehraein, P., Yamada, M. and Tarnowska-Dzidoszko, E. (1975) Quantitative study of dendrites and dendritic spines in Alzheimer's disease and senile dementia. In: G. W. Kreutzberg (Ed.), *Advances in Neurology, Vol. 12*, Raven Press, New York, pp. 453–458.

Ngowyang, G. (1932) Beschreibung einer Art von Spezialzelle in der Inselrinde. *J. Psychol. Neurol.*, 44: 671–674.

Olbrich, H. G. and Braak, H. (1985) Ratio of pyramidal cells versus non-pyramidal cells in sector CA1 of the human Ammon's horn. *Anat. Embryol.*, 173: 105–110.

O'Leary, J. L. (1941) Structure of area striata of the cat. *J. Comp. Neurol.*, 75: 131–164.

Peters, A. (1984) Bipolar cells. In: A. Peters and E. G. Jones (Eds.), *Cerebral Cortex, Vol. 1, Cellular Organization of the Cerebral Cortex*, Plenum Press, New York, pp. 381–407.

Peters, A. and Kara, D. A. (1985a) The neuronal composition of area 17 of rat visual cortex. I. The pyramidal cells. *J. Comp. Neurol.*, 234: 218–241.

Peters, A. and Kara, D. A. (1985b) The neuronal composition of area 17 of rat visual cortex. II. The nonpyramidal cells. *J. Comp. Neurol.*, 234: 242–263.

Powell, T. P. S. (1981) Certain aspects of the intrinsic organization of cerebral cortex. In: O. Pompeiano and C. A. Marsan (Eds.), *Brain Mechanisms and Perceptual Awareness and Purposeful Behavior*, Raven Press, New York, pp. 1–19.

Probst, A., Ulrich, J. and Heitz, P. U. (1982) Senile dementia of Alzheimer's type: astroglial reaction to extracellular neurofibrillary tangles in the hippocampus. An immunocytochemical and electron-microscopic study. *Acta Neuropathol.*, 57: 75–79.

Ribak, C. E. and Anderson, L. (1980) Ultrastructure of the pyramidal basket cells in the dentate gyrus of the rat. *J. Comp. Neurol.*, 192: 903–916.

Rösler, B. and Kemnitz, P. (1983) Relations between the lipofuscin contents and the numerical density of organelles in the pyramidal cells of the layer-III and layer-V in the area-10 (Brodmann) of frontal lobe of men at different ages. *J. Hirnforsch.*, 24: 415–424.

Sanides, F. (1962) Die Architektonik des menschlichen Stirnhirns. In: M. Müller, H. Spatz and P. Vogel (Eds.), *Monographen aus dem Gesamtgebiete der Neurologie und Psychiatrie, Vol. 98*, Springer, Berlin, Göttingen, Heidelberg, pp. 1–201.

Sanides, F. and Sanides, D. (1972) The 'extraverted neurons' of the mammalian cerebral cortex. *Z. Anat. Entwicklungsgesch.*, 136: 272–293.

Sass, N. L. (1982) The age-dependent variation of the embedding-shrinkage of neurohistological sections. *Mikroskopie*, 39: 278–281.

Scheibel, A. B. (1981) The gerohistology of the aging forebrain: some structuro-functional considerations. In: S. J. Enna, T. Samorajski and B. Beer (Eds.), *Aging, Vol. 17, Brain Neurotransmitters and Receptors in Aging and Age-related Disorders*, Raven Press, New York, pp. 31–42.

Scheibel, M. E. and Scheibel, A. B. (1978) The methods of Golgi. In: R. T. Robertson (Ed.), *Neuroanatomical Research Techniques*, Academic Press, New York, pp. 89–114.

Schierhorn, H. (1981) Strukturwandel neokortikaler Pyramidenneurone des Menschen während des 5. bis 9. Dezenniums. *Psychiatr. Neurol. Med. Psychol. (Leipz.)*, 33: 664–673.

Schlegelberger, T. and Braak, H. (1982) The packing density of supragranular pigment-laden stellate cells in phylogenetically older and newer portions of the human telencephalic cortex. *J. Hirnforsch.*, 23: 49–54.

Schroeder, K. (1939) Eine weitere Verbesserung meiner Markscheidenfärbemethode am Gefrierschnitt. *Z. Ges. Neurol.*, 166: 588–593.

Schwartzkroin, P. A. and Kunkel, D. D. (1985) Morphology of identified interneurons in the CA 1 regions of guinea pig hippocampus. *J. Comp. Neurol.*, 232: 205–218.

Sloper, J. J. (1973) An electron microscopic study of the neurons of the primate motor and somatic sensory cortices. *J. Neurocytol.*, 2: 351–359.

Sloper, J. J. and Powell, T. P. S. (1978) Gap junctions between dendrites and somata of neurons in the primate sensorimotor cortex. *Proc. R. Soc. Lond. (Biol.)*, 203: 39–47.

Sloper, J. J. and Powell, T. P. S. (1979) An experimental electron microscopic study of afferent connections to the primate motor and somatic sensory cortices. *Phil. Trans. R. Soc. Lond. (Biol.)*, 285: 199–226.

Sloper, J. J., Hiorns, R. W. and Powell, T. P. S. (1979) A qualitative and quantitative electron microscopic study of the primate motor and somatic sensory cortices. *Phil. Trans. R. Soc. Lond. (Biol.)*, 285: 141–171.

Sloper, J. J., Johnson, P. and Powell, T. P. S. (1980) Selective degeneration of interneurons in the motor cortex of infant monkeys following controlled hypoxia: a possible cause of epilepsy. *Brain Res.*, 198: 204–209.

Somogyi, P. and Cowey, A. (1984) Double bouquet cells. In: A. Peters and E. G. Jones (Eds.), *Cerebral Cortex, Vol. 1, Cellular Organization of the Cerebral Cortex*, Plenum Press, New York, pp. 337–360.

Tömböl, T. (1974) An electron microscopic study of the neurons of the visual cortex. *J. Neurocytol.*, 3: 525–531.

Tömböl, T. (1984) Layer VI cells. In: A. Peters and E. G. Jones (Eds.), *Cerebral Cortex, Vol. 1, Cellular Organization of the Cerebral Cortex*, Plenum Press, New York, pp. 479–519.

Tomlinson, B. E. and Henderson, G. (1976) Some quantitative cerebral findings in normal and demented old people. In: R. D. Terry and S. Gershon (Eds.), *Neurobiology of Aging*, Raven Press, New York, pp. 183–204.

Tomlinson, B. E., Blessed, G. and Roth, M. (1970) Observations on the brains of demented old people. *J. Neurol. Sci.*, 11: 205–242.

Uemura, E. and Hartmann, H. A. (1978) RNA content and volume of nerve cell bodies in human brain. I. Prefrontal cortex in aging, normal and demented patients. *J. Neuropathol. Exp. Neurol.*, 37: 487–496.

Vogt, O. (1910) Die myeloarchitektonische Felderung des menschlichen Stirnhirns. *J. Psychol. Neurol. (Leipz.)*, 15: 221–232.

Von Braunmühl, A. (1957) Alterserkrankungen des Zentralnervensystems. Senile Involution. Senile Demenz. Alzheimersche Krankheit. In: O. Lubarsch, F. Henke and R. Rössle (Eds.),

Handbuch der Speziellen Pathologischen Anatomie und Histologie. Vol. 13, Part 1 (A), Springer, Berlin, Göttingen, Heidelberg, pp. 337–539.

Von Economo, C. and Koskinas, G. N. (1925) *Die Cytoarchitektonik der Hirnrinde des Erwachsenen Menschen*, Springer, Wien, Berlin, pp. 1–810.

Wall, G. (1975) Dilute performic acid — a versatile and easily to handle oxidant in general histology and histochemistry of structure bound sulphur compounds. *Microsc. Acta*, 77: 60–62.

Werner, L. and Voss, K. (1981) Cytomorphometrical investigation of the albino rat's visual cortex with the automatical picture processing. *Mikroskopie*, 37: 250–251.

Werner, L., Hedlich, A., Winkelmann, E. and Brauer, K. (1979) Versuch einer Identifizierung von Nervenzellen des visuellen Kortex der Ratte nach Nissl- und Golgi-Kopsch-Darstellung. *J. Hirnforsch.*, 20: 121–139.

Werner, L., Voss, K., Seifert, I. and Neumann, E. (1981) Age-related classification of pyramidal and stellate cells in the rat visual cortex: a Nissl study with the 'Morphoquant'. *J. Hirnforsch.*, 22: 397–403.

Werner, L., Wilke, A., Blödner, R., Winkelmann, E. and Brauer, K. (1982) Topographical distribution of neuronal types in the albino rat's area 17: a qualitative and quantitative Nissl study. *Z. Mikrosk. Anat. Forsch. (Leipz.)*, 96: 433–453.

West, C. D. (1979) A quantitative study of lipofuscin accumulation with age in normals and individuals with Down's syndrome, phenylketonuria, progeria and transneuronal atrophy. *J. Comp. Neurol.*, 186: 109–116.

Winfield, D. A., Gatter, K. C. and Powell, T. P. S. (1980) An electron microscopic study of the types and proportions of neurons in the cortex of the motor and visual areas of the cat and rat. *Brain*, 103: 245–258.

Wisniewski, H. M. and Soifer, D. (1979) Neurofibrillary pathology: current status and research perspectives. *Mech. Ageing Dev.*, 9: 119–142.

Discussion

D. F. SWAAB: 1. What did you mean by the Golgi staining being 'non-representative'?

2. Is the distinction between projection neurons and interneurons on the basis of pigment architecture applicable on the rest of the brain as well?

3. Is the volume of the Brodmann area you measured changing in aging and dementia? This might profoundly influence the cell numbers and your conclusions on cell loss, which are based on cell density.

ANSWER: 1. The Golgi Braitenberg technique we used is unpredictable. Certain types of nerve cells tend to impregnate frequently whereas others are stained only rarely. On this account, we would not dare to base a quantitative analysis of percentages of neural types forming the cortex on an analysis of Golgi impregnated material.

2. Of subcortical nuclei, we have studied the dentate nucleus, substantia nigra, some nuclei of the thalamus, the lateral geniculate nucleus, the basolateral amygdaloid complex, the striatum, and the claustrum. The neuronal types present within these structures showed a characteristic pigmentation that facilitated their recognition in combined pigment Nissl preparations. In all of the nuclei studied, the projection cells showed a pigmentation different from that seen in local circuit neurons. I should emphasize, nevertheless, that one always has to demonstrate the correlation between the neuronal type and the pigmentation by means of a Golgi de-impregnation study before starting analyses of pigment Nissl preparations of other portions of the human brain.

3. We didn't measure the volume of Brodmann's area 11.

G. S. ROTH: Are there any functional correlates of age changes in pigment quantity or distribution?

ANSWER: No. There is a slow increase in the amount of pigment with age but this generally does not change the characteristics of the pigmentation. Tangle-bearing neurons show some changes in the location of the pigment, and age-related maganeurite formation leads to a change in pigment distribution as well.

R. D. TERRY: Are you really confident that tangles occur only in pyramidal (i.e. projections) neurons? Does your tangle stain reveal all the tangles?

ANSWER: Yes. We have studied silver-impregnated material rather specifically stained for neurofibrillary tangles counterstained for lipofuscin pigment. Non-pyramidal cells could therefore be distinguished from pyramidal cells. We haven't found neurofibrillary tangles in isocortical non-pyramidal neurons.

R. N. KALARIA: Am I correct in understanding that when you stain for Golgi and then de-impregnate and stain for lipofuscin, pigment and Nissl, are you not looking at a very small percentage of cells in your analysis?

ANSWER: We use Golgi preparations after de-impregnations and counterstaining with aldehyde-fuchsin only to demonstrate that the pigment is a marker of the neuronal type. After having shown this, simple Nissl preparations counterstained for pigment will be sufficient and will allow one to distinguish between the various neuronal types.

D. F. Swaab, E. Fliers, M. Mirmiran, W. A. Van Gool and F. Van Haaren (Eds.)
Progress in Brain Research, Vol. 70.
© 1986 Elsevier Science Publishers B.V. (Biomedical Division)

CHAPTER 13

Cation shifts and excitotoxins in Alzheimer and Huntington disease and experimental brain damage

J. Korf[a], J.-B. P. Gramsbergen[a], G. H. M. Prenen[b] and K. G. Go[b]

Departments of [a]Biological Psychiatry and [b]Neurosurgery, University of Groningen, Groningen, The Netherlands

Introduction

In the present chapter we have attempted to review (1) the significance of cation shifts as an index to cell death and (2) the results obtained by examination of post-mortem brain material of humans showing that cation shifts are highly related to dysfunction of amino acid neurotransmitters.

The integrity of the brain is highly dependent on the availability of oxygen and glucose. In contrast to non-neuronal tissue, cells of the central nervous tissue die within a few minutes in the absence of appropriate nutrients. Although the energy metabolism in vitro has dropped to about 50% of that in vivo, brain slices can only survive for a few hours even if sufficient oxygen and glucose are available (Whittingham et al., 1984).

In tissue culture, brain cells can be kept alive for several weeks, but also in this preparation a lack of nutrients produces rapid cell death (e.g. Rothman, 1984, 1985). Comparable to in vitro condition, short-term hypoxia in vivo will induce irreversible degeneration (Levine, 1960; Pulsinelli and Brierley, 1979).

The question arises as to why central neurons are so easily and irreversibly damaged. In the last decade several factors were proposed to explain this fact. These factors are: (a) the generation of free radicals (Chan et al., 1984; Imaizumi et al., 1984; Watson et al., 1984); (b) formation of free fatty acids (such as palmitic, stearic, oleic and arachidonic acid, e.g. Bazan et al., 1984; Wieloch et al., 1984), leukotrines (peptidolipids formed from arachidonic acid, Moskowitz et al., 1984) or prostaglandins (eicosanoids, Asano et al., 1985); (c) acidosis (by lactic acid, Paljärvi, 1984; Rosner and Becker, 1984); (d) the influx of Ca-ions (Farber, 1981; Meldrum et al., 1982; Siesjö, 1981; Trump et al., 1980; Van Reempts et al., 1983; Van Reempts, 1984); and (e) release of endogenous neurotoxins, such as glutamate or aspartate (Benveniste et al., 1984; Drejer et al., 1985; Simon et al., 1984b). The possible interrelationship of Ca influx and some of the other proposed processes leading to cell death have been discussed by Siesjö (1981).

Several methods have been developed to assess cell death or to trace the event of degeneration or damage to cells. They include classical histological methods, such as silver staining, and methods based on histochemical visualization of pathological brain processes, including NADH-fluorescence (Welsh, 1984). Enzyme or receptor markers can also be used for tracing particular neurons. A recently described example of a marker for cell death is the neuron-specific enolase which appears in the extracellular fluid and cerebrospinal fluid during disintegration of the neuron (Steinberg et al., 1983, 1984). This tracer may also be used to monitor brain degenerative processes in vivo.

Other possible methods to trace neuronal degenerative processes in vivo are those based on modern computer-assisted imaging techniques, which will not be summarized here (see Chapter 5 by Frackowiak).

Cation shifts to monitor experimental cell death

Living cells maintain large gradients of electrolytes over the outer membrane. In mammalian neurons and glia cells such gradients of free ions are approximately estimated to be for K: intracellular 90–100 mM, extracellular 3 mM; for Na: intracellular 30 mM, extracellular 145 mM; for Ca: intracellular 1–10 μM, extracellular 1.2 mM; for Mg: intracellular unknown, extracellular about 1 mM and for Cl: intracellular 10–30 mM, extracellular 130 mM (Hansen, 1985; Pumain and Heinemann, 1985).

When a cell disintegrates there is an influx of Na, Cl and Ca, and an efflux of K and Mg. Such alterations have been demonstrated by using ion-selective electrodes (Hansen, 1978, 1985; Hansen and Zeuthen, 1981). However, if the circulation of the damaged tissue is intact, cellular ion shifts are rapidly followed by a compensation from the periphery. For example, we have observed that within a few minutes after local application of the neurotoxic compound kainate in the rat striatum the contents of Na, Ca, and K had already changed to an extent that Na and Ca per g tissue had increased by more than 20%, whereas K level had decreased by 20% (Korf and Postema, 1984; Korf et al., 1983).

Increase in the uptake of Ca into dying neurons (and glia cells) can be visualized by autoradiography (Dienel, 1984; Jancsó et al., 1984) at light-microscopical level, or by the oxalate/pyroantimonate fixation technique (Korf and Postema, 1984; Simon et al., 1984a; Van Reempts, 1984) at electron-microscopical level. An example of tracing degenerating cells (intoxicated by kainate), using Ca autoradiography is shown in Fig. 1.

In brain, electron microscopical examinations show Ca predominantly in synaptic vesicles and little in mitochondria and nuclei. Following hypoxic/ischemic injury or kainate intoxication, most Ca is found in the cytosol and in newly formed vacuoles. Some Ca is also taken up by mitochondria (Van Reempts, 1984).

In the hippocampus the cells most vulnerable to ischemia are the pyramidal cells of the areas CA_1 and CA_2 (Pulsinelli and Brierley, 1979; Kirino et al., 1984). Either after 30 min ischemia (Simon et al., 1984a) or after 60–120 min seizure activity these cells accumulate more Ca compared to adjacent cells (Meldrum et al., 1982). With electron microscopy a transient accumulation of Ca was seen in mitochondria in pyramidal neurons and in vacuoles of presumably irreversibly damaged neurons (Simon et al., 1984a).

The question arises, whether changes in the cation levels of tissue may be due to a break-down of the blood–brain barrier. It is well established that in the case of ischemic edema two more or less independent phases can be distinguished. The first phase is characterized as cytotoxic edema, during which most of the cation shifts may occur (Ito et al., 1976). A subsequent phase, which is characterized by the opening of the blood–brain barrier, also changes the levels of electrolytes to a minor extent (Ito et al., 1976). Consistent with these different phases are the following observations. In a study in which brain damage was produced by the occlusion of the middle cerebral artery there was no correlation between leakage of Evans blue from the blood circulation into the brain and tissue cation shifts (Gotoh et al., 1985). In the Levine preparation, unilateral occlusion of the common carotid artery of the rat exposed to hypoxic conditions (Levine, 1960), there was also no coincidence of blood–brain barrier opening and shifts in the Na/K ratio (Prenen et al., 1985).

In kainate-intoxicated striata the blood–brain barrier remains virtually intact, despite the large alteration in cation levels (J. Korf and F. Postema, unpublished data). On the other hand, in the instance of blood–brain barrier impairment by a local injection of collagenase, there was no evident damage to neurons, although there was some increase in the ratio of Na/K (Gazendam et al., 1984).

A direct way to monitor translocations of

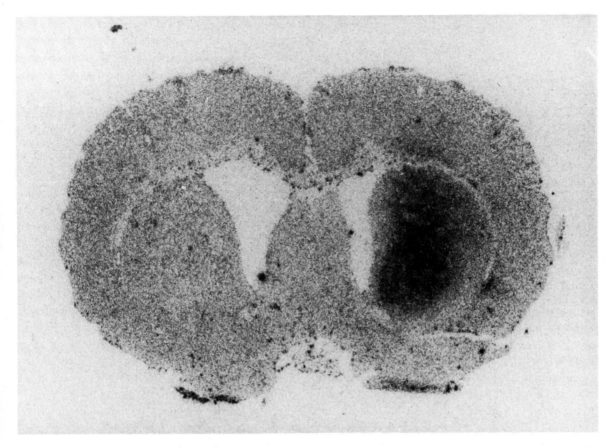

Fig. 1. An autoradiogram of the cerebral distribution of radioactive Ca, administered intravenously 24 h before death. The rats received a unilateral intra-striatal injection of kainate (1 μg in 1 μl) just before labeling. Methods are essentially as those according to Dienel (1984). The black areas include the ipsilateral striatum and a small part of the overlying cerebral cortex and represent sites of high Ca uptake.

electrolytes in the intra- or extracellular space can be performed with ion-selective electrodes (e.g. Hansen, 1985; Pumain and Heinemann, 1985, for reviews). Accordingly, alterations in the concentrations of Ca, K, Na, and Cl have been monitored; e.g. during hypoxia, hypoglycemia and exposure to excitatory compounds such as kainate and glutamate, the influx of Ca, Cl, and Na into nerves and glia cells was increased, whereas K-ions were extruded (Hansen, 1978, 1985; Hansen and Zeuthen, 1981; Ben Ari, 1985; Pumain and Heinemann, 1985). During hypoxia and hypoglycemia these changes were gradual, until the concentration of K in the extracellular fluid rises to 15 mM. Later a rapid and more dramatic alteration in the ion

levels occurs. Apparently a large intracellular space became accessible to the extracellular ions, whereas intracellular K diffuses freely into the extracellular space. These dramatic events coincide and are probably mainly responsible for the generation of changes in a deflection of the interstitial brain potential (Hansen, 1985) and differences in impedance of tissue (Pelligrino et al., 1981). We have measured the deflection of the interstitial brain potential as a measure of cell damage in the striatum, following cardiac arrest produced by the intravenous injection of a saturated solution of $MgCl_2$ in chloral hydrate anesthetized rats. Examples of such recordings are illustrated in Fig. 2. Approximately 2 min following cardiac arrest a

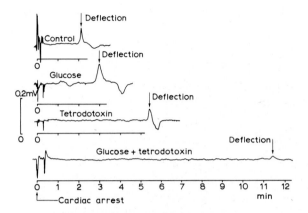

Fig. 2. Brain potentials recorded from the striatum of anesthetized rats, following cardiac arrest. In control (top trace), a positive potential could be recorded between an electrode placed in the striatum and a subcutaneous reference electrode. Pretreatment with either glucose or tetrodotoxin delays the generation of this potential. Combination of glucose and tetrodotoxin (lower trace) dramatically delays as well as decreases striatal potentials (see also Fig. 5).

potential sweep was recorded. The interval between cardiac arrest and the potential sweep was increased when the animals were pretreated intraperitoneally with glucose (30 g·kg^{-1}) or with an intrastriatal injection of tetrodotoxin (TTX, 400 ng) 1 h before death.

Cation shifts in Alzheimer and Huntington disease

Cerebral calcification is known as a cause of cation shifts since the 19th century (for reviews see Löwenthal and Bruyn, 1968). Intracerebral calcification occurs under a variety of circumstances including several diseases affecting the brain such as intoxications, radiation, hypoparathyroidism, and seizures; however, idiopathic calcifications have also been reported. Idiopathic calcification of dentate, pallidum and striatum which occurs frequently has been recognized as striopallidodentate calcinosis or Fahr's disease. The major causes of calcification have been suggested to be an aberrant metabolism of Ca, pathological changes in blood vessels, or increased phosphatase activity (e.g. Brannan et al., 1980). In addition, calcification may also be caused by cell death. In studies

with rats, local application of kainate causes a more than 10-fold increase in the levels of Ca, without any influence on the blood–brain barrier or the circulating levels of Ca (Korf and Postema, 1984).

Cerebral calcifications are often seen together with clinical symptoms, such as mental deterioration, dementia or extrapyramidal dysfunction (Löwenthal and Bruyn, 1968; Boller et al., 1973; Brannan et al., 1980; Smits et al., 1983). However, with computerized tomography, a technique which is sensitive enough to detect calcifications in the brain (Murphy, 1979), cerebral calcinosis can be found before any clinical symptoms emerge.

In post-mortem brain material the accumulation of excessive amounts of calcium has been demonstrated. Most often the Ca deposits are found extracellularly. Ca deposits have been found more frequently in post-mortem brain tissue than in vivo, since even with computerized tomography the relatively mild accumulations of Ca cannot be observed. For instance, the 10-fold increase in Ca contents seen in the rat striatum following kainate injection could not be seen with computerized tomography (J. Korf, unpublished observations). Recently, intracellular accumulation of Ca has been shown in parkinsonism-dementia patients (Garruto et al., 1984). Ca and aluminum were found together in neurons of the pyramidal cell layer of the hippocampus which had also neurofibrillary tangles. In this disease hyperparathyroidism was possibly caused by Ca and Mg deficiency, rather than by genetic factors. Hilal et al. (1985) using nuclear magnetic resonance imaging, have visualized the increase of Na in patients with recent and old strokes. They claimed that ^{23}Na-NMR is more sensitive to detect infarcts, in particular the more recent ones, than computerized tomography (with X-ray absorption).

To further elaborate the possibility that cation shifts may serve as an index for neurodegenerative processes, we analyzed brain tissue of patients who had suffered from Huntington chorea and Alzheimer disease and age-matched controls.

The results and the description of the patients

TABLE I

Cation levels in post-mortem brain tissue of patients with Alzheimer disease, Huntington Chorea and in age-matched controls

Disease and brain area	Number	Age (yr ± SEM)	Post-mortem delay (h ± SEM)	Levels of cations (μmol·g^{-1} ± SEM)			
				Na	K	Ca	Mg
Alzheimer	12	79.1 ± 2.2	40.6 ± 6.4				
hippocampus				94.0 ± 3.1[b]	42.1 ± 1.8[c]	1.8 ± 0.1	4.1 ± 0.2[a]
frontal cortex (BA8)				107.9 ± 6.8	60.1 ± 3.4	1.9 ± 0.1	4.7 ± 0.2
Controls	12	82.6 ± 1.9	55.6 ± 6.5				
hippocampus				77.6 ± 2.7	56.8 ± 2.4	2.0 ± 0.1	4.6 ± 0.1
frontal cortex (BA8)				93.4 ± 3.6	57.2 ± 2.4	2.0 ± 0.1	4.5 ± 0.2
Huntington	13	51.9 ± 9.7	35.6 ± 5.0				
putamen				69.4 ± 2.6[c]	66.8 ± 1.9[c]	1.7 ± 0.1	5.4 ± 0.1[d]
frontal cortex (BA4)				95.3 ± 5.9	58.9 ± 2.0	1.9 ± 0.1	5.3 ± 0.2
Controls	14	53.8 ± 4.6	54.5 ± 3.3				
putamen				52.9 ± 2.8	84.6 ± 2.0	1.8 ± 0.1	5.8 ± 0.1
frontal cortex (BA4)				83.5 ± 4.4	62.0 ± 2.4	2.1 ± 0.3	5.0 ± 0.2

BA8 and BA4: Brodmann area 8 and 4, respectively. Statistical evaluations with ANOCOVA with age and post-mortem delay as covariates: [a]$p < 0.002$; [b]$p < 0.003$; [c]$p < 0.001$; [d]$p < 0.05$, as compared to the appropriate controls.

are summarized in Table I. In the hippocampus of Alzheimer patients Na and K were significantly increased and decreased, respectively. The levels of Ca did not reach significant differences, but the Mg content was lower in the hippocampal tissue. In the cerebral cortex none of the cations were found to be significantly altered. Similar alterations were found in the putamen of Huntington chorea patients. Na content was increased and the Mg and K levels were decreased, while no significant differences were found in the cerebral cortex. The significance of these differences was striking when in the analysis of covariance (ANOCOVA) age and post-mortem delay were taken as covariates. These results emphasized the usefulness of the cations (Na and K but not of Ca) as an index of the extent of brain damage.

Amino acid changes in Huntington chorea and Alzheimer disease

Huntington chorea is a dominant inherited disease (Gusella et al., 1983; Went et al., 1984; for references) of the basal ganglia, of which the deviating DNA molecule has recently been characterized (Gusella et al., 1983). The dysfunction of the γ-aminobutyric acid (GABA) containing neurons in this disease is well established; decreased levels of the amino acid as well as of its synthesizing enzyme, glutamate decarboxylase, have frequently been reported (Bird, 1976; Perry et al., 1973; Spokes et al., 1980).

In the previous section we have described the decreased K and the increased Na levels in the putamen of choreatic patients. If the changes in cation levels are related to neurodegenerative processes in neurotransmitter systems, there should be a correlation between the decrease in GABA and the cation shifts in these patients. Such correlations were indeed detected. As shown in Fig. 3, significant positive correlations were found between K and GABA levels, whereas the correlation was negative between the contents of Na and GABA (Gramsbergen et al., 1986).

With regard to Alzheimer disease the possible role of various neurotransmitters in the pathogene-

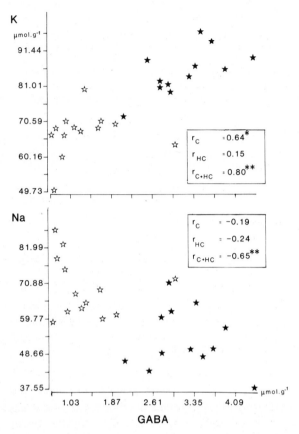

Fig. 3. Relation between the levels of K or Na and those of γ-aminobutyric acid in the putamen of patients who had suffered from Huntington chorea (open asterisks) and non-neurological controls (closed asterisks). Amino acids were determined according to Venema et al. (1983); cations according to Korf and Postema (1984). Significance of the correlations (r) $^{*}p < 0.005$ and $^{**}p < 0.001$.

sis of this disorder has been emphasized. These include acetylcholine, norepinephrine and 5-hydroxytryptamine (Coyle et al., 1983; Pearce et al., 1984). Recently, attention has been paid to the pathological involvement of peptides, such as somatostatin (Morrison et al., 1985; Roberts et al., 1985 for review), and to amino acids (Arai et al., 1984; Greenamyre et al., 1985; Pearce et al., 1984; Tarbit et al., 1980; Zimmer et al., 1984). See also other contributors to this volume.

In addition to the neuropathological changes in the cerebral cortex, the possible role of the hippocampus in dementia has recently been re-

ported (Ball et al., 1985; Hyman et al., 1984). In view of the observed alterations of the cations in the post-mortem hippocampus of Alzheimer patients and the prominent role of amino acids in the hippocampal neurotransmission (Storm-Mathisen, 1977; Fonnum, 1984), we have examined whether there were alterations in glutamate contents and whether those changes were related to cation shifts in Alzheimer disease. In our post-mortem brain material glutamate levels were decreased in the hippocampus, but not in the frontal cortex. There was a significant positive correlation between the glutamate content of the hippocampus and K. The correlation of glutamate and Na was negative, but not statistically significant (Fig. 4; Gramsbergen et al., 1985).

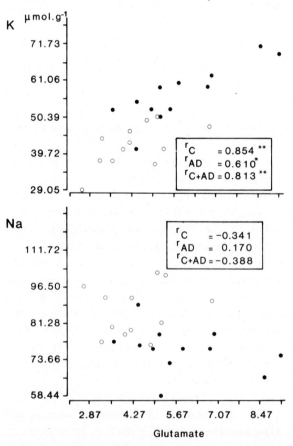

Fig. 4. Relation between cation levels and glutamate content of the hippocampus of controls (closed circles) and Alzheimer patients (open circles). See also legend to Fig. 3.

Our results support the importance of hippocampal pathology, which was emphasized by others (see above). In particular the sub-hippocampal areas such as the CA_1 field and the adjacent subiculum appear to be affected in Alzheimer disease (Hyman et al., 1984). Cross et al. (1984a,b) found decreased 5-hydroxytryptamine receptor binding in the hippocampus of Alzheimer patients. Combining these results with the histopathological observations of Hyman et al. (1984) and our biochemical findings, the possibility emerges that CA_1 pyramidal neurons (which are glutaminergic and contain serotonin receptors) are deficient in Alzheimer disease. Interestingly, CA_1 pyramidal neurons are also very sensitive to anoxia, ischemia and convulsions (e.g. Kirino et al., 1984; Meldrum et al., 1982; Petito and Pulsinelli, 1984; Pulsinelli and Brierley, 1979).

For several neurotransmitter systems it has been shown that denervation induces an increased number of receptors in the target cells. This is also apparent in the case of glutamate innervation of the striatum by the cerebral cortex (Roberts et al., 1982). Increased binding of glutamate, presumably to glutamate receptors, has been found in the caudate nucleus of Alzheimer patients by one group of researchers (Pearce et al., 1984) but not by another (Greenamyre et al., 1985). The latter group, however, observed a decreased number of glutamate binding sites in the cerebral cortex in Alzheimer disease and in the caudate and putamen in Huntington disease. Because of these controversial results (and our own observations), it is not yet clear that cortical glutamate-containing neurons are affected in these diseases, and it is even less certain that cortical pathology is the cause of the possible biochemical alterations in subcortical brain regions.

Possible prevention of neurodegenerative disorders

The pathogenetic factors found responsible for irreversible injury during experimental lesions may guide the search for pharmacological treatments in the prevention of various disorders. Such attempts have obvious clinical relevance in the case of stroke, but — as will be hypothesized below — such an approach may also be of importance in neurodegenerative diseases. Some examples of protective methods are the suppression of formation of free radicals, to alter brain pH and to enhance cerebral blood flow or to block (brain) receptors (Yoshida et al., 1985, Rosner and Becker, 1984; Siesjö, 1981; Simon et al., 1984b; Garcia, 1984). Having in mind cation shifts and amino acid disturbances in certain neurodegenerative diseases such as Alzheimer and Huntington diseases, we shall limit ourselves to these constituents. In living cells excessive influx of Ca and Na or the efflux of K will derange regulatory mechanisms. For instance, neural protease activity and phospholipase activity may become triggered by an increase in the intracellular levels of Ca (Siesjö, 1981; Zimmerman and Schlaepfer, 1984), which may in turn affect the integrity of membranes and skeletons of neurons and glial cells. Indeed in several cases Ca overload has been held responsible for irreversible injury of both peripheral and central cells (Farber, 1981; Meldrum et al., 1982; Siesjö, 1981; Trump et al., 1980; Van Reempts et al., 1983). Not only the enhanced levels of the cation found in damaged tissue, but also reports on the beneficial effects of agents that are capable of blocking Ca entry are in favor of the possible role of Ca in cell death. Neurological recovery of dogs from ischemia has been reported to be improved by nimodipine (Steen et al., 1983) and from brain damage caused by ischemia/hypoxia in rats pretreated with flunarizine (Van Reempts et al., 1983; Dubinsky et al., 1984). These reports are in accordance with the cation hypothesis. Treatment with nimodipine may also reduce occurrence of neurological deficits (such as unconsciousness and disability) in patients with ischemic stroke (e.g. Gelmers, 1984). If the uptake of Ca is reponsible for cell damage, it is understandable why during aging cell loss may occur, since the buffering capacity of mitchondria for intracellular Ca has been diminished during aging (Leslie et al., 1985).

Some observations, however, failed to support

220

the Ca hypothesis. For instance verapamil, another Ca-entry blocker, did hardly protect the brain from hypoxic/ischemic damage (Berger et al., 1984; Dubinsky et al., 1984), although this drug blocks the influx of Ca into cerebral cells following cardiac arrest (Hagberg et al., 1984). However, insufficient penetration of verapamil into the brain cannot be ruled out in this case. In an attempt to reduce the neurotoxicity of kainate, in our own studies, rats were kept on a vitamin D and Ca-deficient diet for 6 weeks before the neurotoxin was applied to the striatum. The shifts in Na and K were similar to those of control rats, but the accumulation of Ca was substantially reduced (Korf and Postema, 1984). Although with such a diet cerebral calcifications may be attenuated or even prevented, degenerative processes do not seem to be influenced. Moreover, pretreatment of rats with high doses of various Ca-entry blockers (including nimodipine, flunarizine, lidoflazine, su-loctidil, ethylenediamine tetra-acetate, $MgSO_4$ or chlorpromazine) failed to modify kainate toxicity (J. Korf and F. Postema, unpublished results). Taken together, all these observations do not justify the intracellular accumulation of Ca as a critical factor in the induction of irreversible damage. Moreover, in cases where Ca-entry blockers are protective, the precise mechanism of action is uncertain, as these drugs may also have a direct effect on membranes (Sihra et al., 1984).

Blockade of Na channels by TTX seems to be more effective in the prevention of cation shifts. Intrastriatal application of TTX (400 ng) delays the occurrence of the deflection of the interstitial electrical potential following cardiac arrest (Figs. 2 and 5). In the striatum of chloral hydrate anesthetized rats the delay was as long as 4 min, compared to 2 min ($p < 0.02$; see Fig. 5) in controls. TTX blocks Na channels, which inhibits spontaneous bioelectrical activities and virtually suppresses the release of all neurotransmitters (Narahashi, 1974). Also the administration of large doses of glucose delays the appearance of the deflection of the brain potential. This protective action of glucose is due to anaerobic glycolysis. Choki et al. (1984) re-

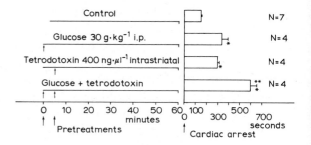

Fig. 5. Cumulative data of the emergence of brain potentials in chloralhydrate anesthetized rats with various treatments given before cardiac arrest. Data obtained with the recording technique shown in Fig. 1. Statistical significances *, $p < 0.005$ compared to control values. **, $p < 0.05$ compared to other treatments. Deflection time in s $\pm$ SEM, number of experiments is as indicated.

ported a high correlation between glucose utilization and K efflux into the extracellular space. Combining glucose and TTX treatment, the time interval between cardiac arrest and potential changes was increased to 9 min (Figs. 1 and 5). Apparently both shortage of energy and the release of neurotransmitters play a concerted role in the disintegration of the nervous membrane.

TTX was not only effective in the above preparation, but also in the procedure, according to Levine, which leads to unilateral ischemic/hypoxic infarction. Local application of TTX in the rat striatum prevented the development of an infarct in the injected area, but not in adjacent brain regions (Fig. 6). This observation shows that the occurrence of an infarct is not only dependent on the cerebral energy stores, but also on action potentials and neurotransmission. Glycolysis may be of importance to maintain the gradients of ions over the cell membrane, although the formation of lactic acid may be harmful (Rosner and Becker, 1984; Siesjö, 1981; Paljärvi, 1984). Therefore, by diminishing the dependency of energy metabolism on the utilization of glucose (by fasting for instance), protection against ischemic/hypoxic insults can be achieved (Kirsch and D'Alecy, 1979; Myles, 1976; Prenen et al., 1985). In this context an interesting observation has been made by Roth et al. (1984). They showed that rats kept on a

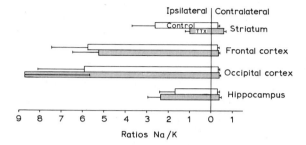

Fig. 6. Ratio of Na/K 24 h after an infarct produced with the Levine procedure. The infarcts were predominantly ipsilateral in the indicated areas. Administration of TTX into the striatum diminished the bilateral differences of Na/K. The differences between the control striatum and TTX-treated striatum ($p < 0.05$) and the adjacent frontal cortex ($p < 0.01$). Number of observations: controls 6; TTX-treated: 9. Bars are mean $\pm$ SEM. Open bars are controls, dotted bars TTX-treated.

restricted diet survive longer and the loss in striatal dopamine receptors during aging was considerably delayed. These receptors are localized at neurons that are highly vulnerable to hypoxia/ischemia (Petito and Pulsinelli, 1984). The loss of dopamine receptors may then point to a gradual dysfunction or degeneration of striatal neurons. Thus, whereas a decreased availability of glucose may offer brain protection, increasing the circulating glucose may lead to more damaging infarcts (Welsh et al., 1980; Welsh, 1984; Rosner and Becker, 1984).

The TTX experiments suggest the importance of neurotransmission in cell damage. They do, however, not indicate the nature of the processes involved. It is well known that certain brain regions and particular nerve cells in these areas are more vulnerable to ischemia/hypoxia than others (Pulsinelli and Brierley, 1979; Petito and Pulsinelli, 1984). Of the endogenous neurotransmitter substances glutamate is both neurotoxic and it is released in large quantities during anoxic or ischemic conditions (Benveniste et al., 1984; Drejer et al., 1985) and during edema formation (Maier-Hauff et al., 1984). Glutamate toxicity in the striatum was greater when the uptake of the amino acid was blocked (McBean and Roberts, 1985). Local application of the glutamate antagonist 2-amino-7-phosphoheptanoic acid (which blocks in

particular the N-methyl-D-aspartate-preferring receptors) prevented damage to hippocampus pyramidal cells in CA_1 and CA_3 regions (Simon et al., 1984b). The question arises whether the possible neurotoxic action and the excitatory effect of glutamate (or similarly acting substances) can be dissociated. Indirect evidence for that is found with electrophysiological studies showing that excitatory amino acids enhanced the uptake of Ca, which was not blocked by TTX (Ben-Ari, 1985; Olney et al., 1984; Pastuszko et al., 1984; Pumain and Heinemann, 1985; Rothman, 1984, 1985). We observed that a pretreatment of the rat striatum with high doses of TTX did not prevent the destructive action of kainate (J. Korf and F. Postema, unpublished observations). Furthermore, there was a lack of correlation between various compounds in neurotoxic as well as in excitatory action (Foster et al., 1984; Notman et al., 1984; Lehman et al., 1985). Recently, several authors supposed that not the influx of Ca, but rather that of Cl (or Na) is pathogenetic (Olney et al., 1984; Rothman, 1984, 1985).

Plaitakis et al. (1982, 1984) described a degenerative neurological disorder associated with a deficiency of glutamate dehydrogenase. In this disease, which is characterized by atypical neurological manifestations (such as extrapyramidal and cerebral dysfunction and peripheral neuropathy), the glutamate levels in the circulation were high, possibly due to low leucocyte contents of the enzyme. The glutamate in the circulation may become neurotoxic when the blood–brain barrier fails. Whether the enzyme deficiency occurs also in the brain is uncertain.

The latter disease, together with our observations in Alzheimer disease supposes a specific dysfunction of glutamate in human neuropathology. A further role of glutamate and aspartate in Alzheimer disease is suggested by the observation that exposure of cultured spinal cells to these amino acids induced neurofibrillary degeneration, very similar to that seen in the senile brain (De Boni and Crapper McLachlan, 1985).

The possibility of the involvement of glutamate

(or other endogenous neurotoxins) in brain damage due to anoxia, ischemia, and possibly in Alzheimer disease, and the protective action of TTX or excitatory amino acid receptor antagonists in some cases, suggest future pharmacological help in neurodegenerative diseases. The dissociation between the excitatory effects and the neurotoxicity of glutamate-related compounds indicates that a blockade of normal physiological events in the process of neurotransmission is not always necessary to prevent pathological changes. In addition, alternative treatments aimed to block selectively certain ion channels may also be worthwhile.

Summary and conclusions

The possible role of excitatory amino acids (glutamate and the related compound kainate) and the influx of cations in experimental animals and human neurodegenerative diseases is discussed. In experimental designs, changes in cations during cell death were detected by measurement of their tissue levels, by autoradiography of Ca, or by recording of interstitial electrical potentials. Cation changes were thus found following local injection of kainate, hypoxic/ischemic infarction (i.e. Levine preparation) and cardiac arrest. Shifts in Na and K (but not in Ca) were also observed in brain tissue postmortally obtained from patients suffering from Huntington chorea and Alzheimer disease.

In post-mortem hippocampal tissue of Alzheimer patients and Huntington chorea putamen we observed a significant increase in Na and a significant decrease in K levels. In the cerebral cortex none of the cations were found to be significantly altered. There was a positive correlation between the contents of glutamate and K in both controls and Alzheimer patients. In the putamen of patients with Huntington chorea a positive correlation was found between K^+ and γ-aminobutyric acid levels, whereas a negative correlation was observed between γ-aminobutyric acid and Na.

These results suggest a possible role for amino acids in the shifts of cations during experimental cell death and neurodegenerative diseases. Early changes in the levels of sodium may also be detected by nuclear magnetic resonance imaging, which may thus become a diagnostic tool for neurodegenerative diseases. Cell death due to excessive activity of glutamate (or another endogenous excitotoxic compound) may be attenuated or prevented by drugs capable of blocking the release of specific receptors of the amino acid. If such a process is involved in neurodegenerative diseases, modification of excitatory neurotransmission by drugs may become of therapeutic value.

Acknowledgements

Technical assistance was given by Mrs. L. Veenma-Van der Duin, Mr. F. Postema and Mr. F. Zuiderveen. Financial support was given by the State University of Groningen, the Dutch Organization for Pure Medical Research, FUNGO, and the J. K. de Cock Stichting. We thank Dr. G. P. Reynolds, MRC Neurochemical Pharmacological Unit, Brain Tissue Bank, Department of Neurological Surgery and Neurology, Addenbrooke's Hospital, Cambridge, UK, who kindly provided the human brain tissue samples. Mr. W. Stadman prepared the Figures and Mrs. W. Van der Meer typed the manuscript.

References

Arai, H., Kobayashi, K., Ichimiya, Y., Kosaka, K. and Iizuka, R. (1984) A preliminary study of free amino acids in the postmortem temporal cortex from Alzheimer-type dementia patients. *Neurobiol. Aging*, 5: 319–321.

Asano, T., Gotoh, O., Koide, T. and Takamyra, K. (1985) Ischemic brain edema following occlusion of the middle cerebral artery in the rat. II. Alteration of the eicosanoid synthesis profile of brain microvessels. *Stroke*, 16: 110–113.

Ball, M. J., Hachinsky, V., Fox, A., Kirshen, A. J., Fisman, M., Blume, W., Kral, V. A. and Fox, H. (1985) A new definition of Alzheimer's disease: a hippocampal dementia. *The Lancet*, i: 14–16.

Bazan, N., Politi, E. and Rodriguez de Turco, E. (1984) Endogenous pools of arachidonic acid — enriched membrane lipids in cryogenic brain edema. In K. G. Go and A. Baethman (Eds.), *Recent Progress in the Study and Therapy of Brain Edema*, Plenum, New York, pp. 203–212.

Ben-Ari, Y. (1985) Limbic seizure and brain damage produced by kainic acid: mechanisms and relevance to human temporal lobe epilepsy. *Neuroscience*, 14: 375–403.

Benveniste, H., Drejer, J., Schoesbou, A. and Diemer, N. H. (1984) Elevation of the extracellular concentrations of glutamate and aspartate in rat hippocampus during transient cerebral ischemia monitored by intracerebral microdialysis. *J. Neurochem.*, 43: 1369–1371.

Berger, J. R., Busto, R. and Ginsberg, M. D. (1984) Verapamil: failure of metabolic amelioration following global forebrain ischemia in the rat. *Stroke*, 15: 1029–1032.

Bird, E. D. (1976) Biochemical studies on gamma-aminobutyric acid metabolism in Huntington's chorea. In H. F. Bradford and C. D. Marsden (Eds.), *Biochemistry and Neurology*, Academic Press, London, pp. 83–90.

Boller, F., Boller, M., Denes, G., Timberlake, W. M., Zieper, I. and Albert, M. (1973) Familial pilalalia. *Neurology*, 23: 1117–1125.

Brannan, T. S., Burger, A. A. and Chaudhary, M. Y. (1980) Bilateral basal ganglia calcifications visualized on CT scan. *J. Neurol. Neurosurg. Psychiat.*, 43: 403–406.

Chan, P. H., Schmidley, J. W., Fishman, R. A. and Longar, S. M. (1984) Brain injury, edema, and vascular permeability changes induced by oxygen-derived free radicals. *Neurology*, 34, 315–320.

Choki, J., Greenberg, J., Sclarsky, D. and Reivick, M. (1984) Correlation between brain surface potassium and glucose utilization after bilateral cerebral ischemia in the gerbil. *Stroke*, 15: 851–857.

Coyle, J. T., Price, D. L. and Delong, M. R. (1983) Alzheimer's disease: a disorder of cortical cholinergic innervation. *Science*, 219: 1184–1190.

Cross, A. J., Crow, T. J., Ferrier, I. N., Johnson, J. A., Bloom, S. R. and Corsellis, J. A. N. (1984a) Serotonin receptor changes in dementia of Alzheimer type. *J. Neurochem.*, 43: 1574–1581.

Cross, A. J., Crow, T. J., Johnson, J. A., Perry, E. K., Perry, R. H., Blessed, G. and Tomlinson, B. E. (1984b) Studies on neurotransmitter receptor systems in neocortex and hippocampus in senile dementia of Alzheimer type. *J. Neurol. Sci.*, 64: 109–117.

De Boni, U. and Crapper McLachlan, D. R. (1985) Controlled induction of paired helical filaments of the Alzheimer type in cultured human neurons, by glutamate and aspartate. *J. Neurol. Sci.*, 68: 105–118.

Dienel, G. A. (1984) Regional accumulation of calcium in post ischemic rat brain. *J. Neurochem.*, 43: 913–925.

Drejer, J., Benveniste, H., Diemer, N. H. and Schoesbou, A. (1985) On the cellular origin of ischemia-induced glutamate release from brain tissue in vivo and in vitro. *J. Neurochem.*, 45, 145–151.

Dubinsky, B., Sierchio, J. N., Temple, D. E. and Ritchie, D. M. (1984) Flunarizine and verapamil: effects on central nervous system and peripheral consequences of cytotoxic hypoxia in rats. *Life Sci.*, 34: 1299–1306.

Farber, J. L. (1981) The role of calcium in cell death. *Life Sci.*, 29: 1289–1295.

Fonnum, F. (1984) Glutamate: a neurotransmitter in mammalian brain. *J. Neurochem.*, 42: 1–11.

Foster, A. C., Collins, J. F. and Schwarcz, R. (1983) On the excitotoxic properties of quinolinic acid, 2,3-piperidine dicarboxylic acids and structurally related compounds. *Neuropharmacol.*, 22: 1331–1342.

Garcia, J. H. (1984) Experimental ischemic stroke: a review. *Stroke*, 15: 5–14.

Garruto, R. M., Fukatsu, R., Yanagihara, R., Gajdusek, D. C., Hook, G. and Fiori, C. E. (1984) Imaging of calcium and aluminium in neurofibrillary tangle-bearing neurons in parkinsonism-dementia of Guam. *Proc. Natl. Acad. Sci. USA*, 81: 1875–1897.

Gazendam, J., Houthoff, H. J., Huitema, S. and Go, K. G. (1984) Cerebral edema formation and blood brain barrier impairment by intraventricular collagenase infusion. In K. G. Go and A. Baethman (Eds.), *Recent Progress in the Study and Therapy of Brain Edema*, Plenum, New York, pp. 159–174.

Gelmers, H. J. (1984) The effects of nimodipine on the clinical course of patients with acute ischemia stroke. *Acta Neurol. Scand.*, 69: 232–269.

Gotoh, O., Asama, T., Koide, T. and Takakura, K. (1985) Ischemic brain edema following ecclusion of the middle cerebral artery in the rat. I: The time courses of the brain water, sodium and potassium contents and blood–brain barrier permeability to ^{125}I-albumen. *Stroke*, 16: 101–109.

Gramsbergen, J. B. P., Veenma-Van der Duin, L., Venema, K. and Korf, J. (1985a) Cationshifts and aminoacids in Alzheimer's disease. In *Proceedings of the IVth World Congress on Biological Psychiatry, September 8–13, 1985. Philadelphia*, abstract, 152.1.

Gramsbergen, J. B. P., Veenma-Van der Duin, L. and Korf, J. (1986) Cerebral cationshifts and amino acids in Huntington's disease. *Arch. Neurol.*, in press.

Greenamyre, J. T., Penney, J. B., Young, A. B., D'Amato, C. J., Hicks S. P. and Shoulson, I. (1985) Alterations in L-glutamate binding in Alzheimer's and Huntington's disease. *Science*, 227: 1496–1499.

Gusella, J. F., Wexler, N. S., Conneally, P. M., Naylor, S. L., Anderson, M. A., Tanzi, R. E., Watkins, P. C., Ottina, K., Wallace, M. R., Sakaguchi, A. Y., Young, A. B., Shoulson, I., Bonilla, E. and Martin, J. B. (1983) A polymorphic DNA marker genetically linked to Huntington's disease. *Nature*, 306: 234–238.

Hagberg, H., Lehmann, A. and Hamberger, A. (1984) Inhibition of verapamil of ischemic Ca^{2+} uptake in rabbit hippocampus. *J. Cereb. Blood Flow Metab.*, 4: 297–300.

Hansen, A. J. (1978) The extracellular potassium concentration in brain cortex following ischemia in hypo- and hyperglycemic rats. *Acta Physiol. Scand.*, 102: 324–329.

Hansen, A. J. (1985) Effect of anoxia on ion distribution in the brain. *Physiol. Rev.*, 65: 101–148.

Hansen, A. J. and Zeuthen, T. (1981) Extracellular ion concentrations during spreading depression and ischemia in the rat brain cortex. *Acta. Physiol. Scand.*, 113: 437–445.

Hilal, S. K., Maudsley, A. A., Ra, J. B., Simon, H. E., Roschmann, P., Wittekoek, S., Cho, Z. H. and Mun, S. K. (1985) In vivo NMR imaging of sodium -23 in the human head. *J. Comp. Ass. Tomogr.*, 9: 1–7.

Hyman, B. T., Van Hoesen, G. W., Damasio, A. R. and Barnes, C. C. (1984) Alzheimer's disease: cell specific pathology isolates the hippocampal formation. *Science*, 225: 1168–1170.

Imaizumi, S., Kayama, T. and Suzuki, J. (1984) Chemiluminescence in hypoxic brain — the first report. *Stroke*, 15: 1061–1065.

Ito, U., Go, K. G., Walker, J. T., Spatz, M. and Klatzo, I. (1976) Experimental cerebral ischemia in mongolian gerbils III. Behavior of the blood brain barrier. *Acta Neuropathol.*, 34: 1–6.

Jancsó G., Karcsú, S., Király, E., Szebeni, A., Tóth, L., Bácsy, E., Joó, F. and Párducz, A. (1984) Neurotoxin induced nerve cell degeneration: possible involvement of calcium. *Brain Res.*, 295: 211–216.

Kirino, T., Tamura, A. and Sano, K. (1984) Delayed neuronal death in the rat hippocampus following transient forebrain ischemia. *Acta Neuropathol.*, 64: 139–147.

Kirsch, J. R. and D'Alecy, L. G. (1979) Effect of altered availability of energy-yielding substrates upon survival from hypoxia in mice. *Stroke*, 10: 288–291.

Korf, J. and Postema, F. (1984) Regional calcium accumulation and cationshifts in rat brain by kainate. *J. Neurochem.*, 43: 1052–1060.

Korf, J., Zoethout, F. A. and Postema, F. (1983) Regional calcium levels in the rat and mouse brain: automated fluorimetric assay and effects of centrally acting drugs. *Psychopharmacology*, 81: 275–280.

Lehmann, J., Ferkany, J. W., Schaeffer, P. and Coyle, J. T. (1985) Dissociation between the excitatory and 'excitotoxic' effects of quinolinic acid analogues on the striatal cholinergic interneuron. *J. Pharmacol. Exp. Ther.*, 232: 873–882.

Leslie, S. W., Chandler, L. J., Barr, E. M. and Farrar, R. P. (1985) Reduced calcium uptake by rat brain mitochondria and synaptosomes in response to aging. *Brain Res.*, 329: 177–183.

Levine, S. (1960) Anoxic-ischemic encephalopathy in rats. *Am. J. Pathol.*, 36: 1–17.

Löwenthal, A. and Bruyn, G. W. (1968) Calcifications of the striopallidodentate system. In P. J. Vinken and G. W. Bruyn (Eds.), *Handbook of Clinical Neurology, Vol. 6*, North-Holland Publ. Co., Amsterdam, pp. 703–723.

Maier-Hauff, K., Lange, M., Schûrer, L., Guggenbichler, Ch., Vogt, W., Jacob, K. and Beathman, A. (1984) Glutamate and free fatty acid concentrations in extracellular vasogenic edema fluid. In K. G. Go and A. Beathman (Eds.), *Recent Progress in the Study and Therapy of Brain Edema*, Plenum, New York, pp. 183–192.

McBean, G. J. and Roberts, P. J. (1985) Neurotoxicity in L-glutamate and DL-threo-3-hydroxyaspartate in the rat striatum. *J. Neurochem.*, 44: 247–254.

Meldrum, B. S., Griffith, T. and Evans, M. (1982) Hypoxia and neural hyperactivity: a clue to mechanisms of brain protection. In A. Wauquier, M. Borgers and W. K. Amery (Eds.), *Protection of Tissues*, Elsevier, Amsterdam, pp. 275–286.

Morrison, J. H., Rogers, J., Scherr, S., Benoit, R. and Bloom, F. (1985) Somatostatin immunoreactivity in neuritic plaques of Alzheimer's patients. *Nature*, 314: 90–92.

Moskowitz, M. A., Kiwak, K. J., Hekimian, K. and Levine, L. (1984) Synthesis of compounds with properties of leukotrienes C_4 and D_4 in gerbil brains after ischemia and reperfusion. *Science*, 224: 886–889.

Murphy, M. J. (1979) Clinical correlations of CT-scans detected calcifications of the basal ganglia. *Am. J. Neurol.*, 6: 507–511.

Myles, W. S. (1976) Survival of fasted rats exposed to altitude. *Can. J. Physiol. Pharmacol.*, 54: 883–886.

Narahashi, T. (1974) Chemicals as tools in the study of excitable membranes. *Physiol. Rev.*, 54: 813–899.

Notman, H., Whitney, R., Jhamandas, K. (1984) Kainic acid evoked release of D-[^{3}H]aspartate from rat striatum in vitro: characterization and pharmacological modulation. *Can. J. Physiol. Pharmacol.*, 62: 1070–1077.

Olney, J. W., Price, M. T., Samson, L., Labruyere, J. (1984) The ionic basis of excitotoxine-induced neuronal necrosis. *Neurosci. Abstracts*, 10, pp. 24, 11.8.

Paljärvi, L. (1984) Brain lactic acidosis and ischemic cell damage: a topographic study with high-resolution light microscopy of early recovery in a rat model of severe incomplete ischemia. *Acta Neuropathol. (Berl.)*, 64: 89–98.

Pastuszko, A., Wilson, D. F. and Erecińska, M. (1984) Effects of kainic acid in rat brain synaptosomes: the involvement of calcium. *J. Neurochem.*, 43: 747–754.

Pearce, B. R., Palmer, A. M., Bowen, D. M., Wilcock, G. K., Esiri, M. M. and Davison, A. (1984) Neurotransmitter dysfunction and atrophy of the caudate nucleus in Alzheimer's disease. *Neurochem. Pathol.*, 2: 221–232.

Pelligrino, D., Almquist, L.-O. and Siesjö, B. K. (1981) Effects of insuline-induced hypoglycemia on intracellular pH and impedance in the cerebral cortex of the rat. *Brain Res.*, 221: 129–147.

Perry, T. L., Hansen, S. and Kloster, M. (1973) Huntington's chorea: a deficiency of gamma-aminobutyric acid in brain. *New Engl. J. Med.*, 288: 337–342.

Petito, C. K. and Pulsinelli, W. A. (1984) Sequential development of reversible and irreversible neuronal damage following cerebral ischemia. *J. Neuropathol. Exp. Neurol.*, 43: 141–153.

Plaitakis, A., Berl, S. and Yahr, M. D. (1982) Abnormal glutamate metabolism in an adult-onset degenerative neurological disorder. *Science*, 216: 193–196.

Plaitakis, A., Berl, S. and Yahr, M. D. (1984) Neurological disorders associated with deficiency of glutamate dehydrogenase. *Ann. Neurol.*, 15: 144–153.

Prenen, G. H. M., Zuiderveen, F., Postema, F., Korf, J. and Go, K. G. (1985) Regional hypoxic ischemic brain damage in the conscious rat: quantification by cationshifts and protection by fasting. *Proceedings of the 26th Dutch Federation Meeting*, Amsterdam, Abstract 268.

Pulsinelli, W. A. and Brierley, J. B. (1979) A new model of bilateral hemispheric ischemia in the anaesthetized rat. *Stroke*, 10: 267–272.

Pumain, R. and Heinemann, U. (1985) Stimulus- and amino-acid-induced calcium and potassium changes in rat neocortex. *J. Neurophysiol.*, 53: 1–16.

Roberts, G. W., Crow, T. J. and Polak, J. M. (1985) Location of neuronal tangles in somatostatin neurons in Alzheimer's disease. *Nature*, 314, 92–94.

Roberts, P. J., McBean, G. J., Sharif, N. A., Thomas, E. M. (1982) Striatal glutamergic functions: modifications following specific lesions. *Brain Res.*, 235: 83–91.

Rosner, M. J. and Becker, D. P. (1984) Experimental brain injury: successful therapy with the weak base, tromethamine. *J. Neurosurg.*, 60: 961–971.

Roth, G. S., Ingram, D. K. and Joseph, J. A. (1984) Delayed loss of striatal dopamine receptors during aging of dietarily restricted rats. *Brain Res.*, 300: 27–82.

Rothman, S. M. (1984) Synaptic release of excitatory amino-acid neurotransmitter mediates anoxic neuronal death. *J. Neurosci.*, 4: 1884–1891.

Rothman, S. M. (1985) The neurotoxicity of excitatory amino acids is produced by passive chloride influx. *J. Neurosci.*, 5: 1483–1490.

Siesjö, B. K. (1981) Cell damage in the brain: a speculative synthesis. *J. Cereb. Blood Flow Metab.*, 1: 155–185.

Sihra, T. S., Scott, I. G. and Nicholls, D. G. (1984) Ionophore A23187, verapamil, protonophores and veratratridine influence the release of gamma-aminobutyric acid from synaptosomes by modulation of the plasma membrane potential rather than the cytosolic calcium. *J. Neurochem.*, 43: 1624–1630.

Simon, R. P., Griffiths, T., Evans, M. C., Swan, J. H. and Meldrum, B. S. (1984a) Calcium overload in selectively vulnerable neurons of the hippocampus during and after ischemia: an electron microscopy study in the rat. *J. Cereb. Blood Flow Metab.*, 4: 350–361.

Simon, R. P., Swan, J. H., Griffiths, T. and Meldrum, B. S. (1984b) Blockade of *N*-methyl-D-aspartate receptors may protect against ischemic damage in the brain. *Science*, 226: 850–852.

Smits, M. G., Gabreëls, F. J. M., Thijssen, H. O. M., 'tLam, R. L., Notermans, S. L. H., Ter Haar, B. G. A. and Prick, J. J. (1983) Progressive idiopathic strio-pallidodentate calcinosis (Fahr's disease) with autosomal recessive inheritance. *Eur. Neurol.*, 22: 58–64.

Spokes, E. G. S., Garnett, N. J., Rossor, M. N. and Iversen, L. L. (1980) Distribution of GABA in post-mortem brain tissue from control, psychotic and Huntington's chorea subjects. *J. Neurol. Sci.*, 48: 303–313.

Steen, P. A., Newberg, L. A., Milde, J. H. and Michenfelder, J. D. (1983) Nimodipine improves cerebral blood flow and neurological recovery after complete cerebral ischaemia in the dog. *J. Cereb. Blood Flow Metab.*, 3: 38–43.

Steinberg, R., Scarna, H., Keller, A. and Pujol, J. F. (1983) Release of neuron specific enolase (NSE) in cerebrospinal fluid following experimental lesions of the rat brain. *Neurochem Int.*, 5: 145–151.

Steinberg, R., Gueniau, C., Scarna, H., Keller, A., Worcel, M. and Pujol, J. F. (1984) Experimental brain ischemia: neuron-specific enolase level in cerebrospinal fluid as an index of neuronal damage. *J. Neurochem.*, 43: 19–24.

Storm-Mathisen, J. (1977) Localization of transmitter candidates in the brain: the hippocampal formation as a model. *Prog. Neurobiol.*, 8: 119–181.

Tarbit, I., Perry, E. K., Perry, R. H., Blessed, G. and Tomlinson, B. E. (1980) Hippocampal free aminoacids in Alzheimer's disease. *J. Neurochem.*, 35: 1246–1249.

Trump, B. F., Berczensky, I. K., Laiho, K. U., Osornio, A. R., Mergner, W. J. and Smith, M. W. (1980) The role of calcium in cell injury. A review. *Scanning Electron Microscopy, Vol. II*: pp. 437–462.

Ulrich, J. (1985) Alzheimer changes in nondementia patients younger than sixty-five: possible early stages of Alzheimer's disease and senile dementia of Alzheimer's type. *Ann. Neurol.*, 17: 273–277.

Van Reempts, J. (1984) The hypoxic brain: histological and ultra structural aspects. *Behav. Brain Res.*, 14: 94–108.

Van Reempts, J., Borgers, M., Van Dael, L., Van Eijndhoven, J. and Van der Ven, M. (1983) Protection with flunarizine against hypoxic ischaemic damage of the rat cerebral cortex. A quantitative morphologic assessment. *Arch. Int. Pharmacodyn. Ther.*, 262: 76–88.

Venema, K., Leever, W., Bakker, O., Haayer, G. and Korf, J. (1983) Automated precolumn derivatization device to determine neurotransmitter and other aminoacids by reversed-phase high performance liquid chromatography. *J. Chromatogr.*, 260: 371–376.

Watson, B. D., Busto, R., Goldberg, W. J., Santiso, M., Yoshida, S. and Ginsberg, M. D. (1984) Lipid peroxidation *in vivo* induced by reversible global ischemia in rat brain. *J. Neurochem.*, 42: 268–274.

Welsh, F. A. (1984) Regional evaluation of ischemic metabolic alterations. *J. Cereb. Blood Flow Metab.*, 4: 309–316.

Welsh, F. A., Ginsberg, M. D., Rieder, W. and Budd, W. W. (1980) Deleterious effect of glucose pretreatment on recovery from diffuse cerebral ischemia in the cat. II. Regional metabolite levels. *Stroke*, 11: 355–363.

Went, L. N., Vegter-Van der Vlis, M. and Bruyn, G. W. (1984) Parenteral transmission in Huntington's disease. *The Lancet*, i: 1100–1102.

Whittingham, T. S., Lust, W. D., Christatkis, A. and Passonneau, J. V. (1984) Metabolic stability of hippocampal slice preparations during prolonged incubation. *J. Neurochem.*, 43: 689–696.

Wieloch, T., Harris, R. J., Symon, L. and Siesjö, B. K. (1984) Influence of severe hypoglycemia on brain extracellular calcium and potassium activities, energy and phospholipid metabolism. *J. Neurochem.*, 43: 160–168.

Yoshida, S., Busto, R., Watson, B. D., Santiso, M. and Goldberg, M. D. (1985) Postischemic cerebral lipid peroxidation in vitro: modification by dietary vitamine E. *J. Neurochem.*, 44: 1593–1601.

Zimmer, R., Teelken, A. W., Trieling, W. B., Weber, W., Weihmayr, T. and Lauter, H. (1984) Gamma-aminobutyric acid and homovanillic acid concentration in CSF of patients with senile dementia of Alzheimer's type. *Arch. Neurol.*, 41: 602–604.

Zimmerman, U.-J. P. and Schlaepfer, W. W. (1984) Calcium-activated neutral protease (CANP) in brain and other tissues. *Prog. Neurobiol.*, 23: 63–78.

Discussion

J. DE GRAAF: When studying cation shifts, isn't it methodologically peculiar to kill the animal with an excessive amount of cation, i.e. Mg^{2+}?

ANSWER: By giving excess of $MgCl_2$ a rapid cardiac arrest is taking place without directly influencing cerebral functions; since $MgCl_2$ does not enter the brain, as far as we have checked with atomic absorption photometry. Accordingly, any drug effects on potential deflections are not contaminated by central action of the drug used to kill the experimented animal.

E. MENA: At least three different types of excitatory amino acid receptor antagonists cause neurodegeneration. Which amino acid receptor do you think is involved in Alzheimer disease (AD)?

ANSWER: At present no conclusive evidence is available. However, in post mortem material of Alzheimer brains the glutamate binding has been reported to be decreased (Greenamyre et al., 1985) in the cerebral cortex or increased (Pearce et al., 1984) in the caudate nucleus. In both cases the nature of the receptor dysfunction has not been determined.

K. IQBAL: Have you measured glutamine and glutamate synthetase levels in the hippocampus of AD patients?

ANSWER: The level of glutaminate was not significantly altered in the cerebral cortex or hippocampus. We have not measured the enzyme.

D. N. VELIS: How does one explain the (relative) survival value of hypoglycemia in the 4-vessel occlusion model in view of your results which show a (relative) survival value of hyperglycemia?

ANSWER: In our preparation using cardiac arrest we have shown that glucose loading attenuates the occurrence of the deflection of the brain potentials. However, in the 4-vessel occlusion model glucose loading is more toxic, because not only energy metabolism is important but also the formation of lactic acid, thus producing acidosis. In the long run, acidosis may accelerate cell death. Accordingly, hypoglycemia may thus prevent acidosis, and the energy source may in fact be compensated by the utilization of keton bodies.

COMMENT: The changes in cation distribution in Alzheimer's, as reported by you, appear to be similar to those occurring in cells following toxicity and under oxidative stress. It is quite possible that oxidative damage may play an etiological role.

ANSWER: Our data indicate the concomitant action of energy metabolism and excitatory neurotransmitter action. Energy metabolism may lead to free radical formation. In addition, Ca-influx may also enhance indirectly free radicals (Siesjö, 1981).

References

Greenamyre, J. T., Penney, J. B., Young, A. B., D'Amato, C. J., Hicks, S. P. and Shoulson, I. (1985) Alterations in L-glutamate binding in Alzheimer's and Huntington's disease. *Science*, 227: 1496–1499.

Pearce, B. R., Palmer, A. M., Bowen, D. M., Wilcock, G. K., Esiri, M. M. and Davison A. (1984) Neurotransmitter dysfunction and atrophy of the caudate nucleus in Alzheimer's disease. *Neurochem. Pathol.*, 2: 221–232.

Siesjö, B. K. (1981) Cell damage in the brain: a speculative synthesis. *J. Cereb. Blood Flow Metab.*, 1: 155–185.

D. F. Swaab, E. Fliers, M. Mirmiran, W. A. Van Gool and F. Van Haaren (Eds.)
Progress in Brain Research, Vol. 70.
© 1986 Elsevier Science Publishers B.V. (Biomedical Division)

CHAPTER 14

Dendritic proliferation in the aging brain as a compensatory repair mechanism

P. D. Coleman[a] and D. G. Flood[b]

[a]*Department of Neurobiology and Anatomy and* [b]*Department of Neurology, School of Medicine and Dentistry, University of Rochester, 601 Elmwood Avenue, Rochester, NY 14642, USA*

Introduction

The degenerative changes in aging brain are well known, and are the aspects that are usually emphasized. Thus, one frequently hears of loss of neurons and declines in transmitter systems as being hallmarks of the aging brain. The view taken here is that just as the brain has certain repair mechanisms that may compensate for damage at earlier stages of the developmental continuum, these mechanisms may remain intact to some decreased degree during the late stages of life, and may be utilized to at least partially compensate for the damage caused by the degenerative changes of the aged brain. We argue that some of the changes taking place in aging brain may well represent attempts by the brain to utilize its residual plastic capacities to compensate for the degenerative changes that accompany aging. Thus, in younger brains axonal sprouting has been seen as a response to experimentally induced injury; and this response has also been found to occur in the aged brain but at a slower rate (e.g., Hoff et al., 1982). Dendritic proliferation similar (but probably slower) to that seen at earlier ages, has also been described in mature animals as a response to experimentally induced injury (e.g., Sumner and Watson, 1971; Standler and Bernstein, 1982; Caceres and Steward, 1983). Although the nature of the dendritic response to injury has not yet been established in aged brain, dendritic proliferation is

seen in regions of brain that show age-related neuronal loss (e.g., Hinds and McNelly, 1977; Buell and Coleman, 1979, 1981; Flood et al., 1985). It has been suggested that this dendritic proliferation may represent a compensatory response to loss of neighbor neurons (Hinds and McNelly, 1977; Buell and Coleman, 1979). In this chapter we will concentrate on alterations in dendritic extent as potential compensatory responses to age-related neuronal loss in selected brain regions, and the apparent breakdown of this compensatory response in Alzheimer's disease and in extreme old age in some brain regions.

Specificity of changes in aging brain

In considering alterations in dendritic extent as compensatory changes, we also examine changes taking place in the surrounding microenvironment of the dendritic trees being considered. In doing this we capitalize on the 'experiments of nature' that present us with a diversity of specific age-related changes in the brain. Diversity is, indeed, the hallmark of the aging central nervous system. The nature of this diversity is such that some brain regions lose neurons with aging (e.g., Brody, 1976; Vijayashankar and Brody, 1979) while other regions do not (e.g., Konigsmark and Murphy, 1970; Monagle and Brody, 1974; Vijayashankar and Brody, 1977). In addition to this regional diversity, regions in which age-related neuronal loss has been demonstrated in one species fail to show such loss in other species. For example, many studies of human cerebral cortex have demonstrated age-related decreases in neuronal density which are interpreted as neuronal loss (e.g., Brody, 1955; Henderson et al., 1980; Anderson et al., 1983; Curcio et al., 1982 for review). On the other hand, recent studies of neuron numbers in aging rodent cortex have failed to find decreased neuron numbers in visual cortex of old F344 rat (Peters et al., 1983) and somatosensory cortex of old C57B1/6 mouse (Curcio and Coleman, 1982). Thus, neuronal loss shows both a region and species specificity. An age specificity has also been demonstrated. For example, the human locus ceruleus does not start to lose neurons until the 7th decade of life (Vijayashankar and Brody, 1979), while the cerebral cortex (Brody, 1955) and substantia nigra (McGeer et al., 1977) show decreased neuronal density by the 3rd decade. Such specificity of neuronal loss has implications for specificity of changes in afferent supply to target areas.

General rationale

Our interest in the aging brain has focused on changes in dendritic extent for two major reasons. (1) Depending on cell type, dendrites may constitute as much as 95% of the receptive surface that a neuron can offer for contact with other neurons (e.g., Schade and Baxter, 1960). Dendrites are, therefore, important determiners of the ability of neurons to operate in a network to receive, process and transmit information. (2) In addition, dendrites are among the more plastic morphological elements in the brain. They respond to alterations in their microenvironment long before the cell body shows any clearly detectable change at the light microscopic level. For example, manipulations which produce no change in neuron numbers such as partial denervation (e.g., Jones and Thomas, 1962), or even reduced (e.g., Coleman and Riesen, 1968) or increased (e.g., Rutledge et al., 1974) afferent activity, have all been shown to affect dendritic extent significantly.

In our studies of dendrites as a function of age the 'experiments of nature' on which we have capitalized have been those which involve change, or lack of change, in certain other neuronal elements in the immediately surrounding microenvironment — the afferent axonal supply and the neighboring cell bodies. Our strategy has been to examine relationships among dendritic extent, afferent axons and closely neighboring neurons with the aim of determining whether there are interactions among these components in the aging brain that are suggestive of repair mechanisms or developmental changes seen during younger ages.

Compensatory dendritic proliferation in human parahippocampal gyrus in normal aging and failure in Alzheimer's disease

Our initial studies of dendritic extent in aging brain focused on the parahippocampal gyrus of the human cerebral cortex (Buell and Coleman, 1979). This region is of particular interest because of its close association with the hippocampal region. In these studies a semi-automated computer video microscope system (Coleman et al., 1977) was used to quantify Golgi-Cox stained dendritic trees on coded slides of layer II pyramidal neurons from samples obtained at autopsy. The average delay between death and fixation of tissue was 12.67 h. The use of the Golgi-Cox method, as opposed to certain rapid Golgi methods, is important since it has been shown that a commonly used rapid Golgi method is particularly sensitive to post-mortem delay to fixation of human tissue. When post-mortem delay exceeds 6 h the rapid Golgi method gives an appearance of grossly atrophied dendritic trees, while the Golgi-Cox method applied to an immediately adjacent block of tissue gives an appearance of extensive, apparently flourishing, dendritic trees (Buell, 1982).

These studies of parahippocampal gyrus indicated that in normal aging, dendritic extent of the average layer II pyramidal neuron increased as age increased. In Alzheimer's disease (AD) the age-related increase in dendritic extent was not seen

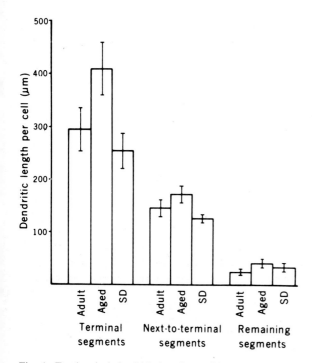

Fig. 1. Total apical dendritic length per. layer II pyramidal neuron from human parahippocampal gyrus in adult (average age 51.2 years), aged (79.6 years) and AD (76.0 years). Centripetal ordering is presented since the terminal and next-to-terminal segments constitute over 90% of the dendritic tree and are the portion of the dendritic tree most sensitive to change in our data. Error bars represent standard error of the mean with n equal to 5, the number of cases in each group. Differences among groups significant at $p < 0.05$ (Kruskal-Wallis one way ANOVA). It is noteworthy that changes in basal dendritic trees of these same neurons were far less pronounced than those seen in apical trees, suggesting that local factors may play an important role in dendritic responses to aging. (From Buell and Coleman, 1979).

(Fig. 1). In fact, the AD group had less extensive dendrites than any group examined. Whether this represents a failure of age-related dendritic proliferation or an actual dendritic regression is not yet clear. However, it is important to note that there was overlap of measures of dendritic extent per cell between some of the severely demented AD cases and the cases that were active and functionally normal up to their final illness. More recent data from our laboratories indicate that this overlap is also seen in other brain regions. This

suggests that the lesser average dendritic extent found in AD is not central to the devastating functional losses of AD, but rather that these losses must be viewed in light of the spectrum of changes in the AD brain in cell numbers, neurotransmitter systems and other parameters.

It should be emphasized that neurons with obviously regressed dendritic trees were seen in all the samples examined. However, these regressing neurons were not sufficiently numerous to negate the contribution to averaged measures made by proliferating neurons. We assume that in human cerebral cortex, neurons with grossly regressing dendrites are often (but perhaps not always — see below) in the process of dying. Since the number of neurons with obviously regressing dendrites apparently did not vary as a function of age, we assume that this sub-population is constantly gaining recruits from the population of surviving, flourishing neurons with proliferating dendritic trees.

In view of the apparently general neuronal fallout found in cerebral cortex of aging human (see Hanley, 1974; Brody, 1976; Curcio et al., 1982 for review) we suggested that the dendritic proliferation found in parahippocampal gyrus was a compensatory response of surviving neurons to the death of their close neighbors (Buell and Coleman, 1979). A similar suggestion has also been made by Hinds and McNelly (1977) with regard to the increased volume fraction of mitral cell dendrites found in the olfactory bulb of aging Sprague-Dawley rats.

Absence of compensatory dendritic proliferation in posteromedial barrel subfield cortex of normally aging mouse

If the hypothesis of dendritic proliferation as a compensatory response to death of neighboring neurons is correct, there should be no dendritic proliferation in brain regions that do not lose neurons with age. The mouse posteromedial barrel subfield (PMBSF) presents an opportune model cortical region that contains a limited number of neurons in well-defined morphological subunits

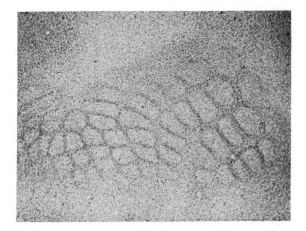

Fig. 2. Barrels in layer IV of posteromedial barrel subfield (PMBSF) of somatosensory cortex of C57Bl/6 mouse. Section was cut tangential to the cortical surface. Nissl stain. There are usually about 35 of the large PMBSF barrels in each hemisphere. The barrels appear in relatively constant configuration from animal to animal. One large barrel of the PMBSF measures approximately 200×300 μm in cross section. Each barrel of the PMBSF is the cortical representation of one large mystacial vibrassa on the opposite side of the animal's snout.

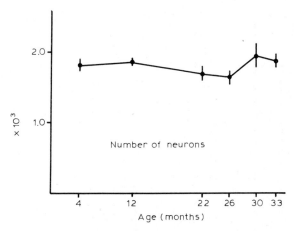

Fig. 3. Neuron numbers from 4 to 33 months of age in barrel C3 of C57Bl/6NNIA mouse PMBSF of somatosensory cortex. Number determined from neuronal density × cross-sectional area × height of layer IV. Error bars are ± 1 SE of the mean. There is no statistically significant age-related change in neuron number. ANOVA: $F(5,19) = 1.12$; $p > 0.05$ (From Curcio and Coleman, 1982).

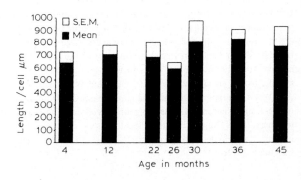

Fig. 4. Total dendritic length per cell of layer IV stellate neurons in PMBSF of C57Bl/6 mouse from 4 to 45 months. There is no statistically significant age-related change in dendritic length. ANOVA: $F(6,14) = 0.83$; $p > 0.05$.

with known functional significance (Fig. 2). It is a cortical region in which it has been possible to estimate total neuron numbers as a function of age. These data (Fig. 3) showed no age-related change in neuron numbers in an identified barrel (C3) of the PMBSF of the C57Bl/6NNIA mouse to 33 months of age (Curcio and Coleman, 1982). Quantitative Golgi-Cox study of single neurons in the PMBSF (Fig. 4) shows no age-related proliferation of dendritic extent (Coleman et al., 1986). These data lead to the corollary hypothesis: in the absence of neuronal loss there will be no significant dendritic proliferation in aged brain.

A large number of questions remain, among them: by what mechanism may neuronal loss induce or allow dendritic proliferation of closely neighboring, surviving neurons? Is this dendritic proliferation sufficient to compensate fully for the loss of dendritic material consequent to death of neighboring neurons? In those regions that show an age-related neuronal loss does this compensatory response continue with increasing age as more

and more neurons are lost, or does the compensatory system eventually collapse, as had been suggested by data from the Sprague-Dawley rat olfactory bulb (Hinds and McNelly, 1977)(Fig. 5)? How can these findings of dendritic proliferation be integrated with other data demonstrating age-related dendritic regression?

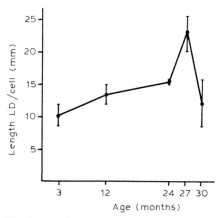

Fig. 5. Age-related changes in the length of large dendrites per mitral cell in olfactory bulb of Sprague-Dawley rat. $F(4,6)=4.82$, $p<0.05$. Error bars are ± 1 SE of the mean. (From Hinds and McNelly, 1977)

Hypothesized mechanisms

The mechanism(s) by which neuronal loss may induce (or permit) dendritic proliferation in surviving neighbors is not known. However, some speculations may be suggested. Death of some of the neurons in a population may present the dendrites of the surviving neurons with reduced competition for afferent supply, which then allows these surviving dendrites to proliferate. This process, illustrated in Fig. 6A, requires that the afferent supply remain sufficiently intact that there are indeed presynaptic elements to be offered for contact with dendrites of the surviving neurons. Another, not mutually exclusive, possibility is that death of neurons may bring about the release of a trophic factor which induces the proliferation of dendrites (Fig. 6B). It is assumed that neuron death leads to an astrocytic reaction in which the astrocytes elaborate a 'growth' factor. It is further assumed that this factor then percolates for some unknown distance through the brain extracellular space to stimulate proliferation of the dendrites of neighboring neurons. At this time it appears possible that this astrocyte-derived factor may be similar to that described by Müller and Seifert (1982), although a variety of other possible factors

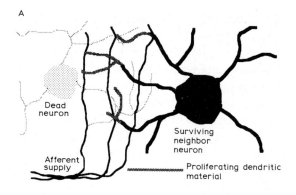

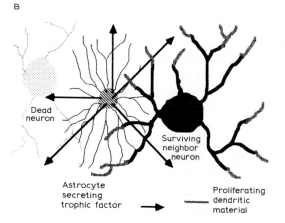

Fig. 6. (A and B). (A) Drawing to represent reduced competition for afferent supply consequent to death of a neuron which then leads to dendritic proliferation by a surviving neighbor neuron. This highly simplified representation ignores complexities of the differential distribution of afferent supply from several sources to different regions of the dendritic tree, as well as the spatial distribution of dying neurons. (B) Representation of secretion of a dendrite trophic or 'growth' factor stimulated by death of an adjacent neuron. Note that in both models dendritic proliferation is assumed to take place at terminal segments of the dendritic tree, both by lengthening and by branching (Buell and Coleman, 1981). Although the data indicate this to be true for neocortical neurons it may not apply to hippocampal neurons (e.g., Duffy and Rakic, 1983).

may also be suggested (e.g., Thoenen and Edgar, 1985).

Is dendritic proliferation in surviving neurons sufficient to compensate for loss of dendritic material?

There are a number of ways in which one may approach the question of the extent to which age-related dendritic proliferation in surviving neurons may compensate for the loss of dendritic material caused by death of neighbor neurons. We have combined data on neuron loss in human dentate gyrus granule cells with our data on age-related changes in dendritic extent of these neurons to arrive at an order of magnitude estimate. Given a neuron *density* loss of 15% of granule cells between 40 and 80 years (Mouritzen Dam, 1979) we can estimate an annual neuronal loss of 0.38%. If we begin at age 52 with a population of 1 000 granule cells (since the total number of granule cells has not been estimated), about four granule cells would die between 52 and 53 years of age. Each of these lost granule cells would have had a total dendritic extent of 784 μm (the average for our middle-aged subjects — see below) resulting in a loss of 3 136 μm in our hypothetical population. Since our data show an increase in *average* dendritic extent from 784 μm to 1 048 μm between 52 and 73 years (see below) we can estimate a growth rate of 12.6 μm per year per cell. Thus the dendritic extent of the remaining 996 neurons would increase by 12 550 μm between ages 52 and 53. The estimated extent of newly formed dendritic material is four times the estimated dendritic extent lost by the death of neurons. It must be cautioned that neuronal *density* changes used here will not be precisely related to changes in absolute numbers of neurons if there are age-related volumetric changes in the human dentate gyrus. In addition, this calculation assumes linear age-related change of the parameters estimated. Also, it only relates to linear extent of dendrites, and is lacking information on thickness of dendrites. Therefore, extent of dendritic surface remains unknown. Furthermore, such an estimate gives no indication of the extent to which newly formed dendritic material in old brains may be making contact with the surrounding neuropil, or what the behavioral significance of this new dendritic material may be. One study in human cerebral cortex suggests no major age-related change in synapse density (Cragg, 1975). However, other studies have found an age-related reduction in synapse density in middle frontal cortex (Huttenlocher, 1979) and in superior frontal cortex but not in mid-temporal cortex (Gibson, 1983).

Collapse of compensatory dendritic proliferation in dentate gyrus of the oldest old

An answer to the question of whether the presumed compensatory dendritic proliferation eventually collapses in the human brain, as had been demonstrated in the rat olfactory bulb (Hinds and McNelly, 1977), is suggested by quantitative studies of dendrites of dentate gyrus granule cells in the aging human brain. In this study (Flood et al., 1985) cases were divided into three groups: 7 middle-aged (MA — average age 52.3 years), 5 old age (OA — average 73.4 years) and 5 very old adults (VOA — average 90.2 years). Tissues were processed using the Golgi-Cox method (Van der Loos, 1956), sections cut at 200 μm, and slides were coded. Fifteen neurons were drawn from each subject using a drawing tube and the dendritic trees were quantified with an Apple II + computer and graphics tablet. Neurons were chosen as usual in our studies of dendrites: (1) soma was in the middle third of the section thickness, (2) dendrites were not obscured by other elements, and (3) no dendrites trailed off as a series of dots. All neurons that satisfied these criteria were noted and numbered, and from this population a random sample of 15 neurons was selected for analysis on the basis of a table of random numbers. Data were summed for the 15 cells within each case to give an average granule cell per case. Results showed an apparent dendritic proliferation between middle age and old age, followed by dendritic regression between old age and very old age (Fig. 7). In very old age both the average and the variance of dendritic tree measures were the smallest of the three age groups. Total dendritic length (TDL) per cell in the oldest old was 57% of TDL in old age and 77% of TDL in middle age. The combination of decrease in both mean and variance of TDL in the VOA cases is an indication of uniform dendritic regression in the oldest old. Dendritic trees in the oldest old, even

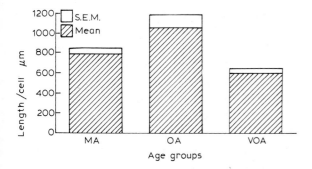

Fig. 7. Total dendritic length per human dentate gyrus granule cell. MA = 7 cases, mean age 52.3 years; OA = 5 cases, mean age 73.4 years; VOA = 5 cases, mean age 90.2 years. There are statistically significant age-related changes. ANOVA: $F(2,14) = 7.32$; $p < 0.01$.

though regressed, are still largely intact and without signs of massive degeneration. Thus, in the dentate gyrus, dendritic proliferation is followed by regression in very old age, unlike the previous report (Buell and Coleman, 1981) of maintained dendritic extent in human parahippocampal gyrus in the oldest old. This comparison emphasizes the regional specificity in the behavior of dendritic extent as a function of age.

Age-related dendritic regression in the rat supraoptic nucleus

Thus far we have emphasized the *proliferative* compensatory dendritic forces in the aging and Alzheimer's disease brain. However, there are also influences on dendrites that are regressive, and these influences cannot be ignored. There are brain regions and ages in which *net* dendritic regression has been seen. These include the human dentate gyrus granule cell very late in life (Flood et al., 1985), the F344 rat supraoptic nucleus (Flood and Coleman, 1983), and the rat cerebellar Purkinje cell (Rogers et al., 1984). Even in regions and at ages in which dendritic regression is not the dominant dendritic behavior — in regions which show net dendritic proliferation — there clearly are cells whose dendritic trees are regressing. We assume that dendritic regression in the aging and AD brain

may be related to a variety of factors. Among these are a regression antecedent to the death of a neuron and regression due to some degree of denervation of the cell in question (i.e., a partial loss of axonal input). Certainly it has long been assumed that neuronal death is preceded by dendritic regression (e.g., Cajal, 1928; Scheibel et al., 1975), and there is no reason to dispute this assumption. However, dendritic regression may be caused by events other than the impending death of the neuron, and this regression need not inevitably precede neuron death. It is now well established that dendritic regression may be induced in the developing or adult brain by surgically produced partial deafferentation (e.g., Jones and Thomas, 1962; Sumner and Watson, 1971; Standler and Bernstein, 1982) or by reduced activity in afferent pathways (e.g., Coleman and Riesen, 1968; Volkmar and Greenough, 1972). We asked whether there is evidence to support the proposition that loss of afferent input seen in many regions of aging brain constitutes a similar regressive influence on the dendrites of the aging brain.

In exploring the possible regressive influence of loss of input on dendritic trees it was important to examine as pure a situation as possible — a region in which denervation-induced regression would not be confused with regression closely antecedent to neuronal death. In other words, a region which does not lose neurons with increasing age. It was also important that the region studied be one in which loss of afferent input had been demonstrated. The supraoptic nucleus (SON) of the F344 rat offered such a model system. It had previously been shown that old female and male Sprague-Dawley rats show no loss of SON neurons (Hsu and Peng, 1978; Peng and Hsu, 1982). We confirmed these findings in the SON of the male F344 rat. In addition, Sladek et al. (1980) had shown a partial loss of noradrenergic input to this region. This loss was particularly pronounced in the ventral region of the SON, the zone into which the dendrites of the magnocellular neurons of the SON project. Data (Flood and Coleman, 1983) on dendritic extent in the SON as a function of age

234

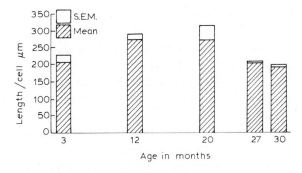

Fig. 8. Dendritic length of neurons in supraoptic nucleus of male F344 rat from 3 to 30 months. There is a statistically significant, approximately 35% decrease in dendritic length between 20 and 27 months. ANOVA: $F(4,14) = 5.01$; $p < 0.02$. There is no age-related loss of neurons in this region to 33 months.

show a 35% decrement in dendritic extent between 20 and 27 months of age (Fig. 8). The loss of noradrenergic input to the ventral region of this nucleus demonstrated previously (Sladek et al., 1980), showed its most dramatic change before 20 months, suggesting that loss of input to a portion of the dendritic tree of these SON cells is followed by dendritic regression in SON neurons.

These data indicate that age-related loss of input may lead to dendritic regression in the aged brain, just as has been demonstrated for earlier periods in the developmental continuum. These data also indicate that age-related dendritic regression need not always be a signal of impending neuronal death.

Summary and conclusions

We have developed a model of two interacting classes of influences on dendritic extent in the aging brain. Loss of neighboring neurons is a proliferative influence in normal aging, at least up to some limit which seems to be exceeded in very old age in some brain regions. This proliferative influence seems to be deficient in Alzheimer's disease. Partial denervation is a regressive influence in the aged brain just as it is during earlier periods in the developmental continuum. There are brain regions in which both of these influences are operating. We suggest that when both influences

are operating on the same cell in the normally aging brain, the final effect on the dendritic tree will be a reflection of the net sum of these two influences. Rat cerebellar Purkinje cells represent one example in which there is both neighbor neuron death (Rogers et al., 1984) and apparent loss of parallel fiber input (Rogers et al., 1981). The net effect on dendritic trees of these cells is regressive (Rogers et al., 1984). Human cerebral cortex is another region showing both loss of neighboring neurons and loss of input resulting from the known widespread loss of cortical neurons (see e.g., Hanley, 1974; Brody, 1976; Curcio et al., 1982 for review). Here the net effect on dendritic trees is proliferative, at least up to some currently undefined limit. Table I provides a set of examples of change (or lack of change) in dendritic extent in aging brain, along with information about changes in cell numbers and axonal input to the cell type under consideration. In this Table, age-related dendritic proliferation is only seen in regions that are known, or presumed, to lose neurons in old age. Dendritic regression is only seen in regions known (or presumed) to lose axonal input during aging. Note that loss of neurons need not inevitably lead to dendritic proliferation in surviving neighboring neurons if loss of axonal input may be sufficiently massive for the regressive influence of partial denervation to overcome the proliferative influence of cell loss. Similar logic also leads to the conclusion that partial denervation need not always lead to dendritic regression if the proliferative stimulus of neighbor neuron death is sufficiently powerful.

The model proposed here should be viewed as providing a working model which is useful for integrating a certain body of information and for suggesting experimental tests of the model. Although it currently appears that the events of neighbor neuron death and partial denervation are important factors in stimulating adaptive changes in dendritic extent of surviving neurons in the aging brain, we can be certain that they are not the only factors. Integrity of the axonal arbor of the neuron, as well as the neuron's impending death,

TABLE I

Summary of concomitant events during aging in a number of model brain regions[a]

Region Region	Neighbor neuron death	Loss of input	Dendrites
1. Mitral cells of Sprague-Dawley rat	+	?	↑
2. Layer II pyramids of human PHG cortex	+?	+?	↑
3. Granule cells of human dentate gyrus	+	+	↑
4. Purkinje cells of Sprague-Dawley rat	+	+	↓
5. Mitral cells of Charles River rat[b]	−	+	↓
6. SON of F344 rat hypothalamus	−	+	↓
7. Stellate cells of mouse PMBSF cortex	−	?	→

[a]The table indicates the probable presence or absence of (1) death of closely neighboring neurons, (2) afferent supply, and (3) the net behavior of dendritic extent in the seven model regions listed. Information such as that represented in this Table suggests hypotheses concerning potentially causal relationships.
[b]Hinds and McNelly, 1981.

are certainly reflected in the dendritic tree. Other events at the cellular and molecular level play major roles in molding the aging brain and may, in fact, be the events that initiate the sequence that results in death of some neurons and adaptations of the surviving neurons.

Acknowledgement

The authors received support from the National Institute on Aging Grants AG 01121 and AG 03644.

References

Anderson, J. M., Hubbard, B. M., Coghill, G. R. and Slidders, W. (1983) The effect of advanced old age on the neurone content of the cerebral cortex. Observations with an automatic image analyser point counting method. *J. Neurol. Sci.*, 58: 233–244.

Brody, H. (1955) Organization of the cerebral cortex. III. A study of aging in the human cerebral cortex. *J. Comp. Neurol.*, 102: 511–556.

Brody, H. (1976) An examination of cerebral cortex and brainstem aging. In R. D. Terry and S. Gershon (Eds.), *Neurobiology of Aging, Aging, Vol. 3*, Raven Press, New York, pp. 177–181.

Buell, S. J. (1982) Golgi-Cox and rapid Golgi methods as applied to autopsied human brain tissue: widely disparate results. *J. Neuropathol. Exp. Neurol.*, 41: 500–507.

Buell, S. J. and Coleman, P. D. (1979) Dendritic growth in the aged human brain and failure of growth in senile dementia. *Science*, 206: 854–856.

Buell, S. J. and Coleman, P. D. (1981) Quantitative evidence for selective dendritic growth in normal human aging but not in senile dementia. *Brain Res.*, 214: 23–41.

Caceres, A. and Steward, O. (1983) Dendritic reorganization in the denervated dentate gyrus of the rat following entorhinal cortical lesions: a Golgi and electron microscopic analysis. *J. Comp. Neurol.*, 214: 387–403.

Cajal, S. Ramon y (1928) *Degeneration and Regeneration of the Nervous System, Vol. 2*, translated and edited by R. M. May, 1959, Hafner Publ., New York, pp. 617–626.

Coleman, P. D. and Riesen, A. H. (1968) Environmental effects on cortical dendritic fields. I. Rearing in the dark. *J. Anat. (London)*, 102: 363–374.

Coleman, P. D., Garvey, C. F., Young, J. H. and Simon, W. (1977) Semiautomatic tracking of neuronal processes. In R. D. Lindsay (Ed.), *Computer Analysis of Neuronal Structures*, Plenum Press, New York, pp. 91–109.

Coleman, P. D. Buell, S. J. Magagna, L., Flood, D. G. and Curcio, C. A. (1986) Stability of dendrites in cortical barrels of C57B1/6N mice between 4 and 45 months. *Neurobiol. Aging*, 7: 101–105.

Cragg, B. G. (1975) The density of synapses and neurons in normal, mentally defective and ageing human brains. *Brain*, 98: 81–90.

Curcio, C. A. and Coleman, P. D. (1982) Stability of neuron number in cortical barrels of aging mice. *J. Comp. Neurol.*, 212: 158–172.

Curcio, C. A., Buell, S. J. and Coleman, P. D. (1982)

Morphology of the aging central nervous system: Not all downhill. In J. A. Mortimer, F. J. Pirozzolo and G. J. Maletta (Eds.), *The Aging Motor System, Advances in Neurogerontology, Vol. 3*, Praeger Publ., New York, pp. 7–35.

Duffy, C. J. and Rakic, P. (1983) Differentiation of granule cell dendrites in the dentate gyrus of the rhesus monkey: a quantitative Golgi study. *J. Comp. Neurol.*, 214: 224–237.

Flood, D. G. and Coleman, P. D. (1983) Age-related changes in dendritic extent of neurons in supraoptic nucleus of F344 rats. *Soc. Neurosci. Abstr.*, 9: 272.12.

Flood, D. G., Buell, S. J., DeFiore, C. H., Horwitz, G. J. and Coleman, P. D. (1985) Age-related dendritic growth in dentate gyrus of human brain is followed by regression in the 'oldest old'. *Brain Res.*, 345: 366–368.

Gibson, P. H. (1983) EM study of the numbers of cortical synapses in the brains of ageing people and people with Alzheimer-type dementia. *Acta Neuropathol. (Berlin)*, 62: 127–133.

Hanley, T. (1974) Neuronal fall-out in the ageing brain: a critical review of the quantitative data. *Age Ageing*, 3: 133–151.

Henderson, G., Tomlinson, B. E. and Gibson, P. H. (1980) Cell counts in human cerebral cortex in normal adults throughout life using an image analysing computer. *J. Neurol. Sci.*, 46: 113–136.

Hinds, J. W. and McNelly, N. A. (1977) Aging of the rat olfactory bulb: growth and atrophy of constituent layers and changes in size and number of mitral cells. *J. Comp. Neurol.*, 171: 345–368.

Hinds, J. W. and McNelly, N. A. (1981) Aging in the rat olfactory system: correlation of changes in the olfactory epithelium and olfactory bulb. *J. Comp. Neurol.*, 203: 441–453.

Hoff, S. F., Scheff, S. W., Bernardo, L. S. and Cotman, C. W. (1982) Lesion-induced synaptogenesis in the dentate gyrus of aged rats. I. Loss and reacquisition of normal synaptic density. *J. Comp. Neurol.*, 205: 246–252.

Hsu, H. K. and Peng, M. T. (1978) Hypothalamic neuron number of old female rats. *Gerontology*, 24: 434–440.

Huttenlocher, P. R. (1979) Synaptic density in human frontal cortex — developmental changes and effects of aging. *Brain Res.*, 163: 195–205.

Jones, W. H. and Thomas, D. B. (1962) Changes in the dendritic organization of neurons in the cerebral cortex following deafferentation. *J. Anat. (Lond.)*, 96: 375–381.

Konigsmark, B. W. and Murphy, E. A. (1970) Neuronal populations in the human brain. *Nature (Lond.)*, 228: 1335–1336.

McGeer, P. L., McGeer, E. G. and Suzuki, J. S. (1977) Aging and extrapyramidal function. *Arch. Neurol. (Chic.)*, 34: 33–35.

Monagle, R. D. and Brody, H. (1974) The effects of age upon the main nucleus of the inferior olive in the human. *J. Comp. Neurol.*, 155: 61–66.

Mouritzen Dam, A. (1979) The density of neurons in the human hippocampus. *Neuropathol. Appl. Neurobiol.*, 5: 249–264.

Müller, H. W. and Seifert, W. (1982) A neurotrophic factor (NTF) released from primary glial cultures supports survival and fiber outgrowth of cultured hippocampal neurons. *J. Neurosci. Res.*, 8: 195–204.

Peng, M. T. and Hsu, H. K. (1982) No neuron loss from hypothalamic nuclei of old male rats. *Gerontology*, 28: 19–22.

Peters, A., Feldman, M. L. and Vaughan, D. W. (1983) The effect of aging on the neuronal population within area 17 of adult rat cerebral cortex. *Neurobiol. Aging*, 4: 273–282.

Rogers, J., Zornetzer, S. F. and Bloom, F. E. (1981) Senescent pathology of cerebellum: Purkinje neurons and their parallel fiber afferents. *Neurobiol. Aging*, 2: 15–25.

Rogers, J., Zornetzer, S. F., Bloom, F. E. and Mervis, R. E. (1984) Senescent microstructural changes in rat cerebellum. *Brain Res.*, 292: 23–32.

Rutledge, L. T., Wright, C. and Duncan, J. (1974) Morphological changes in pyramidal cells of mammalian neocortex associated with increased use. *Exp. Neurol.*, 44: 209–228.

Schade, J. P. and Baxter, C. F. (1960) Changes during growth in the volume and surface area of cortical neurons in the rabbit. *Exp. Neurol.*, 2: 158–178.

Scheibel, M. E., Lindsay, R. D., Tomiyasu, U. and Scheibel, A. B. (1975) Progressive dendritic changes in aging human cortex. *Exp. Neurol.*, 47: 392–403.

Sladek, J. R., Jr., Khachaturian, H., Hoffman, G. E. and Scholer, J. (1980) Aging of central endocrine neurons and their aminergic afferents. *Peptides*, 1, Suppl. 1: 141–157.

Standler, N. A. and Bernstein, J. J. (1982) Degeneration and regeneration of motoneuron dendrites after ventral root crush: Computer reconstruction of dendritic fields. *Exp. Neurol.*, 75: 600–615.

Sumner, B. E. H. and Watson, W. E. (1971) Retraction and expansion of the dendritic tree of motor neurones of adult rats induced in vivo. *Nature (Lond.)*, 233: 273–275.

Thoenen, H. and Edgar, D. (1985) Neurotrophic factors. *Science*, 229: 238–242.

Van der Loos, H. (1956) Une combinaison de deux vieilles méthodes histologiques pour le système nerveux central. *Mschr. Psychiat. Neurol.*, 132: 330–334.

Vijayashankar, N. and Brody, H. (1977) A study of aging in the human abducens nucleus. *J. Comp. Neurol.*, 173: 433–438.

Vijayashankar, N. and Brody, H. (1979) A quantitative study of the pigmented neurons in the nuclei locus coeruleus and subcoeruleus in man as related to aging. *J. Neuropathol. Exp. Neurol.*, 38: 490–497.

Volkmar, F. R. and Greenough, W. T. (1972) Rearing complexity affects branching of dendrites in the visual cortex of the rat. *Science*, 176: 1445–1447.

Discussion

D. F. SWAAB: (1) In AD, the dendritic trees are not much smaller than in healthy controls. May we conclude that the size of the dendritic tree does not give the explanation for Alzheimer's disease or

(2) Could Golgi stain preferentially healthy cells?

ANSWER: Certainly one could conclude that absolute extent of the dendritic tree of surviving neurons does not provide an explanation for the devastating behavioral deficits of Alzheimer's disease. However, if one also considers the probable excess neuronal fall-out in AD in combination with the dendritic deficits the total dendritic loss in the neuropil may well be massive. In addition, as Dr. Roger Williams has suggested, it may be that absolute extent of dendrites may not be as crucial to behavioral deficits as capacity for plastic change in these components of the neuropil. The fact that surviving neurons in the parahippocampal gyrus and dentate gyrus appear to be unable to respond to the death of their neighbors in AD, as they do in early normal aging, suggests that indeed there is a much reduced plastic capability of dendrites in AD.

(2) We believe this kind of relative staining is not taking place since neurons with obviously regressed dendritic trees were stained in our material.

E. FLIERS: (1) Could selective loss of neurons with a relatively small dendritic tree be an alternative explanation for increased average dendritic length in senescence?

(2) Do you have any indication for selectivity of changed catecholamine innervation of supraoptic nucleus neurons with respect to their neurotransmitter content, i.e. vasopressin or oxytocin?

ANSWER: Selective loss of neurons with small dendritic trees is probably not an alternate explanation for our finding of apparent dendritic proliferation in normal aging. We conducted a blind count of numbers of neurons with small dendritic trees in each of our cases and found no relationship between this count and age.

(2) Vasopressin and oxytocin cell bodies are differently distributed in the supraoptic nucleus; one might expect catecholamine innervation of the cell bodies of these two types of neurons to change as the catecholamine fibers shift from the ventral region of the supraoptic nucleus to the dorsal region. In fact, J. Sladek at Rochester has evidence to suggest that this is the case. However, at the present time there is no evidence on this issue with regard to any differential change of catecholamine innervation of the dendrites of these two neuron types.

R. D. TERRY: As to the 'very old' group of humans, were they psychologically intact, and were the hippocampi free of evidence of hypoxia? Also, in addition to dendritic changes in dementia, there is a 35–45% loss of large neurons in neocortex.

ANSWER: Behavior of all cases was studied retrospectively by a psychiatrist based on information obtained from: hospital charts and interviews with doctors, nurses and relatives who were familiar with the patient. All non-demented cases were psychologically intact while all Alzheimer's disease cases were severely demented with a history of progressive dementia. Both non-demented and Alzheimer cases were also screened by a neuropathologist. The 22 cases included in the studies described here were drawn from an initial sample of 115 cases. We judged the hippocampus to be free of evidence of hypoxia on the basis of lack of eosinophilic neurons in H and E sections and absence of distortions of processes in Golgi sections.

H. BRAAK: Layer II pyramidal cells of the entorhinal cortex are — in Alzheimer's disease — particularly prone to develop tangles. May this be a reason why they lose their capability to proliferate their dendrites?

ANSWER: Although there have been no studies examining the relationship between tangles and dendritic extent in individual cells we may draw tentative conclusions from our own studies of dendritic extent in various regions in Alzheimer's disease. Although parahippocampal gyrus shows both tangles and deficient dendritic trees there are other brain regions in which these seem to be dissociated. The subiculum neurons are heavily invested with tangles, yet this region shows little reduction in dendritic trees in Alzheimer's disease (Flood et al., 1985). The dentate gyrus neurons contain very few tangles (R. Williams), yet they show severe deficits of dendritic extent (Buell et al., 1983). It is reasonable to suggest an association between tangles and reduced dendritic extent but we believe current evidence does not support this suggestion.

References

Buell, S. J., DeFiore, C. H., Horwitz, G. J. and Coleman, P. D. (1983) Dendrites of dentate granule cells and hippocampal pyramidal neurons in human aging and dementia. *Soc. Neurosci. Abstr.*, 9: 272.10.

Flood, D. G., Tovey, M. A. and Coleman, P. D. (1985) Dendrites of the subiculum in human aging and Alzheimer's disease. *Soc. Neurosci. Abstr.*, 11: 261.16.

D. F. Swaab, E. Fliers, M. Mirmiran, W. A. Van Gool and F. Van Haaren (Eds.)
Progress in Brain Research, Vol. 70.

CHAPTER 15

Neuronal cell membranes and brain aging

A. B. Oestreicher, P. N. E. De Graan and W. H. Gispen

*Division of Molecular Neurobiology, Rudolf Magnus Institute for Pharmacology and Institute of Molecular Biology,
University of Utrecht, Padualaan 8, 3584 CH Utrecht, The Netherlands*

Introduction

Intercellular communication is one of the characteristic features of neuronal networks. Arrival of a nerve impulse at the presynaptic terminal induces a complex train of events which consists of calcium influx, vesicle membrane and presynaptic membrane fusion, exocytosis of the chemical transmitter, its diffusion across the synaptic cleft and postsynaptic receptor activation followed by receptor-mediated effects on ion channels in the postsynaptic membrane (Krnjevic, 1974). The physico-chemical properties of the participating membranes are of importance for the proper functioning of chemical neurotransmission. In this review we shall discuss some of the molecular events in synaptic membranes that are involved in synaptic functions and that are subject to age-related changes.

Membrane lipid fluidity

Effect of age

The plasma membrane which encloses every cell is more than a passive barrier between cell content and environment. The cell membrane maintains a concentration gradient of the various ions on either side and it serves as a highly selective barrier for chemicals that are of use for cellular metabolism or that are waste products. It is generally accepted that eukaryotic cell membranes consist of a lipid bilayer in which protein molecules float (Alberts et al., 1983). While lipids are providing the basic structure and subserving functions of the membrane, the membrane proteins, that act as the major transport molecules, catalyze membrane-associated chemical reactions and form a cell-specific recognizable outer surface. Membrane proteins are responsible for receiving and transducing chemical messengers from neighboring cells or the intercellular fluid.

The activity and functioning of these proteins in or associated with the membrane are largely determined by the fluidity of their lipid microenvironment (Shinitzky and Henkart, 1979). In general, changes in lipid fluidity affect the lateral migration and the interaction of proteins embedded in the lipid bilayer. Protein displacement across the membrane lipid bilayer may result in changes in their exposure and hence their accessibility to chemicals in and outside the cell (Shinitzky and Henkart, 1979). The fluidity of the lipid bilayer depends on its lipid composition. Notable determinants are the degree of saturation of the fatty acid side chains and the content of cholesterol. During aging, there is a marked increase in the ratio of cholesterol to phospholipids in the membranes of various tissues and, in particular, in the brain (Rouser et al., 1972).

In collaboration with Dr. Hershkowitz, we repeated some of his studies (Hershkowitz, 1983; Hershkowitz et al., 1982) using synaptic plasma membranes (SPM) obtained from brains of 24-

240

months-old male Wistar rats (TNO, Zeist, The Netherlands). Measurements of the mobility of the lipid probe 1,2-diphenyl-1,3,5-hexatriene (DPH) by steady-state fluorescence polarization established that SPM obtained from the brains of old rats were more micro-viscous than those of adult controls (6 months). Regional differences between cerebral cortex and hippocampus were not detected. Since the measurements were performed over a wide temperature range (4–37°C), the data indicated not only the absence of lipid phase transitions in the SPM, but also that in the SPM of the aged rat the decreased lipid fluidity was apparent over the total temperature range tested (Fig. 1; Van Dongen et al., 1983). Therefore, these

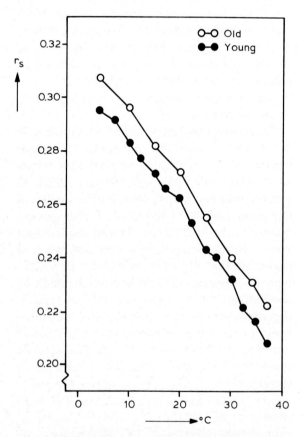

Fig. 1. Steady-state fluorescence anisotropy values of hippocampal SPM as a function of temperature. SPM was prepared from hippocampus from young and old rats. (From Van Dongen et al., 1983)

data are in good agreement with the reports on the age-related increases in micro-viscosity of a crude SPM fraction obtained from mouse forebrain (Hershkowitz, 1983) and rat cerebral cortex and neostriatum (Cimino et al., 1984). The latter study established the diminished lipid fluidity both by means of fluorescence polarization and electron-spin resonance.

Receptors

As reports on the consequences of age-related increases in micro-viscosity of brain membranes are scarce, it is difficult to assess the significance of such membrane changes for synaptic function. Since some receptors may become more exposed with increasing micro-viscosity, while others may be less accessible, one can expect to find diverse rather than uniform effects of aging on neurotransmission, depending on the protein and the functional aspect studied. Likewise, some embedded proteins that are involved in signal transduction may collide more frequently, whereas the interaction of others may be impaired.

Based on their experience with membrane lipid fluidity and the serotonin receptor (Heron et al., 1980), Hershkowitz et al. (1982) selected this receptor for study in relation to aging of brain membranes. They reported that in the SPM obtained from the forebrains of 26-months-old mice there is a 50% reduction in basal serotonin binding, with concomitantly decreased lipid fluidity, in comparison with that observed in membranes obtained from brains of 3-months-old controls. Interestingly, scatchard analysis revealed that the loss of binding was primarily due to a loss of high-affinity binding sites, as the young mouse brain contained both high- and low-affinity sites and the old mouse brain only the low-affinity sites (Hershkowitz et al., 1982). These data are in good agreement with previous studies of these authors in which they show that *in vitro* rigidification of adult mouse brain SPM with cholesterol results in a loss of serotonin binding (Heron et al., 1980).

Cimino et al. (1984) reported that in aging rat

brain cerebral cortex, neostriatum and pineal gland, there is a marked drop in β-adrenergic binding sites, while in the striata of these animals a lower number of dopamine binding sites was observed. Such a loss of striatal dopamine receptors with age has been reported for various animal species as well as man (see Roth et al., 1986).

With respect to the serotonin receptor, it was shown that by *in vivo* treatment of old mice with a known membrane fluidizer AL721 (see below) the number of binding sites became in the order of that seen in the young control mice (Hershkowitz et al., 1982). Chronic treatment of old rats with *S*-adenosyl-L-methionine, a cofactor in phospholipid methylation — a process that increases lipid fluidity (Hirata and Axelrod, 1978) — resulted in a decreased membrane viscosity and an increased β-receptor binding. However, the reduction of putative dopamine receptor sites was not affected by the fluidizing treatment of the old rats (Cimino et al., 1984). This suggests that a decrease in receptor synthesis rather than membrane sequestration, plays a role in the diminishing dopamine receptor availability in old age (Roth et al., 1986), whereas the availability of the other receptors studied seems to be determined by the lipid fluidity of the membrane.

Membrane protein phosphorylation

Post-translational, covalent modification, e.g. phosphorylation, is a common phenomenon in the regulation of the structure and function of membrane proteins. The synaptic membrane is extremely rich in protein kinases and phosphoprotein phosphatases, substrate proteins and receptor-coupled signal transducing systems that mobilize calcium or elevate cAMP, both known modulators of protein kinases (Weller, 1979; Gispen and Routtenberg, 1982). In a series of studies, Hershkowitz et al. (1982) investigated whether membrane lipid fluidity influenced intrinsic membrane protein phosphorylation. If the lipid fluidity of crude mouse brain SPM was decreased (cholesterol) or increased (lecithin) *in vitro*, the phosphorylation of several proteins in the 40–60 kDa molecular weight range was influenced. One of these, a 47 kDa protein, is of special interest because this protein is most likely identical to protein B-50, which seems to play an important role in transmembrane signal transduction (see below). An *in vitro*-induced small decrease in SPM lipid fluidity of about 15% was accompanied by a marked increase in the endogenous phosphorylation of this protein (Hershkowitz, 1983).

When membranes were isolated from brains of old mice, the basal phosphorylation pattern differed from that of young mice only with respect to this 47 kDa/B-50 protein (Hershkowitz, 1983; Hershkowitz et al., 1982). Thus, this protein showed a higher degree of phosphorylation in the more viscous membranes of the aged mice. Why there were no concomitant changes in the phosphorylation of other proteins is unclear. It may suggest that the phosphorylation of this protein is especially sensitive to changes in membrane lipid fluidity that occur under *in vivo* conditions of aging. If, however, cAMP-sensitive phosphorylation was studied, membranes obtained from aged mouse brains responded less to the addition of cAMP in the endogenous phosphorylation assay as compared to that seen in membranes obtained from young mice (Hershkowitz, 1983). Again, the differences in protein phosphorylation could be counteracted by *in vivo* treatment of the old mice with the active lipid extract AL721. The treatment resulted in an increase of the lipid fluidity of the isolated brain membranes, a decrease in the basal phosphorylation level of the 47 kDa protein and an enhancement of the responsiveness of other proteins to cAMP (Hershkowitz, 1983).

Studies with the membrane fluidizer AL721

Based on the assumption that abnormal membrane lipid viscosity is implicated in the etiology of disorders which are relevant to aging (Rouser et al., 1972; Shinitzky, 1984), Shinitzky and coworkers developed a lipid mixture (AL721) from egg yolk that fluidizes membranes. The active ingredients are phospholipids, mainly phosphatidylcholine (Hershkowitz et al., 1982). It was found that old mice and man, both suffering from suppressed immune reactivity, could be effectively treated (per os) with AL721, substantially restoring their immuno-responsiveness (Shinitzky, 1984).

As discussed in the previous paragraph, the *in vivo* treatment of mice with AL721 was also effective in counteracting membrane changes in aging brain. Currently, this group of researchers is testing AL721 in clinical trials that aim to assess the efficacy in improving the condition of geriatric patients (Hershkowitz, 1985).

Signal transduction

Cells function in a coordinated manner by a continuous exchange of signals that are transferred through the plasma membrane from the exterior to the interior and vice versa. External information carried by neurotransmitters, hormones, growth factors and other first messengers, is translated by the constituents of the cell membrane into internal signals, the second messengers. The second messengers, cAMP, cGMP and calcium, govern intracellularly a variety of physiological responses, such as changes in metabolism, neurotransmission and growth, resulting in adaptations to alterations in external environment (Weller, 1979; Nestler and Greengard, 1983, 1984).

In the previous section, marked changes in brain cell membrane lipid fluidity observed during aging have been shown to influence plasma membrane properties. Some of these are directly involved in the homeostatic and communicative functions of the neuronal plasma membrane: i.e. in the processes of signal transduction. Here, we will summarize the features of these processes in general terms, followed by presentation of a model for one particular mechanism, the phosphoinositol-mediated signal transduction and we indicate age-related changes in participating components (Van Dongen et al., 1983).

Recent studies at the level of the plasma membrane in various cell types have resolved in part the train of events occurring in transmembrane signal transduction. Extracellular messengers bind to and activate specific outer membrane receptors. In its activated form, the receptor can interact with one of the types of guanine nucleotide regulatory proteins (N protein) and this complex may activate either a nucleotide cyclase producing cAMP or cGMP as intracellular second messenger (Nestler and Greengard, 1984), or a phosphodiesterase that specifically hydrolyzes polyphosphoinositides associated with intracellular calcium mobilization (Berridge and Irvine, 1984; Nishizuka, 1983).

We will limit our discussion to the latter signalling pathway that mobilizes intracellular calcium using inositol lipids in the transduction mechanism (Michell, 1975; Michell and Kirk, 1981; Downes and Michell, 1982).

Receptor-stimulated inositide metabolism was discovered by Hokin and Hokin (1954), who showed that the incorporation of $[^{32}P]$phosphate into phospholipids in pancreas was stimulated by acetylcholine. Since then the concurrence between calcium mobilization and stimulated inositide turnover has been observed in many types of cells and tissues in response to a wide range of external stimuli (Berridge and Irvine, 1984; Nishizuka, 1984a).

The current view on the signal transduction involving polyphosphoinositides (PPI) is depicted in Fig. 2. In this Fig., the presumed role of the protein B-50 is also illustrated. Agonist-receptor

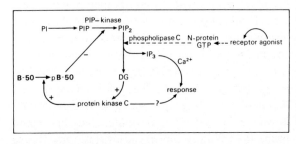

Fig. 2. Working model for the PPI-mediated signal transduction across SPM and for the role of the phosphoprotein B-50 in the feedback response of the PIP_2 turnover. See the text for explanation.

interaction induces phosphodiesteratic cleavage of phosphatidylinositol 4,5-bisphosphate (PIP_2) into inositol 1,4,5-trisphosphate (IP_3) and diacylglycerol (DG). Possibly, a GTP nucleotide-binding protein conveys the information from the occupied receptor to phospholipase C (Cockcroft and Gomperts, 1985). IP_3 has recently been characterized as a second messenger (Berridge, 1983). It leaves the membrane and releases calcium from intracellular stores, most likely calcium that is sequestered in the endoplasmatic reticulum and not that present in mitochondria (Prentki et al., 1984; Berridge and Irvine, 1984). The increased intracellular level of calcium activates various enzyme systems that trigger physiological responses. Nishizuka and colleagues (Nishizuka, 1980, 1983; Takai et al., 1979a; Kishimoto et al., 1980) found that DG greatly increases the affinity of protein kinase C for calcium, thereby activating this enzyme. Therefore, Nishizuka (1984a) has suggested that during inositol lipid-dependent signal transduction, activation by enhanced calcium levels and enhanced protein phosphorylation catalyzed by protein kinase C probably act separately as well as synergistically in the control of a wide range of cellular events. Studies in our laboratory indicated that the degree of phosphorylation of the membrane protein B-50, a substrate of protein kinase C, may act as a negative feedback control in the receptor-mediated PPI response: enhancement of the phosphorylation of B-50 by protein kinase C inhibits PIP kinase. Consequently, less PIP_2 will be available for the receptor-induced breakdown of IP_3 and DG (Gispen et al., 1985a).

The role of the phosphoprotein B-50

Phosphorylation and properties

B-50 (apparent molecular weight 48 kDa, isoelectric point 4.5) is a nervous tissue-specific (Kristjansson et al., 1982), membrane-bound protein with several sites for phosphorylation (Zwiers et al., 1985). The protein was discovered in the course of studies on the neurochemical mechanism of

action of behaviorally active peptides. Zwiers et al. (1976) observed, while screening membrane protein phosphorylation, that in SPM isolated from rat brain the endogenous phosphorylation of several proteins including B-50 was dose-dependently inhibited by ACTH peptides and not affected by cAMP or cGMP (Wiegant et al., 1978). It turned out that ACTH did not influence the activity of protein phosphatases and ATP-ases of SPM, but inhibited a particular membrane protein kinase. B-50 and its protein kinase were purified by extraction from rat brain membranes, DEAE-cellulose column chromatography, ammonium-sulfate precipitation (ASP) and two-dimensional electrophoresis (Zwiers et al., 1980). Aloyo et al. (1982, 1983) demonstrated that the B-50 protein kinase, being an ACTH-sensitive, nucleotide-independent protein kinase, is indistinguishable from calcium- and lipid-activated protein kinase C, isolated by Inoue et al. (1977; Nishizuka, 1984b; Kuo et al., 1980; Takai et al., 1979b). Recent studies on brain membrane protein phosphorylation in several laboratories have indicated that the B-50 protein may be identical to protein γ-5 (Gower and Rodnight, 1982), protein 47 kDa (Hershkowitz et al., 1982), protein P54p (Mahler et al., 1982) and protein F_1 (Routtenberg, 1982; Routtenberg et al., 1985).

In the nervous system there is a rapid PPI turnover, particularly in non-myelin membranes (Gonzalez-Sastre et al., 1971). Parallel to the studies on the effects of peptides on protein phosphorylation, Jolles et al. (1979) began to investigate whether interaction of ACTH with the neuronal membranes influenced the metabolism of PPI. Examining a partially purified preparation of B-50 and B-50 kinase (the ASP fraction of Zwiers et al., 1980), Jolles et al. (1980) discovered that when the lipid PIP and [γ-^{32}P]ATP were added as substrates, $ACTH_{1-24}$ in concentrations of 10^{-7} to 10^{-4}M stimulated the conversion of PIP to PIP_2, while simultaneously inhibiting the [^{32}P]-incorporation in B-50. Thus, this ASP fraction contained a protein kinase as well as a PIP kinase. The ASP fraction was checked for related enzyme activities and was found to be devoid of phospho-diesteratic and protein phosphatase activity. Interestingly, a link between the B-50 and PIP kinase appeared to exist. When, in this ASP fraction, B-50 was prephosphorylated for increasing reaction times, and thereafter PIP was added, the amount of PIP_2 formed was inversely correlated with the extent of B-50 phosphorylation (Jolles et al., 1980). Next, Jolles et al. (1981a) demonstrated that also in rat brain membranes $ACTH_{1-24}$ affected simultaneously both protein and PPI metabolism. The structure-activity profile for the effect of the neuropeptide on B-50 phosphorylation and PIP_2/phosphatidic acid formation was similar (Jolles et al., 1981b). These and other findings led to the hypothesis that PPI metabolism in SPM is regulated by the degree of phosphorylation of B-50.

By several approaches we have tried to test the proposed feedback regulation as summarized in Fig. 2. The following evidence was recently collected:

(1) Affinity-purified anti-B-50 immunoglobulins (IgGs) or $ACTH_{1-24}$ added to SPM markedly and specifically inhibited the B-50 phosphorylation and concomitantly enhanced the [^{32}P]-labelling of PIP_2 several-fold. Control IgGs added in equal amounts were without effect (Oestreicher et al., 1983a).

(2) An inverse relationship between B-50 phosphorylation and [^{32}P]-labelling of PIP_2 was observed in a study on the effect of incubation with $5 \cdot 10^{-4}$M dopamine of rat hippocampal slices. The phosphorylation assays were carried out by 'post-hoc' phosphorylation of the SPM prepared from dopamine-treated and control slices. The effects were reversed when the antagonist haloperidol was added during the incubation of the hippocampal slices, indicating that a receptor-mediated process was involved (Jork et al., 1984).

(3) The proposed regulation of PIP kinase was tested in a system of reconstituted components. When B-50 preparations enriched in either the highly phosphorylated components or the dephosphorylated forms (Zwiers et al., 1985) were examined for their effect on the activity of the purified PIP kinase (45 kDa, isoelectric point 5.8; Van Dongen et al.,

1984), it was found that using equal amounts of both B-50 preparations, only the phosphorylated forms decreased significantly the conversion of PIP to PIP_2 (Van Dongen et al., 1985).

These findings support the proposal that B-50 phosphorylation regulates the activity of PIP kinase. Since these proteins and B-50 kinase can be extracted together from the neuronal membrane, they may occur in a complex in the presynaptic plasma membrane (see below).

Currently, we are interested in the interaction of B-50 and PIP kinase in the signal transduction cycle in relation to development, maturation and aging of neural tissue. Previously, it has been demonstrated that after birth inositol lipid kinases reach an activity peak around the time of myelination (Salway et al., 1968; Eichberg and Hauser, 1969; Shaik and Palmer, 1976; Uma and Ramakrishnan, 1983).

We found that the absolute levels of phosphatidylinositol (PI), PIP and PIP_2 in SPM from forebrain of 24-months-old male rats did not differ from those of 6 months old (Van Dongen et al., 1983). However, it should be kept in mind that the total level of PPI in the membrane itself may be a rather meaningless figure. The amount associated with receptor-mediated signal transduction is of much more relevance. When the influence of age was studied on the turnover of the PPI, it was revealed that the activity of the PIP kinase was specifically decreased in membranes prepared from old rat hippocampus (Van Dongen et al., 1983). This observation and that of Hershkowitz (1983), who demonstrated that the endogenous phosphorylation of specifically the 47 kDa/B-50 protein is high in membranes from old mouse brains, again supports the notion that the B-50 phosphorylation may regulate the activity of PIP kinase (Gispen et al., 1985a).

Does the localization of B-50 in rat brain change during maturation and aging?

Earlier studies on the distribution of B-50 were carried out with adult rat nervous tissue. Kristjansson et al. (1982) demonstrated that B-50 is localized exclusively in rat brain particulate fractions and is not detectable by phosphorylation, two-dimensional gel electrophoresis and immunochemical analysis in non-nervous tissues. The immunohistochemical localization of B-50 was studied in paraffin-embedded sections of cerebellum and hippocampus of the adult rat (inbred Wistar strain, TNO, Zeist, The Netherlands), by means of a rabbit antiserum raised against purified B-50 using the peroxidase-antiperoxidase (PAP) method (Oestreicher et al., 1981). The findings were that B-50 immunoreactivity (BIR) appeared to be concentrated in neuropil-rich brain areas (Oestreicher et al., 1981). In contrast, the white matter and the cell bodies were virtually without immunostaining.

Sörensen et al. (1981) analyzed various subcellular fractions of adult rat brain by endogenous phosphorylation and concluded that B-50 is mainly associated with the presynaptic membrane. Recently, we used immuno electron microscopy for detection of the binding of affinity-purified anti-B-50 IgGs by means of protein-A-coated gold particles, and demonstrated that in the adult hippocampus *in situ*, B-50 is predominantly localized at presynaptic sites of nerve terminals and associated with the inner face of the plasma membrane (Oestreicher et al., 1983b; Gispen et al., 1985b). In order to support this ultrastructural localization, we examined the subcellular sites of B-50 in isolated intact and post-sectioned synaptosomes. When ultra-thin cryosections were first cut from aldehyde-fixed synaptosomes so that the interior of the synaptosomes was exposed to the immuno reagents and then processed for immuno electron microscopy, BIR was detected close to the SPM, at the cytoplasmic face. In contrast, pre-embedding immunostaining of the intact synaptosomes followed by fixation and processing for electron microscopic analysis resulted in micrographs devoid of any immunolabelling (Gispen et al., 1985b). This led us to conclude that B-50 is located at the inner face of the cell membrane, being not accessible to the antibodies when the synaptosomal membrane is not ruptured. In the experiments on the *in situ* labelling of the hippocampus some of the nerve terminals were found to be devoid of BIR. The observation of the absence of immunostaining from some synapses raises many questions, for example whether B-50 is associated selectively with specific populations of nerve terminals involved in certain transmitter and signalling systems.

In view of the restricted localization in hippocampal neurons of adult rat, the question arose whether the localization of B-50 differed as a function of age. Previously, we had demonstrated that in 8-days-old rats, B-50 was one of the prominent proteins in neural membranes that had become labelled after intracranial injection of radiolabelled orthophosphate (Oestreicher et al., 1982). Employing affinity-purified anti-B-50 antibodies (Oestreicher et al., 1983a), we showed in a comparative immunocytochemical study (Oestreicher et al., 1983b) of brain regions in the 8-days-old and adult rat that BIR was distributed throughout the rat brain in regions rich in synaptic contacts. In addition, in the developing brain BIR was also observed in outgrowing axons, probably present in their growth cones (De Graan et al., 1985a).

After finding that the site of localization of B-50 is dependent on the stage of differentiation and growth of the neurons in various brain regions (Oestreicher and Gispen, 1986), we started to explore immunocytochemically changes in the location of B-50 in the hippocampus of young adult and senescent rats (BN strain, obtained from REP Institutes, GO-TNO, Rijswijk, The Netherlands) in more detail. The distribution of BIR in the neuropil areas of the stratum oriens and the stratum moleculare lacunosum of CA1 was rather similar (Fig. 3). However, a conspicuous difference was revealed in the hippocampus of the 27-months-old rat, in which BIR appeared to be present in 'aggregates' at the periphery of the cell body or as 'particulate' material unevenly distributed in the cytosol of the pyramidal neurons of CA3. The same BIR deposits were seen to a

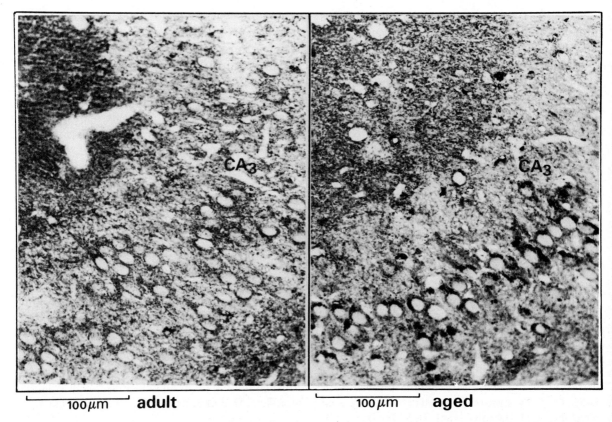

100 μm **adult**   100 μm **aged**

Fig. 3. Distribution of B-50 immunoreactivity (BIR) in the CA3 field of the hippocampus of young adult (left) and senescent (right) rats. The procedures used to perfuse and fix the brains, to obtain the tissue sections and to perform the immunocytochemistry are described in detail in a recent study by Oestreicher and Gispen (1986). Sections were cut from the rat brains perfused with fixative, containing 2% paraformaldehyde, 0.1% dimethylsulfoxide, 0.5% glutaraldehyde in phosphate-buffered saline at pH 7.4, post-fixed and impregnated with paraffin. 5-μm thick parasagittal sections were incubated with anti-B-50 IgGs and the immunoreaction was detected by the PAP method. The micrographs show that small dot-like deposits of BIR are present in the stratum radiatum of the young and senescent hippocampus. The density of the BIR deposits diminishes at the proximal side of the innervation of the apical dendrites of the pyramidal neurones (left and right). Mainly, in the CA3 of the young (left), but also in the old (right) rats, unstained thin dendrites and unstained pyramidal neurons appear to be outlined by small punctuate BIR, probably present in presynaptic terminals of afferents terminating on their membrane (Gispen et al., 1985b). In addition, in the senescent rat (right), there are conspicuous, relatively large deposits of BIR close to the neuronal membrane of the pyramidal cells. This BIR appears to be either in the cytosol of the pyramidal neurons or outside adjoining the perikaryal membrane. Similar sized deposits of BIR are hardly seen in the stratum pyramidale of the young adult rat (left). In both, blood capillaries are unstained.

lesser extent in the pyramidal neurons of CA1, CA2 and CA4. Such a distribution of BIR was much less prominent in the sections of the hippocampus of 4-weeks-old rats. As immunocyto-chemical control we examined sections of the young adult and aged rat hippocampus with two other antisera to immunostain the structural markers myelin and astrocytes. The results did not

display marked qualitative differences, in contrast to those of the immunostaining pattern of B-50 (Fig. 3).

At present, the significance of this age-related change in cellular B-50 localization is unclear. It is tempting to conclude that it relates to the diminu-tion of synaptic plasticity as seen in the hippocam-pus of aged rats (see below). Further work is in progress to gain insight into the nature and precise cellular localization of these BIR deposits around pyramidal cells in the CA3 layer of the hippocampus of old rats.

Distribution of B-50 determined by radioimmunoassay

In order to study the effect of age on B-50 in a more quantitative manner, we developed a sensitive radioimmuno assay (RIA) using anti-B-50 IgGs to measure B-50 (0.1–10 ng) in small amounts of rat brain tissue (5–400 μg wet weight). The tracer was prepared by phosphorylating purified B-50 with carrier-free [γ-^{32}P]ATP, catalyzed by purified protein kinase C. With this RIA we have determined the B-50 content of various brain regions of the adult Wistar rat. We found the following distribution pattern: septum > periaqueductal gray > cerebral cortex > hippocampus > cerebellum > medulla spinalis. The septum contained 80 μg B-50/g wet weight tissue (Oestreicher et al., 1985). This regional distribution pattern shows a fair agreement with the previously reported pattern of distribution of the endogenous B-50 phosphorylation in SPM isolated from the same brain areas (Kristjansson et al., 1982). Furthermore, these data confirm our earlier suggestion that regional differences in the endogenous B-50 phosphorylation reflect differences in the presence of B-50 rather than that of protein kinase C (Kristjansson et al., 1982). Holmes and Rodnight (1981) reported on the ontogeny of substrate proteins for protein kinases in rat brain membrane fractions. They found that the maximum phosphorylation of the 48-kDa protein γ-5 was reached 15 days after birth and from then declined to the adult level. This decline may arise from several age-related changes. We found that the B-50 content in total brain, measured by RIA during postnatal development of the rat, was high after birth and decreased to a lower adult level. That B-50 levels in rat change with age is shown for specific brain regions in Fig. 4. The B-50 content of the septum, cortex cerebri and hippocampus diminishes by 40–50% in 28-months-old rats, in comparison to

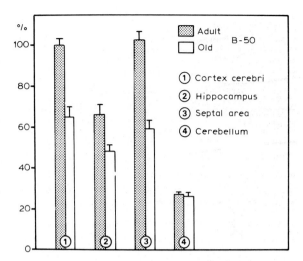

Fig. 4. RIA of B-50 levels in homogenates of various brain regions of young and old rats. The brain regions were dissected from groups of three animals. The B-50 content (84 μg/mg wet weight tissue) of the septum of the young rat has been taken as the reference level (100%). The RIA was carried out as described by Oestreicher et al. (1985). Data represent the mean of triplicate assays, SEM < 5%. Student's t test was applied for the comparison of young versus old rats. The differences found in brain regions: 1, cortex cerebri; 2, hippocampus and 3, septal area, were significant to $p < 0.05$.

that of 2-months-old, young adult rats. Surprisingly, the content of the cerebellum remained unaltered. The causes and consequences of the changes of the levels of B-50 in various brain regions with the age of the rat are unknown. From another field of study concerned with outgrowth and sprouting of axons (Pfenninger et al., 1983; Katz et al., 1985) the suggestion came that protein F_1 may be a growth-associated protein, since its synthesis is stimulated by growth and regeneration. A decrease of B-50, probably identical to F_1, during maturation and aging might reflect a diminished synthesis of some membrane proteins in response to altered requirements for growth associated with synaptic plasticity.

Synaptic plasticity and membrane fluidity

A synaptic system shows plasticity when its response to a certain electrical stimulus is a function of previous experience. This type of plasticity can be observed when a set of fibers is electrically stimulated by a series of brief pulses at relatively high frequencies, i.e. a tetanus. After such a tetanus, the corresponding synapses may present an enhancement in their responses to test stimuli for a period of time that may last from hours to even days. This phenomenon is called long-term potentiation (LTP). It has been considered as the physiological substrate for information storage in the brain (Bliss, 1979; Bliss and Dolphin, 1982; Lopes da Silva et al., 1982a; Eccles, 1983; Voronin, 1983; Teyler and Discenna, 1984). However, the way of stimulation used to experimentally induce LTP is necessarily a prolonged synchronous volley of impulses applied to a relatively large number of fibers. Yet, it may be assumed that in the normal functioning brain similar types of processes, although in a much less widespread way, take place: the scale at which this would occur, however, is so minute that such processes cannot be put in evidence by using the methods available. It may be pointed out that the consolidation of cognitive memory involves repeated recall; in a similar way one may assume that enduring LTPs may be established as a consequence of repeated reinforcements of the type of synaptic processes described here (Eccles, 1983).

LTP is essentially a synaptic phenomenon since it has been clearly demonstrated that it does not correspond to a generalized increase in the excitability of the neurons involved. Indeed, LTP stays restricted to the synapses being stimulated and is not transferred heterosynaptically (Andersen et al., 1977). However, some studies report that under certain conditions generalized changes in the excitability of the post-synaptic membrane may occur (Lynch et al., 1977).

There is still controversy on whether LTP consists of a pre- or a post-synaptic phenomenon, or a combination of both. Evidence in favor of a presynaptic locus is mainly based on experimental findings of transmitter release during LTP and on changes in the phosphorylation and activity of pyruvate dehydrogenase (PDH; Browning et al.,

1982) and in the phosphorylation of B-50/F_1 and the 52-kDa protein (De Graan et al., 1985b; Routtenberg et al., 1985). Skrede and Malthe-Sörensen (1981) found that LTP in the CA1 field of the hippocampal slices is accompanied by a long-lasting increase in the resting release of previously accumulated D-[^{3}H]aspartate. *In vivo*, using the push-pull cannula technique, Dolphin et al. (1982) and Lynch et al. (1984) have shown that LTP in the fascia dentata of the rat hippocampus is accompanied by a prolonged release of glutamate. Voronin (1983) reported that LTP studied in hippocampal slices is related to an increase in the mean number of transmitter quanta released per presynaptic action potential. More experimental evidence for a presynaptic locus is provided by the recent investigation of Dolphin (1983), who showed that a tetanus to the perforant path *in vivo*, during a period where the glutamate antagonist γ-D-glutamylglycine was applied, was able to induce LTP, whose expression was masked until the antagonist was removed.

Against a presynaptic locus of LTP appear to be the experiments of Dunwiddie et al. (1978), who used the glutamate antagonist D,L-2-amino-4-phosphonobutyric acid (APB) to block synaptic transmission in the CA1 field in hippocampal slices, and showed that a tetanus applied under these conditions did not cause LTP even after the antagonist has been washed out.

Regarding the postsynaptic hypothesis of LTP, the main argument emerges from the work of Baudry and Lynch (1979; Lynch and Baudry, 1984), who reported that the number of glutamate receptor binding sites increased during LTP and that this increase was dependent on calcium. They interpret these findings as indicating that a membrane-bound enzyme, calpain, is activated by the influx of calcium provoked by the tetanization, and acts on the cytoskeletal protein fodrin which lines the inner surface of the neuronal membrane. In this way a fodrin lattice would be disrupted which would uncover glutamate receptors on the postsynaptic membrane. Such a mechanism could explain the morphological changes in the shape of dendritic spines as reported in the CA1 field, on *in vitro* hippocampal slices (Lee et al., 1981) and on *in vivo* hippocampus (Lee et al., 1980), and by Chang and Greenough (1984). Fifková and Van Harreveld (1977) found an increased spine surface area after potentiation in fascia dentata, but could not determine a change in shape. Desmond and Levy (1983) reported an increase in the number of large spine profiles in the region of high synaptic activation in the fascia dentata. There remain discrepancies between the morphological data related to LTP obtained from fascia dentata and CA1.

The possibility of both pre- and postsynaptic events being responsible for LTP has been put forward (cf. Lopes da Silva et al., 1982a). Eccles (1983) proposed a unifying hypothesis which assumes that the primary event is an increased sensitivity of the postsynaptic membrane and that, secondary this would induce an increased output of transmitter from the presynaptic terminals by means of a trophic action across the synaptic cleft. A further clarification of pre- and postsynaptic events in LTP may be expected by combining physiological, biochemical and electron microscopical techniques. It may be advanced that LTP is most likely a phenomenon of the whole synaptic system and that it corresponds to changes at both sides of the synapse (De Graan et al., 1985b).

Irrespective of the pre- or postsynaptic locus of LTP, it is clear that the participating synaptic membranes undergo profound functional changes that occur in parallel or that maintain the observed adaptive synaptic response. In view of the marked decrease in membrane lipid fluidity seen in the hippocampus of old rats, presumably impairing synaptic plasticity, it is of interest to note that there is a growing body of evidence to suggest that the aged rat has a lower capacity to generate LTP after tetanic stimulation of hippocampal fiber networks both *in vivo* and *in vitro*. For instance, Landfield et al. (1981) consistently showed that hippocampal synapses in aging rats exhibit a decline in their ability for frequency potentiation, whereas many, but not all, other neurophysiological properties appear normal. It now seems clear that this potentiation deficit is due to specific impairment of synaptic function (Landfield, 1983). Similar age-related impairments after repetitive stimulation were reported by Tielen et al. (1983). They reported that in slices obtained from the hippocampus of senescent rats tetanic stimulation did not result in the generation of LTP as normally seen in slices from hippocampus of young rats. As shown in Table I, there is no change in the amplitude of the population spike characteristics for LTP in senescent rats, during the time after the tetanus that the LTP develops in adult rat

TABLE I

LTP of the population spike of CA1 in young and senescent rats. Population spikes are expressed as percentages (mean ± SEM) of the amplitude of pre-tetanus period (−1′−0′). The two-tailed significance levels of the percentages with respect to the general pre-tetanus mean are given in column p (Student's t test)

Pre-tetanus ($n = 33$, periods: 10′−9′, 5′−4′, 1′−0′) 101 ± 2

Post-tetanus	young ($N = 17$)	p	senescent ($N = 16$)	p
1′−2′	121 ± 11	ns	99 ± 3	ns
3′−4′	137 ± 16	0.05	100 ± 5	ns
5′−6′	133 ± 13	0.05	98 ± 5	ns
7′−8′	131 ± 15	ns	99 ± 6	ns
9′−10′	139 ± 17	0.05	100 ± 6	ns

From Tielen et al., 1983.

hippocampal slices (Lopes da Silva et al., 1982b). It is tempting to assume that impaired functioning of the membranes of those synapses that are affected by repetitive stimulation, is causing this impaired synaptic plasticity.

Summary and conclusions

In the present paper some aspects of neuronal membrane function that are affected by aging have been reviewed. There is increasing evidence to suggest that the age-related increase in the microviscosity of SPM may cause diminution of transmembrane signal transduction and synaptic plasticity. Especially the protein kinase C substrate protein B-50 seems of interest as its degree of phosphorylation exerts a feedback control in receptor-mediated membrane events. Its degree of phosphorylation, its brain localization and content seem to undergo specific alterations during the lifespan of the rat. As an example of impaired synaptic plasticity, the reduced responsiveness of hippocampal networks of aged rats to tetanic stimulation was discussed. Although the precise molecular mechanism of action of LTP is unknown, the impaired lipid fluidity as found in these membranes most likely negatively influences the capacity of these membranes to generate the post-tetanic response.

As shown previously, *in vivo* and *in vitro* induced decreases in membrane lipid fluidity can be restored by *in vivo* and *in vitro* treatment with membrane fluidizers concomitantly normalizing some of the impaired membrane functions originating from the decrease in membrane lipid fluidity. These observations suggest that certain diseases that are parallelled by increases in membrane microviscosity may be therapeutically approached at the level of the membrane lipid fluidity of the cells that are involved in the disease process. Likewise, it may be that part of the loss of plasticity of brain tissue in old age may effectively be counteracted by treatment with membrane fluidizers. Further research should address the efficacy of such treatment in improving brain function in the elderly.

References

Alberts, B., Bray, D., Lewis, J., Raff, M., Roberts, K. and Watson, J. D. (1983) *Molecular Biology of the Cell*, Garland Publ. Inc., New York, London, pp. 256–314.

Aloyo, V. J., Zwiers, H. and Gispen, W. H. (1982) B-50 protein kinase and kinase C in rat brain. In W. H. Gispen and A. Routtenberg (Eds.), *Brain Phosphoproteins: Characterization and Function, Progress in Brain Research, Vol. 56*, Elsevier Biomedical Press, Amsterdam, pp. 303–315.

Aloyo, V. J., Zwiers, H. and Gispen, W. H. (1983) Phosphorylation of B-50 protein by calcium-activated, phospholipid-dependent protein kinase and B-50 protein kinase. *J. Neurochem.*, 41: 649–653.

Andersen, P., Sunderberg, S. H., Sveen, O. and Wigstrøm, H. (1977) Specific-long-lasting potentiation of synaptic transmission in hippocampal slices. *Nature (Lond.)*, 266: 736–737.

Baudry, M. and Lynch, G. (1979) Regulation of glutamate receptors by cations. *Nature (Lond.)*, 282: 748–750.

Berridge, M. J. (1983) Rapid accumulation of inositol trisphosphate reveals that agonists hydrolyse polyphosphoinositides instead of phosphatidylinositol. *J. Biochem.*, 212: 849–858.

Berridge, M. J. and Irvine, R. F. (1984) Inositol trisphosphate, a novel second messenger in cellular signal transduction. *Nature (Lond.)*, 312: 315–321.

Bliss, T. V. P. (1979) Synaptic plasticity in the hippocampus. *Trends Neurosci.*, 2: 42–45.

Bliss, T. V. P. and Dolphin, A. C. (1982) What is the mechanism of long-term potentiation in the hippocampus? *Trends Neurosci.*, 5: 289–290.

Browning, M., Baudry, M. and Lynch, G. (1982) Evidence that high frequency stimulation influences the phosphorylation of pyruvate dehydrogenase and that the activity of this enzyme is linked to mitochondrial calcium sequestration. In W. H. Gispen and A. Routtenberg (Eds.), *Brain Phosphoproteins: Characterization and Function, Progress in Brain Research, Vol. 56*, Elsevier Biomedical Press, Amsterdam, pp. 317–338.

Chang, F. L. F. and Greenough, W. T. (1984) Transient and enduring morphological correlates of synaptic and efficacy change in the rat hippocampal slices. *Brain Res.*, 309: 35–46.

Cimino, M., Vantini, G., Algeri, S., Curatla, G., Pezzoli, C. and Stramentinoli, G. (1984) Age-related modification of dopaminergic and β-adrenergic receptor system: restoration to normal activity by modifying membrane fluidity with S-adenosylmethionine. *Life Sci.*, 34: 2029–2039.

Cockcroft, S., Gomperts, B. D. (1985) Role of the guanine nucleotide binding protein in the activation of polyphosphoinositide phosphodiesterase. *Nature*, 314: 536–543.

De Graan, P. N. E., Van Hooff, C. O. M., Tilly, B. C., Oestreicher, A. B., Schotman, P. and Gispen, W. H. (1985a)

Phosphoprotein B-50 in nerve growth cones from fetal rat brain. *Neurosci. Lett.*, 61: 235–241.

De Graan, P. N. E., Lopes da Silva, F. H. and Gispen, W. H. (1985b) The role of hippocampal phosphoproteins in long-term potentiation. In R. L. Isaacson and K. H. Pribram (Eds.), *The Hippocampus, Vol. 3*, Plenum Press, New York, in press.

Desmond, N. L. and Levy, W. B. (1983) Synaptic correlates of associative potentiation/depression: an ultrastructural study in the hippocampus. *Brain Res.*, 265: 21–30.

Dolphin, A. C. (1983) The excitatory amino acid antagonist γ-D-glutamylglycine masks rather than prevents long-term potentiation of the perforant path. *Neuroscience*, 10: 377–383.

Dolphin, A. C., Errington, M. L. and Bliss, T. V. P. (1982) Long-term potentiation of the perforant path in vivo is associated with increased glutamate release. *Nature (Lond.)*, 297: 496–498.

Downes, C. P. and Michell, R. H. (1982) Phosphatidylinositol 4-phosphate and phosphatidylinositol-4,5-biphosphate: lipids in search of a function. *Cell Calcium*, 3: 467–502.

Dunwiddie, T., Madison, D. and Lynch, G. (1978) Synaptic transmission is required for initiation of long-term potentiation. *Brain Res.*, 150: 413–417.

Eccles, J. C. (1983) Calcium in long-term potentiation as a model for memory. *Neuroscience*, 10: 1071–1081.

Eichberg, J. and Hauser, G. (1969) Polyphosphoinositide biosynthesis in developing rat brain homogenates. *Ann. NY Acad. Sci.*, 165: 784–789.

Fifková, E. and Van Harreveld, A. (1977) Long-lasting morphological changes in dendritic spines of dentate granular cells following stimulation of the entorhinal area. *J. Neurocytol.*, 6: 211–230.

Gispen, W. H. and Routtenberg, A. (Eds.) (1982) *Brain Phosphoproteins: Characterization and Function, Progress in Brain Research, Vol. 56*, Elsevier Biomedical Press, Amsterdam.

Gispen, W. H., Van Dongen, C. J., De Graan, P. N. E., Oestreicher, A. B. and Zwiers, H. (1985a) The role of phosphoprotein B-50 in phosphoinositide metabolism in brain synaptic plasma membranes. In J. E. Bleasdale, G. Hauser and J. Eichberg (Eds.), *Inositol and Phosphoinositides*, Humana Press, Dallas, pp. 399–413.

Gispen, W. H., Leunissen, J. L. M., Oestreicher, A. B., Verkleij, A. J. and Zwiers, H. (1985b) Presynaptic localization of B-50 phosphoprotein: the ACTH sensitive protein kinase substrate involved in rat brain polyphosphoinositide metabolism. *Brain Res.*, 328: 381–385.

Gonzalez-Sastre, F., Eichberg, J. and Hauser, G. (1971) Metabolic pools of polyphosphoinositides in rat brain. *Biochim. Biophys. Acta*, 248: 96–104.

Gower, H. and Rodnight, R. (1982) Intrinsic protein phosphorylation in synaptic plasma membrane fragments from the rat. *Biochim. Biophys. Acta*, 716: 45–52.

Heron, D. S., Shinitzky, M., Hershkowitz, M. and Samuel, D. (1980) Lipid fluidity markedly modulates the binding of serotonin to mouse brain membranes. *Proc. Natl. Acad. Sci. USA*, 77: 7463–7467.

Heron, D. S., Shinitzky, M. and Samuel, D. (1982) Alleviation of drug withdrawal symptoms by treatment with a potent mixture of natural lipids. *Eur. J. Pharmacol.*, 83: 253–263.

Hershkowitz, M. (1983) Mechanisms of brain aging — the role of membrane fluidity. *Dev. Neurol.*, 7: 85–99.

Hershkowitz, M. (1985) Press Release, The Weizmann Institute of Science, Rehovot, Israel, June 9, 1985.

Hershkowitz, M., Heron, D., Samuel, D. and Shinitzky, M. (1982) The modulation in synaptic protein phosphorylation and receptor binding in synaptic membranes by changes in lipid fluidity: implications for ageing. In W. H. Gispen and A. Routtenberg (Eds.), *Brain Phosphoproteins: Characterization and Function, Progress in Brain Research, Vol. 56*, Elsevier Biomedical Press, Amsterdam, pp. 419–434.

Hirata, F. and Axelrod, G. (1978) Enzymatic methylation of phosphatidylethanolamine increases erythrocyte membrane fluidity. *Nature (Lond.)*, 275: 219–220.

Hokin, M. R. and Hokin, L. E. (1954) Effects of acetylcholine on phospholipids in the pancreas. *J. Biol. Chem.*, 209: 549–558.

Holmes, H. and Rodnight, R. (1981) Ontogeny of membrane-bound protein phosphorylating systems in the rat. *Dev. Neurosci.*, 4: 79–88.

Inoue, M., Kishimoto, A., Takai, Y. and Nishizuka, Y. (1977) Studies on a cyclic nucleotide-independent protein kinase and its proenzyme in mammalian tissues. *J. Biol. Chem.*, 252: 7610–7616.

Jolles, J., Wirtz, K. W. A., Schotman, P. and Gispen, W. H. (1979) Pituitary hormones influence polyphosphoinositide metabolism in rat brain. *FEBS Lett.*, 105: 110–114.

Jolles, J., Zwiers, H., Van Dongen, C. J., Schotman, P., Wirtz, K. W. A. and Gispen, W. H. (1980) Modulation of brain polyphosphoinositide metabolism by ACTH-sensitive protein phosphorylation. *Nature (Lond.)*, 286: 623–625.

Jolles, J., Zwiers, H., Dekker, A., Wirtz, K. W. A. and Gispen, W. H. (1981a) Corticotropin-(1-24)-tetracosapeptide affects protein phosphorylation and polyphosphoinositide metabolism in rat brain. *Biochem. J.*, 194: 283–291.

Jolles, J., Bär, P. R. and Gispen, W. H. (1981b) Modulation of brain polyphosphoinositide metabolism by ACTH and beta-endorphin: structure-activity studies. *Brain Res.*, 224: 315–326.

Jork, R., De Graan, P. N. E., Van Dongen, C. J., Zwiers, H., Matthies, H. and Gispen, W. H. (1984) Dopamine-induced changes in protein phosphorylation and polyphosphoinositide metabolism in rat hippocampus. *Brain Res.*, 291: 73–81.

Katz, F., Ellis, L. and Pfenninger, K. H. (1985) Nerve growth cones isolated from fetal rat brain. III. Calcium-dependent protein phosphorylation. *J. Neurosci.*, 5: 1402–1411.

Kishimoto, A., Takai, Y., Mori, T., Kikkawa, U. and

Nishizuka, V. (1980) Activation of calcium and phospholipid-dependent protein kinase by diacylglycerol, its possible relation to phosphatidyl-inositol turnover. *J. Biol. Chem.*, 255: 2273–2276.

Kristjansson, G. I., Zwiers, H., Oestreicher, A. B. and Gispen, W. H. (1982) Evidence that the synaptic phosphoprotein B-50 is localized exclusively in nerve tissue. *J. Neurochem.*, 39: 371–378.

Krnjevic, K. (1974) Chemical nature of synaptic transmission in vertebrate. *Physiol. Res.*, 54: 418–540.

Kuo, J. F., Andersson, R. G. G., Wise, B. C., Mackerlova, L., Salomonsson, I., Brackett, M. L., Katoh, N., Shoji, M. and Wrenn, R. W. (1980) Calcium-dependent protein kinase: widespread occurrence in various tissues and phyla of the animal kingdom and comparison of effects of phospholipid, calmodulin and trifluoperazine. *Proc. Natl. Acad. Sci. USA*, 77: 7039–7043.

Landfield, P. W. (1983) Mechanisms of altered normal function during aging. *Dev. Neurol.*, 7: 51–71.

Landfield, P. W., Braun, L. D., Pitler, T. A., Lindsey, J. D. and Lynch, G. (1981) *Neurobiol. Aging*, 2: 265.

Lee, K. S., Schottler, F., Oliver, M. and Lynch, G. (1980) Brief bursts of high-frequency stimulation produce two types of structural change in rat hippocampus. *J. Neurophysiol.*, 44: 247–258.

Lee, K. S., Oliver, M., Schottler, F. and Lynch, G. (1981) Electron microscopic studies of brain slices: the effect of high-frequency stimulation on dendritic ultrastructure. In G. Kerkut and H. V. Wheal (Eds.), *Electrical Activity in Isolated Mammalian C.N.S. Preparations*, Academic Press, New York, pp. 189–212.

Lopes da Silva, F. H., Bär, P. R., Tielen, A. M. and Gispen, W. H. (1982a) Plasticity in synaptic transmission and changes of membrane-bound protein phosphorylation. In R. M. Buys, P. Pévet and D. F. Swaab (Eds.), *Chemical Transmission in the Brain, Progress in Brain Research, Vol. 55*, Elsevier Biomedical Press, Amsterdam, pp. 369–377.

Lopes da Silva, F. H., Bär, P. R., Tielen, A. M. and Gispen, W.H. (1982b) Changes in membrane phosphorylation correlates with long-lasting potentiation in rat hippocampal slices. In W. H. Gispen and A. Routtenberg (Eds.), *Brain Phosphoproteins: Characterization and Function, Progress in Brain Research, Vol. 56*, Elsevier Biomedical Press, Amsterdam, pp. 339–345.

Lynch, G. S. and Baudry, M. (1984) The biochemistry of memory: a new and specific hypothesis. *Science*, 224: 1057–1063.

Lynch, G. S., Dunwiddie, T. and Gribkoff, V. (1977) Heterosynaptic depression: a post-synaptic correlate to long-term potentiation. *Nature (Lond.)*, 266: 737–739.

Lynch, M., Errington, M. L. and Bliss, T. V. P. (1984) Sustained increase in release of endogenous glutamate associated with long-term potentiation of the perforant path in the anaesthetized rat. *Neurosci. Lett.*, Suppl. 18, S194.

Mahler, H. R., Kleine, L. P., Ratner, N. and Sörensen, R. G. (1982) Identification and topography of synaptic phosphoproteins. In W. H. Gispen and A. Routtenberg (Eds.), *Brain Phosphoproteins: Characterization and Function, Progress in Brain Research, Vol. 56*, Elsevier Biomedical Press, Amsterdam, pp. 27–48.

Michell, R. H. (1975) Inositol phospholipids and cell surface receptor function. *Biochim. Biophys. Acta*, 415: 81–148.

Michell, R. H. and Kirk, C. J. (1981) Why is phosphatidylinositol degraded in response to stimulation of certain receptors? *Trends Pharmacol. Sci.*, 2: 86–89.

Nestler, E. G. and Greengard, P. (1983) Protein phosphorylation in the brain. *Nature (Lond.)*, 305: 583–588.

Nestler, E. G. and Greengard, P. (1984) *Protein Phosphorylation in the Nervous System*, John Wiley and Sons Ltd., New York.

Nishizuka, Y. (1980) Three multifunctional protein kinase systems in transmembrane control. *Mol. Biol. Biochem. Biophys.*, 32: 113–135.

Nishizuka, Y. (1983) Phospholipid degradation and signal translation for protein phosphorylation. *TIBS*, 8: 13–16.

Nishizuka, Y. (1984a) The role of protein kinase C in cell surface signal transduction and tumor promotion. *Nature (Lond.)*, 308: 693–697.

Nishizuka, Y. (1984b) Turnover of inositol phospholipids and signal transduction. *Science*, 1365–1370.

Oestreicher, A. B. and Gispen, W. H. (1986) Comparison of the immunocytochemical distribution of the phosphoprotein B-50 in the cerebellum and hippocampus of immature and adult rat brain. *Brain Res.*, 375: 267–269.

Oestreicher, A. B., Zwiers, H., Schotman, P. and Gispen, W. H. (1981) Immunohistochemical localization of a phosphoprotein (B-50) isolated from rat brain synaptosomal plasma membranes. *Brain Res. Bull.*, 6: 145–153.

Oestreicher, A. B., Zwiers, H., Gispen, W. H. and Roberts, S. (1982) Characterization of infant rat cerebral cortical membrane proteins phosphorylated in vivo: identification of the ACTH-sensitive phosphoprotein B-50. *J. Neurochem.*, 39: 683–692.

Oestreicher, A. B., Van Dongen, C. J., Zwiers, H. and Gispen, W. H. (1983a) Affinity-purified anti-B-50 protein antibody: Interference with the function of the phosphoprotein B-50 in synaptic plasma membranes. *J. Neurochem.*, 41: 331–340.

Oestreicher, A. B., Zwiers, H., Leunissen, J. L. M., Verkleij, A. J. and Gispen, W. H. (1983b) Localization of B-50 in rat brain studied by immuno light and electron microscopy. *J. Neurochem.*, Suppl. 41, S95.

Oestreicher, A. B., Dekker, L. V. and Gispen, W. H. (1985) A radioimmunoassay (RIA) for the phosphoprotein B-50: distribution in rat brain. *Neurosci. Lett.*, Suppl. 22, S560.

Pfenninger, K. H., Ellis, L., Johnson, H. P., Friedman, L. and Somlo, S. (1983) Nerve growth cones isolated from fetal rat brain: subcellular fractionation and characterization. *Cell*, 35: 573–584.

Prentki, M., Biden, T. J., Janjic, D., Irvine, R. F., Berridge, M. J. and Wollheim, C. B. (1984) Rapid mobilization of Ca^{2+} from rat insulinoma microsomes by inositol-1,4,5-trisphosphate. *Nature (Lond.)*, 309: 562–564.

Roth, G. S., Henry, J. M. and Joseph, J. A. (1986) The striatal dopaminergic system as a model for modulation of altered neurotransmitter action during aging: effects of dietary and neuroendocrine manipulations. In D. F. Swaab, E. Fliers, M. Mirmiran, W. A. Van Gool and F. P. A. J. Van Haren (Eds.), *Aging of the Brain and Alzheimer's Disease, Progress in Brain Research, this volume*, Elsevier Biomedical Press, Amsterdam, pp. 473–484.

Rouser, G., Kitchensky, G., Yamamoto, A. and Baxter, C. F. (1972) Lipids in the nervous system of different species as a function of age: brain, spinal cord peripheral nerves, purified whole cell preparations and subcellular particulates: regulatory mechanisms and membrane structure. *Adv. Lipid Res.*, 10: 26–360.

Routtenberg, A. (1982) Brain phosphoproteins and behavioral state. In W. H. Gispen and A. Routtenberg (Eds.), *Brain Phosphoproteins: Characterization and Function, Progress in Brain Research, Vol. 56*, Elsevier Biomedical Press, Amsterdam, pp. 349–374.

Routtenberg, A., Lovinger, D. M. and Steward, P. (1985) Selective increase in phosphorylation state of a 47 kDa protein (F$_1$) directly related to long-term potentiation. *Behav. Neural Biol.*, 43: 3–11.

Salway, J. G., Harwood, J. L., Kai, M., While, G. L. and Hawthorne, J. N. (1968) Enzymes of phosphoinositide metabolism during rat brain development. *J. Neurochem.*, 15: 221–226.

Shaik, N. A. and Palmer, F. B. St. C. (1976) Deposition of lipids in the developing central and peripheral nervous systems of the chicken. *J. Neurochem.*, 26: 597–603.

Shinitzky, M. (1984) Membrane fluidity in malignancy: adversative and recuperative. *Biochim. Biophys. Acta*, 738: 251–261.

Shinitzky, M. and Henkart, P. (1979) Fluidity of cell membranes: current concepts and trends. *Int. Rev. Cytol.*, 60: 121–147.

Skrede, K. K. and Malthe-Sörensen, D. (1981) Increased resting and evoked release of transmitter following repetitive electrical tetanization in hippocampus: a biochemical correlate to long-lasting synaptic potentiation. *Brain Res.*, 208: 436–441.

Sörensen, R. G., Kleine, L. P. and Mahler, H. R. (1981) Presynaptic localization of phosphoprotein B-50. *Brain Res. Bull.*, 7: 57–61.

Takai, Y., Kishimoto, A., Iwasa, Y., Kawahara, Y., Mori, T.

and Nishizuka, Y. (1979a) Calcium-dependent activation of a multifunctional protein kinase by membrane phospholipids. *J. Biol. Chem.*, 254: 3692–3695.

Takai, Y., Kishimoto, A., Iwasa, Y., Kawahara, Y., Mori, T., Nishizuka, Y., Tamura, A. and Fukii, T. (1979b) A role of membranes in the activation of a new multifunctional protein kinase system. *Biochem. J.*, 86: 575–578.

Teyler, T. J. and Discenna, P. (1984) Long-term potentiation as a cardiate mesmonic device. *Brain Res. Rev.*, 7: 15–28.

Tielen, A. M., Mollenvanger, W. J., Lopes da Silva, F. H. and Hollander, C. F. (1983) Neuronal plasticity in hippocampal slices of extremely old rats. *Dev. Neurol.*, 7: 73–83.

Uma, S. and Ramakrishnan, C. V. (1983) Studies on polyphosphoinositides in developing rat brain. *J. Neurochem.*, 40: 914–916.

Van Dongen, C. J., Hershkowitz, M., Zwiers, H., De Laat, S. and Gispen, W. H. (1983) Lipid fluidity and phosphoinositide metabolism in rat brain membranes of aged rats: effects of ACTH (1-24). *Dev. Neurol.*, 7: 101–114.

Van Dongen, C. J., Zwiers, H. and Gispen, W. H. (1984) Purification and partial characterization of the phosphatidylinositol 4-phosphate kinase from rat brain. *Biochem. J.*, 223: 197–203.

Van Dongen, C. J., Zwiers, H., De Graan, P. N. E. and Gispen, W. H. (1985) Modulation of the activity of purified phosphatidylinositol 4-phosphate kinase by phosphorylated and dephosphorylated B-50 protein. *Biochem. Biophys. Res. Commun.*, 8: 1219–1227.

Voronin, L. L. (1983) Long-term potentiation in the hippocampus. *Neuroscience*, 10: 1051–1069.

Weller, M. (1979) *Protein Phosphorylation. The Nature, Function and Metabolism of Proteins, which contain covalently bound Phosphorus*, PION Ltd., London.

Wiegant, V. M., Zwiers, H., Schotman, P. and Gispen, W.H. (1978) Endogenous phosphorylation of rat brain synaptosomal plasma membranes in vitro: methodological aspects. *Neurochem. Res.*, 3: 443–453.

Zwiers, H., Veldhuis, D., Schotman, P. and Gispen, W. H. (1976) ACTH, cyclic nucleotides and brain protein phosphorylation in vitro. *Neurochem. Res.*, 1: 669–677.

Zwiers, H., Schotman, P. and Gispen, W. H. (1980) Purification and some characteristics of an ACTH-sensitive protein kinase and its substrate protein in rat brain membranes. *J. Neurochem.*, 34: 1689–1699.

Zwiers, H., Verhaagen, J., Van Dongen, C. J., De Graan, P. N. E. and Gispen, W. H. (1985) Resolution of rat brain synaptic phosphoprotein B-50 into multiple forms by two-dimensional electrophoresis: evidence for multi-site phosphorylation. *J. Neurochem.*, 44: 1083–1090.

Discussion

R. D. TERRY: Did the PAP reaction with anti-B-50 display a cytoplasmic or a plasma membrane localization of B-50 in the aged hippocampus?

W. H. GISPEN: Presently we cannot be sure about the exact localization of the B-50 in the hippocampus of aged rats. The data strongly suggest, however, that there occurs an age-related redistribution of B-50-like material over the life-span of the rat. Further ultra-localization experiments are necesssary before final conclusions can be drawn.

R. S. WILLIAMS: Is B-50 also on lysosome membranes? Could the apparently paradoxical increase in cytoplasmic staining with anti-B-50 in region CA3 of hippocampus in very old rats be due to lysosomal staining of lipofuscin pigment as it accumulates there in old age?

W. H. GISPEN: From what we know of the cellular distribution of B-50 in the adult rat brain using subcellular fractionation techniques, B-50 is primarily associated with cell and vesicle membranes and not found in fractions enriched in lysosomes (Sörensen et al., 1981; Kristjansson et al., 1982; Gispen et al., 1985b).

D. F. SWAAB: How can you explain the discrepancy between the drop in B-50 in the assay in the hippocampus of old animals and the accumulation of stained material in this structure as shown by immunocytochemistry?

W. H. GISPEN: The immunocytochemical techniques show profound effects of age on the regional distribution of B-50. However, the local accumulation of B-50 in or around hippocampal pyramidal cells is not in disagreement with a drop in total B-50 content of the whole hippocampus as measured by RIA.

T. SCHUURMAN: How can it be explained (theoretically) that with increased membrane fluidity some receptor types are more available in the membrane, whereas other receptors have a lower availability?

W. H. GISPEN: This depends on the structure and microenvironment of the receptor. Some are pulled out of the membrane, others stay inside with increasing fluidity. There is no general rule. Every receptor type has to be studied separately.

R. RAVID: How do you explain that the changes in fluidity and responses of membranes with age are purely restricted to the protein systems like B-50?

W. H. GISPEN: I do not think that the effect of changes in membrane lipid fluidity will be limited to proteins like B-50 in particular. As more will be known about the function of other membrane proteins more effects of changes in the microviscosity will become apparent as is already the case in many nonneuronal cell types.

J. KORF: Are the coupling proteins located inside the membrane as was shown in the presented models?

W. H. GISPEN: The exact localization of the proteins involved in the signal transduction is not entirely known. It seems reasonable, however, to assume that regulatory proteins that couple receptors to catalytic subunits at the inside of the membrane are in part inverted into the lipid bilayer. Therefore, it can be assumed that lipid fluidity may affect the function of such proteins.

References

Gispen, W. H., Leunissen, J. L. M., Oestreicher, A. B., Verkleij, A. J. and Zwiers, H. (1985b) Presynaptic localization of B-50 phosphoprotein: the ACTH sensitive protein kinase substrate involved in rat brain polyphosphoinositide metabolism. *Brain Res.*, 328: 381–385.

Kristjansson, G. I., Zwiers, H., Oestreicher, A. B. and Gispen, W. H. (1982) Evidence that the synaptic phosphoprotein B-50 is localized exclusively in nerve tissue. *J. Neurochem.*, 39: 371–378.

Sörensen, R. G., Kleine, L. P. and Mahler, H. R. (1981) Presynaptic localization of phosphoprotein B-50. *Brain Res. Bull.*, 7: 57–61.

D. F. Swaab, E. Fliers, M. Mirmiran, W. A. Van Gool and F. Van Haaren (Eds.)
Progress in Brain Research, Vol. 70.
© 1986 Elsevier Science Publishers B.V. (Biomedical Division)

CHAPTER 16

Aging and circadian rhythms

W. A. Van Gool and M. Mirmiran

Netherlands Institute for Brain Research, Amsterdam, The Netherlands

Introduction

Circadian rhythms, i.e. rhythmic changes with a periodicity of approximately 24 hours, can be observed in organisms ranging from protozoans to humans (Aschoff, 1981). The notion that these temporal variations are a significant dimension of biological organization has gained much support over the last decades. Pittendrigh (1960) emphasized the importance of the temporal dimension in stating that circadian rhythms are a fundamental feature of all living systems. This observation implicates that it is not sufficient to consider only spatial characteristics in biology (Halberg, 1960). As paraphrased by Edmunds (1983): the 'right' substance (e.g. a neurotransmitter) should not only be at the 'right' place in the 'right' amount, but all of this should also happen at the 'right' time. In addition to the classical concept of homeostasis, i.e. the maintenance of a constant internal milieu, it is now recognized that the functional integrity of living organisms also depends on the maintenance of intricate temporal relations between various oscillating variables at a cellular level as well as at the level of organs and organ-systems. Within this framework, Samis (1968) hypothesized that the gradual and progressive deterioration of functional potential, which is the ubiquitous hallmark of aging, is the result of the loss of co-ordination among the many interdependent oscillating systems. Furthermore, Pittendrigh and Daan (1974) contended, independently from Samis, that a decay of circadian organization may be involved in the

preprogrammed physiological deterioration that limits lifespan.

In this chapter these hypotheses are explored in the light of recent experimental data from both animal and human studies. Present knowledge about the circadian system and its organization will be summarized first. Thereafter, an overview will be given of chronobiological studies in which 'age' or 'dementia' has been treated as independent variable. Subsequently the relevance of taking circadian variations into account in gerontology is discussed, and finally an attempt is made to indicate possible fruitful future directions of research related to aging and circadian rhythms.

Circadian rhythms

General considerations

Rotations of the earth result in a periodically changing environment. In such an environment it would be inappropriate for an organism to retain its internal organization and its behavioral activity at a constant level (Aschoff, 1981; Moore-Ede et al., 1982). Being synchronized with changes in illumination, temperature and humidity for instance, circadian rhythms appear to be an optimal adaptation to environmental periodicity. The very stable light-dark cycle plays in fact an important role in the entrainment of circadian rhythms. Although a specific and constant phase relation between the solar day and these rhythms is maintained, circadian rhythms are not considered to be readily induced by the periodic changes in the environment. Numerous chronobiological studies in which the environmental conditions were rigorously controlled showed the majority of the 24-h rhythms to be endogenously controlled (cf. Aschoff, 1981). Recently, the circadian period of the *Neurospora crassa* conidiation rhythm has even been shown to be normal when the fungus was on a space mission (Sulzman et al., 1984). Thus the exogenous influence of the subtle 24-h fluctuations of many geophysical variables, which are difficult to control in experiments on earth, is not necessary for the expression of endogenous circadian rhythms.

Pittendrigh (1960) summarized the major empirical generalizations about circadian rhythms in stating that they are ubiquitous, endogenous, innate, precise, light-intensity dependent and that they occur at both cell and whole organism levels of organization. Examples of the latter are the highly stable and well-documented sleep-wakefulness and body temperature rhythms. Fluctuations in such global functions implicate that elaborate regulatory strategies would be necessary to counterbalance rhythmic processes in order to establish an absolutely non-rhythmic function, as Moore-Ede et al. (1982) pointed out in their comprehensive monograph. Such non-rhythmic functions are, in general, extremely rare and rhythms can be found in parameters ranging from the mitosis frequency in the pinna epidermis to the number of leucocytes in the blood. In this chapter we will mainly focus on various aspects of brain function which vary during the 24 h of the day. We will assume these rhythms to be endogenously controlled, rather than exogenously driven, although this has not yet been proven for every rhythm which will be referred to.

Circadian rhythms in neurobiology

Rhythmic variations of 'classical' neurotransmitters such as serotonin (Quay, 1964; Friedman and Walker, 1968; Scheving et al., 1968; Héry et al., 1972; Walker et al., 1980; Semba et al., 1984),

dopamine (Bobillier and Mouret, 1971; Cahill and Ehret, 1981), norepinephrine (Friedman and Walker, 1968; Manshardt and Wurtman, 1968; Reis et al., 1968; Cahill and Ehret, 1981; Semba et al., 1984; Aldegunde et al., 1984; Schweiger et al., 1985) and acetylcholine (Hanin et al., 1970; Mohan and Radha, 1977) have been documented in various areas of the brain. Levels of serotonin (Garrick et al., 1983), norepinephrine (Perlow et al., 1978), vasopressin, oxytocin, dynorphin (Perlow et al., 1982; Schwartz et al., 1983a; Reppert et al., 1981a, 1984) and melatonin (Reppert et al., 1981b) vary rhythmically in the cerebrospinal fluid (CSF). All these rhythms are possibly related to variations in synthesizing and degrading enzymes of the respective substances such as tyrosine hydroxylase, tyrosine aminotransferase (Cahill and Ehret, 1981), tryptophan hydroxylase (Kan et al., 1977; Cahill and Ehret, 1981), monoamine oxydase (Owasoyo et al., 1984), acetylcholine esterase (Mohan and Radha, 1977) and N-acetyltransferase (Klein and Weller, 1970; Binkley et al., 1973; Mefford et al., 1983).

In addition to circadian fluctuations in releasing factors controlling anterior pituitary hormone release, hypothalamic concentrations of neuroactive substances such as vasopressin (Kafka et al., 1983a; Noto et al., 1983), dynorphin (Przewlocki et al., 1983) bombesin, cholecystokinin, neurotensin, substance P, and vasoactive intestinal polypeptide, change periodically as well (Nicholson et al., 1983). Furthermore, Nicholson et al. (1983) showed that the basal release of cholecystokinin and neurotensin from the hypothalamus depends on the time of day, whereas release of substance P, bombesin, and vasopressin, only varied significantly with time in the presence of high concentrations of potassium. In addition to variations in content and release of neuroactive substances, significant periodic changes occur at the receptor site as well (Kafka et al., 1983b). At present, daily rhythms have been documented in the number of receptors for: acetylcholine (muscarine) (Kafka et al., 1983b), serotonin (Bruinink et al., 1983), epinephrine (α- and β-adrenergic) (Kafka et al., 1981, 1983b,

1985), dopamine (Kafka et al., 1983b; Naber et al., 1980), opioids (Kafka et al., 1983b; Naber et al., 1981), adenosines (Virus et al., 1984) and benzodiazepines (Kafka et al., 1983b, 1985). Recent data indicate that changes in muscarine receptors merely reflect circadian alterations in affinity of agonists for receptors rather than true changes in receptor density (Mash et al., 1985). A similar phenomenon may play a role at other receptor sites as well.

In addition to the obvious sleep-wakefulness cq. rest-activity rhythms, numerous other behavioral rhythms can be observed in both animals and humans. Some speculations have been made on correlations between these rhythms and the aforementioned variations in neuroactive substances. Daily vasopressin variations in the CSF were implicated in both the 24-h rhythm in retention of one-trial passive avoidance tasks (Reppert et al., 1981a; Schwartz et al., 1983a) and the rhythm in reproductive behavior in rats (Södersten et al., 1983). The latter behavioral rhythm has also been suggested to be linked to the melatonin rhythm (Tamarkin et al., 1985). Dopaminergic circadian rhythms were hypothesized to be connected to motor activity cycles (Bruinink et al., 1983) whereas opiate-receptor rhythms are considered to be consistent with rhythmicities in food intake (Kavaliers and Hirst, 1985), aversive thermal response, and morphine-induced analgesia (Kavaliers and Hirst, 1983).

In the context of aging and dementia it is interesting to note the circadian organization of performance efficiency. In animal experiments, retention of active and passive avoidance as well as retention following one-trial appetitive training was shown to vary with time of day (Holloway and Wansley, 1973a,b; Wansley and Holloway, 1975). Human performance on a variety of tasks is also subject to daily variations of significant magnitude. Time-of-day effects have been described for performance on serial reactions, calculation, vigilance, card- and letter-sorting tasks (Blake, 1967). The same holds true for recall of meaningful material (Folkard et al., 1977), digit span (cf. Folkard and

Monk, 1983), reaction time, information processing rate, and eye-hand tracking capacity (Freivalds et al., 1983). Circadian rhythms in human performance do not simply reflect sleep-wakefulness rhythms or the course of changes in arousal, nor do they all have the same relation to the time of day (Folkard and Monk, 1983). Desynchronization techniques showed that rhythms of alertness in humans may even, quite counter-intuitively, dissociate from the sleep-wakefulness rhythm (Folkard et al., 1985). Cognitively complex tasks such as verbal reasoning usually have shorter free-running periods than simple repetitive tasks (e.g. serial search), suggesting that they are under different oscillatory control (Monk et al., 1984).

Organization of circadian rhythms

For reasons which are to be discussed below, it is widely accepted that the suprachiasmatic nuclei (SCN) are a major component of the mammalian circadian system (Rusak and Zucker, 1979; Moore, 1983). The SCN display a distinct circadian rhythm in metabolic (Schwartz et al., 1980, 1983b) and electrophysiological activity, which is independent of their afferent connections or the ambient light-dark conditions (Inouye and Kawamura, 1979, 1982). Groos and Hendriks (1982) have shown this SCN rhythm in electrophysiological activity even to persist in *in vitro* explants, from which a periodically varying vasopressin release can be measured as well (Earnest and Sladek, 1984). These experiments suggest that the SCN may comprise an endogenous oscillator. A pacemaker function of the SCN is suggested by studies in which complete lesions of the SCN were shown to result in a loss of circadian rhythms in drinking and locomotor activity (Stephan and Zucker, 1972), sleep-wakefulness (Ibuka et al., 1975, Eastman et al., 1984), body temperature (Eastman et al., 1984), adrenal corticosterone (Moore and Eichler, 1972), and a number of adrenergic and benzodiazepine receptors (Kafka et al., 1985). Furthermore, *in vivo* stimulation of the SCN by electrical (Rusak and Groos, 1982) or pharmacological means such as carbachol (Zatz and Herkenham, 1981), or neuropeptide Y (Albers and Ferris, 1984), results in phase shifts of overt behavioral rhythms.

The entrainment of the circadian pacemaker inside the SCN is mediated by a light-responsive subpopulation of cells in these nuclei. Groos and Mason (1980) have shown that these cells have characteristics which are consistent with such a function; that is, they appear to be specialized for luminance coding rather than for image processing (cf. Groos and Meijer, 1985). Visual information reaches the SCN via both the direct retino-hypothalamic projection (Moore, 1973) and a retinofugal projection, which reaches the SCN mainly via the intergeniculate leaflet of the ventral lateral geniculate (Pickard, 1982, 1985). The latter projection appears to comprise neuropeptide Y containing fibers (Harrington et al., 1984). A possible role for this projection in entrainment is suggested by studies in which direct release of neuropeptide Y in the SCN (Albers and Ferris, 1984) or electrical stimulation of the intergeniculate leaflet (Meijer et al., 1984) resulted in phase shifts of the circadian cycle. The retino-hypothalamic projection itself, however, appears to be sufficient for entrainment, since bilateral lesions of the lateral geniculate nucleus did not affect entrainment (Dark and Asdourian, 1975; Zucker et al., 1976).

At present, little is known about the way in which the SCN convey their driving influence upon regulatory mechanisms underlying respective overt circadian rhythms. It can be assumed that variations in neurotransmitter levels mentioned above, play a role in such a process. Circadian sleep-wakefulness rhythms can only be eliminated by circular cuts around the SCN or by selectively cutting the caudal SCN efferents to the median eminence (Yamaoka, 1978; cf. also Groos, 1983) while they are not affected by interruption of the SCN-pineal pathway nor by pinealectomy (Rusak and Zucker, 1979). The pineal gland is believed to be involved in mediating the effects of photoperi-

odic changes upon the reproductive cycle (Tamarkin et al., 1985).

Although the SCN are commonly accepted as a major part of the circadian system, they are not generally considered to represent the exclusive, singular clock controlling circadian rhythms. Phenomena such as internal desynchronization between various rhythms, as described in humans under conditions of temporal isolation (Aschoff, 1965; Wever, 1979), splitting into different components of temperature rhythms (Fuller et al., 1979), and desynchronization between circadian temperature and activity rhythms in squirrel monkeys (Gander et al., 1985), indicate that the SCN do not comprise the only oscillator in mammals (Moore-Ede, 1983). This notion is also supported by experiments in which SCN lesions have been shown not to abolish food anticipatory rhythms in rats (Stephan, 1981), body temperature rhythms in squirrel monkeys (Fuller et al., 1981), and cortisol rhythms in rhesus monkeys (Reppert et al., 1981b). The localization of the other putative oscillator(s), however, is at present not known (Moore-Ede, 1983). The SCN encompass one functional unity essential for the manifestation of many overt circadian rhythms and for the entrainment of these rhythms to the light-dark cycle. Furthermore, they appear to orchestrate other putative oscillators into synchrony.

Aging and circadian rhythms

Animal studies

Recently, Ingram et al. (1982) extensively reviewed the literature on age-related changes in circadian rhythms in laboratory animals. They concluded that circadian rhythmicity is disrupted with aging at various levels of biological organization. The amplitude of the circadian temperature rhythm (Halberg et al., 1955, 1981; Sacher and Duffy, 1978; Yunis et al., 1974) and the amplitude of adrenal corticosterone (Nicolau and Milcu, 1977), serum testosteron (Miller and Riegle, 1982; Simpkins et al., 1981), thyroid-stimulating hormone

(Klug and Adelman, 1979) and melatonin rhythms (Reiter et al., 1981; Tang et al., 1985) are all reduced in senior rats. Variations in plasma progesterone (Simpkins et al., 1981) and corticosterone (Oxenkrug et al., 1984), however, have been reported to be increased in old male rats. Reduced light-dark activity differences have been described in a variety of genetically different strains of aged rats and mice (Peng et al., 1980; Sacher and Duffy, 1978; Wax, 1975; Mosko et al., 1980; Yehuda and Carasso, 1983; Martin et al., 1986; Welsh et al., 1985). Day-night variations in spontaneous, morphine-induced and naloxone-suppressed consummatory behavior also appear to decrease with age (Jakubczak, 1975; Mosko et al., 1980; Peng et al., 1980; Kavaliers and Hirst, 1985), and Peng and Kang (1984) reported even a complete loss of circadian rhythmicity for wheel-running activity in two out of 11 old rats, for feeding behavior in six out of 10, and for drinking behavior in one out of six old rats. Normal light-dark ratios for these three types of behavior were found in all the young control rats. Furthermore, magnitudes of diurnal variations in aversive thresholds and morphine-induced analgesia in mice were both shown to be markedly reduced with aging by Kavaliers et al. (1984).

Long-term sleep-wakefulness recordings in old rats reveal a reduction in the amount of time spent in slow wave sleep (SWS) and desynchronized sleep (DS; i.e. rapid eye movement sleep) (Rosenberg et al., 1979; Van Gool and Mirmiran, 1983; Van Gool and Mirmiran, 1986). Even though the amount of DS over 24 h is clearly reduced, old rats show significantly *more* DS during the first hours of the dark period (Fig. 1). During that short period of the day the aged circadian system seems to overrule the reduced DS-tendency of old rats. The senescence-related reduction of circadian fluctuations in rats is significant for DS, SWS as well as wakefulness, as quantified by a mean-adjusted amplitude measure (Van Gool and Mirmiran, 1986). These findings are consistent with the reported reduction of light-dark ratios in locomotor, consummatory, temperature and endocrine rhythms.

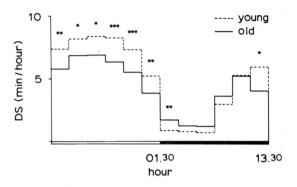

Fig. 1. Amounts of desynchronized sleep (DS) in blocks of 2 h throughout 24 h (12 h light and dark are indicated by the white and black bar, respectively). DS as a mean of 24 h is reduced in old rats ($n=26$, ages 27–31 months) in comparison with young rats ($n=36$, ages 4–7 months). As a result of the concomitant circadian rhythm amplitude reduction, however, old rats show *more* DS in the beginning of the dark period.

Alterations of light-dark ratios do not, of course, necessarily constitute evidence for alterations intrinsic to the circadian timekeeping system itself. For instance, Mistlberger et al. (1983) have pointed out that the amplitude of the circadian sleep-wakefulness rhythm in rats can also be dampened solely by a reduction of the maximum time spent asleep in the light period. Other basic needs such as feeding and drinking must be satisfied before sleep can be resumed, and they can, therefore, be considered to compete with the need for sleep. It is thus feasible that primary senescent changes in feeding and drinking homeostasis for instance, prohibit adequate amounts of sleep during the light period in old rats. A subsequent homeostatic sleep rebound during the dark period, resulting in a reduced light-dark ratio, should then not be taken to reflect senescent changes in the circadian system, but merely alterations in mechanisms regulating food or water intake. However, arguments in favor of interpreting the age-related changes in the light-dark ratios in terms of changes intrinsic to the circadian timekeeping system during aging can be presented.

Not only the amplitude but also another important characteristic of circadian rhythms, the period, appears to be changed in senescence as well. In a study initiated to elucidate the stability or lability of free-running pacemakers Pittendrigh and Daan (1974) recorded rest-activity rhythms in *Mesocricetus aureatus*, *Peromyscus maniculatus*, and *Peromyscus leucopus*. The freerunning period of the circadian pacemaker was determined with an interval of about 14 months in individual rodents. In this way the period of the circadian pacemaker was shown to become systematically shorter as the rodents aged in 21 out of the 25 animals used in their study (Pittendrigh and Daan, 1974). It was concluded that changes in circadian organization may be an important concomitant of aging. In a later study by the same investigators old mice (*Mus musculus*) also tended to have shorter freerunning periods than young mice, although this intergroup difference did not reach statistical significance, which was attributed to the small sample size and the range of interindividual variation (Pittendrigh and Daan, 1976). Wax (1977) also observed circadian period changes with aging, but in her cross-sectional study, in which mice of different ages were allowed to select their own light-dark schedules, an increase in the length of the circadian period was found. There appeared to be no conspicuous age effect on circadian period length in cockroaches (*Lecophaea maderiae*) (Page and Block, 1980), sparrows (*Passer domesticus*) (Eskin, 1971), ground squirrels (*Ammospermophilus leucurus*), or in kangeroo rats (*Dipodomys merriami*) (Kenagy, 1978). Wax's study allowed for analysis of interactions between the genetic background of the mice strains and the age-related changes in various behavioral rhythms. It was concluded that genetic differences diminish with age, and that the data support the concept of enhanced desynchronization between various rhythms in old age. In discussing the discrepancy with the data of Pittendrigh and Daan (1974), Wax (1977) pointed to differences in the species and relative ages of the animals selected for study, and, perhaps most important: to the differences in experimental procedure (longitudinal vs. cross-sectional; recording of rest-activity vs. light-dark selection rhythms). To our knowledge there are only two other longitudinal studies in which the period length of a free-running rhythm was studied in relation to age. Similar to Pittendrigh and Daan, Rietveld et al. (1985) made long-term recordings in individual animals of a free-running behavioral rhythm. In accordance with the findings of Pittendrigh and Daan, registrations of food intake of — initially — 12 albino rats, revealed a systematic decrease of the circadian period length in the four rats that were still alive after 26 months. A 1-year-long record of locomotor activity made in a blind hamster by Davis and Menaker (1980) also showed a gradual and consistent shortening of the period of the pacemaker underlying this circadian rhythm.

Age-related changes in the sensitivity to light may explain the reduced light-dark ratios of overt circadian variations, since Wax (1977) found the magnitude of age-related differences to be dependent on the level of illumination. Changed sensory capacities or altered sensitivity to subtle environmental changes may therefore play a role in the observed amplitude changes of biological rhythms in old age. Alleged visual impairments can, however, not readily account for the shortening of the period of free-running rhythms, observed in constant darkness (Pittendrigh and Daan, 1974) and in blinded animals (Davis and Menaker, 1980; Rietveld et al., 1985). Neither can the combination of changes in period length and reductions of circadian amplitude easily be reconciled with the idea that only the coupling between the central pacemaker(s) and overt rhythms is impaired in old age. Reductions in circadian fluctuations have been reported for endocrine, temperature, sleep-wakefulness, as well as for various other behavioral rhythms. Although these rhythms may not all be completely independent, they are probably not linked to the central pacemaker through a single, common effector pathway. Therefore, identical changes of the coupling between the central pacemaker(s) and the numerous effector mechanisms, resulting in similar changes in all the various overt rhythms, would have to be hypothesized in order to explain the generality of the finding of altered light-dark ratios in senescence. Such concerted changes in different effector pathways are not very likely to occur. At present it seems, therefore, more reasonable to suspect that some central part of the circadian timekeeping system has been changed in old age.

Unfortunately, little is known about the central nervous system (CNS) correlates of the senescence-related changes in circadian rhythms. Mohan and Radha (1977) have reported that the relative amplitude variation of the acetylcholine level is reduced in the cerebrum and cerebellum of old rats, and increased in the superior colliculi. Walker (1980) related the arrest of estrous cycles in aged female rats to the lack of a circadian rhythm of serotonin content in the hypothalamus. Age-associated reductions in hypothalamic catecholamine content have also been implicated in altered circadian patterns of gonadotropin secretion (Bremner et al., 1983). Age-related changes in reproductive behavior coincide with histological and ultrastructural changes in the pineal gland (Bondareff, 1965; Johnson, 1980; Allen et al., 1982; Boya and Calvo, 1984). These morphological findings in aged rats are accompanied by marked reductions of the nocturnal pineal melatonin concentration (Reiter et al., 1981; Hoffmann et al., 1985), the pineal β-adrenergic receptor density (Greenberg and Weis, 1978) and the oxygen consumption of *in vitro* pineal explants (Walker, 1978). Furthermore, Tang et al. (1985) have shown that light-dark ratios for the pineal serotonin and 5-hydroxyindoleacetic acid were not changed in old rats, whereas pineal dopamine and norepinephrine showed reduced light-dark ratios in senescence. Similarity between the circadian corticosterone rhythm in aged and pinealectomized rats was taken to indicate that age-related changes in the pineal structure and function are involutional (Oxenkrug et al., 1984).

At present there are no direct indications of senescence-related structural or functional changes in the SCN of experimental animals. Age-related reductions have not been found in the volume of the SCN in 31–33-months-old Brown-Norway rats

as compared to 6–8-months-old rats (Roozendaal et al., in preparation). In addition, the number of neurons in the SCN appears not to change significantly with age in Long-Evans rats (Peng et al., 1980). Only the moderately decreased vasopressin innervation of the dorsomedial hypothalamic nucleus (Fliers et al., 1985), which originates in the SCN (Hoorneman and Buijs, 1982), suggests changes in the SCN of old rats.

Human studies

Circadian rhythms have been extensively studied in humans under both entrained as well as free-running conditions. However, 'age' was only treated as an independent variable in a few studies. Probably the most thorough experiment was conducted by Weitzman et al. (1982), who studied young adult and elderly males (ages 23–30 and 53–70 years, respectively) living under conditions of temporal isolation for 3–8 weeks. The results of this study supported the idea that the neural substrate underlying circadian oscillations changes with age. In elderly subjects a decrease of both the amplitude and period of the body temperature rhythm was found, in contrast to Wever's (1979) results showing no significant correlation between age and period of the circadian temperature rhythm. Furthermore, Weitzman et al. (1982) showed an increase of the frequency and duration of arousals from sleep and, although no significant change of the period of the sleep-wake rhythm was found, the findings were consistent with survey data indicating that aging leads to a phase advance of the main sleep episode relative to clock time (Tune, 1969). Similar to Weitzman et al.'s (1982) data, reductions of the extent of temperature fluctuations were reported in various other studies (Scheving et al., 1974; Leutz, 1984), sometimes accompanied by indications of a phase advance of the circadian temperature rhythm (Leutz, 1984). Reinberg et al. (1980) showed, in a study on elderly oil refinery operators, that a low amplitude of the circadian temperature rhythm is associated with poor tolerance to shift-work. Recently Prinz et al.

(1984) reported the absence of apparent age effects on circadian temperature amplitude. The interpretation of this latter study, however, is hampered by the fact that temperature recordings were not made in young controls, but data from the literature served as the source of reference. Various other investigators (Cahn et al., 1968; Wever, 1979; Nicolau et al., 1983) reported to have made temperature recordings in elderly subjects as well, but unfortunately they did not report measures of amplitude of the rhythm systematically.

The age-related reduction of the circadian temperature rhythm as reported by Weitzman et al. (1982), Scheving et al. (1974) and Leutz (1984) coincides with a reduction or even a complete disappearance of the circadian rhythm amplitudes for the following hormones: aldosterone (Nelson et al., 1980; Cugini et al., 1982; Pasqualetti et al., 1983), renin (Pasqualetti et al., 1983), testosterone (Bremner et al., 1983), growth hormone (Carlson et al., 1972; Finkelstein et al., 1972; Murri et al., 1980), thyroid-stimulating hormone (Barreca et al., 1985), and estradiol (Nelson et al., 1980). Circadian variations of plasma epinephrine appear not to change with age, while a disproportionate night-time increase of norepinephrine levels in elderly subjects of 62–80 years of age correlated significantly with poor sleep (Prinz et al., 1979). Stern et al. (1984) also did not observe the nocturnal decrease of norepinephrine plasma level which is normal in young subjects. In addition, Iguchi et al. (1982) have reported a 85% reduction of the normal nocturnal increase of melatonin levels in a group of aged subjects, consistent with data from a study by Touitou et al. (1981).

The amplitude of the circadian plasma cortisol rhythm was also found to be decreased in subjects over 70 years of age (Milcu et al., 1978; Colucci et al., 1975). A tendency towards a complete disappearance of cortisol rhythms was noted in the four oldest subjects studied by Milcu et al. (1978) (ages 91–100). In addition to the reduction in amplitude, a phase advance of the peak cortisol level was also observed in the same study (Milcu et al., 1978), which is in agreement with recent findings showing

a significant negative correlation between age and time of the maximum, nadir, and acrophase of the cortisol circadian rhythm (Sherman et al., 1985). However, these data remain controversial since other groups reported no significant age-related changes in the circadian organization of adrenocortical function (Jensen and Blichert-Toft, 1971; Serio et al., 1970; Krieger et al., 1971; Colucci et al., 1975; Touitou, 1982; Prinz and Halter, 1983). The data on a possible phase advancement of the daily cortisol rhythm are consistent with findings of Lakatua et al. (1984), and should perhaps be related to the report of Nicolau et al. (1983) who studied circadian rhythms in 18 blood constituents in elderly, and also found indications of phase advancement in old age. Levels of luteinizing hormone and prolactin appear to show increased circadian variations in elderly subjects (Murri et al., 1980; Nelson et al., 1980), although prolactin levels did not appear to change in a study by Touitou (1982).

Other circadian rhythms which are changed in senescence are the urinary excretion of water and electrolytes (Lobban et al., 1963; Lobban and Tredre, 1967; Scheving et al., 1978) and the excretion of epinephrine and nor-epinephrine (Descovich et al., 1974). In a review of the chronobiology of aging, Casale and de Nicola (1984) state furthermore that senescence is accompanied by a loss of circadian rhythmicity for the leukocyte number, serum γ-glutamyltransferase, lactate dehydrogenase, choline esterase, ferritin and some lipid fractions which normally can be shown to exhibit circadian variations in adulthood.

The regular alternation of wakefulness and sleep is a key example of circadian rhythmicity. Sleep disorders in the elderly have, therefore, been suggested to be, at least in part, manifestations of changed circadian timekeeping in general, expressing itself as a temporal redistribution of sleep (Miles and Dement, 1980; Weitzman et al., 1982). In this section only the temporal patterning of sleep will be discussed; an extensive review of the literature on aging and all aspects of sleep can be found in a comprehensive monograph by Miles and Dement (1980). Sleep in old age can best be characterized by stating that elderly people show a reduced tendency to sleep at night and have more difficulty to remain awake during daytime. This observation can be taken to reflect a dampening of the circadian sleep-wakefulness rhythm. The reduced nocturnal sleep tendency in elderly is reflected in all-night polygraphic sleep recordings which reveal a reduced total sleep time (Feinberg and Carlson, 1968; Březinová, 1975; Webb, 1982a; Hayashi and Endo, 1982), an increased sleep latency (Feinberg et al., 1967; Hayashi and Endo, 1982; Webb and Schneider-Helmert, 1984), and an increase in both the number and duration of arousals from sleep (Agnew et al., 1967; Kahn and Fisher, 1969; Murri et al., 1980; Webb, 1982a,b; Bixler et al., 1984; Webb and Schneider-Helmert, 1984). The development of an objective measure of sleepiness at Stanford, i.e. the multiple sleep latency test allowed for the investigation of daytime sleepiness as a function of age. Carskadon et al. (1980) showed that the range of daytime sleep latencies in elderly would be considered pathological and associated with severe performance impairments in young subjects (cf. Miles and Dement, 1980). Various other reports show that the amount of daytime sleep is indeed high in the aged, as determined either by 24-h recordings (Prinz et al., 1982) or by subjective sleep reports (Tune, 1969; Webb et al., 1981). Of course, all of this does not necessarily imply that circadian rhythms are changed in aged humans, since daytime napping in old age, for instance, also may be merely the result of a reduced social pressure to stay awake (Tune, 1968; Webb and Swinburne, 1971; Wever, 1975). Increased wakefulness at night should thus perhaps be considered a simple homeostatic consequence of increased daytime sleep. Studies carried out under conditions of temporal isolation, in which also the social environment is controlled, could resolve this issue but, to our knowledge, only one of these studies has been carried out in subjects of different ages without reporting nap frequency or duration (Weitzman et al., 1982). However, the results from this study show that the excess of

arousals from nocturnal sleep in elderly subjects as compared with young subjects is preserved even when physical and social environmental cues are the same in both age groups, suggesting that, if increased nocturnal awakenings are indeed the result of increased daytime sleep, the young also nap less than the elderly when living under similar conditions. It thus appears that disturbed sleep at night and increased daytime sleep are not exclusively a reflection of changed social conditions in the aged. Zepelin, as cited by Miles and Dement (1980), has also reported that among men the number of daytime naps increases with age irrespective of the employment status. In women, however, nap tendency was negatively correlated with being full-time employed.

There are only a few systematic studies of circadian rhythms in dementia. Sleep patterns in elderly patients suffering from Alzheimer's disease (AD) are severely disturbed. A marked fragmentation of the diurnal sleep-wake pattern was found in AD in Prinz et al.'s (1982) study in which 24-h registrations were made in AD patients and age-matched controls. Daytime sleep showed about a 10-fold increase and nocturnal sleep was severely fragmented (e.g. 20 vs. 10 awakenings from sleep), while AD patients and controls had equal total amounts of sleep as measured over 24 h (Prinz et al., 1982). Although day-night cycles could still be recognized in the 24-h recordings made in hospitalized AD patients by Allen et al. (1983), numerous daytime naps occurred in the AD patients in this study as well. In accordance with these findings Feinberg et al. (1969) showed patients suffering from a 'chronic brain syndrome' to exhibit more and longer awakenings during nocturnal sleep than elderly in good health. Data from Loewenstein et al. (1982) suggest, however, that the decrements of AD sleep do not occur in less severely impaired and younger AD patients. Referring to unpublished observations of their own group, Casale and de Nicola (1984) state that circadian rhythms seem to be particularly affected in AD. However, not every parameter exhibiting a circadian rhythm is affected in AD. Gross changes in adrenocortical function (Sugai and Fujita, 1984) and nocturnal melatonin release (Touitou, 1982) do not appear to be associated with AD.

The amplitude of a circadian rhythm is believed to reflect directly the stability of such a rhythm (Wever, 1979). Changes in the amplitude of temperature, endocrine and sleep-wakefulness rhythms in old age, therefore, may represent alterations in circadian timekeeping. However, numerous factors, not necessarily related to the circadian rhythm itself but merely related to other aspects of aging, may influence overt rhythms in the elderly. For instance, increased nycturia in congestive heart failure, or sleep-related respiratory disturbances sometimes underly insufficient nocturnal sleep, thus inducing a homeostatic sleep rebound during the subsequent day. Altered light/dark ratios of sleep and wakefulness may therefore be indirectly related to various pathological states. Changes in the cardiorespiratory system however, cannot by themselves account for the generality of the finding of altered circadian rhythms. In analogy to animal experimental data, age-related changes have been described for hormonal, temperature, as well as behavioral rhythms in humans. Furthermore, not only amplitude measures are changed but also the period of the relatively stable oscillator underlying temperature rhythms is changed in aged humans (Weitzman et al., 1982). The fact that the internal synchronization of various circadian rhythms appears to be changed in addition to alterations in the respective rhythm itself, also points to the circadian rhythm generating system as the site of origin of age-related changes in overt rhythms. Dissociation of the normally observed intricate synchrony between various circadian rhythms seems to occur more frequently in the elderly (Cahn et al., 1968; Wever, 1979) and was shown to be associated with depression (Cahn et al., 1968), a state frequently observed in the aged.

The SCN are believed to encompass a functional unity which plays an important role in the generation, entrainment, and coordination of circadian rhythms. Recent immunocytochemical studies on the human hypothalamus by Swaab et al. (1985) (cf. Fliers and Swaab, 1986), therefore, point to a possible morphological correlate of the changed circadian rhythms in aging and AD. Total SCN cell number was reduced by 45% and 75% in old age and AD, respectively. It was noted that the alterations in the SCN occur at a later age than the changes in circadian rhythms. Thus, the observed cell loss may only be a late correlate of functional changes appearing much earlier (Swaab et al., 1985). This may also explain the negative findings with respect to morphological changes in the SCN of old rats reported so far (Peng et al., 1980).

Possible implications of circadian rhythm alterations in senescence

Methodological implications for gerontological studies

In addition to changes in many different functional systems themselves, temporal patterning as a principle of biological organization appears to be changed during aging and in AD. This imposes some special constraints upon research into these issues. In gerontology, time-of-day effects should not be taken into account for the sake of methodological sophistication per se. The comparison of variables subject to circadian variation can be carried out perfectly, even while the time dimension is ignored, if the temporal organization of the variable under study is identical in the populations that are compared. A large body of data reviewed in this paper suggests, however, that the functional characteristics of the circadian timekeeping system are markedly changed in aging and AD. For example, in Fig. 1 it is illustrated that old rats spent significantly more time in DS than young animals, at the beginning of the dark period. An experiment in which measurements would have been restricted to this short period of time would have arrived at conclusions which are not valid for the entire 24-h period. DS times are clearly reduced in old rats, although concomitant changes in temporal organization may suggest otherwise at some time points.

With respect to data on sleep and wakefulness or body temperature it is obvious that circadian variations should be taken into account. In studying variables of which circadian variations are less prominent or less known, such as for instance, levels of neuroactive substances in the brain or CSF, number of binding sites for various agonists, levels of hormones in plasma, or levels of performance, exactly the same difficulties may be encountered if measurements are taken at only one point in time. Studies treating 'age' or 'pathologic state' (AD) as independent variable commonly ignore this methodological implication of age-related changes in the circadian rhythm generating system. A perfect example of the confusion which can thus arise was given by Bremner et al. (1983), who demonstrated that the observation of significant age-related reductions of plasma testosterone levels in man depends on the time of day that samples are taken. Testosterone levels were higher in young men between 2 a.m. and 1 p.m, while during the rest of the day testosterone levels in young men did not differ significantly from those in the old. Thus, the controversy which existed in the literature on this issue (Harman and Tsitouras (1980) reporting no decrease in afternoon samples, while a clear-cut reduction of testosterone levels was found in morning samples of old men by Stearns et al. (1974), was solved. Nelson et al. (1980) suggested that the controversy with respect to age-related changes in serum prolactin levels should be attributed to a similar phenomenon, since prolactin levels only exhibit an age-related reduction between 10 a.m. and 4 p.m. Yet another example of this methodological pitfall was given by Pauly (1983). With data taken from the work of Halberg and colleagues it was illustrated that single time-point sampling could have resulted in the observation of either no difference with age, a significant increase or decrease of plasma aldosterone levels, depending on the time of sampling. This observation essentially represented a reduced circadian amplitude, since the 24-h mean of plasma aldosterone did not change with age (Pauly, 1983). It can therefore be concluded that it is imperative to include time-of-day effects when studying the effects of aging, since temporal patterning of the function of various systems appears to be changed in senescence, irrespective of possible changes in these functional systems themselves.

Speculations on the functional significance of circadian rhythm alterations

Alterations of circadian amplitude, period, phase position and synchrony were discussed in previous sections of the present paper. Even though some of these aging effects may be quantitatively small, it is conceivable that even subtle alterations (e.g. in phase relation or coordination between respective rhythms) may result in gross deleterious functional changes in an oscillating system (Pittendrigh and Daan, 1974). In this section possible functional consequences of age-related changes in circadian rhythms will be explored in a speculative way, without suggesting to present any sort of definitive argument.

Interestingly, the magnitude of the amplitude of the circadian activity rhythm is positively related to subsequent survival time in rats (Martin et al., 1986). Several experimenters have noticed that a, sometimes pronounced, circadian rhythm dissociation precedes death in rodents (Wax and Goodrick, 1978; Albers et al., 1981; Rietveld et al., 1985). Life expectancy in flies is shortened when they live in an environment with a non-24-h time structure. Pittendrigh and Minis (1972) reduced lifespan, as measured in days to 50% survival of the initial population, by about 5% to 18% when fruit flies (*Drosophila melanogaster*) were reared under constant light conditions or conditions simulating either a 21-h or 27-h day. Similar reductions of survival in non-24-h days can be observed in blowflies (*Phormia terranovae*) (Aschoff et al., 1971), and the lifespan of the rotifer (*Asplanchna brightwelli*) (Sawada and Enesco, 1984) is also sensitive to manipulation of the normal 24-h light-dark regimen. Disorder of the circadian system is believed to be a key factor for this shortening of life in blowflies (Von Saint Paul and Aschoff, 1978), since repeated phase shifts by advancing or delaying the onset of light have the same effect (Aschoff et al., 1971). Using various paradigms of phase shifting, Hayes and Cawley (1977) also found a significant reduction of lifespan in five out of seven experimental groups of codling moths (*Laspeyresia pomonella*). Thus, in various species there appears to be a relation between undisturbed circadian synchrony and survival.

Subjects suffering from circadian desynchronization may not only live shorter, but their level of performance may also be affected. In accordance with data of Davies et al. (1974), Tapp and Holloway (1981) reported that rats subjected to a phase shift of either +6, –6, or 12 h show profound performance deficits on retention of a passive avoidance task. Fekete et al. (1985) recently replicated and extended this work, showing that the performance deficit diminished gradually as a function of the time between the phase shift and the exposure to experimental contingencies. Furthermore, extinction of active avoidance behavior was facilitated by phase shifting, whereas social and explorative behavior were not conspicuously affected after the shifts. It was concluded, therefore, that disruption of circadian rhythms may induce retrograde amnesia without affecting innate behavioral patterns (Fekete et al., 1985). This contention could be studied in more detail by also using other strategies for interfering with normal circadian organization (e.g. SCN lesions) and by also testing in other behavioral paradigms, since the passive avoidance procedure has been shown not necessarily to be an adequate procedure to study memory processes (Van Haaren and Van de Poll, 1984).

The findings in animal studies with respect to the effects of phase shifts are in accordance with data obtained in aerospace medicine. Circadian desynchrony in humans caused by transmeridian flights is associated with deficits in reaction and decision times and with decrements in psychomotor performance (Hauty and Adams, 1966; Klein et al., 1972). Colquhoun (1984) described a statistically significant correlation between the degree of post-flight disruption of the temperature rhythm and the loss of performance speed on a calculation test. Susceptibility to phase shifts appears to be age-dependent: in a study on crews on long-haul transmeridian routes Preston (1973) showed that the older an airline pilot gets, the greater the cumulative sleep loss becomes. Worsening of health with increasing age is reported to be more pronounced in night-shift than in day workers, whereas investigations of cardiovascular, pulmonar, neurological and psychiatric disorders did not reveal direct negative effects of shiftwork (cf. Folkard et al., 1984). Increased industrial accidents have been considered as a possible consequence of shiftwork (Folkard et al., 1984), and there are some indications that the phase shift of millions of humans in spring after the light-saving time change affects levels of performance as well. Monk (1980) reported an increase of the number of traffic accidents as a possible indicant of circadian desynchrony after such a nationwide time shift in England. Data from Holland also show a tendency for the number of traffic casualties to be increased on the day following the 1-h phase shift in comparison to normal days (Fig. 2). Thus, as Moore-Ede et al. (1982) pointed out, presumably even small decrements in psychomotor performance as a result of circadian desynchrony can affect the outcome of traffic accidents in a negative way.

In an experiment not primarily designed to study age effects, a 79-years-old subject was shown to lack significant rhythmicity in two of three performance tests in contrast to the younger subjects (Monk et al., 1984). An indication of increased differences between the periods of the verbal reasoning rhythm and the sleep-wakefulness and temperature rhythm was noticed as well (Monk et al., 1984). It is tempting to speculate on possible relations between the performance deficits during aging and in AD and the changes of biological rhythms which accompany these conditions.

The correlations between circadian desynchronization and depression (Cahn et al., 1968) and between low amplitude of the circadian temper-

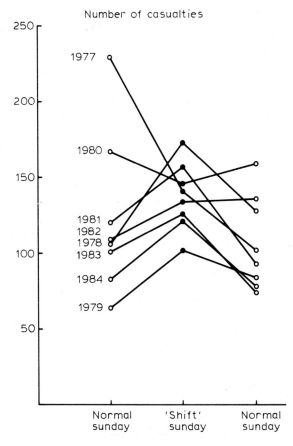

Fig. 2. Number of traffic casualties (ordinate) on three subsequent Sundays at the time of the light-saving time change in the years 1977–1984 (source: F. Mullenders, CBS, Heerlen The Netherlands). There is a tendency towards an increase in the number of traffic casualties on Sundays of the weekend in which the nation-wide 1-h phase-shift takes place. Eight 'shift' Sundays (●) tested against 16 pooled 'normal' Sundays (○) of the weeks immediately preceding or following the shift week, revealed: $p = 0.0537$ (Mann-Whitney test, groups 8/16, $U = 32.5$).

ature rhythm in elderly and poor tolerance to shift-work (Reinberg et al., 1980), point to other possible functional correlates of circadian rhythm alterations in senescence. Furthermore, Fuller et al. (1978) showed that internal desynchronization of circadian rhythms results in an impairment of body temperature homeostasis in squirrel monkeys. It was suggested that effective thermoregulation requires precise internal synchronization, thus indicating still another possible functional correlate of age-related changes in the circadian timekeeping system. Collins et al. (1977) confirmed in both a cross-sectional and longitudinal design, that the thermoregulatory capacity is markedly impaired in old people. The incidence of accidental hypothermia is indeed high in old age. In a series of 23 cases of hypothermia (< 32 degrees Celcius), all patients were over 55 years of age and in eight patients mental impairment or senility was diagnosed in addition to hypothermia (Duguid et al., 1961).

Practical implications for the clinical approach towards elderly and demented subjects

Most chronobiological experiments in gerontology have been purely descriptive. Thus, functional implications of disturbed circadian rhythmicity in senescence are not yet obvious. Practical consequences of changed circadian timekeeping for every-day life on geriatric wards can therefore only be suggested in a very tentative way. In this section it will, nevertheless, be attempted to draw some preliminary conclusions from basic research for the clinical approach towards geriatric patients.

A subject of major practical importance in this context may be the prescription of hypnotics among elderly. Survey data reveal that elderly frequently complain of 'insomnia'. Almost 90% of subjects aged 60–80 years report to be dissatisfied with sleep (cf. Miles and Dement, 1980; Reynolds et al., 1985). Dutch survey data reveal that 98% of the patients presenting a sleep complaint almost automatically receive a sedative-hypnotic drug (Van den Hoofdakker and Goettsch, 1979). Prevalence of hypnotic use is also high in residential homes for elderly (> 60%). Since 1980, there is even a tendency towards increased hypnotic usage, although considerable variations among various homes were observed (from over 60% to 0%) in a survey by Gilleard et al. (1984). Some of the undesired effects of hypnotics (exacerbation of sleep-related respiratory disturbances, rebound insomnia, reduction of daytime alertness, and interactions with other drugs) are potentially harmful, especially in a geriatric population. The elimination half-life of various benzodiazepines is prolonged in old age, whereas possible changes in receptor-site sensitivity in the brain cannot be excluded as a cause of increased sensitivity to toxicity in elderly (Castleden et al., 1977; Hicks et al., 1981). The frequency of adverse reactions after hypnotic ingestion such as CNS depression is indeed considerably higher in the elderly (Greenblatt et al., 1977; Greenblatt and Allen, 1978). In a prospective, but not randomized study the use of hypnotics and tranquillizers was even found to be statistically associated with an excess of nocturnal deaths (Kripke et al., 1979; Kripke and Garfinkel, 1984). The desirability of high hypnotic consumption among elderly should, therefore, be seriously questioned.

It appears reasonable to assume that, among other factors, altered circadian rhythms affect sleep patterns in elderly. Weitzman et al.'s (1982) experimental data, for instance, support the interpretation of early morning arousals as a reflection of phase advance of the daily main sleep period. Hypnotics or sedative drugs do not affect circadian rhythms as such. In addition to being potentially harmful, a large proportion of hypnotic prescriptions may, therefore, be considered non-rational as well. A non-pharmacologic approach towards elderly insomniacs has been suggested to be more appropriate (Miles and Dement, 1980; Weitzman et al., 1982; Reynolds et al., 1985). Correction of poor sleep hygiene (e.g. irregular sleep-waking schedules, use of alcohol, nicotine, or caffeine before bed-time), relaxation therapy, and adjustment of the social environment to the senescent sleep-wake pattern rather than vice versa, are all potentially beneficial. Such measures can, in addition, be expected to have no or only a few side effects. Adjustment of the social environment may have special significance for the institutionalized elderly. Kripke et al. (1982) stated that the "notion that people should remain awake all day and sleep soundly all night is more derived from Puritan ethics than from scientific data". Within a similar

context, routine prescription of hypnotics has been said to be for the benefit of the nursing staff rather than for the elderly patient (cf. Miles and Dement, 1980). However, it may also be that 'prophylactic' (Miles and Dement, 1980) hypnotic prescriptions merely reflect a need which itself is caused by inadequate manpower planning by health authorities. Day-night ratios of nursing staff manpower reflect light-dark ratios of normal adult sleep, which is restricted to the night. Light-dark differences, however, are considerably smaller in the senescent sleep-wakefulness or rest-activity pattern. Manpower planning in geriatric institutional settings could therefore be scaled more adequately to the needs of its population by relatively increasing the presence of nursing staff during the night. In combination with more clinical awareness of the peculiarities of sleep in elderly, this measure may reduce the frequency of hypnotic prescriptions, which are merely aimed at nocturnal quiescence on geriatric wards.

Summary and directions for future research

Organization in the dimension 'time' is a pervasive characteristic of living systems. The circadian timekeeping system appears to be changed during aging in both animals and humans (Miles and Dement, 1980; Ingram et al., 1982). Gerontology should take this observation into account and thus move beyond classical homeostatic concepts (Halberg and Nelson, 1978). Simple biometry in which only comparisons are made with static, 'normal' young, reference values may not be adequate to describe age-related changes.

As a result of the growing interest in gerontology, the number of functional systems for which age-related changes are described is continuously increasing. In contrast to some other systems sensitive to the effects of aging, the circadian timekeeping system is directly implicated in the organization of various important physiological functions. Characteristics of circadian rhythms have been documented extensively (cf. Aschoff, 1981; Moore-Ede et al., 1982), and recent studies indicate that even the molecular descriptions of a gene related to circadian timekeeping comes within our scope (Bargiello et al., 1984). The reduction in SCN cell number found in old age and even stronger in AD (Swaab and Fliers, 1985) represents a possible morphological correlate of circadian rhythm alterations in old age. At present, data on functional changes in the aged CNS underlying the altered characteristics of overt circadian rhythms in senescence, are not available. The functional integrity of the SCN, as a major part of the circadian rhythm generating system, is, however, open to study with current neurobiological techniques. An entrainable circadian clock, for instance, could be shown to oscillate in the SCN during fetal development of the rat (Reppert and Schwartz, 1983, 1984). Furthermore, in young and adult animals functional aspects of these nuclei have been characterized by metabolic (Schwartz et al., 1980, 1983b), electrophysiological (Inoue and Kawamura, 1979; Groos and Mason, 1980; Groos and Hendriks, 1982; Inoue and Kawamura, 1982; Rusak and Groos, 1982; Groos and Meijer, 1985), and neurochemical methods (Zatz and Herkenham, 1981; Albers and Ferris, 1984; Earnest and Sladek, 1984). Similar studies carried out in 'old age' may reveal functional impairments of a neural substrate related to circadian timekeeping. Animal and human experiments directed at possible correlations between circadian synchrony on one hand and depression, levels of performance on cognitive tasks, thermoregulatory capacity, or disturbed sleep patterns on the other, may reveal functional correlates of circadian rhythm alterations in senescence and AD.

Numerous descriptive data are consistent with hypotheses as formulated by Samis (1968) and Pittendrigh and Daan (1974). Temporal organization as an important dimension of living systems suffers indeed from senescent deterioration. The neural mechanisms underlying the altered time structure and the extent to which the decay of circadian organization affects adaptive capabilities in old age and AD remain, however, to be determined.

Acknowledgements

Research of the authors was supported by the 'Stimuleringsfonds Gerontologie' (SOOM-grant 83.111, Project 830804). We are indebted to J. H. Meijer and S. Daan for valuable suggestions on early drafts of this chapter and to F. Mullenders for supplying the data on traffic casualties.

References

Agnew, H. W., Jr., Webb, W. B. and Williams, R. L. (1967) Sleep patterns in late middle aged males: an EEG study. *Electroencephalogr. Clin. Neurophysiol.*, 3: 168–171.

Albers, H. E. and Ferris, C. F. (1984) Neuropeptide Y: role in the light-dark cycle entrainment of hamster circadian rhythms. *Neurosci. Lett.*, 50: 163–168.

Albers, H. E., Gerall, A. A. and Axelson, J. F. (1981) Circadian rhythm dissociation in the rat: effects of long-term constant illumination. *Neurosci. Lett.*, 25: 89–94.

Aldegunde, M., Arneaz, E., Miguez, I. and Fernandez, P. (1984) Variations in monoamine contents in discrete brain regions and their concomitance with plasma corticosteroids during the day. *Int. J. Neurosci.*, 24: 233–238.

Allen, D. J., DiDo, L. J. A., Gentry, E. R. and Ohtani, O. (1982) The aged rat pineal gland as revealed in SEM and TEM. *Age*, 5: 119–126.

Allen, S. R., Stähelin, H. B., Seiler, W. O. and Spiegel, R. (1983) EEG and sleep in aged hospitalized patients with senile dementia: 24-h recordings. *Experientia*, 39: 249–255.

Aschoff, J. (1965) Circadian rhythms in man. *Science*, 148: 1427–1432.

Aschoff, J. (Ed.) (1981) *Biological Rhythms. Handbook of Behavioral Neurobiology, Vol. 4*, Plenum Press, New York, 1981.

Aschoff, J., Von Saint Paul, U. and Wever, R. (1971) Die Lebensdauer von Fliegen unter dem Einfluss von Zeit-Verschiebungen. *Naturwissenschaften*, 58: 574.

Bargiello, T. A., Jackson, F. R. and Young, M. W. (1984) Restoration of circadian behavioral rhythms by gene transfer in *Drosophila. Nature (Lond.)*, 312: 752–754.

Barreca, T., Franceschini, R., Messina, V., Bottaro, L. and Rolandi, E. (1985) 24-Hour thyroid-stimulating hormone secretory pattern in elderly men. *Gerontology*, 31: 119–123.

Binkley, S., MacBride, S. E., Klein, D. C. and Ralph, C. L. (1973) Pineal enzymes: regulation of avian melatonin synthesis. *Science*, 181: 273–275.

Bixler, E. O., Kales, A., Jacoby, J. A., Soldatos, C. R. and Vela-Bueno, A. (1984) Nocturnal sleep and wakefulness: effects of age and sex in normal sleepers. *Int. J. Neurosci.*, 23: 33–42.

Blake, M. J. F. (1967) Time of day effects on performance in a range of tasks. *Psychonom. Sci.*, 9: 349–350.

Bobillier, P. and Mouret, J. R. (1971) The alterations of the diurnal variations of brain tryptophan, biogenic amines and 5-hydroxyindolic acetic acid in the rat under limited time feeding. *Int. J. Neurosci.*, 2: 271–282.

Bondareff, W. (1965) Electron microscopic study of the pineal body in aged rats. *J. Gerontol.*, 20: 321–327.

Boya, J. and Calvo, J. (1984) Structure and ultrastructure of the aging rat pineal gland. *J. Pineal Res.*, 1: 83–89.

Bremner, W. J., Vitiello, M. V. and Prinz, P. N. (1983) Loss of circadian rhythmicity in blood testosterone levels with aging in normal men. *J. Clin. Endocrinol. Metab.*, 56: 1278–1281.

Březinová, V. (1975) The number and duration of the episodes of the various EEG stages of sleep in young and older people. *Electroencephalogr. Clin. Neurophysiol.*, 39: 273–278.

Bruinink, A., Lichtensteiger, W. and Schlumpf, M. (1983) Ontogeny of diurnal rhythms of central dopamine, serotonin and spirodecanone binding sites and of motor activity in the rat. *Life Sci.*, 33: 31–38.

Cahill, A. L. and Ehret, C. F. (1981) Circadian variations in the activity of tyrosine hydroxylase, tyrosine aminotransferase, and tryptophan hydroxylase: relationship to the catecholamine metabolism. *J. Neurochem.*, 37: 1109–1115.

Cahn, H. A., Folk, G. E. and Huston, P. E. (1968) Age comparison of human day-night physiological differences. *Aerosp. Med.*, 39: 608–610.

Carlson, H. E., Gillin, J. C., Gordon, P. and Snyder, F. (1972) Absence of sleep related growth hormone peaks in aged normal subjects and acromegaly. *J. Clin. Endocrinol. Metab.*, 34: 1102–1104.

Carskadon, M. A., Van Den Hoed, J. and Dement, W. C. (1980) Insomnia and sleep disturbances in the aged. Sleep and daytime sleepiness in the elderly. *J. Geriatr. Psychiat.*, 13: 135–151.

Casale, G. and de Nicola, P. (1984) Circadian rhythms in the aged: a review. *Arch. Gerontol. Geriatr.*, 3: 267–284.

Castleden, C. M., George, C. F., Marcer, D. and Hallett, C. (1977) Increased sensitivity to nitrazepam in old age. *Br. Med. J.*, i: 10–12.

Collins, K. J., Dore, C., Exton-Smith, A. N., Fox, R. H., MacDonald, I. C. and Woodward, P. M. (1977) Accidital hypothermia and impaired temperature homeostasis in the elderly. *Br. Med. J.*, I: 353–356.

Colquhoun, W. P. (1984) Effects of personality on body temperature and mental efficiency following transmeridian flight. *Aviat. Space. Environm. Med.*, 55: 493–496.

Colucci, C. F., D'Alessandro, B., Bellastella, A. and Montalbetti, N. (1975) Circadian rhythm of plasma cortisol in the aged (cosinor method). *Gerontol. Clin.*, 17: 89–95.

Cugini, P., Scavo, D., Halberg, F., Schramm, A., Pusch, H. J.

and Francke, H. (1982) Methodologically critical interactions of circadian rhythm, sex, and aging characterize serum aldosterone and the female adrenopause. *J. Gerontol.*, 37: 403–411.

Dark, J. and Asdourian, D. (1975) Entrainment of the rat's activity rhythm by cyclic light following lateral geniculate nucleus lesion. *Physiol. Behav.*, 15: 295–301.

Davies, J. A., Navaratnam, V. and Redfern, P. H. (1974) The effect of phase-shift on the passive avoidance response in rats and the modifying action of chlordiazepoxide. *Br. J. Pharmacol.*, 51: 447–451.

Davis, F. C. and Menaker, M. (1980) Hamsters through time's window: temporal structure of hamster locomotor rhythmicity. *Am. J. Physiol.*, 239: R149–R155.

Descovich, G. C., Kühl, J. F. W., Halberg, F., Montalbetti, N., Rimondi, S. and Ceredi, C. (1974) Age and catecholamine rhythms. *Chronobiologia*, 1: 163–171.

Duguid, H., Simpson, R. G. and Stowers, J. M. (1961) Accidental hypothermia. *Lancet*, II: 1213–1219.

Earnest, D. J. and Sladek, C. D. (1984) Circadian rhythm in vasopressin release from rat suprachiasmatic explants in vitro. *Soc. Neurosci. Abstr.*, 10: 500.

Eastman, C. I., Mistlberger, R. E. and Rechtschaffen, A. (1984) Suprachiasmatic nuclei lesions eliminate circadian temperature and sleep rhythms in the rat. *Physiol. Behav.*, 32: 357–368.

Edmunds, L. N. (1983) Chronobiology at the cellular and molecular levels: models and mechanisms for circadian timekeeping. *Am. J. Anat.*, 168: 389–431.

Eskin, A. (1971) Some properties of the system controlling the circadian activity rhythm of sparrows. In M. Menaker (Ed.), *Biochronometry*, Washington, D. C., pp. 55–80.

Feinberg, I. and Carlson, V. R. (1968) Sleep variables as a function of age in man. *Arch. Gen. Psychiat.*, 18: 239–250.

Feinberg, I., Koresko, R. L. and Heller, N. (1967) EEG sleep patterns as a function of normal and pathological aging in man. *J. Psychiat. Res.*, 5: 107–144.

Fekete, M., van Ree, J. M., Niesink, R. J. M. and de Wied, D. (1985) Disrupting circadian rhythms in rats induces retrograde amnesia. *Physiol. Behav.*, 34: 883–887.

Finkelstein, J. W., Roffwarg, H. P., Boyar, R. M., Kream, J. and Hellman, J. (1972) Age-related change in the twenty-four-hour spontaneous secretion of growth hormone. *J. Clin. Endocrinol. Metab.*, 35: 665–670.

Fliers, E. and Swaab, D. F. (1986) Neuropeptide changes in aging and Alzheimer's disease. In D. F. Swaab, E. Fliers, M. Mirmiran, W. A. Van Gool and F. Van Haaren (Eds.), *Aging of the Brain and Alzheimer's Disease, Progress in Brain Research, Vol. 70.*, Elsevier, Amsterdam. this volume, pp. 141–152.

Fliers, F., De Vries, G. J. and Swaab, D. F. (1985) Changes with aging in the vasopressin and oxytocin innervation of the rat brain. *Brain Res.*, 348: 1–8.

Folkard, S. and Monk, T. H. (1983) Chronopsychology:

circadian rhythms and human performance. In A. Gale and J. Edwards (Eds.), *Physiological correlates of human behavior, Vol. II*, Academic Press, London, 57–78.

Folkard, S., Monk, T. S., Bradbury, R. and Rosenthall, J. (1977) Time of day effects in school children's immediate and delayed recall of meaningful material. *Br. J. Psychol.*, 68: 45–50.

Folkard, S., Minors, D. S. and Waterhouse, J. M. (1984) Chronobiology and shift work: current issues and trends. *Chronobiologia*, 12: 31–54.

Folkard, S., Hume, K. I., Minors, D. S., Waterhouse, J. M. and Watson, F. L. (1985) Independence of the circadian rhythm in alertness from the sleep/wake cycle. *Nature (Lond.)*, 313: 678–679.

Freivalds, A., Chaffin, D. B. and Langolf, G. D. (1983) Quantification of human performance circadian rhythms. *Am. Ind. Hyg. Assoc. J.*, 44: 643–648.

Friedman, H. H. and Walker, C. A. (1968) Circadian rhythms in rat mid-brain and caudate nucleus biogenic amine levels. *J. Physiol. (Lond.)*, 197: 77–85.

Fuller, C. A., Sulzman, F. M. and Moore-Ede, M. C. (1978) Thermoregulation is impaired in an environment without time cues. *Science*, 199: 794–795.

Fuller, C. A., Sulzman, F. M. and Moore-Ede, M. C. (1979) Circadian control of thermoregulation in the squirrel monkey *(Saimiri sciureus)*. *Am. J. Physiol.*, 236: R153–R161.

Fuller, C. A., Lydic, R., Sulzman, F. M., Albers, H. E., Tepper, B. and Moore-Ede, M. C. (1981) Circadian rhythm of body temperature persists after suprachiasmatic lesions in the squirrel monkey. *Am. J. Physiol.*, 241: R385–R391.

Gander, P. H., Lydic, R., Albers, H. E. and Moore-Ede, M. C. (1985) Forced internal desynchronization between circadian temperature and activity rhythms in squirrel monkeys. *Am. J. Physiol.*, 248: R567–R572.

Garrick, N. A., Tamarkin, L., Taylor, P. L. and Murphy, D. L. (1983) Light and propanolol suppress the nocturnal elevation of serotonin in the cerebrospinal fluid of rhesus monkeys. *Science*, 221: 474–476.

Gilleard, C. J., Smits, C. and Morgan, K. (1984) Changes in hypnotic usage in residential homes for the elderly: a longitudinal study. *Arch. Gerontol. Geriatr.*, 3: 223–228.

Greenberg, L. H. and Weis, B. (1978) Beta-adrenergic receptors in the aged rat brain: reduced number and reduced capacity of pineal gland to develop supersensitivity. *Science*, 201: 61–63.

Greenblatt, D. J. and Allen, M. D. (1978) Toxicity of nitrazepam in the elderly: a report from the Boston collaborative drug surveillance program. *Br. J. Clin. Pharmacol.*, 5: 407–413.

Greenblatt, D. J., Allen, M. D. and Shader, R. I. (1977) Toxicity of high-dose flurazepam in the elderly. *Clin. Pharmacol. Ther.*, 21: 355–361.

Groos, G. (1983) Regulation of the circadian sleep-wake cycle. In Koella, W. P. (Ed.) *Sleep 1982*, Karger, Basel pp. 19–29.

Groos, G. and Hendriks, J. (1982) Circadian rhythms in electrical discharge of rat suprachiasmatic neurones recorded in vitro. *Neurosci. Lett.*, 34: 283–288.

Groos, G. and Mason (1980) The visual properties of the rat and cat suprachiasmatic neurones. *J. Comp. Physiol.*, 135: 349–356.

Groos, G. A. and Meijer, J. H. (1985) Effects of illumination on suprachiasmatic nucleus electrical discharge. In R. J. Wurtman, M. J. Beum and J. T. Pottf, Jr. (Eds.), *The Medical and Biological Effects of Light. Ann NY Acad. Sci.*, 453: 134–146.

Halberg, F. (1960) The 24-hour scale: A time dimension of adaptive functional organization. *Perspect. Biol. Med.*, 3: 491–527.

Halberg, F. and Nelson, W. (1978) Chronobiologic optimization of aging. In H. V. Samis and S. Capobianco (Eds.), *Aging and Biological Rhythms. Adv. Exp. Med. Biol. Vol. 108*: pp. 5–56.

Halberg, F., Bittner, J. J., Gully, R. J., Albrecht, P. G. and Brackney, E. L. (1955) 24-Hour periodicity and audiogenic convulsions in I mice of various ages. *Proc. Soc. Exp. Biol. Med.*, 88: 169–173.

Halberg, J., Halberg, E., Regal, P. and Halberg, F. (1981) Changes with age characterize circadian rhythm in telemetered core temperature of stroke prone rats. *J. Gerontol.*, 36: 28–30.

Hanin, I., Massarelli, R. and Costa, E. (1970) Acetylcholine concentrations in rat brain: diurnal oscillations. *Science*, 170: 341–342.

Harman, S. M. and Tsitouras, P. D. (1980) Measurement of sex steroids, basal luteinizing hormone, and Leydig cell response to human choriogonadopin. *J. Clin. Endocrinol. Metab.*, 51: 35–40.

Harrington, M. E., Nance, D. M. and Rusak, B. (1984) NPY-like immunoreactivity in the geniculo-suprachiamatic tract. *Soc. Neurosci. Abstr.*, 10: 502.

Hauty, G. T. and Adams, T. (1966) Phase shifts of the human circadian system and performance deficit during the periods of transition: I. East-west flight. *Aerospace Med.*, 37: 668–674.

Hayashi, Y. and Endo, S. (1982) All-night polygraphic recordings of healthy aged persons: REM and slow-wave sleep. *Sleep*, 5: 277–283.

Hayes, D. K. and Cawley, B. M. (1978) Phase shifting and life span in the codling moth, *Laspeyresia pomonella (L)*. In H. V. Samis and S. Capobianco (Eds.), *Aging and Biological Rhythms. Adv. Exp. Med. Biol. Vol. 108*: 97–100.

Héry, F., Rouer, E. and Glowinsky, J. (1972) Daily variations of serotonin metabolism in the rat brain. *Brain Res.*, 43: 445–465.

Hicks, R., Dysken, M. W., Davis, J. M., Lesser, J., Ripecky, A. and Lazarus, L. (1981) The pharmacokinetics of psychotropic medication in the elderly: a review. *J. Clin. Psychiat.*, 42: 374–385.

Hoffmann, K., Illnerová, H. and Vanêck, J. (1985) Comparison of pineal melatonin rhythms in young and old Djungerian hamsters (*Phodopus sungorus*) under long and short photoperiods. *Neurosci. Lett.*, 56: 39–43.

Holloway, F. A. and Wansley, R. A. (1973a) Multiple retention deficits at periodic intervals after passive avoidance learning. *Science*, 180: 208–210.

Holloway, F. A. and Wansley, R. A. (1973b) Multiple retention deficits after active and passive avoidance learning. *Behav. Biol.*, 9: 1–14.

Hoorneman, E. M. D. and Buijs, R. M. (1982) Vasopressin fiber pathways in the rat brain following suprachiasmatic nucleus lesioning. *Brain Res.*, 243: 235–241.

Ibuka, N., Inouye, S. T. and Kawamura, H. (1975) Analysis of sleep-wakefulness rhythms in male rats after suprachiasmatic lesions and ocular enucleation. *Brain Res.*, 122: 33–47.

Iguchi, H., Kato, K. I. and Ibayashi, H. (1982) Age-dependent reduction in serum melatonin concentrations in healthy human subjects. *J. Clin. Endocrinol. Metab.*, 55: 27–29.

Ingram, D. K., London, E. D. and Reynolds, M. A. (1982) Circadian rhythmicity and sleep: effects of aging in laboratory animals. *Neurobiol. Aging*, 3: 287–297.

Inouye, S. T. and Kawamura, H. (1979) Persistence of circadian rhythmicity in a mammalian hypothalamic 'island' containing the suprachiasmatic nucleus. *Proc. Natl. Acad. Sci. USA*, 76: 5962–5966.

Inouye, S. T. and Kawamura, H. (1982) Characteristics of a circadian pacemaker in the suprachiasmatic nucleus. *J. Comp. Physiol.*, 146: 153–160.

Jakubczak, L. F. (1975) Re-entrainment of food intake of mature and old rats to the light-dark cycle. *Bull. Psychonom. Soc.*, 6: 491–493.

Jensen, H. K. and Blichert-Toft, M. (1971) Serum corticotrophin, plasma cortisol and urinary excretion of 17-ketogenic steroids in the elderly (age group: 66–94 years). *Acta Endocrinol. (Copenh.)*, 66: 25–34.

Johnson, J. E. (1980) Fine structural alterations in the aging rat pineal gland. *Exp. Aging Res.*, 6: 189–211.

Kafka, M. S., Wirz-Justice, A. and Naber, D. (1981) Circadian and seasonal rhythms in alpha- and beta-adrenergic receptors in the rat brain. *Brain Res.*, 207: 409–419.

Kafka, M. S., Benedito, M. A., Zerbe, R. L. and Jacobowitz, D. M. (1983a) Circadian rhythm in argenine vasopressin concentration in the rat suprachiasmatic nucleus. *Soc. Neurosci. Abstr.*, 9: 1068.

Kafka, M. S., Wirz-Justice, A., Naber, D., Moore, R. Y. and Benedito, M. A. (1983b) Circadian rhythms in the rat brain neurotransmitter receptors. *Fed. Proc.*, 42: 2796–2801.

Kafka, M. S., Marangos, P. J. and Moore, R. Y. (1985) Suprachiasmatic nucleus ablation abolishes circadian rhythms in rat brain neurotransmitter receptors. *Brain Res.*, 327: 344–347.

Kahn, E. and Fisher, C. (1969) The sleep characteristics of the normal aged male. *J. Nerv. Ment. Dis.*, 148: 477–494.

Kan, J. P., Chouvet, G., Héry, F., Debilly, G., Mermet, A., Glowinski, J. and Pujol, J. F. (1977) Daily variations of various parameters of serotonin metabolism in the rat brain. I. Circadian variations of tryptophan-5-hydroxylase in the raphe nuclei and the striatum. *Brain Res.*, 123: 125–136.

Kavaliers, M. and Hirst, M. (1983) Daily rhythms of analgesia in mice: effects of age and photoperiod. *Brain Res.*, 279: 387–393.

Kavaliers, M. and Hirst, M. (1985) The influence of opiate agonists on day-night feeding rhythms in young and old mice. *Brain Res.*, 326: 160–167.

Kavaliers, M., Hirst, M. and Teskey, G. C. (1984) Aging and daily rhythms of analgesia in mice: effects of natural illumination and twilight. *Neurobiol. Aging*, 5: 111–114.

Kenagy, G. J. (1978) Seasonality of endogenous circadian rhythms in a diurnal rodent *Ammonspermophilus leucurus* and a nocturnal rodent *Dipodomys merriami*. *J. Comp. Physiol.*, 128: 21–36.

Klein, D. C. and Weller, J. E. (1970) Indole metabolism in the pineal gland: a circadian rhythm in *N*-acetyltransferase. *Science*, 169: 1093–1095.

Klein, K. E., Wegmann, H. M. and Hunt, B. (1972) Desynchronization of body temperature and performance circadian rhythm as a result of outgoing and homegoing transmeridian flights. *Aerospace Med.*, 43: 119–132.

Klug, T. I. and Adelman, R. C. (1979) Altered hypothalamic-pituitary regulation of thyroptropin in male rats during aging. *Endocrinology*, 104: 1136–1142.

Krieger, D., Allen, W., Rizzo, F. and Krieger, H. (1971) Characterization of the normal temporal pattern of plasm corticosteroid levels. *J. Clin. Endocrinol. Metab.*, 32: 266–284.

Kripke, D. F. and Garfinkel, L. (1984) Excess nocturnal deaths related to sleeping pill and tranquiliser use. *Lancet*, I: 99.

Kripke, D. F., Simons, R. N., Garfinkel, L. and Hammond, E. C. (1979) Short and long sleep and sleeping pills. *Arch. Gen. Psychiat.*, 36: 103–116.

Kripke, D. F., Ancoli-Israel, S. and Okudaira, N. (1982) Sleep apnea and nocturnal myoclonus in the elderly. *Neurobiol. Aging*, 3: 329–336.

Lakatua, D. J., Nicolau, G. Y., Bogfan, C., Petrescu, E., Sackett-Lundeen, L. L., Irvine, P. W. and Haus, E. (1984) Circadian endocrine time structure in humans above 80 years of age. *J. Gerontol.*, 39: 648–654.

Lobban, M. C. and Tredre, B. E. (1967) Diurnal rhythms of excretion and of body temperature in aged subjects. *J. Physiol. (Lond.)*, 188: 48P–49P.

Lobban, M., Tredre, B., Elithorn, A. and Bridges, P. (1963) Diurnal rhythms of electrolyte excretion in depressive illness. *Nature (Lond.)*, 199: 667–669.

Leutz, M. J. (1984) Circadian temperature rhythms in healthy young and old men. *Sleep Res.*, 13: 222.

Loewenstein, R. J., Weingartner, H., Gillin, J. C., Kaye, W., Erbert, M. and Mendelson, W. B. (1982) Disturbances of sleep and cognitive functioning in patients with dementia. *Neurobiol. Aging*, 3: 371–377.

Manshardt, J. and Wurtman, R. J. (1968) Daily rhythm in the

noradrenaline content of rat hypothalamus. *Nature (Lond.)*, 217: 574–575.

Martin, J. R., Fuchs, A., Bender, R. and Harting, J. (1985) Altered light-dark activity difference with aging in two rat strains. *J. Gerontol.*, 4: 2–7.

Mash, D. C., Flynn, D. D., Kalinoski, L. and Potter, L. T. (1985) Circadian variations in radioligand binding to muscarine receptors in rat brain dependent upon endogenous agonist occupation. *Brain Res.*, 331: 35–38.

Mefford, I. N., Chang, P., Klein, D. C., Namboodiri, M. A. A., Sugden, D. and Barchas, J. (1983) Reciprocal day/night relationship between serotonin oxidation and N-acetylation products in the rat pineal gland. *Endocrinology*, 113: 1582–1586.

Meijer, J. H., Rusak, B. and Harrington, M. E. (1984) Geniculate stimulation phase shifts hamster circadian rhythms. *Soc. Neurosci. Abstr.*, 10: 507.

Milcu, S. M., Bogdan, C., Nicolau, G. Y. and Crista, A. (1978) Cortisol circadian rhythm in 70–100-year-old subjects. *Rev. Roum. Med. Endocrinol.*, 16: 29–38.

Miles, L. E. and Dement, W. C. (1980) Sleep and aging. *Sleep*, 3: 119–220.

Miller, A. E. and Riegle, G. D. (1982) Temporal patterns of serum luteinizing hormone and testosterone and endocrine response to luteinizing hormone releasing hormone in aging male rats. *J. Gerontol.*, 37: 522–528.

Mistlberger, R. E., Bergmann, B. M., Waldenar, W. and Rechtschaffen, A. (1983) Recovery sleep following sleep deprivation in intact and suprachiasmatic nuclei-lesioned rats. *Sleep*, 6: 217–233.

Mohan, C. and Radha, E. (1978) Circadian rhythms in the central cholinergic system in aging animals. In H. V. Samis, and S. Capobianco, (Eds.), *Aging and Biological Rhythms, Adv. Exp. Med. Biol.*, 108: 275– 300.

Monk, T. H. (1980) Traffic accident increases as a possible indicant of desynchronosis. *Chronobiologia*, 7: 527–529.

Monk, T. H., Weitzman, E. D., Fookson, J. E. and Moline, M. L. (1984) Circadian rhythms in human performance efficiency under free-running conditions. *Chronobiologia*, 11: 343–354.

Moore, R. Y. (1973) Retinohypothalamic projection in mammals: a comparative study. *Brain Res.*, 49: 403–409.

Moore, R. Y. (1983) Organization and function of central nervous system oscillator: the suprachiasmatic hypothalamic nucleus. *Fed. Proc.*, 42: 2783–2789.

Moore, R. Y. and Eichler (1972) Loss of the circadian corticosterone rhythm following suprachiasmatic lesions in the rat. *Brain Res.*, 42: 210–206.

Moore-Ede, M. C. (1983) The circadian timing system in mammals: two pacemakers preside over many secondary oscillators. *Fed. Proc.*, 42: 2802–2808.

Moore-Ede, M. C., Sulzman, F. M. and Fuller, C. A. (1982) *The Clocks that Time Us*. Harvard University Press, Cambridge.

Mosko, S. S., Erickson, G. F. and Moore, R. Y. (1980) Dampened circadian rhythms in reproductively senescent female rats. *Behav. Neural Biol.*, 28: 1–14.

Murri, L., Barreca, T., Cerone, G., Massetani, R., Gallamini, A. and Baldassarre, M. (1980) The 24-h pattern of human prolactin and growth hormone in healthy elderly subjects. *Chronobiologia*, 7: 87–92.

Naber, D., Wirz-Justice, A., Kafka, M. S. and Wehr, T. A. (1980) Dopamine receptor binding in rat striatum: ultradian rhythm and its modification by chronic imipramine. *Psychopharmacology*, 68: 1–5.

Naber, D., Wirz-Justice, A. and Kafka, M. S. (1981) Circadian rhythm in rat brain opiate receptor. *Neurosci. Lett.*, 21: 45–50.

Nelson, W., Bingham, C., Haus, E., Lakatua, D. J., Kawasaki, T. and Halberg, F. (1980) Rhythm-adjusted age effects in a concomitant study of twelve hormones in blood plasma of women. *J. Gerontol.*, 35: 512–519.

Nicholson, S. A., Adrian, T. E., Bacarese-Hamilton, A. J., Gillham, B., Jones, M. T. and Bloom, S. R. (1983) 24-Hour variation in content and release of hypothalamic neuropeptides in the rat. *Regul. Peptides*, 7: 385–397.

Nicolau, G. Y. and Milcu, S. (1977) Circadian rhythms of corticosterone and nucleic acids in the rat adrenals in relation to age. *Chronobiologia*, 4: 136.

Nicolau, G. Y., Haus, E., Lakatua, D. J., Bogdan, C., Popescu, M., Petrescu, E., Sackett-Lundeen, L., Swoyer, J. and Adderley, J. (1983) Circadian periodicity of the results of frequently used laboratory tests in elderly subjects. *Rev. Roum. Med.-Endocrinol.*, 21: 3–21.

Noto, T., Hashimoto, H., Doi, Y., Nakajima, T. and Kato, N. (1983) Biorhythm of arginin-vasopressin in the paraventricular, supraoptic and suprachiasmatic nuclei of rats. *Peptides*, 4: 875–878.

Owasoyo, J. O., Gipson, K. D., Soliman, K. F. and Walker, C. A. (1984) Circadian variation in the monoamine oxidase activity of specific rat brain areas. *J. Interdisc. Cycle Res.*, 15: 163–168.

Oxenkrug, G. F., McIntyre, I. M. and Gershon, S. (1984) Effects of pinealectomy and aging on the serum corticosterone circadian rhythm in rats. *J. Pineal Res.*, 1: 181–185.

Pasqualetti, P., Acitelli, P., Casale, R., Festuccia, V., Giusti, A., Di Lauro, G. and Natali, G. (1983) Plasmatic renin activity, aldosterone and aging: chronobiological study. *Chronobiologia*, 10: 403–404.

Pauly, J. E. (1983) Chronobiology: Anatomy in time. *Am. J. Anat.*, 168: 365–388.

Page, T. L. and Block, G. D. (1980) Circadian rhythmicity in the cockroach: effects of age, sex, and prior light history. *Physiol. Entomol.*, 5: 271–282.

Perlow, M., Ebert, M. H., Gordon, E. K., Ziegler, M. G., Lake, C. R. and Chase, T. N. (1978) The circadian variation of catecholamine metabolism in the subhuman primate. *Brain Res.*, 139: 101–113.

Perlow, M. J., Reppert, S. M., Artman, H. A., Fisher, D. A.,

Seif, S. M. and Robinson, A. G. (1982) Oxytocin, vasopressin, and estrogen-stimulated neurophysin: daily patterns of concentration in cerebrospinal fluid. *Science*, 216: 1416–1418.

Peng, M. T. and Kang, M. (1984) Circadian rhythms and patterns of running-wheel activity, feeding and drinking behaviors of old male rats. *Physiol. Behav.*, 33: 615–620.

Peng, M. T., Jiang, M. J. and Hsü, H. K. (1980) Changes in running-wheel activity, eating and drinking and their day/night distributions throughout the life span of the rat. *J. Gerontol.*, 35: 339–347.

Pickard, G. E. (1982) The afferent connections of the suprachiasmatic nucleus of the golden hamster with emphasis on the retinohypothalamic projection. *J. Comp. Neurol.*, 211: 65–83.

Pickard, G. E. (1985) Bifurcating axons of retinal ganglion cells terminate in the hypothalamic suprachiasmatic nucleus and the intergeniculate leaflet of the hypothalamus. *Neurosci. Lett.*, 55: 211–217.

Pittendrigh, C. S. (1960) Circadian rhythms and the circadian organization of living systems. *Cold Spring Harbor Symp. Quart. Biol.*, 25: 159–182.

Pittendrigh, C. S. and Daan, S. (1974) Circadian oscillations in rodents: a systematic increase of their frequency with age. *Science*, 186: 548–550.

Pittendrigh, C. S. and Daan, S. (1976) A functional analysis of circadian pacemakers in nocturnal rodents. *J. Comp. Physiol.*, 106: 223–252.

Pittendrigh, C. S. and Minis, D. (1972) Circadian systems: Longevity as a function of circadian resonance in *Drosophila melanogaster*. *Proc. Natl. Acad. Sci. USA*, 69: 1537–1539.

Preston, F. S. (1973) Further sleep problems in airline pilots on world-wide schedules. *Aerospace Med.*, 44: 775–782.

Prinz, P. N. and Halter, J. B. (1983) Sleep disturbances in the elderly: neurohormonal correlates. In M. Chase and E. D. Weitzman (Eds.), *Sleep Disorders Basic and Clinical Research. Adv. Sleep Res.*, 8: 463–488.

Prinz, P. N., Halter, J., Benedetti, C. and Raskind, M. (1979) Circadian variation of plasma catecholamines in young and old men: Relation to rapid eye movement and slow wave sleep. *J. Clin. Endocrinol. Metab.*, 49: 300–303.

Prinz, P. N., Peskind, E. R., Vitaliano, P. P., Raskind, M. A., Eisdorfer, C., Zemcuznikov and Gerber, C. J. (1982) Changes in the sleep and waking EEGs of nondemented and demented elderly subjects. *J. Am. Geriat. Soc.*, 30: 86–93.

Prinz, P. N., Christie, C., Smallwood, R., Vitaliano, P., Bokan, J., Vitiello, M. V. and Martin, D. (1984) Circadian temperature variation in healthy aged and in Alzheimer's disease. *J. Gerontol.*, 39: 30–35.

Przewlocki, R., Lasón, W., Konecka, A. M., Gramsch, C., Herz, A. and Reid, L. D. (1983) The opioid peptide dynorphin, circadian rhythms, and starvation, *Science*, 219: 71–73.

Quay, W. B. (1964) Circadian and estrous rhythms in pineal melatonin and 5-hydroxy indole-3-acetic acid. *Proc. Soc. Exp. Biol. Med.*, 115: 710–713.

Reinberg, A., Andlauer, P., Guillet, P. and Nicolai, A. (1980) Oral temperature, circadian rhythm amplitude, ageing and tolerance to shift-work. *Ergonomics*, 23: 55–64.

Reis, D. J., Weinbren, M. and Corvelli, A. (1968) A circadian rhythm of norepinephrine regionally in cat brain: its relationship to environmental lighting and to regional diurnal variations in brain serotonin. *J. Pharmacol. Exp. Ther.*, 164: 135–145.

Reiter, R. J., Craft, C. M., Johnson Jr., J. E., King, T. S., Richardson, B. A., Vaughan, G. M. and Vaughan, M. K. (1981) Age-associated reduction in nocturnal pineal melatonin levels in female rats. *Endocrinology*, 109: 1295–1297.

Reppert, S. M. and Schwartz, W. J. (1983) Maternal coordination of the fetal biological clock in utero. *Science*, 220: 969–971.

Reppert, S. M. and Schwartz, W. J. (1984) The suprachiasmatic nuclei of the fetal rat: characterization of a functional circadian clock using 14C-labeled deoxyglucose. *J. Neurosci.*, 4: 1677–1682.

Reppert, S. M., Artman, H. G., Swaminathan, S. and Fisher, D. A. (1981a) Vasopressin exhibits a rhythmic daily pattern in cerebrospinal fluid but not in blood. *Science*, 213: 1256–1257.

Reppert, S. M., Perlow, M. J., Ungerleider, L. R., Mishkin, M., Tamarkin, L., Orloff, D. G., Hoffmann, H. J. and Klein, D. C. (1981b) Effects of damage to the suprachiasmatic area of the anterior hypothalamus on the daily melatonin and cortisol rhythms in the rhesus monkey. *J. Neurosci.*, 1: 1414–1425.

Reppert, S. M., Schwartz, W. J., Artman, H. G. and Fisher, D. A. (1983) Comparison of the temporal profiles of vasopressin and oxytocin in the cerebrospinal fluid of the cat, monkey and rat. *Brain Res.*, 261: 341–345.

Reppert, S. M., Perlow, M. J., Artman, H. G., Ungerleider, L. G., Fisher, D. A. and Klein, D. C. (1984) The circadian rhythm of oxytocin in primate cerebrospinal fluid: effects of destruction of the suprachiasmatic nuclei. *Brain Res.*, 307: 384–387.

Reynolds, C. F., Kupfer, D. J., Hoch, C. C. and Sewitch, D. E. (1985) Sleeping pills for the elderly: are they ever justified? *J. Clin. Psychiat.*, 46: 9–12.

Rietveld, W. J., Boon, M. E., Korving, J. and Schravendijk, K. (1985) Circadian rhythms in elderly rats. *J. Interdiscipl. Cycle Res.*, 16: 154.

Rosenberg, R. S., Zepelin, A. M. and Rechtschaffen, A. (1977) Sleep in young and old rats. *J. Gerontol.*, 34: 525–532.

Rusak, B. and Groos, G. (1982) Suprachiasmatic stimulation phase shifts rodent circadian rhythms. *Science*, 215: 1407–1409.

Rusak, B. and Zucker, I. (1979) Neural regulation of circadian rhythms. *Physiol. Rev.*, 59: 449–526.

Sacher, G. A. and Duffy, P. H. (1978) Age changes in rhythms of energy metabolism, activity, and body core temperature in *Mus* and *Peromyscus*. In H. V. Samis and S. Capobianco (Eds.), *Aging and Biological Rhythms, Adv. Exp. Med. Biol. Vol. 108*: 105–124.

Samis, H. V. Jr. (1968) Aging: loss of temporal organization. *Perspect. Biol. Med.*, 3: 95–102.

Sawada, M. and Enesco, H. (1984) The effect of light, dark or altered circadian cycle on the lifespan of the rotifier *Asplanchna brightwelli*. *Exp. Gerontol.*, 19: 335–343.

Scheving, L. E., Harrison, W. H., Gordon, P. and Pauly, J. E. (1968) Daily fluctuation (circadian and ultradian) in biogenic amines of the rat brain. *Am. J. Physiol.*, 214: 166–173.

Scheving, L., Roig, C., Halberg, F., Pauly, F. and Hand, E. (1974) Circadian variations in residents of a 'senior citizens' home. In L. Scheving, F. Halberg and J. Pauly (Eds.), *Chronobiology*, Igaku Shoin, Tokyo, pp. 353–357.

Scheving, L. E., Pauly, J. E. and Tsai, T. H. (1978) Significance of the chronobiological approach in carrying out aging studies. In: H. V. Samis and S. Capobianco (Eds.), *Aging and Biological Rhythms, Adv. Exp. Med. Biol. Vol. 108*: 57–96.

Schwartz, W. J., Davidsen, L. C. and Smith, C. B (1980) In vivo metabolic activity of a putative circadian oscillator, the rat suprachiasmatic nucleus. *J. Comp. Neurol.*, 189: 157–167.

Schwartz, W. J., Coleman, R. J. and Reppert, S. M. (1983a) A daily vasopressin rhythm in rat cerebrospinal fluid. *Brain Res.*, 263: 105–112.

Schwartz, W. J., Reppert, S. M., Eagan, S. M. and Moore-Ede, M. C. (1983b) In vivo metabolic activity of the suprachiasmatic nuclei: a comparative study. *Brain Res.*, 274: 184–187.

Schweiger, U., Warnhoff, M. and Pirke, K. M. (1985) Norepinephrine turnover in the hypothalamus of adult male rats: alteration of circadian patterns by semistarvation. *J. Neurochem.*, 45: 706–709.

Semba, J. I., Toru, M. and Mataga, N. (1984) Twenty-four hour rhythms of norepinephrine and serotonin in nucleus suprachiasmatic, raphe nuclei, and locus coeruleus in the rat. *Sleep*, 7: 211–218.

Serio, M., Piolanti, P., Romano, S., De Magistris, L. and Guisti, G. (1970) The circadian rhythm of plasma cortisol in subjects over 70 years of age. *J. Gerontol.*, 25: 95–97.

Sherman, B., Wysman, C. and Pfohl, B. (1985) Age-related changes in the circadian rhythm of plasma cortisol in man. *J. Clin. Endocrinol. Metab.*, 61: 439–443.

Simpkins, J. W., Kalra, P. S. and Kalra, S. P. (1981) Alterations in daily rhythms of testosterone and progesterone in old male rats. *Expl. Aging Res.*, 7: 25–32.

Södersten, P., Henning, M., Melin, P. and Lundin, S. (1983) Vasopressin alters female sexual behavior by acting on the brain independently of alterations in blood pressure. *Nature (Lond.)*, 301: 608–610.

Stearns, E. L., MacDonnel, J. A., Kaufman, B. J., Padua, L., Lucman, T. S., Winter, J. S. D. and Faiman, C. (1974) Declining testicular function with age, hormonal and clinical correlates. *Am. J. Med.*, 57: 761–766.

Stephan, F. K. (1981) Limits of entrainment to periodic feeding in rats with suprachiasmatic lesions. *J. Comp. Physiol.*, 143: 401–410.

Stephan, F. K. and Zucker, I. (1972) Circadian rhythms in drinking behavior and locomotor activity of rats are eliminated by hypothalamic lesions. *Proc. Natl. Acad. Sci. USA*, 69: 1583.

Stern, N., Beahm, E., Sowers, J., McGinty, D., Eggena, P., Littner, M., Nyby, M. and Catania, R. (1984) The effect of age on circadian rhythm of blood pressure, catecholamines, plasma renin activity, prolactin and corticosteroids in essential hypertension. In M. A. Weber and J. I. M. Drayer (Eds.), *Ambulatory blood pressure monitoring*. Steinkopf, Darmstadt/ Springer-Verlag, New York, pp. 157–162.

Sugai, Y. and Fujita, H. (1984) Circadian rhythm of plasma aldosterone in older patients with dementia under forced bed rest. *Kitakanto Med. J.*, 34: 445–450.

Sulzman, F. M., Ellman, D., Fuller, C. A., Moore-Ede, M. C. and Wassmer, G. (1984) *Neurospora* circadian rhythms in space: a reexamination of the endogenous-exogenous question. *Science*, 225: 232–234.

Swaab, D. F., Fliers, E. and Partiman, T. S. (1985) The suprachiasmatic nucleus of the human brain in relation to sex, age and senile dementia. *Brain Res.*, 342: 37–44.

Tamarkin, L., Baird, C. J. and Almeida, O. F. X. (1985) Melatonin: a coordinating signal for mammalian reproduction? *Science*, 7 227: 714–720.

Tang, F., Hadjiconstantinou, M. and Pang, S. F. (1985) Aging and diurnal rhythms of pineal serotonin, 5-hydroxyindoleacetic acid, norepinephrine dopamine and serum melatonin in the male rat. *Neuroendocrinology*, 40: 160–164.

Tapp, W. N. and Holloway, F. A. (1981) Phase shifting circadian rhythms produces retrograde amnesia. *Science*, 211: 1056–1058.

Touitou, Y. (1982) Some aspects of the circadian time structure in the elderly. *Gerontology* 28 (Suppl. 1): 53–67.

Touitou, Y., Fevre, M., Lagoguey, M., Carayon, A., Bogdan, A., Reinberg, A., Beck, H., Cesselin, F. and Touitou, C. (1981) Age- and mental health-related circadian rhythms of plasma levels of melatonin, prolactin, luteinizing hormone and follicle-stimulating hormone in man. *J. Endocrinol.*, 91: 467–475.

Tune, G. S. (1968) Sleep and wakefulness in normal human adults. *Br. Med. J.*, 2: 269–271.

Tune, G. S. (1969) Sleep wakefulness in 509 normal human adults. *Br. J. Med. Psychol.*, 42: 75–80.

Van den Hoofdakker, R. H. and Goettsch, H. (1979) Slapeloosheid bij bejaarden, *Pharmac. Weekbl.*, 114: 1131–1146.

Van Gool, W. A. and Mirmiran, M. (1983) Age-related changes in the sleep-pattern of male adult rats. *Brain Res.*, 279: 394–398.

Van Gool, W. A. and Mirmiran, M. (1986) Effects of aging and housing in an enriched environment upon sleep-wake patterns in rats. *Sleep*, 9: 335–347.

Van Haaren, F. and Van de Poll, N. E. (1984) The effects of a choice alternative on sex differences in passive avoidance behavior. *Physiol. Behav.*, 32: 211–215.

Von Saint Paul, U. and Aschoff, J. (1978) Longevity among blowflies *Phormia terraenovae* R. D. kept in non-24-hour light-dark cycles. *J. Comp. Physiol.*, 127: 191–195.

Virus, R. M., Baglajewski, T. and Radulovacki, M. (1984) Circadian variation of [3H]N6-(L-phenylisopropyl)adenosine binding in rat brain. *Neurosc. Lett.*, 46: 219–222.

Walker, R. F. (1980) Serotonin circadian rhythm as a pacemaker for reproductive cycles in the female rat. In: F. Brambilla and D. de Wied (Eds.), *Progress in Psychoneuroendocrinology*, Elsevier/North Holland, Amsterdam, pp. 591–600.

Walker, R. F., McMahon, K. M. and Pivorun, E. B. (1978) Pineal gland structure and respiration as affected by age and hypocaloric diet. *Exp. Gerontol.*, 13: 91–99.

Wansley, R. A. and Holloway, F. A. (1975) Multiple retention deficits following one-trial appetitive training. *Behav. Biol.*, 14: 135–149.

Wax, T. M. (1975) Runwheel activity patterns of mature-young and senescent mice. The effect of constant lighting conditions. *J. Gerontol.*, 30: 22–27.

Wax, T. M. (1977) Effects of age, strain, and illumination intensity on activity and self-selection of light-dark schedules in mice. *J. Comp. Physiol. Psychol.*, 91: 51–62.

Wax, T. M. and Goodrick, C. L. (1978) Nearness to death and wheelrunning behavior in mice. *Exp. Gerontol.*, 13: 233–236.

Webb, W. B. (1981) Patterns of sleep in healthy 50–60 year old males and females. *Res. Commun. Psychol. Psychiat. Behav.*, 6: 133–140.

Webb, W. B. (1982a) The measurement and characteristics of sleep in older persons. *Neurobiol. Aging*, 3: 311–319.

Webb, W. B. (1982b) The sleep of older subjects fifteen years later. *Psychol. Rep.*, 50: 11–14.

Webb, W. B. and Schneider-Helmert, D. (1984) A categorical approach to changes in latency, awakening, and sleep length in older subjects. *J. Nerv. Ment. Dis.*, 172: 291–295.

Webb, W. B. and Swinburne, H. (1971) An observation of sleep of the aged. *Percept. Motor Skills*, 32: 895–898.

Weitzman, E. D., Moline, M. L., Czeisler, C. A. and Zimmerman, J. C. (1982) Chronobiology of aging: temperature, sleep-wake rhythms and entrainment. *Neurobiol. Aging*, 3: 299–309.

Welsh, D. K., Richardson, G. S. and Dement, W. C. (1985) Age differences in the circadian pattern of sleep and wakefulness in the mouse. *Sleep Res.*, 14: 82.

Wever, R. (1975) Die Bedeutung der circadiane Periodiek für den alternden Menschen. *Verh. Dtsch. Ges. Pathol.*, 59: 160–180.

Wever, R. (1979) *The Circadian System of Man*. Berlin-Heidelberg-New York: Springer Verlag.

Yamaoka, S. (1978) Participation of the limbic-hypothalamic structures in circadian rhythm of slow wave sleep and paradoxical sleep in the rat. *Brain Res.*, 151: 255–268.

Yehuda, S. and Carasso, R. L. (1983) Changes in the circadian rhythms of thermoregulation and motor activity in rats as a function of aging: effects of d-amphetamine and a-MSH. *Peptides*, 4: 865–869.

Yunis, E. J., Fernandes, G., Nelson, W. and Halberg, F. (1974) Circadian temperature rhythms and aging in rodents. In I. E. Scheving, F. Halberg, and J. E. Pauly (Eds.), *Chronobiology*, Igaku Shoin, Tokyo, pp. 358–363.

Zatz, M. and Herkenham, M. A. (1981) Intraventricular carbachol mimics the phase-shifting effect of light on the circadian rhythm of wheel-running activity. *Brain Res.*, 212: 234–238.

Zucker, I., Rusak, B. and King, R. G. (1976) Neural basis for circadian rhythms in rodent behavior. In A. H. Riesen and R. F. Thompson (Eds.), *Advances in Psychobiology, Vol. III*, Wiley & Sons, New York, pp. 35–74.

Discussion

D. M. GASH: Have studies shown any long-term effects on neurotransmitter systems by the loss of circadian rhythms?

W. A. VAN GOOL: I am not aware of any studies concerning the effects of SCN lesions or phase shifts upon neurotransmitter levels. There has been a study on the effects of sleep deprivation, thus interfering with at least one overt rhythm, upon circadian receptor rhythms (Wirz-Justice et al., 1981). In this study only minor differences in receptor rhythms were found between sleep-deprived and control rats. Recently, SCN ablation was shown to result in the loss of circadian variations in a number of adrenergic and benzodiazepine receptors in rat brain (Kafka et al., 1985).

G. S. ROTH: You certainly make a good point for studying the effects of diurnal rhythms on various age-dependent functional differences. However, I think we need to make a practical distinction between attempts to eliminate primary causes and attempts to deal with the results of these causes. I would argue that age differences in function are worthy of study, regardless of the time at which they occur. Certainly if Samis' hypothesis (1968) is correct, it offers an interesting possible explanation for the causes of age-associated dysfunction. On the other hand, if the hypothesis is incorrect, then we need to examine events close to the changes in the functions themselves. Thus, we come back to the discussion on the need to strike a balance between studies of etiology and attempts to devise a therapy for the manifestation of aging, dementia, and other CNS deterioration.

W. A. VAN GOOL: I agree with you that age-differences in itself, such as in the dopaminergic system for instance, can be worthwhile studying, irrespective of the time-point at which they occur. However, for a proper overall interpretation of the findings it is mandatory to take temporal variations into account, since (1) numerous parameters of brain function vary in the course of time and (2) temporal organization as such appears to be changed in old age. These arguments refer to experimental findings and they are not affected by the degree of validity of Samis' hypothesis. With respect to your last point, in which you referred to future therapies, my guess is that it may turn out to be problematic to devise an optimal therapy if circadian rhythm alterations are completely ignored because they may imply, for instance, that the substance which is to be suppleted is deficient only at a specific point in time.

H. VAN CREVEL: Could the disruption of circadian sleep rhythms in old age and dementia be due, partly, to the 'de-structuring' of daily activity? Could this be tested in animals or human subjects?

W. A. VAN GOOL: Alterations of the structure of every-day life caused by reduced social constraints may indeed play a role in changed sleep patterns in aged humans. Changes in temperature and endocrine rhythms can thus be hypothesized to result from those changes in the sleep-wakefulness rhythm. However, Weitzman et al.'s (1982) study in which the environment was controlled showed that also when adults and elderly are isolated from temporally patterned social cues, age-differences in sleep patterns and temperature rhythms are preserved. Also data from animal experiments in which both young and old rodents were isolated from exogenous influences suggest that age-related differences in circadian rhythms are, at least in part, due to alterations intrinsic to the aged organism itself.

References

Kafka, M. S., Marangos, P. J. and Moore, R. Y. (1985) Suprachiasmatic nucleus ablation abolishes circadian rhythms in rat brain neurotransmitter receptors. *Brain Res.*, 327: 344–347.

Samis, H. V. Jr. (1968) Aging: loss of temporal organization. *Perspect. Biol. Med.*, 3: 95–102.

Weitzman, E. D., Moline, M. L., Czeisler, C. A. and Zimmerman, J. C. (1982) Chronobiology of aging: temperature, sleep-wake rhythms and entrainment. *Neurobiol. Aging*, 3: 299–309.

Wirz-Justice, A., Tobler, I., Kafka, M. S., Naber, D., Marangos, P. J., Borbély, A. A. and Wehr, T. A. (1981) Sleep deprivation: effects on circadian rhythms of rat brain neurotransmitter receptors. *Psychiat. Res.*, 5: 67–76.

D. F. Swaab, E. Fliers, M. Mirmiran, W. A. Van Gool and F. Van Haaren (Eds.)
Progress in Brain Research, Vol. 70.
© 1986 Elsevier Science Publishers B.V. (Biomedical Division)

CHAPTER 17

Neuronal cytoskeleton in aging and dementia

K. Iqbal*, I. Grundke-Iqbal and H. M. Wisniewski

New York State Office of Mental Retardation and Developmental Disabilities, Institute for Basic Research in Developmental Disabilities, 1050 Forest Hill Road, Staten Island, NY 10314, USA

Introduction

The cytoskeleton of a normal mature neuron is composed of three types of fibrils, the microtubules, the neurofilaments and the microfilaments. One of the cellular and molecular changes with aging, the mechanism of which remains unknown to date, is the formation of argentophilic intracellular neurofibrillary tangles in selected neurons of the aged human brain. These extraordinary neurofibrillary changes are seen in great abundance in several adult and late life dementias, especially the Alzheimer disease/senile dementia of the Alzheimer type (AD/SDAT) (for review see Iqbal and Wisniewski, 1983). The Alzheimer neurofibrillary tangles (ANT) are composed of paired helical filaments (PHF). Bundles of these PHF are also found in the dystrophic neurites of the neuritic (senile) plaque, the second leading histopathological lesion of AD/SDAT. Together these two lesions, the ANT and the plaques, both of which contain the PHF, are the histopathological hallmark of AD/SDAT (Terry, 1963; Terry et al., 1964; Kidd, 1964); occasionally either tangles of 15 nm straight filaments or these filaments admixed with PHF have been observed in a few AD/SDAT cases (Shibayama and Kitoch, 1978; Yagishita et al., 1981). The number of ANT and plaques correlates positively with the degree of psychomet-

ric deficiency in the affected patients (Tomlinson et al., 1970), but their origin and role in disease are not understood. The number of tangles and plaques does not appear to be interdependent because in some cases there are numerous tangles and very few plaques, and vice versa. Therefore, each of these lesions is of importance on its own and the understanding of its pathogenetic mechanisms may enhance our understanding of the disease. In this chapter the morphology and the biochemistry of the neurofibrillary changes and their analogs in animal models are discussed.

Cytoskeleton of a normal neuron

The normal neurofibrils are microtubules, neurofilaments and microfilaments. Microtubules of the neuron are apparently identical to those in glial cells and all eukaryotic cells (Olmsted and Borisy, 1973). Each microtubule measures 20–24 nm in diameter, has a well-defined lumen of about 15 nm and short side arms. The protein subunit of microtubules is tubulin, a heterodimeric protein. The apparent molecular weights (mol. wts.) of human brain tubulin monomers are 56 000 for α and 53 000 for β. These tubulin monomers are acidic and differ slightly in amino acid composition and tryptic and cyanogen bromide peptide maps (Feit et al., 1971; Iqbal et al., 1977a). About

---

*Address all correspondence to Khalid Iqbal, PhD, NYS Institute for Basic Research in Developmental Disabilities, 1050 Forest Hill Road, Staten Island, New York 10314, USA

80–85% of microtubule protein is tubulin, most of the remaining 15–20% protein is of two groups of microtubule-associated proteins (MAPS), one group of about 225 kDa (kilodalton) to 350 kDa, called high molecular weight proteins and the other of about 68 kDa, called 'tau'; by sodium dodecyl sulfate-polyacrylamide gel electrophoresis (SDS-PAGE) tau resolves into several polypeptide bands corresponding to 55 kDa–68 kDa. In the absence of MAPS, microtubules assembled in vitro do not have side arms (Dentler et al., 1975; Murphy and Borisy, 1975). Tau is believed to be required for the in vitro assembly of tubulin into microtubules (Weingarten et al., 1975). In vitro assembled brain microtubules contain as contaminants small amounts of several brain proteins (Iqbal et al., 1977a). The function of microtubules in brain is not yet clearly established but they are believed to be involved in the movement of cytoplasmic constituents, especially in axoplasmic flow.

The neurofilaments are the intermediate filaments of the neuron. They are linear, 9–10 nm in diameter and have side arms. They are found sparsely in the cell body, moderately in the dendrites and most abundantly in the axon. Like microtubules, neurofilaments can be made to undergo in vitro disassembly-assembly cycles (Iqbal et al., 1981). However, the conditions for disassembly and assembly of neurofilaments are different from those of microtubules. Neurofilaments are biochemically different from intermediate filaments of other cell types and are made up of a triplet of about 70-kDa, 160-kDa and 200-kDa polypeptides that are apparently unique to nerve cells (Hoffman and Lasek, 1975; Schlaepfer, 1977; Soifer et al., 1981). Neurofilaments isolated from CNS contain varying amounts of a 50-kDa polypeptide which is believed to be mostly the glial fibrillary acidic protein, the major protein of astroglial filaments (Eng et al., 1971). The function of neurofilaments is not yet understood. They may act as a part of the force-generating mechanism in axoplasmic transport, and as a cytoskeletal element in the preservation of cell asymmetry.

Brain microfilaments, like those in muscle, are 5 nm in diameter and are made up of actin, the 45-kDa polypeptide (Berl et al., 1973).

Cytoskeletal alterations in AD/SDAT

Morphology

PHF are morphologically unlike any of the normal neurofibrils. Each PHF is a pair of filaments, 10–13 nm in diameter wound helically around each other at regular intervals of 80 nm (Kidd, 1963; Wisniewski et al., 1976, 1984). Each PHF is made up of eight protofilaments; in longitudinal section only four protofilaments are seen, the other four are hidden behind. The substructure of PHF is different from normal neurofilaments in that the globules making the PHF protofilaments are larger (32 Å ± 4 vs. 20 Å ± 3) and the longitudinal bars are longer (47 Å ± 6 vs. 27 Å ± 2) than those in neurofilaments (Wen and Wisniewski, 1984; Wisniewski and Wen, 1985).

In neurons undergoing neurofibrillary changes, PHF appear to gradually become more densely packed and take over greater proportions of cell space displacing cytoplasmic organelles. It remains unclear whether accumulations of PHF lead to cell death. It is also unknown whether the affected cells can recover. Maintenance of synaptic contact has been observed in situations where pre- and post-synaptic processes are filled with PHF, suggesting that a certain degree of function might persist in these affected synapses.

Topography

ANT are found mostly in cerebral cortex, especially in the hippocampal pyramidal neurons of Sommers sector and in small pyramidal neurons in the outer laminae of fronto-temporal cortex. They have not been observed in cerebellum, spinal cord, peripheral nervous system or extraneuronal tissues. In addition to ANT, PHF are found as bundles in the dystrophic neurites of the senile plaques and, less frequently, as individual fibrils and small bundles in the neuropil.

Neurofibrillary changes in conditions other than AD/SDAT

In addition to AD and SDAT which are believed to be the same disease with a different age of onset, PHF are also found in great abundance in Guam parkinsonism dementia complex, dementia pugilistica, postencephalitic parkinsonism and adults with Down syndrome (for review see Iqbal et al., 1977b; Wisniewski et al., 1979). The ANT have also been reported in small numbers in several cases of subacute sclerosing panencephalitis (SSPE) and in rare cases of Hallervorden-Spatz disease and juvenile neurovisceral lipid storage disease (see Table I). The PHF in these different human conditions are morphologically identical to that in AD/SDAT and antisera to PHF isolated from AD/SDAT brain label PHF in aged brain, Down syndrome and AD/SDAT cases (Grundke-Iqbal et al., unpublished observations). Thus, the accumulation of PHF is associated with normal aging, viral infection, chromosomal disorders and metabolic abnormalities. However, PHF of the Alzheimer type have never been observed in any aged animal species or have they been produced experimentally in animals.

The neurofibrillary changes in human disorders are not always of the Alzheimer type, i.e. made up of PHF. For instance, in progressive supranuclear palsy (PSP) neurons of some of the same areas which contain tangles of PHF in Alzheimer brain have neurofibrillary tangles of 15-nm straight filaments (Tellez-Nagel and Wisniewski, 1973). These tangles of 15-nm filaments in PSP are sometimes admixed with PHF (Ghatak et al., 1980). The 15-nm filaments might cross-react immunochemically with PHF since antisera to PHF label some PSP tangles at light microscopic level in tissue sections (Grundke-Iqbal et al., 1983).

In sporadic motor neuron disease, vincristine neuropathy and infantile neuroaxonal dystrophy in humans, the neurofibrillary changes are of 10-nm intermediate filament type. The 10-nm intermediate filament type neurofibrillary changes have been experimentally induced in animals with

TABLE I

Conditions and type of neurofibrillary changes

Condition	PHF	10-nm filament
Human		
aged persons	+[a]	
Alzheimer presenile and senile dementia	+[b]	
Guam parkinsonism dementia	+[b]	
dementia pugilistica	+[b]	
Down syndrome	+[b]	
post encephalitic parkinsonism	+[b]	
subacute sclerosing panencephalitis (SSPE)	+[c]	
Hallervorden-Spatz disease	+[c]	
progressive supranuclear palsy (PSP)	+[d]	+, 15 nm
sporadic motor neuron disease		+
vincristine neuropathy		+
infantile neuroaxonal dystrophy		+
Animal		
aged Rhesus monkey	**	
chronic alcohol treated rat	**	
whip spider	**	
aluminum encephalomyelopathy		+
spindle inhibitor encephalopathy		+
lathyrogenic encephalopathy (IDPN)		+
vitamin E deficiency		+
copper deficiency		+
retrograde and wallerian degeneration		+

[a]Small numbers of tangles.
[b]Numerous tangles.
[c]Small number of tangles and in a few cases only.
[d]Tangles of 15-nm straight filaments some of which are admixed with various amounts of PHF.
**PHF found in these conditions have different dimensions from that of Alzheimer dementia.

aluminum, mitotic spindle inhibitors like colchicine, vinblastine and podophyllotoxin, various nitrates and acrylamide. The aluminum-induced filamentous accumulation is apparently specific to the nervous system, while in case of the mitotic spindle inhibitors similar changes occur in a wide range of cell types. In all of these intoxications, the filaments formed are morphologically identical to normal neurofilaments. These filaments induced with various agents have not yet been isolated and characterized. The neurofilamentous tangles induced with aluminum, colchicine, vinblastine and vincristine have been shown to immunostain with an antiserum to the 70-kDa neurofilament polypeptide, but not with an antiserum to the 160-kDa neurofilament polypeptide (Dahl and Bignami, 1978; Dahl et al., 1980). Unlike PHF, both normal neurofilaments and the aluminum-induced filaments do not produce in polarized light the characteristic green birefringence after staining with congo red.

Biochemistry of PHF

PHF are stable in both fresh and frozen autopsy tissue and are resistant to solubilization in aqueous buffer in the absence of detergents or denaturants. There are two general populations of tangles, ANT I and II (Iqbal et al., 1984). ANT I and II are readily soluble and insoluble, respectively, on treatment with 2% SDS at room temperature for 3–5 minutes. ANT II are, however, soluble on sonication and heating in 1% SDS or extraction in formic acid.

PHF isolated under non-denaturing conditions are not highly purified (Iqbal et al., 1974). A 50-kDa PHF polypeptide has been identified by SDS-PAGE of these PHF-enriched preparations in comparison with identically treated normal brains (Iqbal et al., 1974; Grundke-Iqbal et al., 1979b). This 50-kDa PHF polypeptide is distinct from but has significant homologies with normal neurofibrous polypeptides and it cross-reacts with brain microtubules (Iqbal et al., 1978; Grundke-Iqbal et al., 1979a).

Highly purified PHF are isolated from autopsied tissue by a combination of sucrose density gradient centrifugation and SDS treatment of enriched preparations of neuronal cell bodies (Grundke-Iqbal et al., 1981; Iqbal et al., 1984). PHF isolated by heating the whole chopped tissue with SDS and β-mercaptoethanol according to Ihara et al. (1983), are less purified and are made insoluble most likely with this harsh detergent treatment (Iqbal et al., 1985).

PHF isolated by SDS treatment have a heterogeneous polypeptide pattern by SDS-PAGE; the polypeptide profile consists of several bands with a size difference of less than 5 kDa between adjacent bands. The most prominent PHF polypeptide bands are in the 45 kDa–62 kDa region. These PHF polypeptides are labelled on Western blots both with monoclonal and polyclonal antibodies to PHF, raised against isolated PHF as the immunogen (Grundke-Iqbal et al., 1984, 1985b; Wang et al., 1984). Furthermore, the PHF staining antibodies in the anti-PHF sera are absorbed with these PHF polypeptides cut out and extracted from the SDS-polyacrylamide gel. Neurofilament polypeptides identically extracted from the gel, do not absorb the ANT staining antibodies in the anti-PHF sera. While native PHF are resistant to proteolysis, PHF isolated by SDS-treatment are readily digested with proteases. Solubility of PHF in detergents and denaturants and their proteolysis demonstrate that, contrary to the report of Selkoe et al. (1982), PHF cannot be polymers of polypeptides cross-linked with γ-glutamyl-ε-lysine.

Relationship between PHF and normal neurofibrous proteins

The exact relationship between PHF and normal neurofibrous proteins is not clear. The polypeptide patterns of PHF do not show the presence of either neurofilament triplet or tubulin by SDS-PAGE and by Western blots of the PHF polypeptides developed with both monoclonal and polyclonal antibodies to PHF (Iqbal et al., 1984; Grundke-Iqbal et al., 1984, 1985b). However, some but not all antisera to brain microtubules (Grundke-Iqbal et al., 1979b, 1985a; Iqbal et al., 1980; Yen et al., 1981), neurofilaments and monoclonal antibodies to neurofilaments (Ishii et al., 1979; Gambetti et al., 1980, 1983; Dahl et al., 1982; Anderton et al., 1982), label PHF.

The cross-reactivity between neurofilaments and PHF appears to be due to a phosphorylated epitope shared between the two fibrils (Cork et al., 1985). In case of microtubules, the cross-reactivity with PHF is due to microtubule-associated proteins tau and not tubulin (Iqbal et al., 1980; Yen et al., 1981; Grundke-Iqbal et al., 1985a,b, 1986a,b). Anti-microtubule sera label on immunoblots some of the same PHF polypeptides identified with antisera to PHF and monoclonal antibodies to PHF (Grundke-Iqbal et al., 1985a,b); affinity-purified antibodies to tubulin do not label any PHF polypeptides on the immunoblots. The tangle-reactive antisera to microtubules, when preabsorbed with PHF polypeptides, do not label tangles. Furthermore, the tangle-staining antibodies both in the anti-PHF and anti-microtubule sera are not absorbed with neurofilaments, tubulin, actin, myosin, desmin, vimentin or keratin.

Relationship between PHF and plaque amyloid

The relationship between PHF (ANT) and plaque amyloid is summarized in Table II. Both PHF and amyloid are congophilic, and because of this common staining property a close relationship between the two lesions has been suggested by some investigators. It has been shown that this property is most likely due to β-pleated sheet structure (Glenner et al., 1974), and this conformation can be induced in many unrelated polypep-

TABLE II

Relationship between PHF and plaque amyloid

Characteristic	PHF	Amyloid
Fibril diameter (nm)	10–22	7
Congophilia	+	+
Argentophilia	+	−
Periodic acid Schiff (PAS)	−	+
Solubility in SDS	+	−
Mol. wt. (SDS-PAGE)	45 kDa–62 kDa	4 kDa
Reaction with anti-PHF sera	+	rare
Reaction with anti-amyloid[a]	−	+

[a]Antisera to two synthetic peptides consisting of first 10 and 24 amino residues of amyloid protein (Glenner et al., 1984).

tides which will then in turn become congophilic. PHF and amyloid fibrils are different ultrastructurally and in several staining properties other than with congo red and thioflavin S. Anti-PHF sera which label PHF do not by and large label plaque amyloid. To date, we have observed immunostaining of plaque amyloid in only 1/20 AD/SDAT cases studied. Furthermore, neither are PHF-staining antibodies in the anti-PHF sera absorbed with the synthetic amyloid polypeptide (24 amino acid residue), nor these antisera label the amyloid polypeptide on western blots (Grundke-Iqbal et al., unpublished data). Antisera to a synthetic peptide, consisting of first 10 amino acid residues of the amyloid polypeptide, label plaque amyloid but not the PHF (Glenner et al., 1984). According to Shirahama et al. (1982), both ANT and plaque amyloid are immunostained with a commercially available anti-prealbumin serum. These findings have not been reproduced (Alafuzoff et al., 1985; Stam and Eikelenboom, 1985).

Relationship between PHF and scrapie associated fibrils (SAF) or prion rods

Scrapie-associated fibrils (SAF) (Merz et al., 1981) or prion rods (Prusiner et al., 1982) are seen in vitro in scrapie-infected brain homogenates fractionated by treatment with proteases and detergents; the SAF are not seen in situ. These fibrils have been recently isolated and scrapie infectivity has been reported to be associated with them (Diringer et al., 1983; Prusiner et al., 1982, 1983). Since like PHF and plaque amyloid, SAF are congophilic, Prusiner et al. (1983) have proposed that SAF is the infectious agent and that AD/SDAT might be caused by a transmissible agent similar to scrapie. However, it should be pointed out here that congophilia is an indication of β-pleated sheet conformation and can be induced in unrelated polypeptides (Glenner et al., 1974). Furthermore, SAF are most likely amyloid fibrils which are formed in vitro during tissue fractionation and are not the scrapie agent; Wisniewski et al. (1985) have shown the reactivity of anti-SAF

TABLE III

Relationship between PHF and scrapie-associated fibrils

Characteristic	Tangles (PHF)	SAF (Pr)
Fibril diameter (nm)	10–22	5–14
Congophilia	+	+
Argentophilia	+	−
PAS	−	Prob. +
Solubility in SDS	+	+
Mol. wt. (SDS-PAGE)	45 kDa–62 kDa	25 kDa–30 kDa
Reaction with anti-PHF	+	−
Reaction with anti-SAF	−	+

serum with plaque amyloid in scrapie-infected animals. SAF and PHF are distinct from each other in morphology, polypeptide composition and immunochemical cross-reactivity (see Table III). Furthermore, while SAF are observed in Creutzfeldt-Jakob disease (Merz et al., 1983) they are not seen in AD/SDAT.

Animal models

To date there is no true animal model for AD/SDAT or the Alzheimer PHF. As stated above in this article, none of the animals develop Alzheimer PHF. The aluminum-induced neurofibrillary changes most commonly employed as an animal model have different topography and are of 10-nm straight filaments; these fibrils do not cross-react immunochemically with PHF. The other commonly referred animal model is scrapie-infected animals. These scrapie animals do not develop any intraneuronal neurofibrillary changes but some of the host and agent strain combinations develop varying numbers of neuritic plaques and amyloid deposits. However, firstly these changes are far fewer than those in AD/SDAT and secondly there is no cross-reactivity between scrapie amyloid deposits and AD/SDAT plaque amyloid (Wisniewski et al., 1985).

Summary and discussion

PHF have, by SDS-PAGE, a heterogeneous polypeptide composition which might vary from 2–3 major bands in the 45 kDa–62 kDa area to a ladder of polypeptides with mol. wt. difference of less than 5 kDa between the adjacent bands. This protein composition of isolated PHF is different from that of neurofilaments, microtubules, plaque amyloid and scrapie-associated fibrils. Although a number of normal brain polypeptides have been shown to cross-react immunochemically with PHF, only the presence of microtubule-associated proteins tau in PHF has been demonstrated to date.

Antibodies to PHF appear to be only partially absorbed with brain microtubules, suggesting that PHF might contain some antigenic determinants in addition to those in the microtubule-associated proteins. It is this modification of normal brain polypeptide(s) or some additional PHF antigen(s) which is probably required for the formation of PHF. PHF might be a product of derepression of some previously repressed genes. Alternatively and most probably, no new proteins are synthesized but posttranscriptional or posttranslational modifications take place in the affected neurons leading to the formation of PHF. These biochemical events might be initiated in the neuron by a variety of insults to the CNS including viral infection and chromosomal or metabolic abnormalities. The nature of these biochemical events which lead to the formation of PHF is not understood. One of these biochemical changes might be a shift towards β-pleated conformation of the polypeptides involved in the assembly of PHF.

To date the evidence for biochemical relationship between PHF and plaque core amyloid is minimal. Both of these lesions are congophilic, producing characteristic green birefringence in polarized light. Physicochemical studies of the amyloid fibrils from systemic amyloidosis have shown that they are made of proteins consisting of polypeptide chains arranged in β-pleated sheet conformation. Furthermore it has been shown that the synthetic polypeptide, poly-1-lysine, and synthetic insulin and glucagon fibers, when converted to their β-form, produce green birefringence in polarized light after congo red staining identical to that of amyloid fibrils (Glenner et al., 1974). The optical properties of congo red stained fibrillar proteins thus appear to be dependent on the β-pleated sheet formation, and this property is shared under appropriate conditions by a number of chemically unrelated proteins. Therefore, PHF though chemically might be unrelated to amyloid are most likely made of β-pleated protein fibrils. Furthermore, PHF under non-denaturing conditions are insoluble and are resistant to proteolysis, a characteristic of β-pleated sheet fibrils. This property should lead to the accumulation of fibrils made from such proteins which is indeed the case with PHF.

Acknowledgements

Studies reviewed in this article from our laboratory were made possible by assistance from Tanweer Zaidi, Yunn-Chyn Tung, Nasim Ali, Nora Lagmay and Maureen Quinlan. We would also like to acknowledge the help of summer students, Sabah Zaidi, Ambreen Qureshi, Karen Katz, Cara Della Ventura, Steve Teblitz and Kenneth Steinberg. Patricia Calimano typed the manuscript.

This work was supported in part by the National Institutes of Health Grants NS 17487, AG 05892, AG/NS 04220 and NS 18105.

References

Alafuzoff, T., Adolfsson, R., Grundke-Iqbal, I. and Winblad, B. (1986) Blood–brain barrier (BBB) in Alzheimer dementia and in nondemented elderly: an immunocytochemical study. *Acta Neuropathol. (Berl.)*, in press.

Anderton, B. H., Breinburg, D., Downes, M. J., Green, P. J., Tomlinson, B. E., Ulrich, J. and Wood, J. N. (1982) Monoclonal antibodies show that neurofibrillary tangles and neurofilaments share antigenic determinants. *Nature*, 298: 84–86.

Berl, S., Puszkin, S. and Nicklas, H. J. (1973) Actomyosin-like protein in brain. *Science*, 179: 441–443.

Cork, L. C., Altschuler, R. J., Struble, R. G., Casanova, M. F., Price, D. L., Sternberger, N. and Sternberger, L. (1985) Changes in the distribution of phosphorylated neurofilaments in Alzheimer's disease. *J. Neuropathol. Exp. Neurol.*, 44: Abst. 183.

Dahl, D. and Bignami, A. (1978) Immunochemical cross-reactivity of normal neurofibrils and aluminum-induced neurofibrillary tangles. Immunofluorescence study with anti-neurofilament serum. *Exp. Neurol.*, 58: 74–80.

Dahl, D., Bignami, A., Bich, N. T. and Chi, N. H. (1980) Immunohistochemical characterization of neurofibrillary tangles induced by mitotic spindle inhibitors. *Acta Neuropathol. (Berl.)*, 51: 165–168.

Dahl, D., Selkoe, D. J., Pero, R. T. and Bignami, A. (1982) Immunostaining of neurofibrillary tangles in Alzheimer's senile dementia with a neurofilament antiserum. *J. Neurosci.*, 2: 113–119.

Dentler, W. L., Granett, S. and Rosenbaum, J. L. (1975) Ultrastructural localization of the high molecular weight proteins associated with in vitro assembled brain microtubules. *J. Cell Biol.*, 65: 237–241.

Diringer, H., Gelderblom, H., Hilmert, H., Ozel, M., Edelbluth, C. and Kimberlin, R. H. (1983) Scrapie infectivity, fibrils and low molecular weight protein. *Nature*, 306: 476–478.

Eng, L. F., Vanderhaegen, J. J., Bignami, A. and Gerstl, B. (1971) An acidic protein isolated from fibrous astrocytes. *Brain Res.*, 28: 351–354.

Feit, H., Slusarek, L. and Shelanski, M. L. (1971) Heterogeneity of tubulin subunits. *Proc. Natl. Acad. Sci. USA*, 68: 2028–2031.

Gambetti, P., Velasco, M. E., Dahl, D., Bignami, A., Roessmann, U. and Sindely, S. D. (1980) Neurofibrillary tangles in Alzheimer disease; an immunohistochemical study. In L. Amaducci, A. N. Davison and P. Antuono (Eds.), *Aging, Vol. 13, Aging of the Brain and Dementia*, Raven Press, New York, pp. 55–63.

Gambetti, P., Shecket, G., Ghetti, B., Hirano, A. and Dahl, D. (1983) Neurofibrillary changes in human brain. An immunocytochemical study with a neurofilament antiserum. *J. Neuropathol. Exp. Neurol.*, 42: 69–79.

Ghatak, N. R., Nochlin, D. and Hadfield, M. G. (1980) Neurofibrillary pathology in progressive supranuclear palsy. *Acta Neuropathol. (Berl.)*, 52: 73–76.

Glenner, G. G. and Wong, C. W. (1984) Alzheimer's disease: initial report of the purification and characterization of a novel cerebrovascular amyloid protein. *Biochem. Biophys. Res. Commun.*, 120: 855–890.

Glenner, G. G., Eanes, E. G., Bladen, H. A., Linke, R. P. and Termine, J. D. (1974) β-Pleated sheet fibrils: a comparison of native amyloid with synthetic protein fibrils. *J. Histochem. Cytochem.*, 22: 1141–1158.

286

Glenner, G. G., Wong, C. W., Quaranto, V. and Eanes, E. D. (1984) The amyloid deposits in Alzheimer's disease: their nature and pathogenesis. *Appl. Pathol.*, 2: 357–369.

Grundke-Iqbal, I., Johnson, A. B., Terry, R. D., Wisniewski, H. M. and Iqbal, K. (1979a) Alzheimer neurofibrillary tangles: production of antiserum and immunohistological staining. *Ann. Neurol.*, 6: 532–537.

Grundke-Iqbal, I., Johnson, A. B., Wisniewski, H. M., Terry, R. D. and Iqbal, K. (1979b) Evidence that Alzheimer neurofibrillary tangles originate from neurotubules. *Lancet*, I: 578–580.

Grundke-Iqbal, I., Iqbal, K., Merz, P. and Wisniewski, H. M. (1981) Isolation and properties of Alzheimer neurofibrillary tangles. *J. Neuropathol. Exp. Neurol.*, 40: 312.

Grundke-Iqbal, I., Iqbal, K., Tung, Y. C., Wang, G. P. and Wisniewski, H. M. (1984) Alzheimer paired helical filaments: immunochemical identification of polypeptides. *Acta Neuropathol. (Berl.)*, 62: 259–267.

Grundke-Iqbal, I., Iqbal, K., Tung, Y. C., Wang, G. P. and Wisniewski, H. M. (1985a) Alzheimer paired helical filaments: crossreacting polypeptide(s) present normally in brain. *Acta Neuropathol. (Berl.)*, 66: 52–61.

Grundke-Iqbal, I., Wang, G. P., Iqbal, K., Tung, Y. C. and Wisniewski, H. M. (1985b) Alzheimer paired helical filaments: identification of polypeptides with monoclonal antibodies. *Acta Neuropathol. (Berl.)*, 68: 279–283.

Grundke-Iqbal, I., Iqbal, K., Quinlan, M., Tung, Y-C., Zaidi, M. S. and Wisniewski, H. M. (1986) Microtubule-associated protein tau: a component of Alzheimer paired helical filaments. *J. Biol. Chem.*, 261: 6084–6089.

Grundke-Iqbal, I., Iqbal, K., Tung, Y-C., Quinlan, M., Wisniewski, H. M. and Binder, L. I. (1986) Abnormal phosphorylation of the microtubule associated protein tau in Alzheimer cytoskeletal pathology. *Proc. Natl. Acad. Sci., USA*, 83: 4913–4917.

Hoffman, P. N. and Lasek, R. J. (1975) The slow component of axonal transport. Identification of major structural polypeptides of the axon and their generality among mammalian neurons. *J. Cell Biol.*, 66: 351–356.

Ihara, I., Abraham, C. and Selkoe, D. J. (1983) Antibodies to paired helical filaments in Alzheimer's disease do not recognize normal brain proteins. *Nature*, 304: 727–730.

Iqbal, K. and Wisniewski, H. M. (1983) Neurofibrillary tangles. In: B. Reisberg, (Ed.), *Alzheimer's Disease, The Standard Reference*, The Free Press, New York, pp. 48–56.

Iqbal, K., Wisniewski, H. M., Shelanski, M. L., Brostoff, S., Liwnicz, B. H. and Terry, R. D. (1974) Protein changes in senile dementia. *Brain Res.*, 77: 337–343.

Iqbal, K., Grundke-Iqbal, I., Wisniewski, H. M. and Terry, R. D. (1977a) On neurofilament and neurotubule proteins from human autopsy tissue. *J. Neurochem.*, 29: 417–424.

Iqbal, K., Wisniewski, H. M., Grundke-Iqbal, I. and Terry, R. D. (1977b) Neurofibrillary pathology: an update. In K.

Nandy and L. Sherwin (Eds.), *The Aging Brain and Senile Dementia*, Plenum, New York, pp. 209–227.

Iqbal, K., Grundke-Iqbal, I., Wisniewski, H. M. and Terry, R. D. (1978) Chemical relationship of the paired helical filaments of Alzheimer's dementia to normal human neurofilaments and neurotubules. *Brain Res.*, 142: 321–332.

Iqbal, K., Grundke-Iqbal, I., Johnson, A. B. and Wisniewski, H. M. (1980) Neurofibrous proteins in aging and dementia. In L. Amaducci, A. N. Davison and P. Antuono (Eds.), *Aging, Vol. 13, Aging of the Brain and Dementia*, Raven Press, New York, pp. 39–48.

Iqbal, K., Merz, P., Grundke-Iqbal, I. and Wisniewski, H. M. (1981) Studies on mammalian neurofilaments isolated by in vitro assembly-disassembly. *J. Neuropathol. Exp. Neurol.*, 40: 315.

Iqbal, K., Zaidi, T., Thompson, C. H., Merz, P. A. and Wisniewski, H. M. (1984) Alzheimer paired helical filaments: bulk isolation, solubility and protein composition. *Acta Neuropathol.*, 62: 167–177.

Iqbal, K., Grundke-Iqbal, I. and Wisniewski, H. M. (1985) Solubility of Alzheimer paired helical filaments in sodium dodecyl sulfate. *Trans. Am. Soc. Neurochem.*, 16: 165.

Ishii, T., Haga, S. and Tobutake, S. (1979) Presence of neurofilament protein in Alzheimer's neurofibrillary tangles (ANF); an immunofluorescent study. *Acta Neuropathol. (Berl.)*, 48: 105–112.

Kidd, M. (1963) Paired helical filaments in electron microscopy of Alzheimer's disease. *Nature*, 197: 192–193.

Kidd, M. (1964) Alzheimer's disease. An electron microscopical study. *Brain*, 87: 307–320.

Merz, P. A., Sommerville, R. A., Wisniewski, H. M. and Iqbal, K. (1981) Abnormal fibrils from scrapie-infected brain. *Acta Neuropathol. (Berl.)*, 54: 63–74.

Merz, P. A., Sommerville, R. A., Wisniewski, H. M., Manuelidis, L. and Manuelidis, E. (1983) Scrapie-associated fibrils in Creutzfeldt-Jakob disease. *Nature*, 306: 474–476.

Murphy, D. B. and Borisy, G. G. (1975) Association in high molecular weight proteins with microtubules and their role in microtubule assembly in vitro. *Proc. Natl. Acad. Sci. USA*, 72: 2696–2700.

Olmsted, J. B. and Borisy, G. G. (1973) Microtubules. *Ann. Rev. Biochem.*, 42: 507–540.

Prusiner, S. B., Bolton, D. C., Groth, D. F., Bowman, K. A., Cochran, S. P. and McKinley, M. P. (1982) Further purification and characterization of scrapie prions. *Biochemistry*, 21: 6942–6950.

Prusiner, S. B., McKinley, M. P., Bowman, K. A., Bolton, D. C., Bendheim, P. E., Groth, D. F. and Glenner, G. (1983) Scrapie prions aggregate to form amyloid-like birefringent rods. *Cell*, 35: 349–358.

Schlaepfer, W. W. (1977) Immunological and ultrastructural studies of neurofilaments isolated from rat peripheral nerve. *J. Cell Biol.*, 74: 226–240.

Selkoe, D. J., Ihara, Y. and Salazar, F. J. (1982) Alzheimer's disease: insolubility of partially purified paired helical filaments in sodium dodecyl sulfate and urea. *Science*, 215: 1243–1245.

Shibayama, H. and Kitoch, J. (1978) Electron microscopic structure of the Alzheimer's neurofibrillary changes in case of a typical senile dementia. *Acta Neuropathol. (Berl.)*, 41: 229–234.

Shirahama, T., Skinner, M., Westermark, P., Rubinow, A., Cohen, A. S., Brun, A. and Kemper, T. L. (1982) Senile cerebral amyloid. Prealbumin as a common constituent in the neuritic plaque, in the neurofibrillary tangle and in the microangiopathic lesion. *Am. J. Pathol.*, 107: 41–50.

Soifer, D., Iqbal, K., Czosnek, H., DeMartini, J., Sturman, J. A. and Wisniewski, H. M. (1981) The loss of neuron-specific proteins during the course of Wallerian degeneration of optic and sciatic nerve. *J. Neurosci.*, 1: 461–470.

Stam, F. C. and Eikelenboom, P. (1985) Immunopathological study of cerebral senile amyloid. Congophilic angiopathy and senile plaques. In F. C. Rose (Ed.), *Interdisciplinary Topics on Gerontology, Vol. 19, Modern Approaches to the Dementias, Part 1*, S. Karger, Basel, pp. 127–130.

Tellez-Nagel, I. and Wisniewski, H. M. (1973) Ultrastructure of neurofibrillary tangles in Steele-Richardson-Olszewski syndrome. *Arch. Neurol.*, 29: 324–327.

Terry, R. D. (1963) The fine structure of neurofibrillary tangles in Alzheimer's disease. *J. Neuropathol. Exp. Neurol.*, 22: 629–642.

Terry, R. D., Gonatas, N. K. and Weiss, M. (1964) Ultrastructural studies in Alzheimer's presenile dementia. *Am. J. Pathol.*, 44: 269–297.

Tomlinson, B. E., Blessed, G. and Roth, M. (1970) Observations on the brains of demented old people. *J. Neurol. Sci.*, 11: 205–242.

Wang, G. P., Grundke-Iqbal, I., Kascsak, R. J., Iqbal, K. and Wisniewski, H. M. (1984) Alzheimer neurofibrillary tangles: monoclonal antibodies to inherent antigen(s). *Acta Neuropathol. (Berl.)*, 62: 268–275.

Weingarten, M. D., Lockwood, A. H., Hwo, S.Y. and Kirschner, M. W. (1975) A protein factor essential for microtubule assembly. *Proc. Natl. Acad. Sci. USA*, 72: 1858–1862.

Wen, G. Y. and Wisniewski, H. M. (1984) Substructures of neurofilaments. *Acta Neuropathol. (Berl.)*, 64: 339–343.

Wisniewski, H. M. and Wen, G. Y. (1985) Substructures of paired helical filaments from Alzheimer's disease neurofibrillary tangles. *Acta Neuropathol. (Berl.)*, 66: 173–176.

Wisniewski, H. M., Narang, H. K. and Terry, R. D. (1976) Neurofibrillary tangles of paired helical filaments. *J. Neurol. Sci.*, 27: 173–181.

Wisniewski, H. M., Merz, P. A. and Iqbal, K. (1984) Ultrastructure of paired helical filaments of Alzheimer's neurofibrillary tangle. *J. Neuropathol. Exp. Neurol.*, 43: 643–656.

Wisniewski, H. M., Merz, P. A., Kascsak, R. J., Rubenstein, R., Carp, R. I. and Lassmann, H. (1985) Crossreactivity of SAF protein and scrapie amyloid plaques. *J. Neuropathol. Exp. Neurol.*, 44: Abst. 169.

Wisniewski, K., Jervis, G. A., Moretz, R. C. and Wisniewski, H. M. (1979) Alzheimer neurofibrillary tangles in diseases other than senile and presenile dementia. *Ann. Neurol.*, 5: 288–294.

Yagishita, S., Itoh, Y., Nan, W. and Amano, N. (1981) Reappraisal of the fine structure of Alzheimer's neurofibrillary tangles. *Acta Neuropathol. (Berl.)*, 54: 239–246.

Yen, S. C., Gaskin, F. and Terry, R. D. (1981) Immunocytochemical studies of neurofibrillary tangles. *Am. J. Pathol.*, 104: 77–89.

Discussion

R. D. TERRY: (1) Could the rare side arms on paired helical filaments (PHF) account for the immunoreactivity with anti-microtubule-associated protein (MAP)?

(2) Even if there is no product-precursor relation between PHF and core amyloid, could there not be a functional relationship by way of PHF interference with axonal flow inducing dystrophic terminals and, subsequently, plaques?

ANSWER: (1) Yes, it is possible but I think it is most likely that the staining of PHF polypeptides on western blots with the anti-microtubule serum is with polypeptides making the PHF and not just the side arms. Do not forget that the isolated PHF employed for western blots were SDS-treated which might have removed all the 'side arm' polypeptides during this procedure; we do not see any side arms on the isolated PHF. Secondly, the anti-microtubule serum labels almost all the same bands as labelled with both, the monoclonal and the polyclonal antibodies to PHF. The differences in the relative staining intensity of different bands between these different antibodies is most likely due to their affinity to different antigenic determinants of the same PHF polypeptide or polypeptides.

(2) The answer is yes, it is possible, but only where tangles lead to the formation of plaques. I believe that such a sequence of events might not be true i.e., the formation of plaques might not be dependent on the presence of tangles, e. g. (i) cases of AD/SDAT with numerous plaques and minimal number of tangles, (ii) plaques in scrapie animals which never show tangles, and (iii) Guam parkinsonism dementia cases which show numerous neurons with neurofibrillary tangles of the Alzheimer type but no plaques.

E. MENA: You showed that the amyloid plaques were not dissolved by SDS treatment. Also, synaptic junctions are resistant to solubilization by SDS. Do you ever see these structures contaminating your preparation of PHF?

ANSWER: In order to minimize contamination of PHF with plaque amyloid cores our strategy has been to first isolate neuronal cell bodies and only then treat them with SDS, followed by refractionation of PHF by sucrose density gradient centrifugation. Synaptic junctions are not the only other component which are insoluble in SDS. For instance, lipofuscin is also insoluble by SDS treatment employed in our isolation procedure. That is why we employ the sucrose gradient step following the detergent treatment to remove the remaining SDS-insoluble contaminants.

C. A. MAROTTA: What was the significance of anti-MAP staining of PHF, since MAP staining was not apparent? What is the relationship to your previously reported 50kDa PHF protein?

ANSWER: The 50kDa polypeptide is recognized both by the anti-microtubule and anti-PHF antisera. We do not see high molecular weight MAPS bands but the tau polypeptides which are in the 45 kDa–62 kDa region are labelled. Staining of PHF with anti-microtubule sera is absorbed out with MAPS-tau.

D. F. SWAAB: Is it possible that the fact that PHF were isolated by SDS and the tissue was fixed by formalin lead to three-dimensional structural differences that make e.g., that the plaque is rarely staining?

ANSWER: This is unlikely, because our anti-PHF sera label PHF not only in formalin-fixed tissue sections but also in unfixed isolated neurons with neurofibrillary tangles, SDS-treated isolated tangles and PHF polypeptides on western blots of SDS-PAGE of isolated PHF. Furthermore, anti-microtubule sera raised against non-detergent treated microtubules which label PHF, do not label plaque core amyloid. The rare staining of amyloid cores with the anti-PHF serum is most likely due to contaminating antibodies because (i) titration of the antiserum to a dilution which still labels PHF, does not label plaque amyloid and (ii) the anti-PHF serum preabsorbed with synthetic amyloid peptide labels PHF but not amyloid cores.

Etiological factors and animal models

D. F. Swaab, E. Fliers, M. Mirmiran, W. A. Van Gool and F. Van Haaren (Eds.)
Progress in Brain Research, Vol. 70.
© 1986 Elsevier Science Publishers B.V. (Biomedical Division)

CHAPTER 18

DNA damage, DNA repair and the genetic basis of Alzheimer's disease

C. Kidson and P. Chen

Queensland Institute of Medical Research, Bramston Terrace, Brisbane, Australia, 4006

Introduction

Alzheimer's disease (AD) most often occurs as single, sporadic cases in given families. However, in a minority of cases one or more affected relatives are recorded and some kindreds display many affected individuals. Classically, familial clustering may reflect either genetic determinants of disease or common exposure to environmental causative factors. Where a pattern consistent with Mendelian dominant inheritance is observed it is traditional to consider the existence of a predominantly genetic basis. This is presumed in truly familial Alzheimer's disease (Cook et al., 1979). An issue of great uncertainty is whether all AD has a genetic component, with familial AD simply representing the end of a spectrum of increasing genetic determination. Whatever the genetic component, there is no reason to exclude environmental triggers or even causative pathogens, a lesson learned from studies of the behaviour of slow viruses in the aetiopathogenesis of sporadic and familial Creutzfeldt-Jakob disease (Gajdusek and Gibbs, 1975).

The high frequency of AD is an important consideration in assessing possible genetic components. Conservative estimates placing the incidence of severe dementia at more than 5% among individuals over 65 (Ward et al., 1977) put this disease group in a high-incidence category. If there were a single gene predisposing to AD its fre-

quency would need to be very high indeed. If such a gene were homozygous recessive in behaviour, consonant with sporadic disease, the heterozygote frequency would have to be extraordinarily high. A dominant gene of limited penetrance would still have a very high frequency. It would be difficult to envisage such gene frequencies unless they were advantageous in earlier life, prior to their expression as dementia, or unless they were irrelevant in earlier life and had accumulated in human populations by genetic drift. Given the apparent universality of AD, the idea of drift is difficult to sustain.

In reality it is most unlikely that AD is due to a single gene. A more complex pattern would appear to fit the available data. In a study of 125 patients with histologically proven AD Heston et al. (1981) found that in 60% of cases the index patients were not associated with other cases in the family. Where secondary cases did occur the disease onset was often earlier and the course more rapid. It was rare to find secondary cases where symptoms of dementia first appeared over 70 years of age. When the proband and a parent are affected, nearly half the siblings eventually become demented, consistent with autosomal dominant inheritance. Quite possibly there is a range of subtypes of AD with different genetic backgrounds. Biochemical heterogeneity would thus not be surprising, reflecting genetic heterogeneity.

A number of studies have examined HLA associations with AD in an attempt to identify genetic markers, with reports of increased frequencies of HLA-B7, HLA-CW3 and DR4 (Henschke et al., 1978; Walford and Hodge, 1980). Another study (Reed et al., 1983), involving 44 patients and 100 controls, suggested that the relative risk for individuals carrying HLA-AW30, B14 or B13, might be increased. This conclusion was based on the finding of shared HLA-AW30 in a sib pair in one family and of HLA-B13 and B14 in a sib pair in a second family. However, no general phenotype associations were found. Thus, while HLA associations might be attractive in relation to slow virus theories (Harris, 1982), the data so far do not permit general conclusions vis à vis genetic markers on chromosome 6 in relation to AD.

More direct approaches to genetic analysis of AD are now available. The use of restriction fragment length polymorphism analysis employing random or, potentially, specific chromosome DNA probes should yield marker information in familial AD pedigrees just as it has for Huntington's disease (Gusella et al., 1983). This information may or may not shed light on the more prevalent sporadic AD.

Chromosomes in Alzheimer's disease

A number of studies has examined karyotypes of cells from patients with AD, with variable results. Nielson (1970) reported increased aneuploidy in six AD patients compared with age- and sex-matched controls. Mark and Brun (1973) reported no aneuploidy increase in eight AD patients while Ward et al. (1979) found increased aneuploidy in five familial AD cases and five of eight sporadic AD cases. Martin et al. (1981) reported increased hypodiploidy with age but no differences between AD cases and matched controls. Likewise White et al. (1981) found no increase in aneuploidy or chromosome aberrations in seven familial and five sporadic AD cases or their relatives compared with matched controls. In contrast, Buckton et al. (1983) reported increased aneuploidy in AD patients similar to that observed in a group of controls 20 years older. Clearly no general conclu-

sion can be reached on the basis of these conflicting data at this time. At best, a wide spectrum of variability may exist, or may relate to other undefined characteristics of patient populations.

Bergener and Jungklaass (1972) reported large acentric chromosomes in AD, while Nordenson et al. (1980) reported chromosome fragments in ten sporadic AD cases compared with matched controls. Fragments have also been reported in a small percentage of AD cells by Fischman et al. (1984). These authors also found a small increase in sister chromatid exchanges in AD cells. The suggestion has been made on the basis of these studies that the 'fragments' observed may represent chromosomes that have undergone premature centromere division and that such an event would be consistent with a basic disturbance of tubular function, e.g. a defective tubular protein leading to aberrant function of the spindle mechanism (Fischman et al., 1984).

Another facet of AD in this broad context is the association between AD and Down's syndrome. Most individuals with Down's syndrome over 40 develop AD-like neuropathology (Ellis et al., 1974; Ball and Nuttall, 1980; Williams and Matthysse, 1986). From the viewpoint of AD, the occurrence of trisomy 21 is, in turn, higher than expected in the general population, as are myeloproliferative disorders (Heston, 1976). Thus, there is more than a suggestion that factors leading to chromosome non-dysjunction may be operative in the arena of AD.

DNA damage and repair in AD/SDAT

Both the scattered chromosome data and broad theories of aging have led to studies concerned with the response of cells from AD patients to DNA-damaging agents. Thus, Hirsch et al. (cited by Fischman et al., 1984) reported a high rate of chromosomal breakage and a retardation of the cell cycle in lymphocytes treated with bleomycin, from five AD patients. Fischman et al. (1984) reported decreased mitotic indices, prolongation of the cell cycle and increased levels of sister chromatid exchanges in cells from AD patients compared with controls, in the presence of the DNA cross-linking agent mitomycin C. There is one report of increased susceptibility of AD cells to the effects of a DNA alkylating agent (Tarone et al., 1983). Robbins et al. (1983) and Kidson et al. (1983) have reported sensitivity of AD cells to ionizing radiation.

Although the available data published so far are somewhat cursory in nature and should be seen primarily as the basis for further, more detailed studies, some authors have proposed (Robbins et al., 1983; Robbins, 1983; Robison and Bradley, 1984) that DNA damage on a background of genetic sensitivity is a primary cause of AD. The broader concept of DNA damage as a ubiquitous cause of the aging process itself has had considerable support (see Gensler and Bernstein, 1981). The concept of aging as representing the cumulative effects of DNA damage is attractive in some respects, carrying as it does the implication of a substantial element of stochasticity in the aging of individuals. However, it is also difficult to escape the evidence of a major role of genetic programming in the aging process, for species do tend to have well-defined life-span ranges (Sohal, 1986). There seems no good reason to consider genetic programming and accumulation of DNA damage as mutually exclusive, indeed DNA repair capacity may itself be one of a number of genetically programmed events that set the major machinery of the biological time clocks. In this context there is merit in the idea that aging is controlled at the gene regulatory level, with natural selection operating on genes that are beneficial for youth (Cutler, 1975). The point at issue is whether there is a general relationship between aging and DNA damage, and whether genetic sensitivity to DNA damage accentuates the situation in AD/SDAT, perhaps playing a causative role in the genesis of the underlying neuropathology.

To tackle this question requires rather more detailed information than is presently available in published reports. We have recently examined lymphocytes (T cells) and lymphoblastoid cell lines (B cells) from a series of 15 unrelated sporadic AD cases with respect to response to ionizing radiation.

Sensitivity to DNA radiation damage was assessed by cell survival, cell clongenicity and induced chromosome aberrations, all of which methods gave reasonable agreement. There was a range of sensitivities exhibited by AD cells, with the majority showing significantly greater sensitivity than cells from age-matched control donors. It is important, however, to note that some AD cells were quite indistinguishable from the controls. In hybrids formed between AD and control cells, radiosensitivity was in the control range, consistent with recessive gene expression, in keeping with studies on ataxia-telangiectasia (A-T) (Chen et al., 1984). This finding was somewhat surprising, in view of the above arguments about gene frequencies. However, the gene dosage effects observed in A-T hybrids (Chen et al., 1984) if applied to these AD results imply that it is not possible to distinguish between homozygous recessive and heterozygous gene expression by such hybrid analyses. The possibility must therefore be kept in mind that the radiosensitive AD phenotype could reflect a heterozygous gene locus. Expression in diploid cells could be governed by the nature of the other allele in this case and might well be variable. Hybrids between different AD cell lines in most, but not all cases gave complementation, raising the possibility of different complementation groups and hence of different gene loci associated with radiosensitivity, again by analogy with A-T (Chen et al., 1984).

These findings open the door for extensive analysis of the number and nature of the genes conveying cellular radiosensitivity in sporadic AD. It is expected that the preliminary evidence of heterogeneity will be confirmed. Whether such an association is causal is another question, but the association is too impressive to be ignored as a component in the overall equation.

In studies on one extensive pedigree with familial AD we have found ionizing cellular radiosensitivity in all affected individuals available for study and in a proportion of their first degree relatives (unpublished data). Such a correlation is consistent with a dominant association of both cellular phenotype and disease. Such a pedigree can be subjected to restriction fragment length polymorphism analysis to obtain further marker associations. Taken together, the sporadic and familial AD data suggest the possibility that some cellular phenotypic features may be present across the spectrum of the disease complex, even though not all cases exhibit the same phenotype.

Sensitivity to DNA damage in other neurodegenerative syndromes

Association of genetic sensitivity to DNA damaging agents, specifically to ionizing radiation, and neuronal degeneration is not limited to AD. The prototype of ionizing radiation-sensitive neurodegenerative disease in man is ataxia-telangiectasia. Although radiosensitivity has become accepted as one of the diagnostic criteria of A-T, we and others (unpublished data) have come across patients with normal cellular radiation sensitivity whose clinical signs otherwise fit this syndrome. Thus, even in A-T the precise role of the radiosensitive phenotype is not certain. Even without taking this subgroup into account, an impressive feature of this rare autosomal recessive disorder is the underlying genetic heterogeneity. There are at least four complementation groups (Chen et al., 1984) and possibly many more. All appear to share a defect in control of DNA replication (Houldsworth and Lavin, 1980; Edwards and Taylor, 1980), while some may exhibit anomalous DNA repair (Paterson et al., 1982). This heterogeneity underscores the large number of gene loci that we expect to be necessary for regulation of DNA manipulation in man (Kidson, 1980).

To date, sensitivity to DNA damage by one or more agents has been reported in at least some cases of a number of neurodegenerative disorders (Table I). Discussion of some of the data is found in Robbins (1983) and Kidson et al. (1983). In no case in the studies we have done ourselves have we found an absolute association between disease and

TABLE I

Neurodegenerative syndromes associated with sensitivity to DNA damage

Ataxia-telangiectasia (Taylor et al., 1975)
Huntington's disease (Moshell et al., 1980; Chen et al., 1981)
Parkinson's disease (Robbins, 1983)
Friedreich's ataxia (Chamberlain and Lewis, 1982)
Alzheimer's disease (Robbins, 1983; Kidson et al., 1983)
ALS-PD of Guam (Kidson et al., 1983)

sensitivity, even for Huntington's disease, the classical example of Mendelian dominant inheritance (Chen et al., 1981). Tempting as it is to ponder causal association (Robbins, 1983) we feel this is premature on the basis of current evidence. However, it is of great interest that there does indeed appear to be an unexpectedly frequent association between sensitivity to DNA damage and a number of quite different neurodegenerative diseases.

In all the syndromes listed in Table I the pathological process may be initiated in somewhat select groups of specific neurons, no matter how global the ultimate pathology. Coyle et al. (1983) proposed that the neurons of the nucleus basalis of Meynert (NbM) undergo degeneration early in the pathogenesis of AD. These neurons are a major source of cholinergic innervation of the cerebral cortex and related structures and appear to play an important role in cognitive functions, including memory. Although recent data (Gottfries, 1986; Fliers and Swaab, 1986) suggest that more widespread lesions are present in AD, there does appear to be a degree of selectivity involved with respect to cell loss in the NbM. If sensitivity to radiation damage of DNA per se were in any way related to the cause of AD or other syndromes in this group, there would have to be an explanation of *selectivity* of neuron subsets in the initiation of the degenerative cascade.

It is also important to note that Down's syndrome cells are sensitive to radiation (Lambert et al., 1976), although there is a need for a large random series of Down's syndrome cases to be studied in detail. This observation is fascinating given the relationship between Down's syndrome and AD discussed above, and raises the interesting question of whether this Down's syndrome phenotype is a primary feature of the causal events leading to non-dysjunction or whether it is secondary to the trisomy 21.

Interpretation of data on sensitivity to DNA damage

Although the two are popularly associated, sensitivity to DNA damage and defective DNA repair mechanisms are not necessarily synonymous (Kidson, 1980). There is little doubt that defective repair is operative in many cases but anomalous DNA replication could lead to sensitivity (Houldsworth and Lavin, 1980; Edwards and Taylor, 1980) as could anomalous DNA recombination (Kidson, 1979). The interrelationships between genes controlling various facets of DNA manipulation is complex but is at least partly understood in *E. coli* (Little and Mount, 1982). Here there is a sophisticated degree of coordinate control of a range of gene functions involved in DNA replication, repair, generalized recombination and site-specific recombination as well as mutagenesis and cell division via the *lexA-recA* system. While little is understood at this level in man, it would indeed be surprising if some useful facets of coordinate control were not evolutionarily conserved.

Thus, a phenotype measured as sensitivity to DNA damage could reflect any one of a vast range of genotypes in this broad class. Indeed, the primary effect of the underlying mutation may be to modify an important function such as DNA site-specific recombination, with sensitivity to DNA damage as a side issue. The inference from this concept is important, namely that DNA damage per se is a useful assay tool but may play little or no part in the genesis of pathology associated with this class of polymorphic mutants. Such an interpretation shifts the focus towards development and differentiation events in addition to DNA damage.

It should be stressed that assays of the type used in this field are not particularly sensitive nor specific enough to be sufficiently discriminatory among all different phenotypes. Gene probes are clearly needed. Modification of phenotype by different alleles in the case of heterozygous mutations or by complex gene interactions such as are known in *E. coli* might be expected to lead to variability of the type observed. Coupled with the heterogeneity introduced by multiple gene loci associated with a particular clinical syndrome, as evidenced by multiple complementation groups, the extent of variability noted is not surprising. The associations of mutations affecting DNA manipulation with several neurodegenerative syndromes must be taken seriously, whether or not they reflect genetic causation.

DNA manipulation, brain function and neuropathology

We may rightly ask whether there are special features of brain structure, development and maintenance that might render neurons particularly susceptible to effects of mutations influencing DNA manipulation. The brain is far from uniform and comprises cell populations with widely differing features. The mammalian nervous system develops from pluripotent precursor cells into an array of interacting cell networks with different specialized functions. In simplified terms there is a genetically programmed evolution of basic circuitry which is largely completed during embryonic development. Upon this is superimposed further extension of circuit construction which occurs postnatally with learning inputs. The former requires organized patterns of cell division and migration, whilst the latter is virtually devoid of a requirement for neuronal multiplication. In the cerebellum the granule cells continue DNA replication postnatally as they set up specific ramifications in relation to Purkinje cells.

Special features of the mature mammalian nervous system are listed in Table II. Simplistic as this list is, these features underscore the response of the nervous system, including the brain, to cellular

TABLE II

Special features of the mammalian nervous system

Replicative glial cells
Non-replicative neurons
Programmed primary circuitry
Learning-influenced secondary circuits
Neuronal pathway dependence
Neuronal pathway redundancy

---

damage. Extreme redundancy of individual pathways means the neuronal death may be extensive in a particular circuit before clinical signs are evident. Neuronal pathway dependence, on the other hand, means that if one neuron dies, outputs from that cell to other neurons cease, with death of these secondary neurons where they are critically dependent on these informational inputs. The programmed primary circuits are prone to errors in construction during embryonic development, due to inherited or acquired mutations or to other damage, while learning-influenced secondary circuits are subject to a wider set of environmental influences.

Most neurodegenerative diseases of man involve initial death of a relatively select group of neurons in a particular region or regions, followed by dependent pathway degeneration, with the time of clinical expression depending on circuit redundancy. Thus the causative events may occur many years before evident clinical disease is diagnosed and complete degeneration of particular pathways may take decades.

Replicating and dividing neurons are radiosensitive but become relatively resistant to ionizing radiation, for example, once cell division has ceased, whereas many glia retain the capacity to divide along with radiosensitivity (Kidson, 1979). This picture has been verified in broad terms experimentally, both in the postnatal cerebellum and using brain cell cultures. Resistance of neurons to both UV and gamma-radiation increases upon terminal differentiation (Dambergs and Kidson, 1977). While there is probably a diminution of

DNA repair capacity with terminal differentiation (Kidson, 1978, 1979) some repair functions are evidently retained which can cope with UV (Dambergs and Kidson, 1979) and ionizing radiation (Lett et al., 1978) damage. The precise capacity of different mature neuron subsets to repair DNA damage is subject to some controversy (Gensler and Bernstein, 1981).

It must be remembered that some groups of neurons are destined to die as part of the embryonic developmental program, so that there may be subpopulations with grossly different expression of repair functions. At the same time this phenomenon of neuronal death during development reflects the important event of neuronal competition and selection (Purves, 1980), which occurs in both peripheral and central nervous systems. While the mechanisms and criteria for neuronal survival are not known, the process is fundamental to the structure and function of the brain. If we assume that this process is, broadly speaking, under control of genetic systems, some of which relate to the regulation of DNA manipulation, then programmed neuronal degeneration might become unbalanced as the result of mutations in such genetic systems. Conceivably neuronal competition and selection may have mechanistic parallels with immunocyte subset differentiation, which we know to depend in part on critical gene rearrangement events involving DNA recombination (Kidson and Dambergs, 1982).

Against this theoretical background, genetically based anomalies affecting DNA manipulation could have several different classes of effect on the genesis of neurodegenerative pathology.

Thus, unrepaired DNA damage in non-replicative neurons could lead to cell death, while differential expression of DNA repair genes in particular neuron subsets could possibly explain the selectivity of neuronal drop-out in a particular syndrome, e.g. the nucleus basalis in AD. Given the neuronal redundancy factor it could conceivably take considerable time before a critical number of neurons in this subset population was killed leading to dependent-pathway loss of an order that would lead to clinically identifiable functional disturbance. Such a concept would require different mutant genes to affect DNA repair pathways differentially in different neuronal subsets, i.e. a differentiation-related phenomenon.

Another possibility already alluded to above, is that the critical mutations affecting DNA manipulation are more likely to concern DNA recombination, either generalized or site-specific in nature. If gene shuffling/recombination of the kind now known to be essential for the genesis of immunocyte (T and B cell) subsets is also required to generate neuronal subsets during brain development, mutations in appropriate gene loci could result in subtle phenotypic variants. This would be particularly true if a degree of stochasticity were involved in generating approximate numbers and subclasses of neuronal subpopulations, since a quantitative change in the chance element might conceivably lead to neuropathology with a prolonged — and variable — lead time. The anomalous phenotype so produced might have, for example, fewer surface receptors of a particular class, reducing the chances for optimal numbers of stable interneuronal corrections. Neuronal death might then be of the inbuilt time-bomb character, dependent on the precise number and nature of feedback signals required for viability. In the absence of hard data at this juncture it is not profitable to speculate too widely on the specific events that might be involved.

Mature neurons are non-dividing, so that DNA replication-related events would need to operate *in embryo*. What is not known is whether limited site-specific DNA recombination events can occur in neurons in their post-replication phase. The answer to this question would determine the limitations on the period during which anomalous recombination events could occur. Clearly important pathological features of AD, such as structural abnormalities in the paired helical neurofilaments (Ihara et al., 1983) and their accumulation as the classical neurofibrillary tangles, need to be explained appropriately if anomalous DNA manipulation is to be implicated in the aetiopathology of

this disease class. The problem is not to find a pertinent molecular mechanism (e.g. mutation, recombination) but to explain the time-frame and the eventual global distribution of such lesions. The possibility that they are secondary effects rather than primary ones is easier to interpret.

The clinical problem is one of neuropathology of a particular type. However, genetic anomalies will be widely expressed in a variety of somatic cell populations. Thus it is conceivable that host genetics of the type described could affect virus behaviour, either directly (replication, mutation, recombination) or by influence on receptor numbers, availability or specificity. Thus a role for host genetics of this class in slow virus pathogenesis is not beyond conjecture.

Summary and conclusions

In the present context we must ask whether neurodegenerative diseases like AD provide a window on the normal aging process in the brain. Certainly AD, with an incidence of more than 5% among individuals over 65 in some populations, is a major concomitant of aging in a substantial number of people. In this sense its importance lies in the possibilities it opens up for delineation of some gene functions that, when mutant, give rise to exaggerated, rapid brain failure, a phenomenon that occurs more slowly, to a lesser degree, in a larger proportion of the aging human population.

Pursuit of the molecular details of the neurodegeneration-associated radiosensitivity mutants promises to open up new leads in this respect. It will be important to consider the spectrum of activities involved in the genetic control of DNA manipulation rather than assume that we are dealing simply with repair of DNA damage. Since neurons are not required to undergo multiplication, they have a longer time to repair DNA damage than do dividing cells, where fidelity of DNA replication is a high priority. Mature neurons are remarkably resistant to DNA damage, at least that due to ionizing radiation.

There is no doubt that increased sensitivity to

DNA damaging agents such as ionizing radiation is associated with AD in the statistical sense. However, not all individuals with AD exhibit the sensitivity and there is growing evidence for considerable heterogeneity of the underlying mutations. These are recessive in cell hybridization experiments but the latter cannot discriminate between heterozygous and homozygous gene expression. Many different gene loci are probably involved. The central question, whether the resultant phenotypes may be causatively related to AD must remain open at this time, although mechanisms by which they could so operate are conceptually available. A causal role could be at the level of primary neuronal death, neuronal gene expression, neuronal network development and maintenance, or even of host determination of virus behaviour.

The two critical features of AD that would need to be explained in this context are the relative neuronal subset specificity of the initial lesions and the time-frame of development of the neuropathology. These questions and the tantalizing issues of whether genetic sensitivity to DNA damage is a common cohort phenomenon of AD/SDAT, a genetically linked characteristic or an aetiological factor remain for future investigation.

Acknowledgements

Work reported here was supported by the National Health and Medical Research Council of Australia.

References

Ball, M. D. and Nuttall, K. (1980) Neurofibrillary tangles, granulovacuolar degeneration and neuron loss in Down's syndrome: quantitative comparison with Alzheimer dementia. *Ann. Neurol.*, 7: 462–465.

Bergener, M. and Jungklaass, F. K. (1972) Die Alzheimersche Krankheit: ein pathologischer Alterungsvorgang des Gehirns? *Acta Gerontol.*, 2: 359–367.

Buckton, K. E., Whalley, L. J., Lee, M. and Christie, J. E. (1983) Chromosome changes in Alzheimer's presenile dementia. *J. Med. Genet.*, 20: 46–51.

Chamberlain, S. and Lewis, P. D. (1982) Studies of cellular hypersensitivity to ionising radiation in Friedreich's ataxia. *J. Neurol. Neurosurg. Psychiat.*, 45: 1136–1138.

Chen, P., Kidson, C. and Imray, F. P. (1981) Huntington's disease: implications of associated cellular radiosensitivity. *Clin. Genet.*, 20: 331–336.

Chen, P., Imray, F. P. and Kidson, C. (1984) Gene dosage and complementation analysis of ataxia-telangiectasia lymphoblastoid cell lines assayed by induced chromosome aberrations. *Mutat. Res.*, 129: 165–172.

Cook, R. H., Ward, B. E. and Austin, J. H. (1979) Studies in aging of the brain. IV. Familial Alzheimer's disease: relation to transmissible dementia aneuploidy and microtubular defects. *Neurology*, 29: 1402–1412.

Coyle, J. T., Price, D. L. and DeLong, M. R. (1983) Alzheimer's disease: a disorder of critical cholinergic innervation. *Science*, 219: 1184–1190.

Cutler, R. G. (1975) Evolution of human longevity and the genetic complexity governing aging rate. *Proc. Natl. Acad. Sci. USA*, 72: 4664–4668.

Dambergs, R. G. and Kidson, C. (1977) Differential radiosensitivity of mouse embryonic neurons and glia in cell culture. *J. Neuropathol. Exp. Neurol.*, 36: 576–585.

Dambergs, R. G. and Kidson, C. (1979) Quantitation of DNA repair in brain cell cultures: implications for autoradiographic analysis of mixed cell populations. *Int. J. Radiat. Biol.*, 36: 271–280.

Edwards, M. J. and Taylor, A. M. R. (1980) Unusual levels of ADP–ribose and DNA synthesis in ataxia-telangiectasia cells following gamma-ray irradiation. *Nature*, 287: 745–747.

Ellis, W. G., McCullogh, J. R. and Corley, C. L. (1974) Presenile dementia in Down's syndrome: ultrastructural identity with Alzheimer's disease. *Neurology*, 24: 101–106.

Fischman, H. K., Reisberg, B., Albu, P., Ferris, S. H. and Rainer, J. D. (1984) Sister chromatid exchanges and cell cycle kinetics in Alzheimer's disease. *Biol. Psychiat.*, 19: 319–327.

Fliers, E. and Swaab, D. F. (1986) Neuropeptide changes in aging and Alzheimer's disease. In D. F. Swaab, E. Fliers, M. Mirmiran, W. A. Van Gool and F. Van Haaren (Eds.), *Aging of the Brain and Alzheimer's Disease, Progress in Brain Research, this volume*, Elsevier, Amsterdam, pp. 141–152.

Gajdusek, D. C. and Gibbs, C. J. Jr. (1975) Familial and sporadic chronic neurological degenerative disorders transmitted from man to primates. In B. S. Meldrum and C. D. Marsden (Eds.), *Advances in Neurology*, Raven Press, New York, pp. 219–317.

Gensler, H. L. and Bernstein, H. (1981) DNA damage as the primary cause of aging. *Quart. Rev. Biol.*, 56: 279–303.

Gottfries, C. G. (1986) Monoamines and myelin components in aging and dementia disorders. In D. F. Swaab, E. Fliers, M. Mirmiran, W. A. Van Gool and F. Van Haaren (Eds.), *Aging of the Brain and Alzheimer's Disease, Progress in Brain Research, this volume*, Elsevier, Amsterdam, pp. 133–140.

Gusella, J. F., Wexler, N. S., Conneally, P. M., Naylor, S.,

Anderson, M. A., Tanzi, R. E., Watkins, P. C., Ottina, K., Wallace, M. R., Sakaguchi, A. Y., Young, A. B., Shoulson, I., Borrilla, E. and Martin, J. B. (1983) A polymorphic DNA marker genetically linked to Huntington's disease. *Nature*, 306: 234–238.

Harris, R. (1982) Genetics of Alzheimer's disease. *Br. Med. J.*, 284: 1065–1066.

Henschke, P. J., Bell, D. A. and Cape, R. D. T. (1978) Alzheimer's disease and HLA. *Tissue Antigen*, 12: 132–135.

Heston, L. L. (1976) Alzheimer's disease, trisomy 21 and myeloproliferative disorders: association suggesting a genetic diathesis. *Science*, 196: 322–323.

Heston, L. L., Mastri, A. R., Anderson, V. E. and White, J. (1981) Dementia of the Alzheimer type. Clinical genetics, natural history and associated conditions. *Arch. Gen. Psychiat.*, 38: 1085–1090.

Houldsworth, J. and Lavin, M. F. (1980) Effect of ionizing radiation on DNA synthesis in ataxia-telangiectasia cells. *Nucl. Ac. Res.*, 8: 3709–3720.

Ihara, Y., Abraham, C. and Selkoe, D. J. (1983) Antibodies to paired helical filaments in Alzheimer's disease do not recognize normal brain proteins. *Nature*, 304: 727–730.

Kidson, C. (1978) DNA repair in differentiation. In P. C. Hanawalt, E. C. Friedberg and C. F. Fox (Eds.), *DNA Repair Mechanisms*, Academic Press, New York, pp. 761–768.

Kidson, C. (1979) Repair systems and differentiation. In S. Okada, M. Immamura, T. Terashima and Y. Yamagushu (Eds.), *Radiation Research*, Toppan, Tokyo, pp. 627–631.

Kidson, C. (1980) Disease of DNA repair. *Clin. Haematol.*, 9: 141–157.

Kidson, C. and Dambergs, R. G. (1982) Nervous system development and ataxia-telangiectasia. In B. A. Bridges and D. G. Harnden (Eds.), *Ataxia-telangiectasia: a Cellular and Molecular Link between Cancer, Neuropathology and Immune Deficiency*, John Wiley and Sons, Chichester, pp. 373–377.

Kidson, C., Chen, P., Imray, F. P. and Gipps, E. (1983) Nervous system disease associated with dominant cellular radiosensitivity. In E. C. Friedberg and B. A. Bridges (Eds.), *Cellular Responses to DNA Damage*, Alan R. Liss, New York, pp. 721–729.

Lambert, B., Hansson, K., Bui, T. H., Funes–Cravioto, F., Linsten, J., Holmberg, M. and Strausmanis, R. (1976) DNA repair and frequency of X-ray and u.v. light induced chromosome aberrations in leukocytes from patients with Down's syndrome. *Ann. Hum. Genet. (Lond.)*, 39: 293–332.

Lett, J. T., Keng, P. C. and Sun, C. (1978) Rejoining of DNA strand breaks in non-dividing cells irradiated in situ. In P. C. Hanawalt, E. C. Friedberg and C. F. Fox (Eds.), *DNA Repair Mechanisms*, Academic Press, New York, pp. 481–484.

Little, J. W. and Mount, D. W. (1982) The SOS regulatory system of *Escherichia coli*. *Cell*, 29: 11–22.

Mark, J. and Brun, A. (1973) Chromosomal deviations in Alzheimer's disease compared to those in senescence and senile dementia. *Gerontol. Clin.*, 15: 253–258.

Martin, J. M., Kellett, J. M. and Kahn, J. (1981) Aneuploidy in cultured human lymphocytes. II. A comparison between senescence and dementia. *Age Ageing*, 10: 24–28.

Moshell, A. N., Tarone, R. E., Barrett, S. F. and Robbins, J. H. (1980) Radiosensitivity in Huntington's disease: implications for pathogenesis and presymptomatic diagnosis. *Lancet*, 1: 9–11.

Nielson, J. (1970) Chromosomes in senile, presenile and arteriosclerotic dementia. *J. Gerontol.*, 25: 312–315.

Nordenson, L., Adolfsson, R., Bechman, G., Bucht, G. and Winblad, B. (1980) Chromosomal abnormality in dementia of the Alzheimer type. *Lancet*, 1: 481–482.

Paterson, M. C., Smith, P. J., Bech–Hansen, N. T., Smith, B. P. and Middlestadt, M. V. (1982) Anomalous repair in radiogenic DNA damage in skin fibroblasts from ataxia-telangiectasia patients. In B. A. Bridges and D. G. Harnden (Eds.), *Ataxia-telangiectasia: A Cellular and Molecular Link between Cancer, Neuropathology and Immune Deficiency*, John Wiley and Sons, Chichester, pp. 271–289.

Purves, D. (1980) Neuronal competition. *Nature*, 287: 585–586.

Reed, E., Thompson, D., Mareyux, R. and Suciu-Foca, N. (1983) HLA antigens in Alzheimer's disease. *Tiss. Antigens*, 21: 164–167.

Robbins, J. H. (1983) Hypersensitivity to DNA-damaging agents in primary degenerations of excitable tissue. In E. C. Friedberg and B. A. Bridges (Eds.), *Cellular Responses to DNA Damage*, Alan R. Liss, New York, pp. 671– 700.

Robbins, J. H., Otsuka, F., Tarone, R. E., Bromback, R. A., Moshell, A. N., Nee, L. E., Ganges, M. B. and Cayeux, S. J. (1983) Radiosensitivity in Alzheimer disease and Parkinson disease. *Lancet*, 1: 468–469.

Robison, S. H. and Bradley, W. G. (1984) DNA damage and chronic neuronal degenerations. *J. Neurol. Sci.*, 64: 11–20.

Sohal, R. S. (1986) Origin and functional significance of lipofuscin accumulation under normal and pathological conditions. In D. F. Swaab, E. Fliers, M. Mirmiran, W. A. Van Gool and F. Van Haaren (Eds.), *Aging of the Brain and Alzheimer's Disease, Progress in Brain Research, this volume*, Elsevier, Amsterdam, pp. 171–183.

Tarone, R. E., Scudiero, R., Brumback, A., Polinsky, R., Nee, L. E., Clatterbuck, B. E. and Robbins, J. H. (1983) Statistical analysis of the hypersensitivity to *N*-methyl-*N'*-nitro-*N*-nitrosoguanidine (MNNG) in muscular dystrophy (MD) or neurodegeneration. *J. Cell Biochem.*, Suppl. 7B: 209.

Taylor, A. M. R., Harnden, D. G., Arlett, C. F., Harcourt, S. A., Lehmann, A. R., Stevens, S. and Bridges, B. A. (1975) Ataxia-telangiectasia: a human mutation with abnormal radiation sensitivity. *Nature*, 258: 427–429.

Walford, R. L. and Hodge, S. E. (1980) HLA distribution in Alzheimer's disease. In P. I. Terasaki (Ed.), *Histocompatibility Testing 1980*. UCLA Press, Los Angeles, pp. 727–729.

Ward, B. E., Cook, R. H., Robinson, A. and Wang, H. S. (1977) Dementia in old age. In C. E. Wells (Ed.), *Dementia*, F. A. Davis and Co., Philadelphia, pp. 15–26.

Ward, B. E., Cook, R. H., Robinson, A. and Austin, J. H. (1979) Increased aneuploidy in Alzheimer disease. *Am. J. Med. Genet.*, 3: 137–144.

White, B. J., Crandall, C., Goudsmit, J., Morrow, C. H., Alling, D. W., Gajdusek, D. C. and Tijio, J. H. (1981) Cytogenetic studies of familial and sporadic Alzheimer's disease. *Am. J. Med. Genet.*, 10: 77–89.

Discussion

D. M. GASH: Given the observation of the extensive heterogeneity of AD in the age of onset, do your data indicate a difference in radiosensitivity between those individuals with early vs. late appearance of dementia?

ANSWER: Our series of AD patients studied ranges from about 50 to over 70 but the numbers are too few to draw statistically valid conclusions about the quantitative relationship, if any, between sensitivity to DNA damage and age of onset of clinical disease. It is perhaps important here to remember that the genetic heterogeneity inferred from our hybrid experiments would leave open the possibility of different gene products from gene loci in this DNA manipulation class to affect the disease process in different ways, possibly giving different ages of onset. If the relevant mutants are indeed heterozygous, as we suspect, these mutant loci are also open to modification by the second allele, which we would expect to be variant, with great opportunity for variable expressivity consistent with the differing clinico-pathological time course.

D. F. SWAAB: Is it possible that the capability of a neuron to execute DNA repair is dependent on its metabolic state? This might, at least partly, explain the different changes in different systems in the Alzheimer brain.

ANSWER: There are no direct data experimentally or inferentially derived. However, in principle you are right, it is quite possible that there is differential repair capacity of different neuron subsets, perhaps related to their overall metabolic state. If so, mutations in different gene loci coding for different repair enzymes could theoretically explain specificity of response of the different neuron subsets to DNA damage, consistent with a causal role of DNA damage in the pathogenesis of AD. However, we would still expect a high degree of stochasticity with respect to the particular neurons hit by DNA damaging agents and to the particular gene loci that were hit, i.e. random damage. This is not so easy to reconcile with the clinical and pathological patterns seen in AD. Nevertheless, differential repair capability, mutations in different specific repair enzyme genes in different neurodegenerative disorders must remain a formal possibility in interpretation of the data. It is also possible that while other effects on DNA manipulation are more important, the effect of DNA damage may be superimposed. Ataxia-telangiectasia provides an inter-esting parallel: the neuropathology is clearly developmental but these children are clinically radiosensitive, even though DNA damage is not the cause of the disease.

R. D. TERRY: Do not the population statistics of AD rule out the homozygous recessive postulate coming from the hybrid work?

ANSWER: Almost certainly yes. The gene frequencies required for a homozygous recessive model involving a single gene locus would be very large. Since we have observed heterogeneity consistent with multiple gene loci in the hybridization experiments we must assume multiple gene loci are indeed involved in the AD radiosensitive phenotype, which would increase the required gene frequency for this model still further. Thus we favour the heterozygous gene expression interpretation of our data, even though as I have expressed, it is not possible to formally decide between homozygous and heterozygous expression on the basis of the hybrid data per se. By comparison with the well-established data from similar experiments with ataxia telangiectasia homozygotes and heterozygotes crossed with normals it is, however, quite sure that the AD data are consistent with heterozygous gene expression in keeping with the population frequency of AD.

J. VIJG: Would you elaborate a little bit more on how Alzheimer's disease might originate during development, maturation and aging in terms of hypothetical site-specific recombination events in the brain DNA?

ANSWER: The idea that what we measure as sensitivity to DNA damage might reflect side effects of mutant genes governing other facets of DNA manipulation is consistent with *E. coli* genetics. The most appealing facet from the viewpoint of developmental biology is site-specific recombination, such as is well established for T-cell receptor and B-cell immunoglobulin loci. While similar events have yet to be established for specific target genes concerned with brain development, it could make sense if some such classes of molecules were involved in the genesis of basic neural activity, e.g. proteins needed to initiate or consolidate specific groups of synapses. Mutations in genes involved in generating site-specific gene fragment selection or gene rearrangement (cf. oncogene shuffling) would then have a bearing on the accuracy of neural circuit formation, on the stability thereof or on the half-life of particular classes of neurons. This would be predetermined during brain development if it required DNA replication for the recombination events, although we cannot yet rule out the remote possibility that some site-specific DNA recombination events might occur in post-replicative neurons. If we are right about the mutations we measure by increased sensitivity to DNA damage being heterozygous, there will presumably be different gene products arising from the mutant and non-mutant allelic loci. These may be in competition for their phenotypic effects such that, for example, a mixed set of critical synaptic proteins is produced, half normal, half abnormal. This could lead to a functional synapse but one with reduced stability that might fall apart earlier than usual, leading to premature neuronal death.

Many other theoretical examples could be imagined. Selectivity would be expected consistent with the neuropathology. While it does not pay at this point to speculate too much, the concept is useful as one means of reconciliation of the clinical and genetic data, if the observed genetic associations are somehow causally related rather than being simply linked or cohort phenomena. Remember that this avenue of thought presumes that the important genetic effects are concerned with the neurons directly, whereas the same host genetics could lead to virus modification for example. The difficulty with the concept lies in identifying possible gene loci where site-specific recombination might occur relevant to brain differentiation; if we knew that we could test the hypothesis directly.

D. F. Swaab, E. Fliers, M. Mirmiran, W. A. Van Gool and F. Van Haaren (Eds.)
Progress in Brain Research, Vol. 70.
© 1986 Elsevier Science Publishers B.V. (Biomedical Division)

CHAPTER 19

Transcriptional and translational regulatory mechanisms during normal aging of the mammalian brain and in Alzheimer's disease

C. A. Marotta[a,b,c,*], R. E. Majocha[a,c], J. F. Coughlin[a,c,**], H. J. Manz[d], P. Davies[e], M. Ventosa-Michelman[c], W.-G. Chou[f], S. B. Zain[f] and E. M. Sajdel-Sulkowska[a,c]

[a]*Department of Psychiatry, Harvard Medical School, and* [b]*Neurobiology Laboratory, Massachusetts General Hospital, Boston, MA, USA;* [c]*Molecular Neurobiology Laboratory, Mailman Research Center, McLean Hospital, Belmont, MA, USA;* [d]*Department of Pathology, Georgetown University School of Medicine, Washington, DC, USA;* [e]*Department of Pathology, Albert Einstein College of Medicine, Bronx, NY, USA;* [f]*Cancer Center, University of Rochester Medical School, Rochester, NY, USA*

Introduction

Irrespective of the etiology of Alzheimer's disease (AD), increasing evidence supports the hypothesis that basic defects at the level of transcription or translation, or both, may be involved in the pathogenesis of this illness. Recent positron emission tomography studies indicating a substantial decrease in brain protein synthesis in living patients with dementia (Bustany et al., 1983) underscore the importance of molecular biological approaches to the study of AD. Advances in molecular techniques applied to post-mortem human brain tissue demonstrated that this material can be used for direct structural and functional studies of polynucleotides (Marotta et al., 1981a; Sajdel-Sulkowska et al., 1983a). The same procedures were applicable to the post-mortem AD brain (Sajdel-Sulkowska et al., 1983b). This methodological approach appears essential since AD is a uniquely human disorder. Early investigations were carried out on human brain to determine the extent to which RNA survived the post-mortem

interval by measuring the yields and the stimulation of protein synthesis in vitro. Examination of these two parameters appeared germane to the study of an age-related disease since a host of animal experiments, carried out over the past two decades, had indicated that during aging of the mammalian brain, there is a progressive decline in RNA levels and protein-synthesizing capacity. Aspects of these investigations are reviewed in the following sections; subsequently, we discuss macromolecular changes in the AD brain.

RNA content in the aging animal brain

Among the earlier studies, Ringborg (1966) measured the RNA content of rat hippocampal CA3 neurons that were isolated by microdissection. There was an increase in RNA from the fetal value of 19 pg/cell to the newborn value of 24 pg/cell with a further increase in the adult to 110 pg/cell; however, in old rats (36–38 months), the amount of RNA declined to nearly half the adult amount (53 pg/cell). Although Chaconas and

---

*Address for correspondence: Dr. Charles A. Marotta, Mailman Research Center, McLean Hospital, Belmont, MA 02178, USA.
**Present address: New England Deaconess Hospital, Boston, MA 02115, USA.

Finch (1973) observed a slight decline with age in the ratio of RNA/DNA in rat hippocampal homogenates, the values obtained did not reach statistical significance. However, the ratio for striatal RNA/DNA was significantly lower in the senescent animal (28–30 months). The differences between the two reports may reflect vastly different experimental approaches as well as the use of considerably older animals in the earlier study.

One would expect the RNA/DNA ratio to reflect changes in RNA levels since the content of DNA does not significantly alter after the early postnatal period. For example, Adams (1966) measured the DNA and partly fractionated RNA in cerebral cortex from Wistar albino rats. DNA increased up to 18 days and then remained fairly constant. Nuclear and transfer RNA followed a similar course. However, in the oldest rats (225 g) the ribosomal RNA content declined steeply to approximately half the peak value.

Several studies are available concerning the synthesis of total cellular RNA. In the early experiments of Adams (1966) [^{14}C]orotic acid was injected into 4-days-old and adult (200–250 g) rats. The incorporation of labeled precursor was noted to be substantially lower in the adult. Gibas and Harman (1970) isolated rat brain nuclei and examined the incorporation of [^{14}C]ATP into RNA. The level of incorporation attained at 1 month of age declined by 28% at 5 months with little further change at 22 months. Essentially the same results were obtained at low and high ammonium sulfate values, suggesting that RNA polymerase I and II behaved similarly. A more easily interpreted investigation was reported by Benson and Harker (1978). These authors prepared RNA polymerase from C57B1/6J mouse brains and measured the incorporation of [^{3}H]UMP into RNA using denatured calf thymus DNA as a template. The data indicated that under the experimental conditions the RNA polymerase activity did not appear to decrease in the older age group. However, others have shown that the rate of RNA synthesis continues to decrease in aged animals (Semsei et al., 1982; Petricevic et al., 1983).

Different experimental approaches partly account for the differing results. Further direct measurements of RNA polymerases and DNA template activity are required to clarify the relationship between aging and transcription. If the rate of synthesis of RNA cannot fully account for the decline in RNA levels previously noted, then other factors merit attention, viz., processing and degradation.

The synthesis of poly(A +) RNA in the developing rat cortex was investigated after a 5-h pulse of [^{32}P]inorganic phosphate administered intracranially (Berthold and Lim, 1976a). Although the period of labeling was arbitrary, the authors demonstrated that the proportion of the total RNA represented by poly(A +) RNA decreased from 34% in newborn rats to 23% during the interval from 40 to 150 days of age. If verified in further studies, the more rapid decline of mRNA levels relative to total RNA during aging is of particular interest in view of the relationship between brain RNA content and protein synthesis activity, described subsequently. Evidence was also obtained to suggest that the transport of rat forebrain RNA from nucleus to cytoplasm declines during the interval between birth and adulthood (Berthold and Lim, 1976b). Measurements made of nuclear and cytoplasmic RNAs after intracranial injection of [^{32}P]inorganic phosphate indicated that in the young brain a larger fraction of the labeled rRNA and poly(A +) RNA was transported to cytoplasm as compared with the adult.

From 10 days of age to adulthood, significant differences have been noted with respect to polyadenylic acid sequences. DeLarco et al. (1975) found that relative to young rat brain RNA, adult brain RNA exhibited decreased binding to oligo(dT)-cellulose, hybridized to 38% less [^{3}H]poly-(U), and had an average poly(A) length that was 10% shorter. Shortening of poly(A) segments with age is an early observation by Sheiness and Darnell (1973). Although the functional significance of losing poly(A) sequences is not clear, it has been shown that removal of poly(A) from purified mRNA caused a decrease in the translational half-life during in vitro protein synthesis (Doel and Carey, 1976). However, the functional activity is independent of poly(A) length and is, rather, proportional to the mRNA concentration (Cann et al., 1974).

Among other possibilities, the decline in poly(A) sequences may be related to an age-related loss, due to nuclease activity, of previously synthesized poly(A), or to a decline in the synthetic activity of poly(A) polymerase. Polymerase activity was measured in nuclear lysates of developing and maturing rat brains (Richter and Schumm, 1981). Between 8 and 120 days, the enzyme activity declined by 58% and remained at the reduced level until 300 days of age. Since the experiment was carried out on lysates, it cannot be inferred that decreased enzyme activity was related to an age-related loss of poly(A) polymerase. Equally plausible is a decline in the concentration of ATP available for polymerization or the decreased availability of polynucleotide substrates.

Protein synthesis in the aging animal brain

A variety of approaches has been used to investigate the influence of aging on protein synthesis levels in the animal brain. Data on the incorporation of amino acids into proteins in vastly different experimental systems, ranging from crude preparations to those containing highly purified components, have led to a remarkably consistent conclusion, viz., that as the brain ages there is a decline in the level of protein synthesis.

For in vivo protein synthesis studies, Dunlop et al. (1975) suggested the use of high concentrations of certain amino acids in order to minimize variations due to metabolism and precursor pool sizes. Using this approach the same authors demonstrated an age-related decline in protein synthesis during early development (Dunlop et al., 1977). Dwyer et al. (1980) made use of the same procedure to measure the rates of lysine incorporation into protein of rat brain during aging. Synthesis of protein in forebrain declined by 11% between 3 and 10.5 months and declined a further

9% between 16.5 and 22.5 months. The absolute levels of amino acid incorporation of the brain in vitro are not comparable to those of in vivo systems (Fando et al., 1980). Nevertheless, an age-related decline can be demonstrated in slices and fractionated systems. Rat brain slices of varying ages were incubated in enriched medium in the presence of [^{14}C]amino acids. From the perinatal period to one month of age, protein synthesis declined approximately 80% with a further decline of 35% over a period of 20 months (Orrego and Lipmann, 1967). The protein synthesizing activity of the postmitochondrial supernatant from rat brains of increasing ages was measured (Ekstrom et al., 1980). The incorporation of amino acids decreased by 43% between 6 and 14 months and by 56% by 32 months. Other studies have used in vitro systems fractionated into their various components. During development and aging, the decline in protein synthesis has been related to decreased concentration of translationally competent ribosomes and RNA as well as soluble factors (Murthy, 1966; Yamagami et al., 1966; Lerner and Johnson, 1970; Zomzely et al., 1971; Johnson, 1976; Goertz, 1979; Vargas and Castaneda, 1981; Soreq et al., 1983).

From the previous discussion concerning the loss of brain RNA in older animals, it might be expected that the decreased concentration of polysomal RNA would be of significant consequence with respect to protein synthesis rates. Pertinent observations are discussed below.

The contribution of RNA levels to the regulation of protein synthesis

Dunlop et al. (1984) investigated the relationship between total RNA content and protein synthesis in studies designed to distinguish between changes in activity per ribosome vs. changes in concentration of ribosomes as the significant factor related to rates of protein synthesis in the developing brain. From 2 days of age to adulthood the RNA levels of rat brain were measured. These values were compared to protein synthesis rates, previously obtained (Dunlop et al., 1975, 1977), in which large doses of [^{14}C]valine were injected into the rat to maintain a constant specific activity of precursor. It was determined that RNA activity (mg protein synthesized per h per mg RNA) remains unchanged during normal growth and that higher protein synthesis rates in young brain are due to a higher content of ribosomal RNA. Similar results were also obtained by Waterlow et al. (1978) for the interval between 4–6 weeks and 1 year of age. These studies indicate that protein synthesis activity in brain is regulated to a large extent by the content of RNA.

Other investigations have addressed the efficiency of specific mRNAs during translation. Tubulin, the most abundant brain cytoskeletal protein, can be separated into multiple isoelectric forms (Marotta et al., 1978), a number of which correspond to separate mRNAs (Marotta et al., 1979). During early development, from the prenatal period to 1 month, rat brain poly(A +) messenger RNA synthesizes first five forms and then seven forms; at least two of the latter increase while three forms decrease (Gozes et al., 1980). Having established that tubulin heterogeneity at early time points is partly, although not exclusively, controlled at the level of mRNA, it became of interest to examine more aged animals. A fairly comprehensive study that measured mRNA activity as well as tubulin microheterogeneity was carried out on cerebellum by Soreq et al. (1983) who prepared unfractionated RNA from 4-months- and 30-months-old mouse cerebella and measured the translational efficiency of the RNA in the reticulocyte lysate protein synthesizing system (Pelham and Jackson, 1976). Although relatively few proteins are synthesized by unfractionated RNA compared with poly(A +) RNA, the most abundant proteins are detectable on autoradiographs (Sajdel-Sulkowska et al., 1983a). It was found that the translational efficiency of the mRNA in total RNA of the older cerebella was decreased by 40% when compared to the younger preparation. The products of translation were separated by gel fractionation; after autoradiogra-

phy it was observed that there was decreased intensity in the 55 000 molecular weight (mol. wt.) region corresponding to tubulin, whereas actin appeared unchanged. Tubulin microheterogeneity was also altered.

These data demonstrate that age-related protein synthesis changes in CNS tissues can occur at the level of mRNA. Several possible explanations may be considered. Taking into account the results of Dunlop et al. (1984), the mRNA content of the unfractionated RNA may have declined more rapidly that the total RNA fraction. Or, the old mRNA may have failed to initiate protein synthesis as efficiently as the young mRNA, e.g., due to structural modification or partial degradation at the 5'-terminal. In addition, the presence of inhibitors of translation (e.g., double-stranded RNA, RNA of low molecular weight, etc.) cannot be ruled out. At this time all these factors should be the subject of further studies.

Histological investigations of brain cell RNA during human aging and in Alzheimer's disease

A considerable body of data, from a number of different laboratories, have indicated that as the normal human brain ages there occurs a reduction in neuronal RNA and that in AD a further decline in RNA is a consistent finding.

Mann and associates have used a microspectrophotometric method to assess the nucleolar volume and cytoplasmic RNA content of stained tissues from the post-mortem human CNS (Mann and Yates, 1974; Mann et al., 1978). Upon examination of the inferior olivary and dentate nuclei, as well as anterior horn cells, pyramidal cells of the hippocampus and cerebellar Purkinje cells, a decline of 30% was noted in the volume of the nucleolus and a reduction of 10–15% in the content of cytoplasmic RNA by 90 years of age. The nucleolus, a darkly staining region of the nucleus, is the site of genes coding for ribosomal RNA. The size of the nucleolus has been related to the ribosomal RNA content of the cell and indirectly may provide a rough indication of protein synthesis activity

(Watson, 1968). It is of interest to note that Strehler and Chang (1979) found an age-dependent loss of genes coding for ribosomal RNA, as measured by hybridization to [³H]rRNA, in DNA from human hippocampus and cortex.

Oksova (1975) used a cytospectrophotometric procedure to measure the RNA content of cells in layer III of the frontal and temporal cortex of patients with AD. After taking into account the cellular volume it was observed that the AD neuronal RNA content significantly decreased in two areas examined (by 38%, 24%). The additional interesting observation was made that the glial RNA content increased by 13–15%. This finding is consistent with the in vitro protein synthesis studies of Sajdel-Sulkowska et al. (1983b) who observed an overall decline in protein synthesis by AD brain mRNA but an increase in the synthesis of glial fibrillary acidic protein.

The nucleolar volume and RNA content in neurons of the AD brain were decreased in inferior olivary and dentate nuclei, and hippocampal and Purkinje cells of autopsied demented patients, compared to controls of similar age (Mann and Sinclair, 1978). The loss of cytoplasmic RNA was 26–33% and the decline in nucleolar volume ranged from 23–25%. It was particularly interesting to note that cellular areas not usually associated with AD were involved. However, previous studies had indicated a decrease in dendrites and dendritic arborization in Purkinje cells, as well as cortical neurons, in AD (Mehraein et al., 1975). Thus, the belief of some authors that AD cerebellar RNA serves as a suitable normal control for other brain areas that show more obvious pathological changes, is to be questioned. Indeed, Hirano bodies have now been described in cerebellar Purkinje cells in a patient with Alzheimer's disease (Yamamoto and Hirano, 1985).

The above investigation (Mann and Sinclair, 1978) was carried out without regard to whether or not the neurons under scrutiny contained neurofibrillary tangles (NFTs); the neuropathological diagnosis was made on the temporal lobe. However, three separate studies have focused upon RNA content and nucleolar size in tangle vs. non-tangle-containing neurons. The earliest report to investigate morphologic aspects of the genetic apparatus was by Dayan and Ball (1973) who compared the nucleolar diameter of post-mortem temporal lobe neurons with and without NFTs. Cells bearing tangles had significantly smaller nucleoli than adjacent unaffected neurons. Glial cell nuclei were also examined in order to assess incidental effects (e.g., state of hydration of the brain at time of fixation); no significant differences were found between the mean diameters of these nuclei in cases which did or did not show NFTs in cortical neurons. This type of investigation was extended by Mann and Yates (1981) who assessed the relationship between NFTs and nucleolar volume for a large number of autopsied cortical and subcortical areas. It was uniformly observed that the mean nucleolar volume of non-tangle-bearing cells in AD cases was significantly reduced when compared to similar cells from aged controls; and that the nucleolar volume of tangle-bearing cells was significantly reduced even further when compared to their non-tangle-bearing neighbors. Compared with controls the volume of nucleoli in neurons without fibrillary pathology was reduced by 15–40%; however, in the presence of tangles, the relative reduction was in the range of 40–50%.

An elegant study carried out by Uemura and Hartmann (1979) measured the cytoplasmic RNA content of tangle-containing and tangle-free neurons of the post-mortem hippocampus from AD patients at ages 66, 79 and 82. Nerve cell bodies from sections fixed in formalin were excised with a microneedle under phase contrast; 60 neurons with and without NFTs were removed from each specimen. After nuclease digestion the RNA was measured by microspectrophotometry. Statistically significant differences were found with respect to the RNA content of nerve cell bodies free of tangles compared with tangle-containing cells: 41 pg vs. 29 pg, respectively, for the 66- and 79-year-olds. The 82-years-old case had the lowest tangle-free neuronal value, 31 pg; this value approached that for neighboring neurons with neurofibrillary degeneration (28 pg). The neuronal RNA content of a suitable normal control sample was 74 pg. Similar to the aforementioned studies, these data suggest a relatively increased rate of RNA loss coincident with aging and a further decrease in RNA associated with the presence of NFTs.

The consistent results from different laboratories offer convincing evidence for a dramatic decline in nucleolar volume and RNA levels in AD neurons. However, these investigations were subject to criticism concerning the use of post-mortem tissue for investigations of polynucleotides. Although with a suitably large sample size, normal and AD cases can be matched with respect to age, cause of death and post-mortem interval prior to fixation of tissue, other variables such as the effects of a prolonged terminal illness, respiratory functioning and agonal status are less easily controlled. To address these concerns, measurements were made on biopsy tissue. Cytoplasmic RNA content and nuclear and nucleolar volumes were all significantly reduced in nerve cells of the AD temporal cortex (by 43%, 36% and 26%, respectively) examined at diagnostic biopsy when compared to age-matched non-demented controls (Mann et al., 1981a). Values for the similar measurements made on autopsied AD specimens were reduced approximately 40–50% compared with controls. The authors concluded that decreases in the measured values cannot be ascribed solely to post-mortem effects. Although in some cases there may be increased losses after death, these data argue strongly for a decline in macromolecular functioning in the living (and younger) demented patients. The presence of neurofibrillary tangles in biopsied temporal cortex neurons was not associated with a further decline in nucleolar volume (40% vs. 41%, Mann et al., 1981b). However, similar sections from post-mortem cases revealed a 38% decline in nucleolar volume in non-tangle-bearing cells and a further decline to a value of 51% of normal when tangles were present.

The observation that non-tangle-bearing cells from autopsy and biopsy cases had about the same decline in nucleolar volume indicates that agonal state and post-mortem factors per se were not responsible for differences between the two sample sources. The mean age of the biopsied cases was 57 years whereas the autopsy group was 81 years old and had a longer duration of illness. It was inferred that the presence of the NFT for longer periods of time was associated with further nucleolar changes. The possibility that the NFT itself is the causal factor was not clarified by these studies and merits attention. For example, the intraneuronal accumulation of even minute amounts of fibrillary material may have consequences for the turnover of RNA.

Major abnormalities in central cholinergic neurons are a frequent finding in AD (Davies and Maloney, 1976; Perry et al., 1977; White et al., 1977). The nucleus basalis of Meynert (nbM) in the basal forebrain provides the major source of cholinergic innervation to the cortex (Johnson et al., 1979; Wenk et al., 1980; Lehman et al., 1980). In AD, degeneration of cells in the basal nucleus has been documented (Whitehouse et al., 1981); and evidence has accumulated to suggest that changes in cholinergic innervation are closely related to the reduction in choline acetyltransferase and acetylcholine esterase as well as to the development of the neuritic plaque (Struble et al., 1982). At present, however, it is not known whether this degeneration is due to a primary involvement of cell bodies within the nbM or to primary events in the cortex. In addition, little information is available concerning the relationship between cholinergic dysfunction and macromolecular control mechanisms. Using the techniques described earlier, Mann et al. (1984) determined that whereas in normal aging nbM neurons are reduced in number by 30% and their cytoplasmic RNA content and nucleolar volume by 20%, these values are 70% and 40%, respectively, in AD. Younger AD patients exhibited more severe changes than elderly individuals. Neurofibrillary tangles were far more common in the AD cases. It was concluded that reductions in RNA, and consequently of protein synthesis, contribute to the loss of presynaptic cholinergic markers in AD.

The RNA content and neuronal volume of human brain neurons in health and in dementia was reviewed in some detail due to their potential importance to understanding the molecular pathogenesis of AD. The findings can be summarized as follows: (1) during normal aging there is a decline in the neuronal nucleolar volume and cytoplasmic RNA content; (2) in AD, there is a further decline in nucleolar volume and RNA content compared to age-matched controls in all brain areas examined, even those without the obvious pathologic features of AD; (3) biopsied AD cases exhibit the changes noted above, as well as a decrease in nuclear volume, indicating that data derived from autopsied samples cannot be ascribed exclusively to agonal or post-mortem events; (4) when neurofibrillary tangles are present within neurons in postmortem cases, a further decline occurs in nucleolar volume and RNA content; (5) glial RNA appears to be spared or may even increase slightly in AD.

In our earlier discussion of conditions influencing the age-related decrease in brain protein synthesis levels, it was noted that current evidence indicates that a decline in RNA is a significant contributing factor. It has been suggested that decreased nucleolar volume in AD reflects a decline in transcription and thus a reduction in cytoplasmic ribosomal RNA and, consequently, in protein synthesis. The histologic measurements, however, do not indicate whether or not the decrease in RNA is due exclusively to decreased transcription. Indeed, the association between NFTs and an accentuated decline in cytoplasmic RNA content suggests that other factors, in addition to a transcriptional deficit, may be germane to the pathogenesis of dementia. In the following sections we describe the biochemical evidence that confirms a decline in AD cellular RNA and extends the causative factors to include cytoplasmic degradation of RNA.

Biochemical investigations on brain RNA from controls and cases of Alzheimer's disease

Complementing the extensive histochemical and stereometric studies, a number of biochemical investigations have indicated that a reduction in RNA occurs in the AD brain. Thus, Bowen et al. (1977) reported a reduced RNA/DNA ratio in the temporal lobe of one case of AD. Recently, with the availability of rapid RNA purification methods, the levels of RNA that are extractable from the post-mortem human brain are now easily determined (Sajdel-Sulkowska et al., 1983a,b). Guanidinium thiocyanate and sodium dodecyl sulfate, potent denaturants, were used in the preparation of RNA from control and AD cortices by centrifugation through a cesium chloride gradient. These procedures were an improvement over those used in the first reported studies on the preparation of functionally intact polysomes and messenger RNA from the post-mortem human brain (Marotta et al., 1981a,b,c). Results from histological studies on RNA concentrations in AD neurons (Oksova, 1975; Uemura and Hartmann, 1979; Mann et al., 1981a,b) predicted that the yields of RNA from NFT-rich tissues would be unusually low. This prediction was verified using the guanidinium thiocyanate/cesium chloride extraction method. In AD cortical samples containing numerous NFTs, as well as plaques, total cellular RNA decreased by 45% and poly(A+) RNA decreased by 64% compared with control specimens (Sajdel-Sulkowska and Marotta, 1984).

The reduction in AD poly(A+) RNA and of total cellular RNA, consisting predominantly of ribosomal RNA, was independently confirmed by Taylor et al. (1985). These authors prepared total cellular RNA by a guanidinium thiocyanate/cesium chloride procedure and quantified the levels of poly(A+)RNA using [³H]uridine; in addition they measured the levels of ribosomal RNA and preproenkephalin mRNA by means of cloned probes. A significant reduction in all RNA species was observed: a decline of 38% for ribosomal RNA, 44% for poly(A+)mRNA, and 26% for preproenkephalin mRNA.

The lower yields of RNA from NFT-containing tissues of the AD cortex may result from decreased transcription of AD neuronal RNA in cells with or without NFTs, as well as a further reduction in RNA from neurons that contain NFTs for long durations prior to death (Mann et al., 1981b). We examined the possibility that NFT-containing autopsied specimens may have unusually high levels of ribonuclease (RNase) activity. When four control cases were compared to six AD cases, it was observed that whereas the level of acid (lysosomal) ribonuclease was nearly the same for the two groups, the level of alkaline RNase was significantly different. The mean free alkaline RNase activity per milligram of tissue was increased in the AD brains by an average of 87% (Sajdel-Sulkowska and Marotta, 1984).

Alkaline RNase is present in higher concentrations in neurons than glia and is located in both the nucleus and cytoplasm (Franzoni and Garcia Argiz, 1978; Ittel and Mandel, 1979). Neither the nuclear nor cytoplasmic enzyme activity is affected in brain subjected to anoxic or ischemic conditions for at least six hours (Albrecht and Yanagihara, 1979). The activity of the enzyme is modulated by a second protein, alkaline RNase inhibitor (ARI) that has been identified in brain and other organs (Roth, 1958; Shortman, 1961; Roth, 1962; Takahashi et al., 1970; Blackburn et al., 1977). Alkaline RNase activity is normally low due to the ARI and is referred to as free activity. When ARI is inactivated by sulfhydryl-blocking agents, the RNase activity increases and is referred to as total alkaline RNase (Roth, 1958). Para-chloromercuribenzoate (PCMB), a sulfhydryl inhibitor, was added to control and AD cortical homogenates; the control RNase value increased by 133% while the AD value remained essentially unchanged (Sajdel-Sulkowska and Marotta, 1984).

Data from the preceding RNase-ARI study were pooled with a second group of control and AD cases. Cortical samples were obtained from seven controls and eight AD patients; the mean age of controls was 69 years, and of dements was 68 years; the post-mortem intervals were 11 h and 13 h, respectively. As shown in Fig. 1 (upper panel) the AD free RNase activity was significantly higher than controls. Upon addition of PCMB (Fig. 1, lower panel) the inhibitor-bound RNase activity of controls increased by approximately 58% whereas

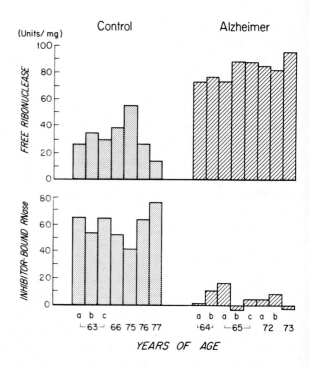

Fig. 1. Ribonuclease activity in cortical specimens from neurologically normal controls and cases of Alzheimer's disease. Upper panel: free brain alkaline RNase activity in the absence of PCMB. Lower panel: the inhibitor-bound RNase activity expressed as the difference between the total activity in the presence of 1 mM PCMB and the free activity. Assays were carried out as previously described (Sajdel-Sulkowska and Marotta, 1984); enzyme activity is expressed in units/mg. One unit of activity is defined as 1 percent hydrolysis of exogenous [^{3}H]RNA per 60 min. Different cases of the same age are indicated by letters. Individual PMI's are as follows: controls: 63a, 6 h; 63b, 8 h; 63c, 15 h; 66, 7 h; 75, 20 h; 76, 7 h; 77, 14 h; Alzheimer cases: 64a, 12 h; 64b, 18 h; 65a, 10 h; 65b, 25 h; 65c, 13 h; 72a, 13 h; 72b, 10 h; 73, 4 h.

AD samples had little residual RNase bound to ARI protein.

These results are consistent with the hypothesis that in tissues with NFTs, a contributing factor to the decline in neuronal RNA levels is increased RNase activity due to decreased inhibition by ARI. This proposed mechanism combined with a possible decline in the transcriptional activity in AD neurons may be sufficient to reduce the RNA levels to quite low values and thus contribute significantly to low protein synthesis rates in AD (see below). It might be expected that in normally functioning cells, increased degradation of RNA may stimulate increased rates of transcription to replenish the supply of polynucleotides. This suggested compensatory mechanism may be compromised in AD. Thus, the interaction of both transcriptional and nucleolytic factors may be of significance to the molecular pathogenesis of AD.

Protein synthesis studies using brain RNA from controls and from cases of Alzheimer's disease

Marotta and associates first demonstrated that human post-mortem brain that is removed within hours after death and stored frozen retains functional polysomes and mRNA (Marotta et al., 1981a,b,c). The subsequent reevaluation by Sajdel-Sulkowska et al. (1983a,b) led to improvements in both the yield and translational activity of poly(A +) RNA during in vitro protein synthesis studies.

In early experiments polysomes were prepared by previously described techniques (Marotta et al., 1979) from three post-mortem brains: cortical tissue was removed from a 51-years-old case of Huntington's disease (HT1) (post-mortem interval, referred to as PMI, 2 h), from a 58-years-old Huntington's disease patient (HT2) who was hypoxic for 4 h before death (PMI, 3 h), and a 78-years-old neurologically normal control (HT3, PMI, 6 h). The yield of polysomes and RNA was 36% less in HT2 compared to HT1 (Marotta et al., 1981a,b). The lower yield may be related to the slightly longer PMI and the pre-mortem hypoxic state of HT2. However, the oldest cortex, HT3, with a PMI twice as long as HT2 had essentially the same yield as the latter. As of this writing, there is no available information on loss of human brain RNA within the first 1 or 2 h after death. Studies subsequently reported used cases with PMI's in the 6–25-h range. The same time interval, 6–25 h, obtained for the study of Naber and Dahnke (1979) who assessed the post-mortem effect on the yield of RNA from neurologically normal brains. Six hours after death samples of frontal cortex,

white matter, cerebellum, thalamus and caudate nucleus were removed and stored in liquid nitrogen while other samples were incubated at 16°C for varying lengths of time up to 25 h. Over this PMI, a significant decrease in the content of extractable nucleic acid was absent.

In the experiments of Marotta et al. (1979), the translational activity of polysomes in the presence of reticulocyte translation factors and [^{35}S]methionine decreased by 52% when HT2 was compared to HT1; the further decline exhibited by HT3, compared to HT2, was only 10%. When examined by one-dimensional polyacrylamide gel electrophoresis (PAGE), the translation products of HT1 were similar in size to native human brain proteins and were as large in size as proteins synthesized by fresh rat cortical polysomes (Figs. 2, 3). Approximately 130 native proteins were visualized by Coomassie Brilliant Blue staining (Fig. 2A) and approximately 250 translation products were observed after autoradiography (Fig. 2B). The most abundant proteins were synthesized by the post-mortem polysomes. The multiple subunits of tubulin and actin were prominent.

Fig. 3 compares the translation products of HT1 and HT3. Over 230 polypeptides were matched to one another on overexposed autoradiographs; few qualitative or quantitative differences were apparent between products from polysomes obtained 2 h or 6 h after death even though the yields of polysomes as well as their efficiency during translation were quite different. The results also demonstrate that in the case of one neurodegenerative disease, Huntington's disease, the abundant cortical polysome translation products appear similar to those of a normal control. The striking reproducibility of the autoradiographs from two cases with dissimilar pre-mortem and post-mortem conditions suggests that the described methods may be quite useful for evaluating the appearance or loss of genetic information.

When mRNA was extracted from the polysomes and translated in a wheat germ homogenate, few polypeptides were detected, and those that were synthesized were predominantly the most abun-

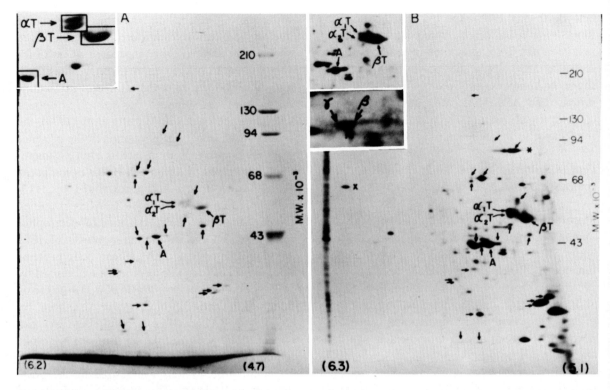

Fig. 2. Two-dimensional gel analysis of human proteins. (A) HT1 native cytoplasmic proteins stained with Coomassie Brilliant Blue. α_1 tubulin (α_1T), α_2 tubulin (α_2T), β tubulin (βT) and actin isomers (A) are indicated. The inset to panel A shows a portion of a gel containing stained rat brain proteins for comparison. (B) Radioactive proteins (2×10^6 cpm) synthesized by HT1 polysomes. Tubulin subunits and actin are indicated. Upper inset: tubulin subunits and actin synthesized by rat cortex polysomes. Lower inset: autoradiograph of human polysome translation products in which the isomeric forms of actin are indicated. The pH values measured for the basic (left) and the acidic (right) ends of the isoelectric focusing gel are listed in parentheses. Arrows designate those proteins present in both panel A and panel B in addition to the cytoskeletal proteins. (From Marotta et al., 1981a)

dant species in lower molecular weight classes (Gilbert et al., 1981). Fine comparisons among RNA preparations do not appear feasible with the wheat germ system. Among the limitations of these preparations are the following: the presence of an endogenous ribonuclease activity (Scheele and Blackburn, 1979); premature termination of poly-peptide chains (Benveniste et al., 1976; Tse and Taylor, 1977); the presence of an endogenous inhibitor (Zagorski, 1978); relatively high levels of proteases (Mumford et al., 1981); and the inability to translate brain mRNA with high efficiency (Mahoney et al., 1976; Giudice and Chaiken, 1979; Matthews and Campagnoni, 1980). In vitro trans-lation of total cellular RNA, rather than poly(A +)

RNA, from brain is particularly inefficient since only the most abundant polypeptides are easily detected on autoradiographs. The use of total RNA, combined with the wheat germ homogenate, which also facilitates translation of abundant species only, appears inadequate for demonstrat-ing subtle variations among RNA preparations.

Taking these factors into consideration, Sajdel-Sulkowska et al. (1983a) prepared RNA from frozen human cortex by the guanidinium thiocyan-ate/cesium chloride procedure. The RNA was twice denatured by heat and detergents and passed through oligo d(T)-cellulose columns to obtain highly purified poly(A +) RNA. The latter was translated in the rabbit reticulocyte translation

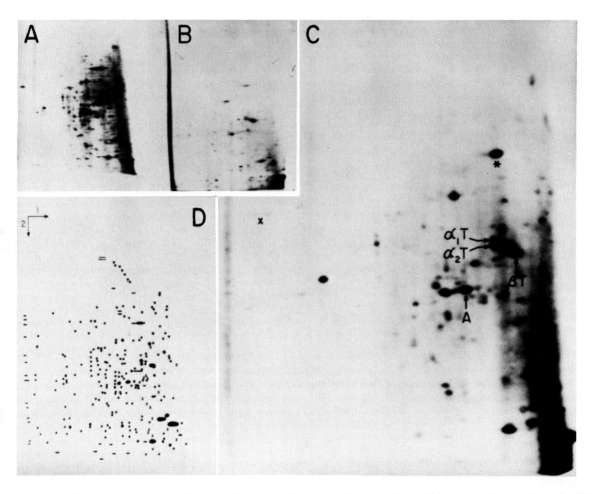

Fig. 3. Two-dimensional separation of human and rat brain polysome translation products. (A) Over-exposed autoradiograph of Fig. 2B showing HT1 translation products; (B) rat cortex polysome translation products (1×10^6 cpm) included for comparison; (C) radioactive products (6×10^5 cpm) synthesized by HT3 polysomes. α_1 tubulin (α_1T), α_2 tubulin (α_2T), β tubulin (βT), and actin (A) are indicated. (D) Sketch showing proteins shared in common between autoradiographs of A and C; the X marks in the panel indicate proteins that were not definitively demonstrated to be present on both autoradiographs. (From Marotta et al., 1981a)

system and stimulated protein synthesis nearly three-fold over endogenous mRNA. Compared with earlier studies (Gilbert et al., 1981) the number of newly synthesized proteins was increased by 30% (Sajdel-Sulkowska et al., 1983a). As shown in Fig. 4, over 300 proteins were separated by two-dimensional PAGE, and size classes up to 130 000 mol. wt. are present as compared to 70 000 mol. wt. in the earlier report (Gilbert et al., 1981). Fig. 4 demonstrates the reproducibility of the methods since no differences

were obvious when translation products of cerebral cortex were compared to those of cerebellum.

The same methods were applied to the post-mortem AD cortex. As shown previously (Sajdel-Sulkowska et al., 1983b; Sajdel-Sulkowska and Marotta, 1985), irrespective of the low yields and possible degradation, the post-mortem AD brain RNA retains functional mRNA that synthesizes numerous proteins. The degree of stimulation of protein synthesis in the reticulocyte system in the presence of [^{35}S]methionine tended to be relatively

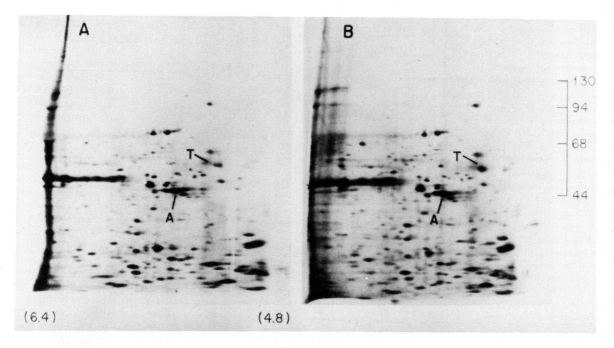

Fig. 4. Two-dimensional PAGE of polypeptides synthesized by poly(A +) RNA from human cerebral cortex and cerebellum. mRNA samples were purified from total cellular RNA as described in the text. After electrophoresis ^{35}S-labeled proteins were transferred to adsorbent membranes; after staining with amido black to visualize molecular weight standards, autoradiographs were prepared. (A) Human cortical mRNA translation products (213 580 dpm); (B) human cerebellar mRNA translation products (169 520 dpm). The tubulin subunits (T) and actin isomers (A) are indicated; pH values are shown in parentheses. (From Sajdel-Sulkowska et al., 1983a)

low; however, even the least efficient preparations stimulated the synthesis of the major cytoskeletal proteins: tubulin, glial fibrillary acidic protein (GFAP) and actin. Actin and GFAP mRNAs were most prominent. This result is consistent with the observation of Oksova (1975) concerning the increase in glial RNA in the AD cortex, and with other reports that demonstrated prominent astrocytic activity in the AD brain (Duffy et al., 1980; Schechter et al., 1981).

The in vitro translation data are of interest from another perspective. The preservation of high levels of AD GFAP mRNA activity suggests that non-specific losses of mRNA did not occur to a significant extent, due to nuclease action as a result of the agonal state, post-mortem processing, or during the procedures used to prepare AD RNA. These results, as well as the extensive histological studies discussed previously, are consistent with

the view that neuronal RNA is lost in the living patient with AD. Transcriptional rates as well as degradative mechanisms deserve further scrutiny in order to clarify the contribution of both processes to brain protein synthesis levels in AD.

Preparation of recombinant DNA using post-mortem Alzheimer's disease brain poly(A +) RNA

The observation that a fraction of the poly(A +) RNA that can be extracted from the post-mortem AD brain remains functionally intact, led us to use this material to construct cDNA expression libraries. As of this writing, preliminary studies have been carried out to assess the template activity of AD mRNA. Poly(A +) RNA was prepared from two normal control cerebral cortices (ages 63 and 76, mean PMI 7 h) and an AD cortex (age 75, mean PMI 16 h). The latter sample was from a specimen with an abundance of NFTs and neuritic plaques. All samples of poly(A+) RNA were shown to have retained protein synthesis activity in the reticulocyte translation system. Using oligo (dT)$_{12-18}$ as a primer, equal amounts of control and AD mRNA samples were reverse transcribed to make single-stranded cDNA by means of avian myeloblastosis virus reverse transcriptase in the presence of the deoxynucleoside triphosphates including α-[^{32}P]CTP. A modified version of the cDNA synthesis method of Gubler and Hoffman (1983) was used. After alkali digestion to remove RNA, the incorporation into cDNA was measured. Control poly(A+) RNA converted 14.7% of the input RNA into single-stranded cDNA, whereas 7% of the AD RNA was transcribed. However, both cDNA samples were 98–100% efficient for the preparation of double-stranded cDNA using the Klenow fragment of DNA polymerase I (in preparation). After sucrose gradient sedimentation, the control DNA was observed to have an average size larger than 5 kb, whereas the AD cDNA was in the 2–3 kb range. The cDNA was treated with R1 methylase to render the cDNA resistant to Eco R1 restriction enzyme; a chemically synthesized R1 linker was added to the cDNA and digested with Eco R1 for use with the lambda gt11 cloning vector (Young and Davis, 1983). The site used for insertion of the cDNA is an Eco R1 cleavage site located within the lacZ region upstream of the β-galactosidase termination codon. Ligated cDNA-lambda gt11 molecules were introduced into E. coli 1088 by a packaging system in vitro. This host carried the hsdR$^-$hsdM$^+$ genotype, thereby preventing the restriction of foreign DNA prior to host modification. Phage-containing inserts generate an inactive β-galactosidase fusion protein that can be detected immunologically.

Although the AD cDNA could be used for the preparation of the recombinant expression vector, the significance of the smaller size of the AD cDNA on the levels of expression is currently under scrutiny. These initial studies will be complemented by the analysis of expression vector libraries prepared from AD poly(A+) RNA obtained after shorter postmortem intervals.

In vivo protein synthesis in Alzheimer's disease patients

Numerous factors affect in vivo protein synthesis levels, e.g., rates of transcription, processing and degradation of RNA, as well as the availability of initiation factors, elongation factors, and energy-supplying mechanisms. An exploration of macromolecular functions that affect the production of protein in the AD brain is of unusual interest because of the in vivo data that have become available. Bustany and associates (Bustany et al., 1981, 1983; Comar et al., 1981) demonstrated that patients with the diagnosis of AD had protein synthesis levels that were 30–58% of normal. The incorporation of [^{11}C]methionine into protein was assessed by positron emission tomography and data were corrected for the size of the endogenous amino acid pool. These results are consistent with the previously described histological and biochemical investigations on AD brain RNA levels and functional activity. However, the other factors listed above merit intensive scrutiny.

Summary and conclusions

Decreased levels of protein synthesis can be demonstrated in living patients with Alzheimer's disease, and the AD post-mortem brain mRNA has diminished capacity to stimulate high levels of protein synthesis in vitro. Although numerous factors may contribute to the observed decline in in vivo functional activity, the concentration of brain RNA appears to be particularly important for regulating the rate of translation. During normal aging, the level of brain RNA decreases. In AD, there appears to be an accelerated general decline in neuronal RNA and a further decrease within neurons containing neurofibrillary tangles. RNA extracted from affected regions supports the limited synthesis of proteins. Although the over-all levels of in vitro synthesis tend to be low, the specific activity of certain proteins, such as GFAP, remains high. These observations may be related, in part, to increased degradation of neuronal RNA with sparing of glial RNA. The level of AD brain alkaline RNase activity is increased due to the loss of inhibitor activity. In our view, these first observations concerning altered regulatory mechanisms in the AD brain do not exclude the possibility that other regulatory factors (e.g., at the level of transcription and post-transcriptional processing) may be relevant to the molecular pathogenesis of Alzheimer's dementia.

Acknowledgements

The studies summarized above were supported by grants to C.A.M. from the American Health Assistance Foundation, the McKnight Foundation, the American Federation for Aging Research and the National Institute on Aging (AG00084, AG02126, AG04522, and AG05134). Several post-mortem brain specimens were obtained from the McLean Hospital Brain Tissue Resource Center, Belmont, MA, courtesy of Dr. Edward D. Bird. Other specimens were the gifts of Dr. Robert D. Terry and Dr. William R. Markesbery. The manuscript was prepared with the skillful assistance of Martha Shea.

References

Adams, D. H. (1966) The relationship between cellular nucleic acids in the developing rat cerebral cortex. *Biochem. J.*, 98: 636–640.

Albrecht, J. and Yanagihara, T. (1979) Effect of anoxia and ischemia on ribonuclease activity in brain. *J. Neurochem.*, 32: 1131–1133.

Benson, R. W. and Harker, C. W. (1978) RNA polymerase activities in liver and brain tissue of aging mice. *J. Gerontol.*, 33: 323–328.

Benveniste, K., Wilczek, J., Ruggieri, A. and Stern, R. (1976) Translation of collagen mRNA in a cell-free system derived from wheat germ. *Biochemistry*, 15: 830–835.

Berthold, W. and Lim, L. (1976a) The metabolism of high molecular-weight ribonucleic acid including polyadenylated species in the developing rat brain. *Biochem. J.*, 154: 517–527.

Berthold, W. and Lim, L. (1976b) Nucleo-cytoplasmic relationships of high molecular weight RNA, including polyadenylated species in the developing rat brain. *Biochem. J.*, 154: 529–539.

Blackburn, P., Wilson, G. and Moore, S. (1977) Ribonuclease inhibitor from human placenta. *J. Biol. Chem.*, 252: 5904–5910.

Bowen, D. M., Smith, C. B., White, P., Flack, R. H. A., Carrasco, L. H., Gedye, J. L. and Davison, A. N. (1977) Chemical pathology of the organic dementias. II. Quantitative estimation of cellular changes in postmortem brains. *Brain*, 100: 427–453.

Bustany, P., Sargent, T., Saudubray, J. M., Henry, J. F. and Comar, D. (1981) Regional human brain uptake and protein incorporation of [^{11}C]-methionine studied in vivo with PET. *J. Cereb. Blood Flow Metab.*, 1: Suppl. 1, S17–S18.

Bustany, P., Henry, J. F., Soussaline, F. and Comar, D. (1983) Brain protein synthesis in normal and demented patients — a study by positron emission tomography with [^{11}C]-L-methionine. In P. S. Magistretti (Ed.), *Functional Radionuclide Imaging of the Brain*, Raven Press, New York, pp. 319–326.

Cann, A., Gambino, R., Bank, J. and Bank, A. (1974) Polyadenylate sequences and biological activity of globin messenger ribonucleic acid. *J. Biol. Chem.*, 249: 7536–7540.

Chaconas, G. and Finch, C. E. (1973) The effect of aging on RNA/DNA ratios in brain regions of the C57BL/6J male mouse. *J. Neurochem.*, 21: 1469–1473.

Comar, D., Bustany, P., Henry, J. F., Sargent, T., Cabanis, E. and Soussaline, F. (1981) Regional brain uptake and metabolism of [^{11}C]-methionine in dementia. *Proceedings of the Third World Congress on Biological Psychiatry (Stockholm)*, Abstract 863.

Davies, P. and Maloney, A. J. F. (1976) Selective loss of cholinergic neurons in Alzheimer's disease. *Lancet*, II, 1403.

Dayan, A. D. and Ball, M. J. (1973) Histometric observations on the metabolism of tangle-bearing neurons. *J. Neurol. Sci.*, 19: 433–436.

DeLarco, J., Abramowitz, A., Bromwell, K. and Guroff, G. (1975) Polyadenylic acid-containing RNA from rat brain. *J. Neurochem.*, 24: 215–222.

Doel, M. T. and Carey, N. H. (1976) The translational capacity of deadenylated ovalbumin messenger RNA. *Cell*, 8: 51–58.

Duffy, P. E., Rappaport, M. and Graf, L. (1980) Glial fibrillary acidic protein and Alzheimer-type senile dementia. *Neurology*, 30: 778–782.

Dunlop, D. S., van Elden, W. and Lajtha, A. (1975) A method for measuring brain protein synthesis rates in young and adult rats. *J. Neurochem.*, 24: 337–344.

Dunlop, D. S., van Elden, W. and Lajtha, A. (1977) Developmental effects on protein synthesis rates in regions of the CNS in vivo and in vitro. *J. Neurochem.*, 29: 939–945.

Dunlop, D. S., van Elden, W. and Lajtha, A. (1984) RNA concentration and protein synthesis in rat brain during development. *Brain Res.*, 294: 148–151.

Dwyer, B. E., Fando, J. L. and Wasterlain, C. G. (1980) Rat brain protein synthesis declines during post-developmental aging. *J. Neurochem.*, 35: 746–749.

Ekstrom, R., Liu, D. S. H. and Richardson, A. (1980) Changes in brain protein synthesis during the life span of male Fischer rats. *Gerontology*, 26: 121–128.

Fando, J. L., Salinas, M. and Wasterlain, C. G. (1980) Age-dependent changes in brain protein synthesis in the rat. *Neurochem. Res.*, 5: 373–383.

Franzoni, L. and Garcia Argiz, C. A. (1978) Rat brain ribonucleases. *Acta Physiol. Lat. Am.*, 28: 185–192.

Gibas, M. A. and Harman, D. (1970) Ribonucleic acid synthesis by nuclei isolated from rats of different ages. *J. Gerontol.*, 25: 105–107.

Gilbert, J. M., Brown, B. A., Strocchi, P., Bird, E. D. and Marotta, C. A. (1981) The preparation of biologically active messenger RNA from human postmortem brain tissue. *J. Neurochem.*, 36: 976–984.

Giudice, L. C. and Chaiken, I. M. (1979) Immunochemical and chemical identification of a neurophysin-containing protein coded by messenger RNA from bovine hypothalamus. *Proc. Natl. Acad. Sci. USA*, 76: 3800–3804.

Goertz, B. (1979) Regulation of protein synthesis during postnatal maturation of mouse brain. *Mech. Aging Dev.*, 10: 261–271.

Gozes, I., deBaetselier, A. and Littauer, U. Z. (1980) Translation in vitro of rat brain mRNA coding for a variety of tubulin forms. *Eur. J. Biochem.*, 103: 13–20.

Gubler, U. and Hoffman, B. J. (1983) A simple and very efficient method for generating cDNA libraries. *Gene*, 25: 263–269.

Ittel, M. E. and Mandel, P. (1979) Ribonuclease activities in various classes of nuclei from bovine cerebrum. *J. Neurochem.*, 33: 521–525.

Johnson, M. V., McKinney, M. and Coyle, J. T. (1979) Evidence for a cholinergic projection to neocortex from neurons in basal forebrain. *Proc. Natl. Acad. Sci. USA*, 76: 5392–5396.

Johnson, T. C. (1976) Regulation of protein synthesis during postnatal maturation of the brain. *J. Neurochem.*, 27: 17–23.

Lehman, J., Nagy, J. I., Atnadja, S. and Fibiger, H. C. (1980) The nucleus basalis magnocellularis. The origin of a cholinergic projection to the neocortex of the rat. *Neuroscience*, 5: 1161–1174.

Lerner, M. P. and Johnson, T. C. (1970) Regulation of protein synthesis in developing mouse brain tissue. Alterations in ribosomal activity. *J. Biol. Chem.*, 245: 1388–1393.

Mahoney, J., Brown, I., Labourdette, G. and Marks, A. (1976) Synthesis of the brain specific S-100 protein in a cell-free system from wheat embryo programmed with poly(A)-containing RNA from rabbit brain. *Eur. J. Biochem.*, 67: 203–208.

Mann, D. M. A. and Sinclair, K. G. A. (1978) The quantitative assessment of lipofuscin pigment, cytoplasmic RNA and nucleolar volume in senile dementia. *Neuropathol. Appl. Neurobiol.*, 4: 129–135.

Mann, D. M. A. and Yates, P. O. (1974) Lipoprotein pigments — their relationship to ageing in the human nervous system. *Brain*, 97: 481–488.

Mann, D. M. A. and Yates, P. O. (1981) The relationship between formation of senile plaques and neurofibrillary tangles and changes in nerve cell metabolism in Alzheimer-type dementia. *Mech. Aging Dev.*, 17: 395–401.

Mann, D. M. A., Yates, P. O. and Stamp, J. E. (1978) The relationship between lipofuscin pigment and ageing in the human nervous system. *J. Neurol. Sci.*, 37: 83–93.

Mann, D. M. A., Neary, D., Yates, P. O., Lincoln, J., Snowden, J. S. and Stanworth, P. (1981a) Alterations in protein synthetic capability of nerve cells in Alzheimer's disease. *J. Neurol. Neurosurg. Psychiat.*, 44: 97–102.

Mann, D. M. A., Neary, D., Yates, P. O., Lincoln, J., Snowden, J. S. and Stanworth, P. (1981b) Neurofibrillary pathology and protein synthetic capability in nerve cells in Alzheimer's disease. *Neuropathol. Appl. Neurobiol.*, 7: 37–47.

Mann, D. M. A., Yates, P. O. and Marcgnicik, B. (1984) Changes in nerve cells of the nucleus basalis of Meynert in Alzheimer's disease and their relationship to ageing and to the accumulation of lipofuscin. *Mech. Aging Dev.*, 25: 189–204.

Marotta, C. A., Harris, J. L. and Gilbert, J. M. (1978) Characterization of multiple forms of brain tubulin subunits. *J. Neurochem.*, 30: 1431–1440.

Marotta, C. A., Strocchi, P. and Gilbert, J. M. (1979) Biosynthesis of heterogeneous forms of mammalian brain tubulin subunits by multiple messenger RNAs. *J. Neurochem.*, 33: 231–246.

Marotta, C. A., Brown, B. A., Strocchi, P., Bird, E. D. and Gilbert, J. M. (1981a) In vitro synthesis of human brain proteins including tubulin and actin by purified postmortem polysomes. *J. Neurochem.*, 36: 966–975.

Marotta, C. A., Strocchi, P., Brown, B. A., Bonventre, J. A. and Gilbert, J. M. (1981b) Gel electrophoresis methods for the examination of human and rat brain fibrous proteins. Application to studies of human brain proteins from postmortem tissue. In E. S. Gershon, S. Matthysse, X. O. Breakefield and R. D. Ciaranello (Eds.), *Genetic Research Strategies for Psychobiology and Psychiatry*, Boxwood Press, Pacific Grove, pp. 39–57.

Marotta, C. A., Strocchi, P., Brown, B. A. and Gilbert, J. M. (1981c) Genetic aspects of mammalian brain macromolecular complexity. In S. W. Matthysse (Ed.), *Psychiatry and the Biology of the Human Brain*, Elsevier, Amsterdam, pp. 71–87.

Matthees, J. and Campagnoni, A. T. (1980) Cell free synthesis of the myelin basic protein in a wheat germ system programmed with brain messenger RNA. *J. Neurochem.*, 35: 867–872.

Mehraein, P., Yamada, M. and Tarnowska-Dzidoszko, E. (1975) Quantitative study of dendrites and dendritic spines in Alzheimer's disease and senile dementia. *Adv. Neurol.*, 27: 549–554.

Mumford, R. A., Pickett, C. B., Zimmerman, M. and Strauss, A. W. (1981) Protease activities present in wheat germ and rabbit reticulocyte lysates. *Biochem. Biophys. Res. Commun.*, 103: 565–572.

Murthy, M. R. V. (1966) Protein synthesis in growing rat tissues. II. Polyribosome concentration of brain and liver as a function of age. *Biochim. Biophys. Acta*, 119: 599–613.

Naber, D. and Dahnke, H. G. (1979) Protein and nucleic acid content in the aging human brain. *Neuropathol. Appl. Neurobiol.*, 5: 17–24.

Oksova, E. E. (1975) Glio-neuronal relationships in the cerebral cortex in senile dementia. *Zh. Neuropathol. Psikhiatr.*, 75: 1026–1030.

Orrego, F. and Lipmann, F. (1967) Protein synthesis in brain slices. *J. Biol. Chem.*, 25: 665–671.

Pelham, H. R. B. and Jackson, R. J. (1976) An efficient mRNA translation system from reticulocyte lysates. *Eur. J. Biochem.*, 67: 247–256.

Perry, E. K., Perry, R. H., Blessed, G. and Tomlinson, B. E. (1977) Necropsy evidence of central cholinergic deficits in senile dementia. *Lancet*, I, 189.

Petricevic, M., Denko, C. W. and Messineo, L. (1983) Age related changes in total DNA and RNA and incorporation of uridine and thymidine in rat brain. *Int. J. Biochem.*, 15: 751–753.

Richter, R. and Schumm, D. E. (1981) Age-associated changes in poly(adenylate) polymerase of rat liver and brain. *Mech. Aging Dev.*, 15: 217–225.

Ringborg, U. (1966) Composition and content of RNA in neurons of rat hippocampus at different ages. *Brain Res.*, 2: 296–298.

Roth, J. S. (1958) Ribonuclease. VIII. Studies on the inactive ribonuclease in the supernatant fraction of rat liver. *J. Biol. Chem.*, 231: 1097–1105.

Roth, J. S. (1962) Ribonuclease. IX. Further studies on ribonuclease inhibitor. *Biochim. Biophys. Acta*, 61: 903–915.

Sajdel-Sulkowska, E. M. and Marotta, C. A. (1984) Alzheimer's disease brain: alterations in RNA levels and in a ribonuclease-inhibitor complex. *Science*, 225: 947–949.

Sajdel-Sulkowska, E. M. and Marotta, C. A. (1985) Functional messenger RNA from the postmortem human brain: comparison of aged normal with Alzheimer's disease. In R. S. Sohal, L. Birnbaum and R. G. Cutler (Eds.), *Molecular Biology of Aging, Gene Stability and Gene Expression*, Raven Press, New York, pp. 243–256.

Sajdel-Sulkowska, E. M., Coughlin, J. F. and Marotta, C. A. (1983a) In vitro synthesis of polypeptides of moderately large size by poly(A)-containing messenger RNA from postmortem human brain and mouse brain. *J. Neurochem.*, 40: 670–680.

Sajdel-Sulkowska, E. M., Coughlin, J. F., Staton, D. M. and Marotta, C. A. (1983b) In vitro protein synthesis by messenger RNA from the Alzheimer's disease brain. In R. Katzman (Ed.), *Banbury Report 15: Biological Aspects of Alzheimer's Disease*, Cold Spring Harbor, pp. 193–200.

Schechter, R., Yen, S.-H. C. and Terry, R. D. (1981) Fibrous astrocytes in senile dementia of the Alzheimer type. *J. Neuropathol. Exp. Neurol.*, 40: 95–101.

Scheele, G. and Blackburn, P. (1979) Role of mammalian RNase inhibitor in cell free protein synthesis. *Proc. Natl. Acad. Sci. USA*, 76: 4898–4902.

Semsei, I., Szeszak, F. and Nagy, I. (1982) In vivo studies on the age-dependent decrease of the rates of total and mRNA synthesis in the brain cortex of rats. *Arch. Gerontol. Geriatr.*, 1: 29–42.

Sheiness, D. and Darnell, J. E. (1973) Polyadenylic acid segment in mRNA becomes shorter with age. *Nature New Biol.*, 241: 265–268.

Shortman, K. (1961) Studies on cellular inhibitors of ribonuclease. I. The assay of the ribonuclease-inhibitor system, and the purification of the inhibitor from rat liver. *Biochim. Biophys. Acta*, 51: 37–49.

Soreq, H., Safran, A. and Eliyahu, D. (1983) Modified composition of major ontogenetically regulated mRNAs and proteins in the cerebellum of old and staggerer mice. *Dev. Brain Res.*, 10: 73–82.

Strehler, B. L. and Chang, M.-P. (1979) Loss of hybridizable ribosomal DNA from human postmitotic tissues during aging. II. Age-dependent loss in human cerebral cortex — hippocampal and somatosensory cortex comparison. *Mech. Aging Dev.*, 11: 379–382.

Struble, R. G., Cork, L. C., Whitehouse, R. J. and Price, D. L. (1982) Cholinergic innervation in neuritic plaques. *Science*, 216: 413–415.

Takahashi, Y., Mase, K. and Suzuki, Y. (1970) Purification and characteristics of RNase inhibitor from pig cerebral cortex. *J. Neurochem.*, 17: 1433–1440.

Taylor, G. R., Carter, G. I., Crow, T. J., Perry, E. K. and Perry, R. H. (1985) Measurement of relative concentrations of RNA in postmortem brains from senile dementia of the Alzheimer type (SDAT) and controls. *J. Neurogenet.*, 2: 177.

Tse, T. P. H. and Taylor, J. M. (1977) Translation of albumin messenger RNA in a cell-free protein-synthesizing system derived from wheat germ. *J. Biol. Chem.*, 252: 1272–1278.

Uemura, E. and Hartmann, H. A. (1979) Quantitative studies of neuronal RNA on the subiculum of demented old individuals. *Brain Res. Bull.*, 4: 301–305.

Vargas, R. and Castaneda, M. (1981) Role of elongation factor 1 in the translational control of rodent brain protein synthesis. *J. Neurochem.*, 37: 687–694.

Waterlow, J. C., Garlick, D. J. and Millward, D. J. (Eds.)

(1978) *Protein Turnover in Mammalian Tissues and in the Whole Body*, Elsevier/North-Holland, New York, pp. 443–479.

Watson, W. E. (1968) Observations on the nucleolar and total cell body nucleic acid of injured nerve cells. *J. Physiol.*, 196: 655–676.

Wenk, H., Bigl, V. and Meyer, U. (1980) Cholinergic projections from magnocellular nuclei of the basal forebrain to cortical areas of rats. *Brain Res.*, 2: 295–315.

White, P., Goodhardt, M. J., Keet, J. P., Hiley, C. R., Carasco, L. H., Williams, L. E. I. and Bowen, D. M. (1977) Neocortical neurons in elderly people. *Lancet*, I, 668–671.

Whitehouse, P. J., Price, D. L., Clark, A. W., Coyle, J. T. and DeLong, M. R. (1981) Alzheimer disease: evidence for selective loss of cholinergic neurons in the nucleus basalis. *Ann. Neurol.*, 10: 122–126.

Yamagami, S., Fritz, R. R. and Rappoport, D. A. (1966)

Biochemistry of the developing rat brain. VII. Changes in the ribosomal system and nuclear RNAs. *Biochim. Biophys. Acta*, 129: 532–547.

Yamamoto, T. and Hirano, A. (1985) Hirano bodies in the perikaryon of the Purkinje cell in a case of Alzheimer's disease. *Acta Neuropathol. (Berl.)*, 67: 167–169.

Young, R. and Davis, R. (1983) Efficient isolation of genes using antibody probes. *Proc. Natl. Acad. Sci. USA*, 80: 1194–1198.

Zagorski, W. (1978) Preparation and characteristics of wheat embryo cell-free extract active in the synthesis of high molecular weight polypeptides. *Anal. Biochem.*, 87: 316–333.

Zomzely, C. E., Roberts, S., Peache, S. and Brown, D. M. (1971) Cerebral protein synthesis. III. Developmental alterations in the stability of cerebral messenger ribonucleic acid-ribosome complexes. *J. Biol. Chem.*, 246: 2097–2103.

Discussion

B. CORDELL: Have you taken into account the data of Hahn et al. (1983) who demonstrated that there exists a major population of unique transcripts which are not polyadenylated which would be excluded from all your studies?

ANSWER: Yes, I know of the work mentioned. The speaker also refers to McLaughlin's work presented in a poster at this meeting which showed no difference in poly A-yields of normals and SDAT patients. However, poly(A −) RNA was only about half as effective in protein synthesis stimulation, similar to the situation for poly(A +) RNA.

E. MENA: Does the mRNA isolated from brains with AD produce any of the pathological protein's characteristics of AD, such as paired helical filament (PHF) proteins?

ANSWER: With suitable antibodies, this question could be probed. However, to be successful the antibody must be directed at an altered apoprotein sequence, not a posttranslationally modified polypeptide.

J. G. GUILLEMETTE: Have you performed complexity studies? What are your neuron to glia ratios? Do you believe that you are looking at abnormal aging?

ANSWER: No, we did not perform complexity studies. We have not yet estimated the neuron to glia ratios in our material. Clearly the glial marker is increased. The one neuronal marker we have tried, antibody to the 70K neurofilament protein was not successful for immunoprecipitation experiments because the antibody was directed to phosphorylated residues. When results for normal aged controls are grouped with the AD data, there is no significant correlation with age.

M. MIRMIRAN: As you have shown, there seems to be a reduction in protein and mRNA in very old controls which get closer to the young AD. Could it be that the reduction you have seen in protein and RNA is a result of general atrophy rather than a specific sign of AD?

ANSWER: The interesting aspect of the protein synthesis levels is that the youngest AD cases resemble the oldest controls. Of course a decreased protein synthesis rate is not unique to AD. However, both the in vitro and in vivo studies (the latter of Bustany et al., 1981) have now demonstrated that a decline in the production of new protein is a significant component of the molecular pathogenesis. Viewed from this perspective, the dramatic reduction in the level of neurotransmitter systems is not too surprising. In my view excessive attention has been paid to measuring enzyme levels and too little has been paid to elucidating the factors that regulate cellular metabolism at the level of transcription and translation.

A. G. UITTERLINDEN: The gel you showed on total RNA isolation from AD/SDAT brain showed the appearance of specific, discrete bands as compared to RNA from an age-matched control. Do you explain this to be due to degradation (which I consider unlikely)? If the latter possibility would hold true how do you relate this finding to the one indicating a dramatic decrease of protein synthesis?

ANSWER: The gel was of poly(A +) RNA, not total RNA. The newly appearing bands may be degradation products or new species or both. We are entertaining both possibilities. If they are new discrete functional mRNAs we should see a huge increase in new bands on the autoradiographs; however, we do not, except for GFAP.

A. G. UITTERLINDEN: Were all of your studies performed on AD/SDAT brain tissue from sporadic and/or familial cases and did you find any differences with regard to both forms in terms of protein synthesis and RNA level?

ANSWER: We have not yet looked at a familial case due to unavailability.

A. G. UITTERLINDEN: Are you extending your studies on the altered activity of the alkaline ribonuclease in AD/SDAT brain tissue to the DNA level and do you think that this finding represents deregulation of a specific gene or that it is part of a more general gene deregulation and represents a secondary (or tertiary, etc.) effect?

ANSWER: We are extending our studies to examine in detail a number of potentially interesting genes, the nuclease inhibitor protein is but one of them. It is extremely unlikely that deregulation of the inhibitor gene is the primary defect; the available literature from model systems suggests that changes in inhibitor activity are secondary to other metabolic events.

References

Bustany, P., Sargent, T., Saudubray, J. M., Henry, J. F. and Comar, D. (1981) Regional human uptake and protein incorporation of [^{11}C]methionine studied in vivo with PET. *J. Cereb. Blood Flow Metab.*, 1, Suppl. 1: S17–18.

Bustany, P., Henry, J. F., Soussaline, F. and Comar, D. (1983) Brain protein synthesis in normal and demented patients — a study by positron emission tomography with [^{11}C]-L-methionine. In P. S. Magistretti (Ed.), *Functional Radionuclide Imaging of the Brain*, Raven Press, New York, pp. 319–326.

Hahn, W. E., Chaudhari, N., Beck, L., Wilber, K. and Peffley, D. (1983) Genetic expression and postnatal development of the brain: some characteristics of nonpolyadenylated mRNAs. *Cold Spring Harbor Symp. Quant. Biol. 48, Pt. 2*, 465–475, Cold Spring Harbor Laboratory, New York.

D. F. Swaab, E. Fliers, M. Mirmiran, W. A. Van Gool and F. Van Haaren (Eds.)
Progress in Brain Research, Vol. 70.
© 1986 Elsevier Science Publishers B.V. (Biomedical Division)

CHAPTER 20

Cell-specific pathology in neural systems of the temporal lobe in Alzheimer's disease

G. W. Van Hoesen[a,b], B. T. Hyman[b] and A. R. Damasio[b]

Departments of [a]Anatomy and [b]Neurology, University of Iowa, Iowa City, IA 52242, USA

Introduction

Alzheimer's disease (AD), once thought to be a rare disorder, has emerged in recent years as a major health risk among the elderly; unmasked so to speak, by increased human longevity, heightened clinical and scientific interest and increased public awareness. Its wake is often prolonged and nearly always devastating for the victim. Innumerable additional health risks accompany the disease (Katzman, 1976). These circumstances alone are sufficient to justify a major medical research effort. However, there are additional reasons that make an understanding of AD a high priority.

For example, in a high percentage of instances, AD is heralded by a memory impairment (Sourander and Sjögren, 1970). This may be complicated by depression and/or other changes in the normal pattern of behavior, but few would dispute the fact that memory dysfunction characterizes the disease from its onset until its termination in death.

The memory impairment seems to follow a progressive history, albeit, one that can vary substantially in tempo. Initially, more immediate memories pertaining to context seem affected. As the disease progresses, a more complete and global amnestic state develops, where all aspects of memory are ravaged. In the latter stages of the illness, even the most familiar generic and rote aspects of learned behaviors may be lost, as well as

self recognition. This invites careful study by the behaviorist, who in longitudinal studies, might find displayed in this illness a slow and particularly well-focused deterioration of a fundamental cognitive process dissected into its elemental components. It also invites clinico-anatomical and neurochemical study on a long-term basis since patterns of pathology and change may emerge that reveal the structural and chemical correlates of memory with identifiable features at each stage of the alterations in memory (Damasio, 1984).

Very much related to the above are other issues that have their roots vested solidly in basic neuroscience research. In the past two decades substantial advances have been made in understanding the anatomy of neural systems for nearly all telencephalic areas thought to play a role in memory (Mishkin, 1982; Van Hoesen, 1985). There has also been substantial progress in terms of understanding the organization of long association, or cortico-cortical connections (Pandya and Kuypers, 1969; Jones and Powell, 1970), in the non-human primate. At the same time a great deal has been learned about cortico-limbic and limbic-cortical connections. The terminal patterns of these projections, as well as the specific cells that give rise to them, are largely now known. Aside for only a few examples (Kemper, 1978), this sizeable body of experimental anatomical knowledge derived from higher primates has not been applied or viewed in the context of the patterns of pathology in

Alzheimer's disease (Hyman et al., 1984a). Since there is a growing body of evidence to support the belief that pathology in Alzheimer's disease is highly cell specific, such comparisons are invited.

The purpose of this chapter is to focus on some major memory-related neural systems of the temporal lobe in the non-human primate and to draw some specific comparisons with the pattern of pathology observed in AD. It is our contention that understanding these neural correlates in AD might lead ultimately to understanding the neural correlates of memory itself.

Materials and methods

The anterior portion of the temporal lobes of 30 patients have been studied (Fig. 1). Included in the tissue block was the temporal polar cortex (Brodmann's area 38), the prepiriform and periamygdaloid cortices (Brodmann's area 51), the entorhinal cortex (Brodmann's area 28), the perirhinal cortex (Brodmann's area 35), the anterior parts of the lateral temporal neocortex (Brodmann's areas 20, 21 and 22), the anterior part of the posterior parahippocampal gyrus (Brodmann's area 36) and the anterior parts of Brodmann's area 37. The entirety of the amygdala and the anterior two-thirds of the hippocampal formation, including the various subicular fields (parasubiculum, presubiculum and subiculum proper) were also included. Twenty-one of the patients had dementia, and nine without dementia were used as controls. Of the 21 with dementia, 16 had pathological changes consistent with a diagnosis of AD. They ranged in age from 59–98 years with a mean age of 78.7 years. Their mean duration of illness was 7.2 years. One patient with dementia (70 yr) had a history of chronic depression, and the brain contained no evidence of infarcts or Alzheimer pathology. The individual was classified as having pseudodementia (depression). Another (57 yr), had a clinical history and pathologic changes consistent with Huntington's chorea. Two patients (95 yr and 75 yr) had histories of multiple infarcts. The more elderly also had neuropathologic changes consistent with AD

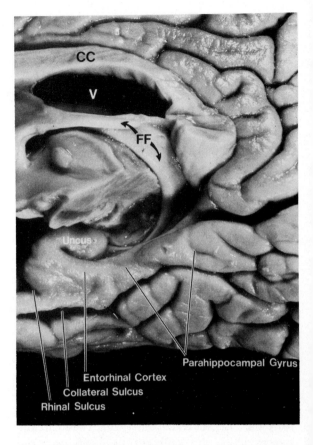

Fig. 1. The medial temporal lobe of the human brain in Alzheimer's disease showing the location of major sulci and the parahippocampal gyrus. The entorhinal cortex is demonstrated in the anterior part of the parahippocampal gyrus. Note the prominent sulci of the temporal lobe and the thinness of the parahippocampal gyrus. CC, corpus callosum; FF, fimbria fornix; V, ventricle.

and was classified as having mixed dementia. The younger did not, and was classified as having multi-infarct dementia. For a fifth patient (98 yr), with dementia, no sufficient material was available to establish a definitive diagnosis of AD and he was classified as probable AD. For the nine non-demented controls six were elderly with a mean age of 78.3 years and a range in age of 70–83 years. Two were in their 5th decades with ages of 53 and 58 years. One was 36 years at the time of death. None died of neurologic causes.

All brains were perfused with 4% formalin.

They were then photographed and the temporal block was dissected. It was soaked overnight in a solution of 4% formaldehyde, 10% sucrose and 10% glycerol. The block was then frozen onto the stage of a large freezing microtome, surrounded by pulverized dry ice and sliced serially at a thickness of 50 μm. At least five 1:10 series of sections were saved for later staining for Nissl substance with thionine, myelin with iron hematoxylin, and for neurofibrillary tangles and neuritic plaques with Congo red, thioflavin-S and silver nitrate. Congo red stained sections were studied under cross-polarized light and thioflavin-S stained sections were studied with the aid of fluorescence illumination (Hyman et al., 1984a). Neurofibrillary tangles and neuritic plaques appear bright yellow against a darker background with both Congo red (Fig. 2) and thioflavin-S under appropriate viewing conditions. All silver-stained sections were studied with both bright and darkfield illumination. Some series of sections were charted with the aid of an X-Y recorder coupled to the movement of the microscope stage and camera lucida methods.

Results

It has been well known for almost three decades that the ventromedial parts of the temporal lobe, and the hippocampal formation in particular, play a critical role in certain key elements of the memory process (Scoville and Milner, 1957). Especially germane are those aspects of memory that pertain to the acquisition of new information. Quite simply, without intact ventromedial temporal structures, new learning in all sensory modalities is precluded, yielding a global amnestic state. We have argued previously that one implication of these observations must be that under normal circumstances, the hippocampal formation should receive as input a rather comprehensive synthesis of cortical information from the sensory and association cortices (Van Hoesen et al., 1972; Van Hoesen and Pandya, 1975; Van Hoesen, 1982). Such connections are now known to exist in several higher mammals and, together with the classic observations of Cajal and Lorente de Nó, they provide a rather comprehensive understand-

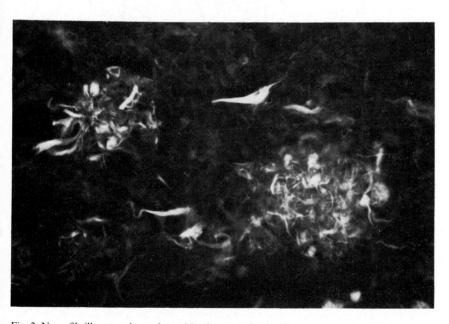

Fig. 2. Neurofibrillary tangles and neuritic plaques stained with Congo red and photographed under fluorescent and cross-polarized conditions.

324

ing of the linkage between the hippocampal formation and the remainder of the cerebral cortex. The major backbone for these connections is summarized in Fig. 3. In brief, it can be stated that the entorhinal cortex is a site of convergence for cortical association input from both modality-specific and multimodal areas. It likewise receives extensive input from other parts of the limbic lobe, which themselves receive association input, and from the amygdala, a limbic structure known to receive sensory inputs related to both the internal and external environments.

The entorhinal cortex, in turn, gives rise to the perforant pathway which conveys entorhinal output to several parts of the hippocampal formation and activates a series of excitatory intrinsic

hippocampal pathways that culminate in hippocampal output. The latter is mediated largely from the subiculum, an allocortical area that is the major recipient of the output from hippocampal intrinsic circuits. It in turn projects back to cortical areas in the temporal lobe, other limbic cortical areas, the amygdala, thalamus, hypothalamus and basal forebrain structures such as the septum, nucleus accumbens and diagonal band nuclei. Many of these project to the association cortices. The subicular cortices thus account for nearly all of the diversity of hippocampal output.

In summary, the majority of hippocampal input and output converges on the entorhinal cortex and subiculum, respectively, making these areas crucial relay and integrative centers. We have therefore

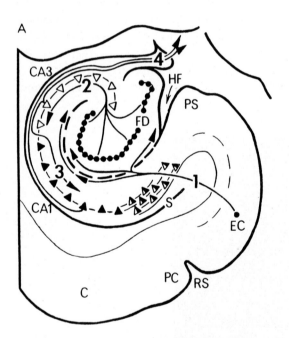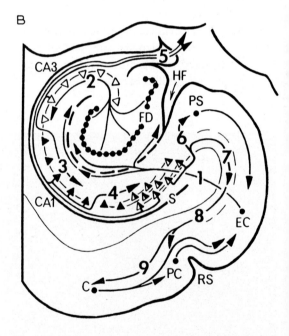

Fig. 3 (A and B). (A) The major connective anatomy of the hippocampal formation in cross-section as revealed by Cajal. Note that the entorhinal cortex (EC) projects via the perforant pathway (1) to the hippocampus (CA1–CA3) and fascia dentata (FD) or dentate gyrus. The latter's output, the mossy fibers (2), terminate on the CA3 pyramids. These give rise to the Schaffer collaterals (3), which terminate on the CA1 pyramids. Axons of CA1–CA3 exit the hippocampal formation via the fimbria fornix (4). (B) depicts a partial update of Cajal's observation. Note that the CA1 pyramids project to the adjacent subiculum (4). This cortex and CA pyramids project to the septum via the fornix, (5), but it is largely subicular projections that course to the anterior thalamus and mammillary bodies. The subicular cortex also projects to several other cortical areas: the presubiculum (PS), the entorhinal cortex (EC), the perirhinal cortex (PC), and other parts of the cortex (C). These are shown schematically in pathways 6–9. The subicular cortices account largely for the diversity of hippocampal output (HF, hippocampal fissure and RS, rhinal sulcus). (From Van Hoesen, 1985)

concentrated our initial studies of the pathology in Alzheimer's disease on the hippocampal formation, and on these areas in particular.

In general, the above sequence of connections suggested by experimental neuroanatomic results of the hippocampal formation in the monkey will be followed in this chapter. We will first review cytoarchitectural and neuropathologic changes due to AD in the entorhinal and perirhinal cortices. Changes in the perforant pathway, which connects the entorhinal cortex to the hippocampus, will be described, followed by examination of the hippocampus itself. The subicular cortices, which give rise to hippocampal output, will follow. Finally, some notes on other structures closely related to these neural systems will be highlighted. In general, there were no significant morphological differences between the younger and more elderly controls, nor between the controls and the patients with dementia due to multiple infarcts, depression, or Huntington's disease. Therefore, we will contrast the morphologic changes due to AD with our observations in these control brains.

Entorhinal and perirhinal cortices

The entorhinal cortex (Brodmann's area 28) in the human brain is an expansive field of periallocortex that dominates the piriform lobe, along the anterior parts of the parahippocampal gyrus (Fig. 1). It is a highly atypical cortex from many viewpoints. For example, layer II is formed by large multipolar, star-shaped neurons that stand out conspicuously in Nissl-stained preparations (Fig. 4A). Moreover, in transverse sections these neurons appear to be aggregated into islands or clusters. However, they actually form a complex mosaic of continuous strips of neurons that form a maze-like arrangement (Braak, 1972). A dense interstitial fiber plexus occupies the intra-strip part of the neuropil. Layer I contains a large number of myelinated and unmyelinated axons coursing parallel to the pia. Layer III is formed by a wide band of medium-sized pyramidal shaped cells, with few departures from that observed in the isocortex. Its

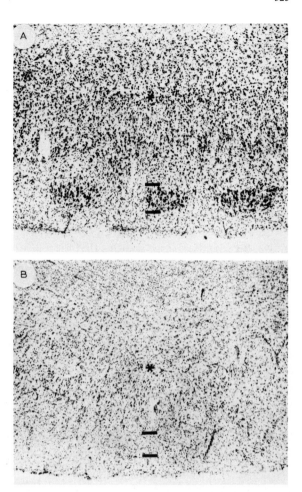

Fig. 4 (A and B). Photomicrographs of Nissl-stained coronal sections of the entorhinal cortex (area 28) of a 70-years-old control (A) and a 71-years-old case of AD (B). In (A), layer II of the entorhinal cortex contains characteristic clusters of large multipolar stellate-shaped neurons and a prominent layer IV. These normal cytoarchitectonal features are largely absent in (B), suggesting a lack of stainable Nissl substance in these two layers, with relative preservation of the adjacent lamina. The approximate location of layer II is marked by bars, and the approximate location of layer IV by an asterisk.

deepest part in certain entorhinal areas is nearly cell-free and is occupied largely by dendritic and axonal processes of more deeply or more superficially located neurons. This forms the so-called lamina dissecans and is a prominent architectural feature of much of the entorhinal cortex. The adjacent cellular layer, that we term layer IV, is formed by a conspicuous population of large multipolar neurons with long apical dendrites that course throughout nearly the full width of the more superficial layers. Layers V and VI are highly multilaminate and composed of many differing cell types. No doubt they could be parcellated into many sub-layers, but their periodic lack of alignment and full differentiation largely precludes this in most species.

In all 16 of the cases of AD we have studied, with varying degrees of dementia but with major alterations in memory functions, the entorhinal cortex is altered greatly. In fact, in Nissl preparations, the islands of large neurons that form layer II are largely absent (Fig. 4B). Likewise, the superficial parts of layer III and layer IV are often altered to a degree that they are undetectable (Fig. 4B). Curiously, with either Congo red or thioflavin-S staining, and microscopic visualization with cross-polarized or fluorescent illumination, these layers seemingly reappear with neurofibrillary tangles marking the location of once viable neurons depleted of ribosomes, rough endoplasmic reticulum, and other cytoplasmic constituents (Fig. 5).

Layer II is uniformly and severely affected by Alzheimer neurofibrillary tangles. The pathology in layer IV is somewhat more variable, but it is often involved as well. Neuritic plaques seem to occur for the most part in layer III, being less dense

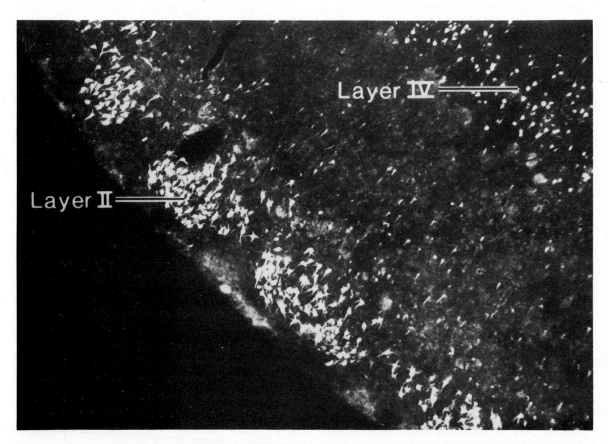

Fig. 5. Photomicrograph of thioflavin-S stained coronal section of the entorhinal cortex from a 60-years-old case of AD. Clusters of thioflavin-S stained neurofibrillary tangles appear when viewed under fluorescent illumination, demonstrating layer II and layer IV. Neurofibrillary tangles are also evident in the most superficial part of layer III. Neuritic plaques appear most frequently in layer III.

in other laminae (Fig. 5). This pattern is most evident in the lateral and intermediate sections of the entorhinal cortex. In the medial entorhinal cortex, the pattern of neurofibrillary tangles resembles that of the adjacent proisocortex, with a line of neurofibrillary tangles in the deep cell layers, predominantly in layer IV.

Using the X-Y recorder to plot the location of neurofibrillary tangles and neuritic plaques visualized under high magnification, we have developed a series of 'maps' of the medial temporal lobe (Fig. 6). The entorhinal cortex can be seen in its mediolateral entirety, and the laminar distribution of neurofibrillary tangles and neuritic plaques described above is readily apparent.

The perirhinal cortex (Brodmann's area 35) is a narrow strip of proisocortex that is interposed between the entorhinal periallocortex and the temporal isocortex. It resembles the latter in overall structure, but its laminar composition departs discernibly. For example, layer II is thicker and accentuated in comparison to the thin and highly differentiated layer II of temporal isocortex. Layer III is comparable to that of the temporal isocortex and the entorhinal periallocortex, but appears less homogenous in terms of cell distribution, and consequently, somewhat patchy. Layer IV of the perirhinal cortex is characterized by small neurons with patchy distribution. In some parts of area 35, it is insipient, disrupting the continuity of the layer. Larger pyramidal neurons are seen occasionally, but they are not as large as those observed in layer IV of the entorhinal cortex. Layers V and VI in Nissl preparations are composed of large neurons with a distinct pyramidal shape, but they are differentiated poorly and appear usually as a dense deeply-stained band of neurons. This departs noticeably from the adjacent well-differentiated layers V and VI of the temporal isocortex and the multilaminate layers V and VI of the entorhinal cortex.

The involvement of perirhinal cortex in AD is more variable than that of the entorhinal cortex. Nonetheless, in patients with severe pathologic changes and a history of profound dementia, the perirhinal cortex is often affected. When it is, there is again an interesting laminar distribution of changes. In Nissl preparations, the major difference in the affected Alzheimer cases is that the zone of deep pyramidal cells in layers V and VI is less well defined. In Congo red and thioflavin-S preparations, these deep neurons appear as a band of neurofibrillary tangles (Fig. 6). In some brains, this band appears to be continuous with the line of tangles in layer II of the adjacent entorhinal cortex. Occasionally, a second band of neurofibrillary tangles is evident in layer II of perirhinal cortex as well. Neuritic plaques occur mainly in layer III.

Perforant pathway zone

The perforant pathway is a major fiber system of the temporal lobe that provides nearly all cortical input to the hippocampal formation. It arises from the large stellate neurons in layer II of the entorhinal cortex, as well as from some of the medium-sized pyramidal neurons of the superficial portion of layer III. The axons of these neurons join to form the angular bundle, then 'perforate' across the subiculum as a cascade of small fascicles. Some of these axons form synapses with the apical dendrites of pyramidal cells of the hippocampus, but a large contingent cross the hippocampal fissure to synapse in a distinctly laminar pattern on the outer dendritic branches of the dentate gyrus granule cells.

Because of our observations in the entorhinal cortex, we have recently examined the cells of origin, the course, and termination zones of the perforant pathway in AD (Hyman et al., 1984b; Van Hoesen et al., 1985). The cells of origin, in layer II and the superficial portion of layer III of the entorhinal cortex, are essentially uniformly affected by neurofibrillary tangles as discussed above. Silver-stained material using the Vogt procedure (1974) shows distinct myelin cuffing and degenerating argyophilic debris throughout the course and terminal zone of the perforant pathway. Finally, there is a line of neuritic plaques that occupies a portion of the molecular layer of the

328

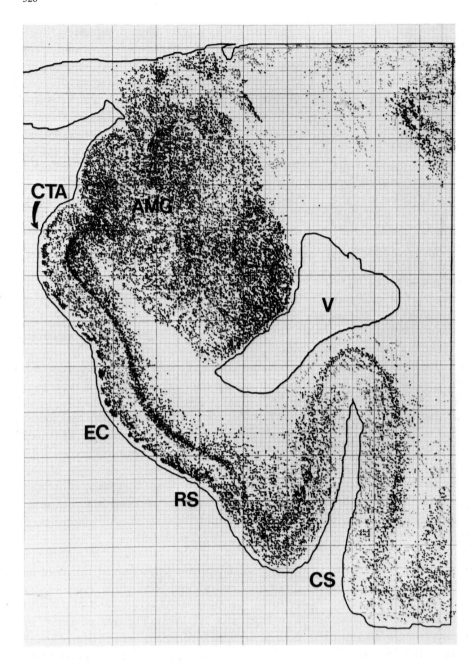

Fig. 6. X-Y plot depicting the location of neurofibrillary tangles (black dots) and neuritic plaques (gray dots) in the medial temporal lobe and adjacent structures in AD. X-Y recorder and camera lucida techniques were used with a thioflavin-S stained section, viewed under fluorescent illumination. The pattern of tangles in layers II and IV of the entorhinal cortex illustrated photographically in Fig. 5 is readily apparent throughout the entire lateral and intermediate entorhinal areas. AMG, amygdala; CTA, cortical transition area; CS, collateral sulcus; EC, entorhinal cortex; RS, rhinal sulcus; V, ventricle.

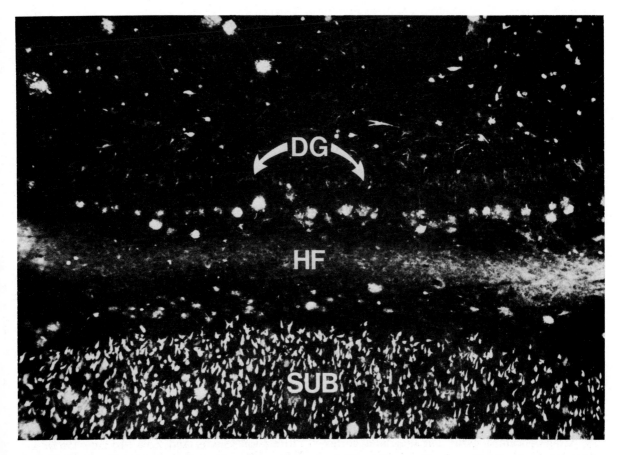

Fig. 7. Distribution of neuritic plaques in the hippocampus. The section is from a 60-years-old patient with AD and was stained with thioflavin-S and viewed under fluorescent illumination. Note the distribution of neuritic plaques in the molecular layer of the dentate gyrus (DG), above the hippocampal fissure (HF), and in the molecular layer of the subiculum (SUB), below the hippocampal fissure. The neurofibrillary tangles in the subiculum are apparent below the hippocampal fissure.

dentate gyrus (Fig. 7), in the expected location of the termination of that portion of the perforant pathway which arises from the lateral and intermediate entorhinal cortex. As seen in Fig. 7, the plaques occur in a laminar arrangement in the outer two-thirds of the molecular layer, and seldom involve the inner one-third of the molecular layer.

Hippocampus and subiculum

The hippocampus forms the rolled-up, medial edge of the temporal cortex and is capped by the dentate gyrus. It consists of several well-defined allocortical subfields. The CA4 neurons are found within the hilum of the dentate gyrus. Proceeding sequentially around Ammon's horn is a narrow layer of CA3 pyramids. They abut the CA1 zone, and the zone of transition is termed CA2. Adjacent to the CA1 pyramids is the subiculum, a somewhat thicker layer of allocortex containing primarily, but not exclusively, pyramidal cells (see Fig. 3 for some of these relationships). Rose's H1 field, and Sommer's sector are alternate terms for areas which largely overlap with the CA1-subicular zone.

In AD, portions of the hippocampus are selectively involved by pathologic changes. In Nissl preparations, the more medial CA1 field has noticeable cell loss. Neurofibrillary tangles invest the CA1 neurons heavily, but are infrequent in the adjacent neurons of CA3. Some tangles are often present in CA4, but their density here and in dentate gyrus granule cells is small in comparison to the involvement of CA1 and the subiculum. The pattern of neuritic plaques in the molecular layer of the dentate gyrus has been described above. In addition, plaques occur primarily in the CA1 pyramidal cell layer and in the molecular layer of the CA1-subiculum zone (Fig. 7).

The subicular cortices lie between the entorhinal cortex and the hippocampus proper. Several subicular subfields can be distinguished in Nissl preparations. The subiculum abuts and joins the CA1 hippocampal zone laterally and is an unusually thick allocortex of several poorly segregated cell types. It occupies the area between CA1 laterally and the presubiculum medially. The presubiculum (area 27) stands out by the presence of the overlying small darkly staining cells that form the lamina principalis externa. Medial to this is Brodmann's area 49, the parasubiculum, which is present largely along the anterior portion of the hippocampal formation. It occupies the crown of the parahippocampal gyrus. The entorhinal cortex, with distinctive clusters of cells in layer II, lies adjacent to the parasubiculum on the ventral surface of the anterior parahippocampal gyrus (Fig. 1).

In the Alzheimer brains, some of the normal cytoarchitectural characteristics of this region are difficult to discern. There is clear neuronal loss in the CA1-subicular zone, while the most medial part of the subiculum and the adjacent lamina principalis externa of the presubiculum stand out as being more preserved. There is however, prominent cellular loss in the medially adjacent parasubiculum.

The cells that appear absent in the Nissl preparations again 'reappear' if one stains for neurofibrillary tangles. Within the subiculum, there is a striking predilection of neurofibrillary tangle involvement in the CA1-subicular zone. The more medial aspect of the subiculum and the presubiculum are often more spared. The parasubiculum is involved heavily, and pathology is especially striking in the superficial lamina of the parasubiculum. These cells provide a strong input to the entorhinal cortex.

The distribution of neuritic plaques in the subicular cortices also seems to respect the cytoarchitecture of the subiculum. They occur mainly in the subiculum-CA1 area and are sparse in the medial subiculum and presubiculum. In addition, neuritic plaques form a prominent band in the deepest part of the molecular layer of the subiculum parallel to the hippocampal fissure (Fig. 7). This zone receives input from the perirhinal cortex, the posterior parahippocampal cortex, and serotinergic projections from the raphe complex. Therefore, this pattern of plaque distribution raises the possibility that neuritic plaques disrupt the terminal zone of additional hippocampal afferents.

Other related structures

The list of structures that seem to play a role in memory has grown in recent years and includes several structures in addition to the hippocampal formation (Squire and Zola-Morgan, 1983). The posterior parahippocampal gyrus, amygdala, certain thalamic nuclei, and mammillary bodies and the nucleus basalis of Meynert must now be included in any discussion of the anatomic basis of memory dysfunction. It is clear that many of these structures are also affected in AD. Moreover, our preliminary observations, and previous reports in the literature, support the fact that this involvement respects the same sort of cellular and regional specificity which we observe in the temporal lobes.

For example, the medial, cortical and basolateral nuclei of the amygdala, as well as the periamygdaloid area and the transitional cortex are all severely affected by neuropathologic changes in AD with relative sparing of adjacent cellular fields (Van Hoesen et al., 1985; Herzog and Kemper, 1980) (Fig. 6). The posterior parahippocampal area (Brodmann's areas 36 and 37) is also affected in a laminar pattern by the neuropathologic changes of AD. In severely affected cases, layer V and, to a lesser extent, layer III of areas 36 and 37 are often invested heavily by neurofibrillary tangles, with few neurofibrillary tangles in other cortical layers.

The topography of Alzheimer pathology in the basal forebrain, thalamus, and hypothalamus has recently been systematically examined by Rudelli et al. (1984). They found that the ventral claustrum, ventral putamen, substantia innominata and septal nuclei consistently contained neuritic plaques. Plaques were also present in a substantial portion of their cases in the thalamus, nucleus basalis of Meynert, and mammillary bodies. In particular, the intralaminar nuclei, the ventral anterior and anterior nuclei, and the ventral lateral and lateral posterior nuclei of thalamus were most heavily affected. Of note, the dorsomedial nucleus was rarely involved by neuritic plaques. Our preliminary observations suggest that certain midline thalamic nuclei with strong connections to the hippocampal formation, including the nucleus reuniens, may be severely affected in AD. In the hypothalamus, the dorsolateral area, including mainly the perifornical portions and the mammillary nuclei, was the region most heavily involved.

The nucleus basalis of Meynert deserves mention. Although it is not always affected heavily by neurofibrillary tangles or neuritic plaques, loss of these cells has been reported in AD (Whitehouse et al., 1982). This is of significance because the majority of these neurons contains cholinergic enzymes and provides the major source of cholinergic input to the cortex (Mesulam and Van Hoesen, 1976; Mesulam and Mufson, 1984). It is well established that cortical levels of acetylcholine drop in AD (Davies and Maloney, 1976), and this may be due to alterations in the nucleus basalis of Meynert.

Discussion

There have been many survey investigations addressing the topography of pathological changes associated with AD (for example, Ball, 1978; Brun and Englund, 1981). In a general sense, the results of these efforts correspond rather well with the memory and cognitive decline associated with this disease. With regard to memory, it is reasonable to believe that alterations in this essential process might be related to temporal lobe pathology, and indeed, this seems clearly to be the case (McLardy, 1973; Kemper, 1978; Burger, 1983; Ball et al., 1985). Temporal structures are nearly always damaged severely and the temporal lobe in general may be more involved than other lobular divisions of the brain (Wilcock, 1983). Within the temporal lobe, memory-related structures like the amygdala, hippocampus and parahippocampal gyrus are common sites to find neurofibrillary tangles, neuritic plaques and cell loss. Hirano bodies and granulovacuolar degeneration are also found in the hippocampus (Hirano and Zimmerman, 1962).

In addition to mapping the topography of pathological changes in Alzheimer's disease, analysis of additional features of cortical anatomy is essential. For example, even within a highly involved area such as the anterior parahippocampal gyrus (entorhinal cortex) not all neurons that form this multi-layered cortex are affected by neurofibrillary tangles (Fig. 5). In fact, our experience indicates that their distribution is rigidly laminar, affecting largely layers II and IV. Similarly, in the hippocampal formation, tangles are found largely in the subiculum and adjacent CA1 sector of the structure, leaving intact the adjacent presubiculum and CA3 and CA4 cells. Thus, the implication is that in addition to a differential topography within the cortex there is also a highly rigid cell-specific pathology even within a pathologically affected area. This may involve one cell layer and not its immediate neighbor, or, as is the case for the hippocampal formation, one field and not a neighboring cellular field.

Of particular interest with respect to memory dysfunction is the fact that the specific pathologic changes affect neurons which are crucial for hippocampal connections. The hippocampus can be considered to be essentially deafferented by the pathologic changes in the entorhinal cortex and perforant pathway. Similarly, the hippocampus is essentially deefferented by the involvement of the subiculum by severe pathologic changes. Interruption of both hippocampal input and output must interfere with normal hippocampal function.

The pattern of pathology in the posterior parahippocampal gyrus may also be of significance because the cells that are specifically affected are important projection neurons. The posterior parahippocampal gyrus appears to be a multimodal staging area that has reciprocal connections to visual, somatic, and auditory association cortices, and which, in turn, also has strong bidirectional projections to both entorhinal cortex and subiculum (Van Hoesen, 1982). Loss of these cells may further compromise the function of the medial temporal lobe structures vital to learning and memory.

The differential topography of pathological changes in AD has important implications for understanding the behavioral changes associated with this illness. But, in addition, it may hold clues for understanding its etiology and pathophysiology as well. For example, in the experimental animal, destruction of the entorhinal cortex leads to a plasticity response in the outer molecular layer of the dentate gyrus (Cotman et al., 1973). The fact that the entorhinal cortex and perforant pathway are affected in AD (Hyman, 1984a,b) has led to the observation that a similar 'plasticity' response occurs in the human hippocampal formation in AD (Geddes et al., 1985; Hyman et al., unpublished observations). This raises the possibility that a portion of the behavioral manifestations of AD is due not only to destructive pathology but also to the brain's response to injury.

The more pervasive cognitive decline observed in AD cannot be separated clearly from the temporal lobe pathology discussed above, or from the memory impairment, but it is likely that pathology in other cortical areas (Terry, 1983) has an additive and devastating effect on higher function. In this regard, there may be specific patterns to the pathologic changes in these regions beyond the temporal lobe. For example, it is not known why neuritic plaques occur with a high frequency in the frontal association cortices, but are relatively rare in the adjacent motor cortices. Similarly, the inferior parietal cortices may be greatly altered, but the adjacent postcentral and superior parietal gyri are much less affected. Initial studies by Pearson et al. (1985) and Rogers and Morrison (1985), suggest that regional and laminar specific patterns of pathology often respect anatomic boundaries and connectional pathways. Our results, along with these sets of data, support the hypothesis that neurofibrillary tangles and neuritic plaques represent pathologic markers for a disease process that respects some, but not other neural systems each of which have a specific connectivity. How affected cells differ from their unaffected neighbors remains unknown, but the distinction between them may allow the formulation and testing of further hypotheses. Certainly cortico-cortical association systems seem involved heavily.

All considered, AD deserves special attention on many counts, but two, in particular, stand out in our minds. The health-related issue of identifying the etiology and treating the illness successfully is manifest in the face of an ever-increasing elderly population (Katzman, 1983). But additionally, the marshalling and recruitment of basic neuroscience effort to this disorder might substantially enhance our understanding of the neural correlates of memory, and be our best bet at ultimately understanding its mechanisms.

Summary and conclusions

A combined analysis of the patterns and cellular specific distribution of pathology in AD has revealed a highly selective involvement of only certain neural systems of the temporal lobe. In large part, the markers of this disorder affect neurons and their axonal processes that in all likelihood interconnect the hippocampal formation with the cerebral cortex, with other parts of the telencephalon such as the basal forebrain, and with a role in memory. Many of the changes affect long associational connections that link one part of the temporal cortex together with other cortical or subcortical parts. In many instances, shorter intrinsic systems are spared. This is particularly apparent in the hippocampal formation where the cells of origin for key intrinsic excitatory linkages between its various parts seem to survive. It is our contention that the diseased neurons of the temporal lobe in AD represent the structural underpinnings for long neural systems that are essential for certain aspects of memory. In their absence, the hippocampal formation is effectively isolated. In this sense, the cellular and laminar specific nature of pathology in AD involves the essential neural elements of a highly complicated behavioral process such as memory.

Acknowledgements

We thank P. Reimann for photographic support, L. Spence for assistance in preparation of specimens and L. Kromer and K. Maskey for excellent technical assistance. Supported by NIH Grants NS 14944, IF21EY5720, and PO NS 19632. We thank Mr. M. Haleem the Yakovlev Collection curator (NINCDS-AFIP contract, Y01-NS-7-0032) for his assistance.

References

Ball, M. J. (1978) Topographic distribution of neurofibrillary tangles and granulo-vacular degeneration in hippocampal cortex of aging and demented patients. A quantitative study. *Acta Neuropathol. (Berl.)*, 74: 173–178.

Ball, M. J., Hachinski, V., Fox, A., Kirshen, A. J., Fishman, M., Blume, W., Kral, V. A. and Fox, H. (1985) A new definition of Alzheimer's disease: A hippocampal dementia. *Lancet*, 1: 14–16.

Braak, H. (1972) Zur Pigmentarchitecktonik der Grobhirnrinde des Menschen. I. Regio entorhinalis. *Z. Zellforsch.*, 127: 407–438.

Brun, A. and Englund, E. (1981) Regional pattern of degeneration in Alzheimer's disease: neuronal loss and histopathological grading. *Histopathology*, 5: 549–564.

Burger, P. C. (1983) The limbic system in Alzheimer's disease. In R. Katzman (Ed.), *Biological Aspects of Alzheimer's Disease, Banbury Report 15*, Cold Spring Harbor Laboratory, pp. 37–44.

Cotman, C. W., Matthews, D. A., Taylor, D. and Lynch, G. (1973) Synaptic rearrangement in the dentate gyrus: histochemical evidence of adjustments after lesions in immature and adult rats. *Proc. Natl. Acad. Sci. USA*, 70: 3473–3477.

Damasio, A. R. (1984) The anatomic basis of memory disorders. *Semin. Neurol.*, 4: 226–228.

Davies, P. and Maloney, A. J. F. (1976) Selective loss of central cholinergic neurons in Alzheimer's disease. *Lancet*, 1: 1403.

Geddes, J. W., Monaghan, D. T., Lott, I. T., Chui, H. C., Kim, R. C. and Cotman, C. W. (1985) Plasticity of hippocampal circuitry in Alzheimer's disease. *Soc. Neurosci.*, 11: 99.

Herzog, A. G. and Kemper, T. L. (1980) Amygdaloid changes in aging and dementia. *Arch. Neurol.*, 37: 625–629.

Hirano, A. and Zimmerman, H. M. (1962) Alzheimer's neurofibrillary changes: a topographic study. *Arch. Neurol.*, 7: 73–88.

Hyman, B. T., Van Hoesen, G. W., Damasio, A. R. and Barnes, C. L. (1984a) Alzheimer's disease: cell-specific pathology isolates the hippocampal formation. *Science*, 225: 1168–1170.

Hyman, B. T., Van Hoesen, G. W. and Damasio, A. R. (1984b) Perforant pathway pathology and the memory impairment of Alzheimer's disease. *Soc. Neurosci.*, 10: 383.

Jones, E. G. and Powell, T. P. S. (1970) An anatomical study of converging sensory pathways within the cerebral cortex of the monkey. *Brain*, 93: 793–820.

Katzman, R. (1976) The prevalence and malignancy of Alzheimer's disease. *Arch. Neurol.*, 33: 217–218.

Katzman, R. (1983) Overview: demography, definitions and problems. In R. Katzman and R. D. Terry (Eds.), *The Neurology of Aging*, F. A. Davis, Philadelphia, pp. 1–14.

Kemper, T. L. (1978) Senile dementia: a focal disease in the temporal lobe. In K. Nandy (Ed.), *Senile Dementia: A Biomedical Approach*, Elsevier/North-Holland, pp. 105–113.

McLardy, T. (1973) Alzheimer tangles and plaques: etiological clues. *IRCS International Research Communications Systems*, October 1973.

Mesulam, M. M. and Mufson, E. J. (1984) Neural inputs into the nucleus basalis of the substantia innominata (Ch4) in the rhesus monkey. *Brain Res.*, 107: 253–374.

Mesulam, M. M. and Van Hoesen, G. W. (1976) Acetylcholinesterase containing basal forebrain neurons in the rhesus monkey project to neocortex. *Brain Res.*, 109: 152–157.

Mishkin, M. (1982) A memory system in the monkey. *Philos. Tran. R. Soc. Lond. (Biol.)*, 298(1089): 83–95.

Pandya, D. N. and Kuypers, H. G. J. M. (1969) Cortico-cortical connections in the rhesus monkey. *Brain Res.*, 13: 13–36.

Pearson, R. C. A., Esiri, M. M., Hiorns, R. W., Wilcock, G. H. and Powell, T. P. S. (1985) Anatomical correlates of the distribution of the pathological changes in the neocortex in

Alzheimer's disease. *Proc. Natl. Acad. Sci. USA*, 83: 4531–4534.

Rogers, J. and Morrison, J. H. (1985) Quantitative morphology and regional and laminar distributions of senile plaques in Alzheimer's disease. *J. Neurosci.*, 5: 2801–2808.

Rudelli, R. C., Ambler, M. W. and Wisniewski, H. M. (1984) Morphology and distribution of Alzheimer neuritic (senile) amyloid plaques in striatum and diencephalon. *Acta Neuropathol. (Berl.)*, 64: 273–281.

Scoville, W. B. and Milner, B. (1957) Loss of recent memory after bilateral hippocampal lesions. *J. Neurol. Neurosurg. Psychiat.*, 20: 11–21.

Sourander, P. and Sjögren, H. (1970) The concept of Alzheimer's disease and its clinical implications. In G. E. W. Wolstenholme and M. E. O'Connor (Eds.), *Alzheimer's Disease and Related Conditions*, Churchill, London, pp. 11–32.

Squire, L. R. and Zola-Morgan, S. (1983) The neurology of memory: the case for correspondence between the findings for human and nonhuman primate. In J. A. Deutsch (Ed.), *The Physiological Basis of Memory, Ch. 6*, Academic Press, New York.

Terry, R. D. (1983) Cortical morphometry in Alzheimer's disease. In R. Katzman (Ed.), *Biological Aspects of Alzheimer's Disease, Banbury Report 15*, Cold Spring Harbor Laboratory, pp. 95–106.

Van Hoesen, G. W. (1982) The primate parahippocampal gyrus: new insights regarding its cortical connections. *Trends Neurosci.*, 5: 345–350.

Van Hoesen, G. W. (1985) Neural systems of the nonhuman primate forebrain in memory. *Ann. NY Acad. Sci.*, 444: 97–112.

Van Hoesen, G. W., Pandya, D. N. and Butters, N. (1972) Cortical afferents to the entorhinal cortex of the rhesus monkey. *Science*, 175: 1471–1473.

Van Hoesen, G. W. and Pandya, D. N. (1975) Some connections of the entorhinal (area 28) and the perirhinal (area 35) cortices of the rhesus monkey. II. Efferent connections. *Brain Res.*, 9: 39–59.

Van Hoesen, G. W., Damasio, A. R. and Hyman, B. T. (1985) Perforant pathway disruption and other temporal lobe pathology in Alzheimer's disease. *Neurology*, 35 Suppl. 1: 219.

Vogt, B. A. (1974) A reduced silver stain for normal axons in the central nervous system. *Physiol. Behav.*, 13: 837–840.

Whitehouse, P. J., Price, D. L., Struble, R. G., Clark, A. W., Coyle, J. T. and DeLong, M. R. (1982) Alzheimer's disease and senile dementia: loss of neurons in the basal forebrain. *Science*, 215: 1237–1239.

Wilcock, G. K. (1983) The temporal lobe in the dementia of Alzheimer's type. *Gerontology*, 29: 320–324.

Discussion

H. G. OLBRICH: (1) Did you observe pathological changes confined either to the entorhinal cortex or the subiculum?

(2) Could you speculate on a certain time course of involvement of various cortical areas?

ANSWER: (1) No, in the 16 cases we have examined, we see pathology in both areas. It may vary in severity, but pathology is always present to some degree in both areas.

(2) This is an important question. The anatomic-pathologic evidence in AD might be consistent with a 'chain' of interconnected neural systems that extend from the association cortices to the hippocampus. Our own results suggest that the entorhinal cortex and subicular pathology occurs early in the illness, but whether this leads ultimately to cell death or other forms of AD pathology in anatomically connected areas elsewhere at a later time in the illness is not something we have studied.

D. GASH: In comparing the age-matched controls with the AD brains, is there a clear-cut dichotomy in the hippocampus between normal aged and AD subjects? Specifically, is there a tendency towards this pathology in normal aging?

ANSWER: In elderly non-demented controls in their 7th decade of life or older it is not unusual to see some evidence of tangles in the entorhinal cortex and subiculum, particularly in thioflavin-S stained material. It does not rival in quantity that seen in AD, even in much younger demented patients.

D. F. SWAAB: As a follow-up of the question of Don Gash, can you give us some more information on the controls, i.e., (1) what is the age range, and (2) is there an increase in pathology with age?

ANSWER: (1) Our controls range in age from the 3rd to the 8th decade.

(2) We have not specifically studied this, but my impression is that there may be a positive correlation. Certainly, the duration of illness in AD seems correlated with severity of pathology.

K. IQBAL (comment): The Alzheimer histopathological changes are generally less in relatively younger cases.

H. BRAAK: Could you comment on the specific targets towards which the large layer IV pyramidal cells of the entorhinal cortex are projecting?

ANSWER: We know on the basis of the classical Golgi studies by Cajal and Lorente de Nó that these cells give rise to a dense axonal plexus that terminates intrinsically in the superficial entorhinal layers. However, several laboratories (e.g., Lohman) have shown, in addition, that they have long projections to the cortex and to other basal forebrain areas. They also give rise to a substantial projection to the amygdala. It would seem reasonable to assume that they would have both a direct influence on cholinergic neurons in the basal forebrain and an indirect influence via the amygdala.

R. N. KALARIA: Correct me please, am I right in understanding that you suggest a high association of memory deficits (in AD) with degeneration, particularly in the hippocampus-parahippocampal gyrus?

ANSWER: Yes, this would be our position. The specific patterns of pathology dissect the key input and output structures of the hippocampal formation. If the connections in man are similar to those of the rhesus monkey, the patterns of pathology would disconnect the hippocampal formation from its major direct cortical, thalamic and hypothalamic sources of input and output. Surely, this would have devastating consequences for certain aspects of memory. Whether it accounts for all aspects of the cognitive decline in AD is quite a separate issue. The memory impairment is only one of many behavioral changes in Alzheimer's disease.

R. D. TERRY: (1) In the 16 AD cases, was the pathology confined to the entorhinal cortex?

(2) How do you interpret absent Nissl staining with many residual tangles seen with thioflavin or Congo red, i.e., are these viable or dead neurons?

ANSWER: (1) No, my point was as follows: brain weight, cortical atrophy, neuritic plaque presence and distribution and basal forebrain pathology in the nucleus basalis of Meynert all vary substantially in our cases. Entorhinal and subicular pathology are present in all of our cases so far, and therefore seem to be far more invariant features of the disease — maybe some of its first pathological manifestations.

(2) The absence of discernible staining in Nissl preparations suggests to me that ribosomes and rough endoplasmatic reticulum are no longer present. The 'ghost-like' re-appearance of these cells with Congo-red and thioflavin-S staining relates only to the persistent abnormal cytoskeleton that remains after cell death. Someone has referred to the tangle-laden image as 'tombstones' marking the former location of a once viable neuron. I favor this interpretation, and simply cannot believe that the images one sees in Congo-red and thioflavin-S stained material represent functionally viable neurons.

L. MRZLJAK: (1) It was shown in the developing human as well as in the infant and adult brain by means of AChE histochemistry that the characteristic islands of the entorhinal area show substantial staining. Have you any evidence for the loss of staining in AD in the island area?

(2) Have you studied the transmitter nature of multipolar large neurons of islands (layer II) area of the entorhinal cortex? Is it your intention to do so?

ANSWER: (1) In the normal adult human brain as well as in some other mammals, the layer II cells of the entorhinal cortex do show a light staining for acetylcholinesterase. There is no evidence of this left in our Alzheimer material.

(2) Glutamate is thought to be the transmitter in the perforant pathway. We have preliminary evidence that suggests that glutamate is non-detectable in the terminal zone of the perforant pathway in the dentate gyrus.

J. M. RABEY: Do you imply when you talk about deafferentiation of the hippocampus, that the process starts *outside the hippocampus* and later on affects this structure, or does the process start at the same time *inside and outside* the hippocampus?

ANSWER: I do not know the answer to your question. We have studied several brains where neurofibrillary tangles are seen largely *outside* the hippocampus in the entorhinal cortex and *inside* the hippocampus in its subiculum subdivision. We have not seen either in isolation. If this represents the usual state of affairs, the hippocampal formation would be both deafferented and deefferented in a significant fashion. The timing in terms of when and where pathology occurs strikes me as an important question to address.

D. F. Swaab, E. Fliers, M. Mirmiran, W. A. Van Gool and F. Van Haaren (Eds.)
Progress in Brain Research, Vol. 70.
© 1986 Elsevier Science Publishers B.V. (Biomedical Division)

CHAPTER 21

The old animal as a model in research on brain aging and Alzheimer's disease/senile dementia of the Alzheimer type

C. F. Hollander[a] and J. Mos[b]

TNO Institute for Experimental Gerontology, Lange Kleiweg 151, P.O. Box 5815, 2280 HV Rijswijk, The Netherlands

Introduction

The aging process should be regarded as a dynamic process which can be studied in mammalian species by essentially two types of investigation, namely, cross-sectional and longitudinal studies. With respect to studies in animals on brain aging and diseases such as the dementias, the method of approach (i.e. longitudinal or cross-sectional) will often be determined by the precise nature of the investigation itself, taking into account the life-span of the species to be studied. For example, studies necessitating highly invasive procedures or those requiring animal tissues for biochemical or morphological analysis, will frequently be cross-sectional in design. Certain behavioral and neurophysiological studies, on the other hand, can be readily carried out in a longitudinal fashion. However, it should be realized that in the case of behavioral studies, due to the repeated testing, one can only compare the test outcome of aged animals with the data obtained from the same animals at younger ages and not with naive animals.

It is generally accepted that the sequence of aging changes in animals resembles that in man, despite the great differences in life-span. However, no known animal model mimics all (or even most) of the behavioral and neuropathological changes of Alzheimer's disease (AD)/senile dementia of the Alzheimer type (SDAT). Investigations have been carried out in old animals of a variety of different species to identify characteristics that in one way or another are similar to the changes typically seen in humans dying with AD/SDAT. Many such characteristics (e.g. plaques, neurofibrillary tangles, nerve cell loss; NAS, 1981) have been identified in aged animals of some species, but none have been identical in all respects to the lesions of AD/SDAT in man (reviewed by NAS, 1981; Mervis, 1983). Wisniewski et al. (1970) have described senile plaques with cerebral amyloidosis in aged dogs. In the rat, by contrast, senile plaques are extremely rare and the occurrence of amyloid in this species is even rarer (Hollander, unpublished observation). It has also to be realized that the evaluation of age-related behavioral and cognitive changes in animals presents problems in itself since one cannot directly apply to animals established test methods used in man. Nevertheless, it is felt worthwhile to increase the effort to develop animal models for studying SDAT. Attention will be focused on the use of old rodents for this purpose.

Mice and rats

In the majority of current gerontological research programs, long-lived, inbred strains of mice and rats are employed. This is primarily because of

---

[a] Present address: Laboratoires MSD CHIBRET, Centre de Recherche, Département d'E.I.M., B.P. 134, 63203 RIOM Cedex, France.
[b] Present address: Duphar B.V., Department of Pharmacology, P.O. Box 2, 1380 AA Weesp, The Netherlands.

their relatively short life-spans, ease of handling in the laboratory and the relatively low costs of production and maintenance of large numbers of rodents as compared to larger laboratory species. Their value in aging research has been recently reviewed by Gibson et al. (1979), by a Committee on Animal Models for Research on Aging, of the Institute of Laboratory Animal Resources, USA (NAS, 1981) and by Hollander et al. (1984). An aged mouse or rat may be defined as one older than the 50% survival age for its strain; it derives from a population exhibiting a more or less rectangular survival curve, in which those that die exhibit multiple pathological changes (Zurcher et al., 1982). For aging research, it is a prerequisite to use animals in good health (Weisbroth, 1972). Specific-pathogen-free (SPF) animals should therefore be used for these studies. The major importance of the SPF status for gerontological research is to avoid the possibility of intercurrent infections terminating the study prematurely. The costs of producing and maintaining SPF rodents add an extra financial burden to already costly experiments. It should be realized that unless the precise nature of the SPF status is specifically stated, the term SPF is rather meaningless since it may vary from one laboratory to another (Hollander and Burek, 1982). However, it is often not realized that not only the health status, but also environmental factors (Clough, 1982) and minor differences in the experimental procedure between laboratories can influence the outcome of a study. Therefore, if animals for experiments are obtained from an outside source, a reasonable adaptation period (i.e. 2 weeks) should be allowed before they are employed in a study at hand.

The need to be informed about the occurrence and distribution of neoplastic and non-neoplastic lesions in mouse and rat strains to be employed in gerontological research has been stressed by several authors (Smith et al., 1973; Cohen and Anver, 1976; Burek, 1978; Anver and Cohen, 1980; Zurcher et al., 1982). It has been shown that multiple pathological lesions, the hallmark of aging in man, also occur in inbred strains of rodents. Some of the lesions are genetically determined (e.g. certain autoimmune disorders, pituitary tumors, see below) and some of them (e.g. degenerative lesions, cysts, etc.) are randomly distributed amongst members of the same inbred strain (Zurcher and Hollander, 1982). In this respect, it is worthwhile mentioning that pituitary tumors are frequently observed in aged rats of different strains. Burek (1978) showed that in the WAG/Rij and BN/BiRij strains these tumors arise shortly before death and are rapidly growing neoplasms. It seems logical to conclude that in randomly selected healthy animals of these strains, these tumors do not interfere with the outcome of a study. However, in other strains of rats, e.g. F344, these tumors may be slow-growing and therefore be present for a long time (Solleveld and McConnell, 1985). Granular cell tumors (granular cell myoblastomas) are the most common primary brain tumors observed in the WAG/Rij and BN/BiRij rat and have also been observed in other rat strains (Burek, 1978). A form of hereditary retinal degeneration occurs in the WAG/Rij rat (Lai et al., 1975). This lesion has been observed in animals of this strain as young as 3 months of age (Hollander et al., 1983). Because the WAG/Rij rat is an albino rat, attention should be drawn to a publication by Creel (1980) concerning the use and misuse of albino animals in biomedical research. Creel summarizes the direct association between hypopigmentation and auditory, visual, metabolic, biochemical and behavioral anomalies. These anomalies affect learning tasks and tests for social behavior. Furthermore, changes in drug metabolism and binding by melanin are also factors that may lead to erroneous extrapolations to the human situation. This warrants a careful selection of the species and strain of rodents to be used and is contrary to the more common practice of using, for sheer convenience, an inbred strain of rodent which is at hand. Provisions have now been made for investigators to obtain old rodents, both in the USA by the NIA and in Europe by EURAGE or the TNO Institute for Experimental Gerontology, which are well characterized along the lines mentioned above.

Lesions of the nucleus basalis in old rats as a model for certain aspects of SDAT

As has been mentioned before, no animal models mimic the complete morphological, neurochemical and clinical features of Alzheimer type dementia. This holds true for various species, from rodents to primates during aging in the natural state or under well-defined laboratory conditions. Regarding the morphological hallmarks of SDAT, some changes such as senile plaque-like structures have been found to occur in old rhesus monkeys and dogs (Wisniewski et al., 1970, 1973). Granulovacuolar degeneration has been little studied, either during aging in the natural state or in experimental animals, while investigations into the lipofuscin accumulation with aging have not resulted in a clear-cut understanding of its possible pathological significance. Attempts have been made to induce the characteristic neurofibrillary tangles seen in human brains by the injection of aluminum salts. The induced tangles are morphologically similar and of similar dimensions, though the experimental filaments are often larger, less prominently twisted and more branched than their counterpart in man (Terry and Peña, 1965). The high mortality in treated animals has not favored its use as an appropriate animal model for SDAT (Crapper and Dalton, 1973a, b; Crapper et al., 1976), although recent investigations reveal new applications for aluminum-induced changes in chronic animal models (Wisniewski et al., 1980, 1982).

Studies on cell numbers, synaptic degeneration, dendritic arborization and spines during aging in various animal species have provided valuable information about the growth and decay of functional connections during aging. Species differences, regional topographic changes and selective neuronal vulnerability or drop-out have been reported. A concise summary of these, sometimes contradictory, findings can be found in Mervis (1983). While animal data form a necessary framework, they do not allow a simple generalization about human aging or human pathological changes. Moreover, the morphological studies on brain aging in animals so far have shed no light on the mechanisms responsible for deterioration of synaptic mechanisms and accelerated cell death.

Advances in the neurochemistry of SDAT revealed the marked decrease in choline acetyl transferase (CAT) activity, a finding that has often been reproduced, leading to the so-called cholinergic hypothesis of dementia (Bartus et al., 1982). By and large, other neurochemical deficits are found mainly in cortical afferents such as noradrenaline, serotonin and neurotensin. Evidence regarding decreased levels of substance P is more controversial. In contrast, the (putative) intrinsic cortical neurotransmitters γ-amino butyric acid (GABA), vasoactive intestinal polypeptide and cholecystokinin octapeptide remain intact, perhaps with the exception of very advanced states of dementia (Candy et al., 1983). Somatostatin, however, is repeatedly reported to be reduced (Candy et al., 1983; Rossor et al., 1984). The recent distinction between early and late onset types of Alzheimer dementia reveals that all deficits are more severe in young individuals, whereas older demented patients show a relatively pure cholinergic deficit (Rossor et al., 1984; Francis et al., 1985). No transmitter has been so closely correlated to behavioral, neuropathological, and clinical parameters of dementia as has acetylcholine, although exclusion of the role of the noradrenaline and serotonin systems would be naive. These findings raise new possibilities for animal models of SDAT by manipulating neurotransmitter function, while the recent progress in the field of brain grafting offers alternatives for non-psychopharmacological amplification of brain function.

Simultaneous developments in monoclonal antibody techniques allowed the unambiguous identification of cholinergic neurons in the brain and the confirmation of previous results obtained by acetyl-cholinesterase staining (Shute and Lewis, 1967; Kimura et al., 1984). The experiments by Coyle and co-workers on the effect of producing lesions in the nucleus basalis in (young) adult rats on the CAT activity in the cortex and hippocampus, revealed that most of the cholinergic activity depends on innervation by the subcortical continuum of cholinergic nuclei of the basal nucleus, the diagonal band of Broca and the septal area. The residual 30% of the CAT activity was thought to be due to intrinsic cholinergic neurons of the cortex (Coyle et al., 1983).

From these findings emerged the hypothesis that lesions of the basal nucleus could be used to study the effects of decreased cortical cholinergic activity. Neurochemical lesions, such as those induced by the excitotoxins kainic acid and ibotenic acid and by the presumed cholinotoxic drug AF64A, as well as electrolytic lesions, have been used to destroy the rather widely dispersed neurons of the basal nucleus. The results of such interventions were a changed sensitivity to cholinergic antagonists (LoConte et al., 1982) and disturbances in memory, measured in active and passive avoidance and spontaneous alternation in a Y maze (LoConte et al., 1982; Lerer and Friedman, 1983; Miyamato et al., 1985). However, several problems were encountered which delayed progress. Unfortunately, only Miyamoto et al. (1985) tested whether recovery of function occurred. Passive avoidance was at least partially restored although extinction was faster than in the sham-operated group. This phenomenon is not sufficiently studied to allow definite conclusions about its magnitude and time course, but it is evident that such a process seriously hampers the use of this model in testing the efficacy of therapeutic modalities. Moreover, it was found that in order to produce demonstrable effects, lesions had to be very large, destroying up to 75% of the cholinergic neurons, which often resulted in a high mortality. The investigator seems to be caught in a dilemma; to cause considerable destruction to reach the limit of the organism's viability, or destroy considerably less and face the consequences of partial or complete recovery. Our own provisional data with young adult rats subjected to kainic acid lesions of the basal nucleus underscore the above dilemma. By analogy with the narrow 'therapeutic range' for

the drug physostigmine (Johns et al., 1983), it seems that the 'experimental range' for cholinergic neural destruction is also very small.

Our aim therefore, is to study the feasibility of using old animals for experimental destruction of the basal nucleus as a more appropriate animal model for SDAT. Several reasons favor this approach. First SDAT is, by nature, superimposed upon normal aging. With the exception of presenile forms, dementing illnesses occur in the phase of life that is characterized by multiple pathological lesions. One example is the coexistence of multi-infarct damage in 15–25% of cases of Alzheimer type dementia in man (Tomlinson et al., 1970). Thus, it is possible that even without overt change in performance by the animals, aging as such decreases adaptive capacities, thereby exacerbating the eventual cholinergic damage by neurochemical lesions. Secondly, the old animals are known to have less 'plasticity' than younger animals (Scheff et al., 1984) and, although the precise mechanisms explaining this decrease are still obscure, this characteristic may be useful in that it may improve the chances of reasonable sized lesions being effective in producing lasting disturbances in memory and cognition.

Experimental studies with old animals, however, demand caution. Not only are the animals very expensive (Hollander et al., 1983) and the chance of spontaneous death greater, but there are also numerous other pitfalls underlying behavioral research with older animals (Rigter, 1983). Caution has to be taken that changes in motivational, perceptual and motor capacities do not lead to erroneous conclusions when measuring performance in various tests. Consequently it is necessary to measure as many parameters as possible, both of spontaneously occurring and acquired behavior (in which the animals serve as their own controls), so that the value of these old animals is effectively exploited. Examples of ways to assess motor dysfunction and learning and memory disorders in old animals together with a discussion on the interpretation appear in a recent conference summary (Ingram and Brennan, 1984). In the design of such studies, it is critical to take steps not only to establish real correlations between the degree of neural damage and behavioral changes, but also to avoid erroneous correlations.

Summary and conclusions

Limitations are existing in employing rodents for studying AD/SDAT, just as in studies on humans, and careful planning is therefore necessary. However, cross-sectional and/or longitudinal studies are more easily conducted in laboratory rodents because of their homogeneity, the possibility to rigorously control their environment, and their limited life-span as compared to the larger laboratory animals (e.g. monkeys, dogs, etc.). Several aspects of husbandry and selection of mice and rats for research on aging in general are depicted. A new approach, employing old rats for studying the possible effect of cholinergic deficits, is proposed insofar as old animals, when lesioned, might have less chance of regeneration and provide a better model for cholinergic changes in AD/SDAT. However, it should be stressed that several species should be employed for studying AD/SDAT and then the results obtained in each species may contribute to solve a part of the puzzle presently encountered in man.

Acknowledgements

We wish to thank Dr. Michael A. Horan for his advice and stimulating discussions in preparing this chapter and Mrs. A. H. Walop for secretarial assistance..

References

Anver, M. R. and Cohen, B. J. (1980) Lesions associated with aging. In H. J. Baker, J. R. Lindsey and S. H. Weisbroth (Eds.), *The Laboratory Rat, Vol. I (14)*, Academic Press, New York, London, pp. 377–399.

Bartus, R. T., Dean, R. L., Beer, B. and Zippa, A. S. (1982) The cholinergic hypothesis of geriatric memory dysfunction. *Science*, 217: 408–417.

Burek, J. D. (1978) *Pathology of Aging Rats. A morphological and experimental study of the age-associated lesions in aging BN/Bi, WAG/Rij and (WAGxBN)F1 rats*, CRC Press, West Palm Beach, FL.

Candy, J., Perry, R., Perry, E., Biggins, A., Thompson, J. and Irving, D. (1983) Transmitter systems in Alzheimer's disease. In W. H. Gispen and J. Traber (Eds.), *Aging of the Brain*, Elsevier Science Publ., Amsterdam, New York, Oxford, pp. 29–48.

Clough, G. (1982) Environmental effects on animals used in biomedical research. *Biol. Rev.*, 57: 487–523.

Cohen, B. J. and Anver, M. R. (1976) Pathological changes during aging in the rat. In M. F. Elias, B. E. Eleftheriou and P. K. Elias (Eds.), *Special Review of Experimental Aging*, EAR Inc., Bar Harbor, ME. pp. 379–403.

Coyle, J. T., Price, D. L. and DeLong, M. R. (1983) Alzheimer's disease: a disorder of cortical cholinergic innervation. *Science*, 219: 1184–1190.

Crapper, D. R. and Dalton, A. J. (1973a) Alterations in short-term retention, conditioned avoidance response acquisition and motivation following aluminum induced neurofibrillary degeneration. *Physiol. Behav.*, 10: 925–933.

Crapper, D. R. and Dalton, A. J. (1973b) Aluminum induced neurofibrillary degeneration, brain electrical activity and alterations in acquisition and retention. *Physiol. Behav.*, 10: 935–945.

Crapper, D. R., Krishnan, S. S. and Quittkat, S. (1976) Aluminium, neurofibrillary degeneration and Alzheimer's disease. *Brain*, 99: 67–80.

Creel, D. (1980) Inappropriate use of albino animals as models in research. *Pharmacol. Biochem. Behav.*, 12: 969–977.

Francis, P. T., Palmer, A. M., Sims, N. R., Bowen, D. M., Davison, A. N., Esiri, M. M., Neary, D., Snowden, J. S. and Wilcock, G. K. (1985) Neurochemical studies of early-onset Alzheimer's disease. *N. Engl. J. Med.*, 313, 7–11.

Gibson, D. C., Adelman, R. C. and Finch, C. (1979) *Development of the rodent as a model system of aging, Book II*, DHEW Publ. No. (NIH) 79–161, Washington, D.C., USA.

Hollander, C. F. and Burek, J. D. (1982) Animal models in gerontology. In A. Viidik (Ed.), *Lectures on Gerontology, Vol. I, Part A (7)*, Academic Press, London, pp. 253–274.

Hollander, C. F., Van Zwieten, M. J. and Zurcher, C. (1983) The aged animal. In W. H. Gispen and J. Traber (Eds.), *Aging of the Brain*, Elsevier Science Publ., Amsterdam, New York, Oxford, pp. 187–196.

Hollander, C. F., Solleveld, H. A., Zurcher, C., Nooteboom, A. L. and Van Zwieten, M. J. (1984) Biological and clinical consequences of longitudinal studies in rodents: their possibilities and limitations. An overview. *Mech. Ageing Dev.*, 28: 249–260.

Ingram, D. K. and Brennan, M. J. (1984) Meeting report. Animal behavioural models in biogerontology. *Neurobiol. Aging*, 5: 63–66.

Johns, C. A., Levy, M. I., Greenwald, B. S., Rosen, W. G., Horvath, T. B., Davis, B. M., Mohs, R. C. and Davis, K. L. (1983) Studies of cholinergic mechanisms in Alzheimer's disease. In R. Katzman (Ed.) *Biological Aspects of Alzheimer's Disease*; *Banbury Report 15*, Coldspring Harbor Laboratory, USA, pp. 435–449.

Kimura, H., McGeer, P. L. and Peng, J. H. (1984) Choline acetyltransferase-containing neurons in the rat brain. In A. Björklund, T. Hökfelt and M. J. Kuhar (Eds.), *Handbook of Chemical Neuroanatomy, Vol. 3*, Elsevier Science Publ., Amsterdam, New York, Oxford, pp. 51–68.

Lai, Y. L., Jacobi, R. O., Jonas, A. M. and Papermaster, D. S. (1975) A new form of hereditary retinal degeneration in WAG/Rij rats. *Invest. Opthalmol.*, 14: 62–67.

Lerer, B. and Friedman, E. (1983) Neurochemical lesion models. In B. Reisberg (Ed.), *Alzheimer's Disease*, The Free Press, New York, pp. 421–427.

LoConte, G., Bartolini, L., Casamenti, F., Marconcini-Pepeu, I. and Pepeu, G. (1982) Lesions of cholinergic forebrain nuclei: changes in avoidance behavior and scopolamine actions. *Pharmacol. Biochem. Behav.*, 17: 933–937.

Mervis, R. (1983) Mammalian pathologic models. In B. Reisberg (Ed.), *Alzheimer's Disease*, The Free Press, New York, pp. 399–420.

Miyamato, M., Shintani, M., Nagaoka, A. and Nagawa, Y. (1985) Lesioning of the rat basal forebrain leads to memory impairments in passive and active avoidance tasks. *Brain Res.*, 328: 97–104.

NAS (National Academy of Sciences) (1981) *Mammalian models for research on aging*. Report of the Committee on animal models for research on aging. Institute of Laboratory Animal Resources, National Research Council, National Academic Press, Washington, DC, USA.

Rigter, H. (1983) Pitfalls in behavioural aging research in animals. In W. H. Gispen and J. Traber (Eds.), *Aging of the Brain*, Elsevier Science Publ., Amsterdam. New York, Oxford, pp. 197–208.

Rossor, M. N., Iversen, L. L., Reynolds, G. P., Mountjoy, C. Q. and Roth, M. (1984) Neurochemical characteristics of early and late onset types of Alzheimer's disease. *Br. Med. J.*, 288: 961–964.

Scheff, S. W., Anderson, K. and DeKosky, S. T. (1984) Morphological aspects of brain damage in aging. In S. W. Scheff (Ed.) *Aging and Recovery of Function in the Central Nervous System*, Plenum Press, New York, London, pp. 57–85.

Shute, C. C. D. and Lewis, R. R. (1967) The ascending cholinergic reticular system: neocortical, olfactory and subcortical projections. *Brain*, 90: 497–521.

Smith, G. S., Walford, R. L. and Mickey, M. R. (1973) Life-span and incidence of cancer and other diseases in selected long-lived inbred mice and their F1 hybrids. *J. Natl. Cancer Inst.*, 50: 1195–1213.

Solleveld, H. A. and McConnell, E. E. (1985) The value and significance of life span and scheduled termination data in long-term toxicity and carcinogenesis studies. *Toxicol. Pathol.*, 13: 128–134.

Terry, R. D. and Peña, C. (1965) Experimental production of neurofibrillary degeneration. *J. Neuorpathol. Exp. Neurol.*, 24: 200–210.

Tomlinson, B. E., Blessed, G. and Roth, M. (1970) Observations on the brains of demented old people. *J. Neurol. Sci.*, 11: 205–242.

Weisbroth, S. H. (1972) Pathogen-free substrates for gerontological research: review, sources, and comparison of barrier-sustained vs. conventional rats. *Exp. Gerontol.*, 7: 417–426.

Wisniewski, H. M., Johnson, A. B., Raine, C. S., Kay, W. J. and Terry, R. D. (1970) Senile plaques and cerebral amyloidosis in aged dogs. A histochemical and ultrastructural study. *Lab. Invest.*, 23: 287–296.

Wisniewski, H. M., Ghetti, B. and Terry, R. D. (1973) Neuritic (senile) plaques and filamentous changes in aged rhesus monkeys. *J. Neuropathol. Exp. Neurol.*, 32: 566–584.

Wisniewski, H. M., Sturman, J. A. and Shek, J. W. (1980) Aluminum chloride induced neurofibrillary in the developing rabbit: a chronic animal model. *Ann. Neurol.*, 8: 479–490.

Wisniewski, H. M., Sturman, J. A. and Shek, J. W. (1982) Chronic model of neurofibrillary changes induced in mature rabbits by metallic aluminum. *Neurobiol. Aging*, 3: 11–22.

Zurcher, C. and Hollander, C. F. (1982) Multiple pathological changes in aging rat and man. *Expl. Biol. Med.*, 7: 56–62.

Zurcher, C., Van Zwieten, M. J., Solleveld, H. A. and Hollander, C. F. (1982) Aging research. In H. L. Foster, J. D. Small and J. G. Fox (Eds.), *The Mouse in Biomedical Research, Vol. IV (2)*, Academic Press, New York, London, pp. 11–35.

Discussion

D. M. GASH: When one critically examines the rat as a model for aging, there are a number of ways to influence longevity — housing conditions, feeding schedule. In addition, there are strain differences. How well then can the rodent be considered as a model of human aging and, more specifically, of aging of the brain?

ANSWER: Under well-controlled conditions, i.e. housing, feeding, nutritional constituents, health, it has been proven in several studies that rodents can be used to study different aspects of the aging process in man. Decline in brain function has been observed employing behavioral tests (De Koning-Verest, 1981; De Koning-Verest et al., 1980). In my opinion, selected questions of brain aging can be addressed in the rat, i.e. what is the value of the cholinergic defect model or the mechanisms underlying it. Manipulation of longevity has not been established beyond doubt.

W. G. M. RAAYMAKERS: We studied learning and memory in a number of inbred strains of rat and we found strain differences. Especially one strain, the BN rat behaves 'a-typical' in aversively motivated situations due to a different unlearned reaction to aversive stimulation, i.e. an increase in activity instead of a decrease.

J. E. PISETSKY: You showed senile histological change in the rat retina; in the human retina no pathological Alzheimer markers have been found. How do you account for the difference?

ANSWER: I do not know. We have not been able to correlate these findings with any easily detectable lesion in the brain and have not undertaken a study to elucidate them.

References

De Koning-Verest, I. F. (1981) *Observations on the Central Nervous System of the Rat: Functional changes in relation to ageing*. Thesis, State University Utrecht, The Netherlands.

De Koning-Verest, I. F., Knook, D. L. and Wolthuis, O. L. (1980) Behavioral and biochemical correlates of aging in rats. In D. G. Stein (Ed.), *The Psychobiology of Aging: Problems and Perspectives*. Elsevier/North-Holland, New York, Oxford, Amsterdam, pp. 177–199.

D. F. Swaab, E. Fliers, M. Mirmiran, W. A. Van Gool and F. Van Haaren (Eds.)
Progress in Brain Research, Vol. 70.
© 1986 Elsevier Science Publishers B.V. (Biomedical Division)

CHAPTER 22

Behavioral and biochemical effects of nucleus basalis magnocellularis lesions: implications and possible relevance to understanding or treating Alzheimer's disease

R. T. Bartus[a,b], C. Flicker[b], R. L. Dean[a], S. Fisher[a], M. Pontecorvo[a] and J. Figueiredo[a]

[a]*Department of Central Nervous System Research, Medical Research Division, Lederle Laboratories, American Cyanamid Company, Pearl River, NY 10965 and* [b]*Department of Psychiatry, New York University School of Medicine, New York University, New York, NY 10016, USA*

Introduction

Because of the size and scope of the problems associated with Alzheimer's disease, the disorder has attracted immense interest in the scientific literature of the last decade. Alzheimer's disease is an age-related neurodegenerative disorder which is clinically characterized by its deleterious effects on higher cognitive function. In the earliest stage the effects may be quite subtle, often indistinguishable from similar deficits in certain types of memory observed in normal, aged subjects. However, the disease progresses insidiously, ultimately destroying the entire intellectual capacity of its victims (Reisberg et al., 1982) and necessitating complete and perpetual institutional care. Annual costs for treatment and care are in excess of 20 billion dollars in the United States alone. The devastating emotional burden and personal loss felt by family members, friends and the patients cannot be properly represented in financial terms. Improvement in other health care areas has been and is expected to continue to rapidly expand the size of the aged sector of the population. The present magnitude of this health care problem, and clear projections for increases in its incidence in the future, demand a concerted effort to determine the nature, etiology and treatment for this and related cognitive impairments in the aged.

Although issues regarding the nature, etiology and treatment of Alzheimer's disease are interrelated, they often require different types of experiments at different levels of analysis. For example, studies of the roles of neurotoxic, genetic, immunological and viral influences in the progression of the disease may be necessary in order to understand the etiology of Alzheimer's disease. At the same time, examination of the development and consequences of neurofibrillary tangles, senile plaques, and possible changes in DNA, RNA, and protein synthesis may help identify the molecular mechanisms responsible for the progressive neuronal damage. Thus, while studies of this type would seem to be invaluable if we are ultimately to prevent or cure the disease, such practical applications of the information obtained are, most likely, some time away. At the same time, serious problems and complications directly related to the primary symptoms of the disease (i.e., severe cognitive deterioration) continue to demand attention. While the relationships between molecular neuropathologic changes and cognitive dysfunction remain obscure and difficult to study, the relationships between the cognitive disturbances and more molar physiologic changes (such as neurotransmitter disturbances) may be more easily established. More importantly, the identification of disturbances in the final common pathways responsible for the cognitive disturbances should suggest effective strategies for more immediate treatment of the disease's major symptomatology. Further, this research may reveal areas of selective vulnerability to the disease which may help expand our understanding of how the etiologic variables produce their progressive damage. In other words, given the increasingly severe medical, economic and emotional problems associated with Alzheimer's disease, much could be gained by developing a better understanding of the factors responsible for its primary symptoms and by pharmacologically reducing the severity of those symptoms. To date, progress in achieving these goals has been severely restricted by: (1) the lack of strong evidence concerning which CNS changes are primarily responsible for the disease's earliest symptoms and (2) the lack of valid and reliable animal models to evaluate treatment alternatives. Research in the last several years has suggested that dysfunctions of cholinergic and certain other brain neurotransmitter systems may play an important role in the cognitive loss. Recent evidence of degeneration of basal forebrain cholinergic neurons in Alzheimer's patients lends additional support to this idea and, as discussed below, provides a potentially unifying framework for further study with animals.

Brief review of evidence supporting the cholinergic hypothesis

Although the neurochemical variables underlying the cognitive loss are as yet undetermined, and are undoubtedly complex, there is extensive evidence suggesting that a dysfunction in central cholinergic transmission contributes significantly to the cognitive impairment in Alzheimer's disease. First, significant changes in cholinergic markers occur in the brains of aged humans and animals (Bartus et al., 1982; Coyle et al., 1983; Kuhar, 1976; Perry et al., 1978; Strong et al., 1980). These changes are accompanied by a decline in memory/cognitive performance (Bartus, 1979; Craik, 1977; Drachman and Leavitt, 1974; Kubanis and Zornetzer, 1981; Lippa et al., 1980). The cholinergic deficits,

and in particular, the decline in choline acetyltransferase (CAT) activity (Bowen et al., 1976; Davies and Maloney, 1976), are exacerbated in Alzheimer's patients. The magnitude of this decline in CAT is correlated with major neuropathological markers, and with the degree of cognitive impairment produced by the disease (Bowen et al., 1976; Perry et al., 1978; Arendt et al., 1984; Mann et al., 1985; Wilcock et al., 1983). Although alterations in other neurotransmitter systems have also been reported (Arai et al., 1984; Benton et al., 1982; Bondareff et al., 1981; Bowen et al., 1983; Davies and Terry, 1981; Gottfries, 1982; Iversen et al., 1983), correlations between these changes and the cognitive deterioration in Alzheimer's disease are not yet as firmly established. In contrast, the decrease in cortical CAT activity in Alzheimer's patients, and its correlation with cognitive deficits, is remarkably consistent and has come to be regarded as a neurochemical hallmark of the disease. Furthermore, pharmacological disruption of the cholinergic system in young, normal animals and humans preferentially induces deficits on learning/memory tasks that mimic those observed in aged and demented subjects (Bartus et al., 1982; Bartus and Johnson, 1976; Drachman and Leavitt, 1974). Moreover, under carefully controlled laboratory conditions, administration of acetylcholinesterase (AChE) inhibitors or cholinergic agonists can reliably improve performance on these same tasks in aged animals, humans, and Alzheimer patients (Bartus et al., 1980a; Bartus and Dean, 1981; Christie et al., 1981; Davis et al., 1982; Drachman and Sahakian, 1980). Although the therapeutic impact of these studies remains uncertain, the data provide considerable support for the hypothesis of an important involvement of the cholinergic system in the cognitive deficits of aging and dementia. Despite the clear treatment implications of this hypothesis, little progress has yet been made in either developing an effective clinical treatment based on the hypothesis, or in rejecting the hypothesis and laying it to rest. Clearly the availability of valid animal models would facilitate these efforts.

On the development of an animal model of Alzheimer's disease

The development of valid animal models would not only improve our ability to test and/or refine the cholinergic hypothesis, but would also (1) provide an important and efficient means of evaluating newly developed pharmacologic agents, (2) offer a convenient means of comparing the effects of cholinomimetics with those of alternative pharmacological approaches, and (3) possibly provide an additional means of studying some of the variables implicated in Alzheimer's disease. However, work in this area is particularly difficult, in part because of problems inherent in accurately measuring memory in animals, and in part because Alzheimer's disease is apparently indigenous only to the human species. Although recent investigations suggest that it may be possible to gain some insight into treatment approaches from the study of normally aged animals (Bartus et al., 1983a,b,c; Bartus and Dean, 1981, 1985), there is little question that greater predictability might be achieved with an animal model that shares more of the neuropathological and neurochemical characteristics found in Alzheimer patients. Earlier attempts to induce neurofibrillary tangles in animals artificially via aluminium (Crapper and Dalton, 1972, 1973) have been disappointing, neither providing greater insight into the nature of the disease nor leading to more effective means of testing drugs to treat its symptoms. Other attempts to produce an animal model through injection of presumed transmissible agents may continue to hold promise, but have so far been equally disappointing (Klatzo et al., 1965; Wisniewski et al., 1975).

More recently, however, evidence of severe deterioration in the nucleus basalis of Meynert in Alzheimer and other demented patients (Whitehouse et al., 1981, 1982; Rogers et al., 1985) has given new momentum to the development of potential animal models of the disease. This formerly obscure brain region is recognized as providing the major extrinsic cholinergic input to the cortex (Johnston et al., 1979), and its degeneration in Alzheimer's disease most likely accounts for the severe loss of cortical CAT activity and other cholinergic markers which characterize the brains from Alzheimer patients. Artificial destruction of this brain region in animals would certainly not be expected to produce an exact model of Alzheimer's disease, including such classic neuropathological features as senile plaques and neurofibrillary tangles. Nevertheless it would provide an animal model that shares many of the other CNS deficiencies associated with the disease, including loss of cortical CAT activity, reduced cortical high-affinity choline uptake, and degeneration of basal forebrain cholinergic neurons. Furthermore, destruction of the homologous brain region in animals provides a means of determining the functional consequences of such nucleus basalis degeneration, thus providing one empirical test of its possible role in the cognitive loss of Alzheimer's disease and other degenerative disorders. If loss of CAT-containing cholinergic neurons in the basal forebrain can be causally linked to a specific decline in memory, then an important explanation for the relationship between the decreases in CAT activity and loss of cognitive function in Alzheimer's patients will be provided. Second, if a significant relationship can be demonstrated between the loss of cholinergic neurons in the basal forebrain and cognitive decline, then it might be possible to use animals with the perturbation as a valid model of the primary neurobehavioral characteristics of Alzheimer's disease. Such an animal model might greatly facilitate the search for alternative pharmacological approaches and help reduce the number of candidates for human testing.

Unfortunately, despite a substantial body of evidence that implicates cholinergic neurotransmission in the control of memory and cognitive performance, there exist little experimental data that can be used to predict the functional consequences of degeneration or lesion of basal forebrain nuclei. Historically, studies remotely related to this question have destroyed the medial septal nucleus, which provides the primary extrinsic cholinergic input to the hippocampus. Animals with lesions of the medial septal nucleus (which represents part of the basal forebrain complex) have been shown to be impaired on a variety of learning and discrimination tasks (see Gray and McNaughton, 1983 for a recent review). However, only a few studies (e.g., Thomas, 1972) have specifically examined the effects of septal lesions on memory performance especially as the deficits relate to human cognitive loss. Moreover, most studies have utilized electrolytic lesions, thereby confounding the experimental manipulation with damage to fibers of passage.

Neurobehavioral studies of the nucleus basalis magnocellularis

Recently, a diffuse cluster of large, cholinesterase-reactive neurons in the ventromedial corner of the rat globus pallidus has been accepted as being homologous to the human nucleus basalis of Meynert (Fibiger, 1982; Johnston et al., 1979, 1981; Lehmann et al., 1980). Designated the nucleus basalis magnocellularis (NBM) (Fibiger, 1982), considerable evidence now indicates that it provides a major source of the extrinsic cholinergic input to the neocortex of the rat. An acetylcholinesterase-reactive fiber pathway originating in this region and terminating in the cerebral cortex was first described by Shute and Lewis (1967). Since that time cells in the NBM staining positively for acetylcholinesterase (AChE) have been shown to be labelled by retrograde transport of cortically injected horseradish peroxidase (Lehmann et al., 1980; Mesulam and Van Hoesen, 1976; Mesulam et al., 1983). Cortical ablation likewise produces retrograde degeneration of this neuronal population (Das, 1971; Lehmann et al., 1980). Furthermore, electrolytic or neurotoxic lesions of the NBM substantially reduce cortical choline acetyltransferase (CAT) activity, AChE activity, ACh release, and choline uptake (Johnston et al., 1979, 1981; Kelly and Moore, 1978; Lehmann et al., 1980; LoConte et al., 1982; Pedata et al., 1982;

Wenk et al., 1980). Finally, neurons in the rat sensorimotor cortex exhibit responsivity to acetylcholine iontophoresis and NBM stimulation, partial blockade of responses by cholinergic antagonists, and supersensitivity to ACh after NBM lesions (Edstrom and Phillis, 1980; Lamour et al., 1982). In summary, although there are almost certainly other externally and internally derived contributions, the NBM appears to be the major source of neocortical acetylcholine in the rodent (Johnston et al., 1981).

The identification of this homologous, cholinergic-projecting site therefore provides an opportunity to evaluate the relationship between basal forebrain cholinergic degeneration and behavior. Although only a handful of studies have been performed to date, almost exclusively employing lesion techniques in rats, some interesting generalizations are nevertheless beginning to emerge.

In one early study, rats with ibotenic acid lesions in the NBM were compared to sham-lesioned rats on a battery of four psychomotor tasks designed to assess the effects of the lesions on reflexes, balance, strength, endurance, coordination, and other motor functions (Flicker et al., 1983). Specifically, a wire-hanging task, inclined screen, rod-walking task, and a series of plank-walking tasks were used. None of these tests of psychomotor performance revealed consistent effects of the lesions. A test of shock sensitivity likewise failed to reveal any lesion effects. However, on two learning/memory tasks, significant effects of the NBM lesions were observed (Flicker et al., 1983). More specifically, the lesioned rats were mildly impaired in the acquisition of a one-way active avoidance task but did not differ from control animals on extinction of the task. Most severely impaired, however, was retention of a passive avoidance task, in which the lesioned rats exhibited deficits at both 1-h and 24-h retention intervals as shown in Fig. 1.

This study confirmed the passive avoidance deficit reported earlier (LoConte et al., 1982) following unilateral destruction of these neurons and adjacent fibers of passage. Moreover, it demonstrated a greater vulnerability to the effects

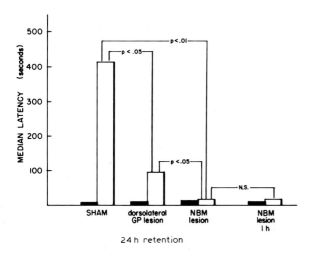

Fig. 1. Passive avoidance retention. Median latencies to enter the shock chamber of the passive avoidance apparatus for rats with nucleus basalis magnocellularis (NBM) lesions ($n=9$), dorsolateral globus pallidus lesions ($n=10$), and sham-operated controls ($n=10$). On the training trial (left columns) the animals received a 3-s 1.0-mA footshock upon entering the rear chamber. All animals were tested for retention 24 h later (right columns) except for the fourth group of NBM-lesioned rats ($n=5$), which was tested 1 h after training. Compared to the sham group, the lesioned animals exhibited significantly shorter latencies to enter the shock chamber on the retention trial (with no differences observed on the training trial). Between-group p values are presented, based upon Mann-Whitney U tests. (From Flicker et al., 1983)

of NBM lesions on certain learning/memory tasks, relative to tasks involving other, non-mnemonic behavioral measures. More recent studies have also demonstrated a more robust effect on tasks requiring reversal of a previously learned habit as well (Dubois et al., 1985; Lerer et al., 1985).

Although the effects of lesions in the NBM on multiple-trial, active avoidance tasks have been mixed (LoConte et al., 1982; Miyamoto et al., 1985; Flicker et al., 1983; Lerer et al., 1985), clear and consistent deficits have been reported on the single-trial passive avoidance paradigm (Flicker et al., 1983; Bartus et al., 1985b, c; Friedman et al., 1983; LoConte et al., 1982; Altman et al., 1985; Miyamoto et al., 1985). It may be noteworthy that this finding parallels observations in aged rodents (Gold and McGaugh, 1975; Lippa et al., 1980;

Bartus et al., 1983a). Later studies testing NBM-lesioned rats on the passive avoidance paradigm demonstrated a very steep, temporal retention gradient (Altman et al., 1985; Miyamoto et al., 1985), suggesting that the deficit may be partly due to a disturbance in memory. At the same time, however, the passive-avoidance procedure is recognized to be a relatively crude behavioral paradigm. Not only are its results often open to multiple, alternative interpretations, but even when an ideal experimental design is employed, most authorities agree that the procedure only provides a rough index of memory ability (Bartus et al., 1983a; Bartus and Dean, 1985; Heise, 1981, 1984). Thus, additional work characterizing the effects of nucleus basalis lesions in more sophisticated paradigms would be valuable. Certainly, information from such studies would help establish, with greater certainty, the role this cholinergic nucleus may play in mediating behaviors requiring intact memory, and the possible effects degeneration of this brain region may have on behavior in numerous degenerative diseases. For these reasons, we conducted a more elaborate rodent experiment to evaluate further the question of the memory loss following NBM destruction.

This study used an eight-choice, radial arm maze in an effort to provide more detailed information regarding the memory deficits produced by destroying cholinergic neurons in the basal forebrain. This task and procedure offered many advantages over the passive avoidance procedure, including the use of positive (food) reinforcement, wider range of performance scores (with eight choices), greater ability to control and manipulate independent variables, and multiple use of subjects (i.e., providing a repeated measures experimental design), for greater reliability. Following an initial acclimatization period, rats were trained to obtain food reinforcement in the eight-arm, radial maze (Olton, 1978; Olton and Samuelson, 1976) by visiting the goal boxes of each of the eight arms only once per test session (see Fig. 2). Repeat visits to an arm were never reinforced and were scored as errors. Following several months of training on the

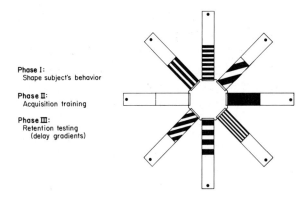

Phase I:
Shape subject's behavior

Phase II:
Acquisition training

Phase III:
Retention testing
(delay gradients)

Fig. 2. Schematic outline of series of training/testing conditions employed for the radial arm maze paradigm. A scale drawing of the maze appears as an insert.

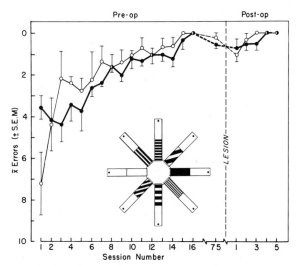

Fig. 3. Acquisition and steady-state performance of the radial arm maze task, as depicted by the mean number of errors to successfully complete all 8 choices in the maze. Repeat reponses to any arm previously entered within the session are not reinforced and are scored as errors. Ability to perform accurately is generally acknowledged to require both reference and working memory. Note the lack of effect of nucleus basalis lesions (solid circles) on performance of this acquired behavior (compared to sham lesion, open circles). (From Bartus et al., 1985c)

task, all rats established near-perfect performance (Fig. 3), demonstrating that they could (a) accurately perform the task on a daily basis according to unchanging reinforcement contingencies, and (b) remember accurately the trial-unique aspects of the task, involving which of the arms had been visited within the brief time periods of the session. By conventional definitions, these two skills demonstrated appropriate 'reference memory' and 'working memory', respectively (Honig, 1978; Olton, 1978; Olton et al., 1979, 1980). Following this initial training, the rats were tested on a modification of this paradigm, in which their ability to remember recent, trial-unique events was further challenged by inserting a series of retention intervals between the fourth and fifth choice in certain sessions (see Fig. 2). The rats were allowed to enter, in any order, each of four pre-selected arms to obtain food reinforcement. Plexiglas doors blocked access to the other four arms. After completing four choices, the rat was removed from the maze and temporarily returned to its home cage for a specified, variable retention interval, ranging from 15 min to 24 h. When the retention interval expired, the rat was returned to the maze, with all eight arms now unobstructed, and given the opportunity to obtain additional food reinforcement from the four previously obstructed arms (i.e., those which had not been visited earlier in the session).

With very short intervals, all rats performed the task perfectly, entering only the four remaining arms that had not been visited in the earlier session. However, as the duration of the retention interval was gradually increased (in a counterbalanced manner), the number of errors (i.e., repeat visits to a previously entered arm) increased correspondingly (Fig. 4). Thus, the pre-operative rats exhibited a time-related performance gradient on this procedure, presumably reflecting a progressive decay in ability to remember recent events.

Following the establishment of the memory performance gradient, the rats were divided into two groups, with one receiving sham lesions and the other ibotenic acid lesions of the NBM. Two weeks following surgery the rats were retested on the radial arm maze task. The animals with NBM lesions not only retained their initial training skills to negotiate the eight arm maze to earn food, but were also unimpaired in their ability to accurately

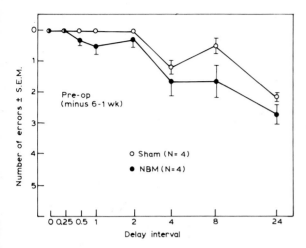

Fig. 4. Time-dependent retention gradients established in the radial arm maze by rats to be given nucleus basalis (shaded circles) and sham lesions (open circles), providing an index of recent memory ability. The gradients were established by allowing access to only 4 of the 8 arms (randomly predetermined each session) before the delay interval. Following variable delay intervals, all 8 arms were made available to assess the animals' ability to remember which arms had been visited earlier in the session. Data depicted here were collected 1–6 weeks prior to surgery. (From Bartus et al., 1985)

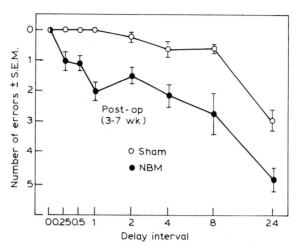

Fig. 5. Time-dependent retention gradients (as described in Fig. 4) generated 3 to 7 weeks following surgery. Note significant effect of NBM lesion (shaded circles) when delay interceded selection of first 4 and last 4 arms. (From Bartus et al., 1985c)

visit each of the eight arms only once during control (no delay) sessions (Fig. 3). This lack of effect of the NBM lesion of retention of, or ability to perform, the more basic requirements of the radial arm maze, contrasts markedly with the effects of NBM lesions on learning the radial arm maze. In this latter case, clear, post-operative deficits in acquisition of the radial arm maze have been reported, suggesting an important role of the NBM on mediating spatial behaviors, and possibly working memory (Dubois et al., 1985; Murray and Fibiger, 1985). However, when a delay condition was added to the radial arm maze procedure, requiring that the rats remember which of the arms had been visited in the recent past, a profound, time-related deficit in the lesion group was revealed (Fig. 5). In other words, little or no effect of the lesion was observed when very short retention intervals were interposed between the selection of the first four arms and the remaining four arms, but progressively greater effects of the lesion were

observed as the retention interval was lengthened. This time-related deficit suggested that destruction of cholinergic neurons in the nucleus basalis of rats may somewhat selectively interfere with performance requiring memory for recent events, while sparing both memory for more immediate events and reference memory (Honig, 1978; Olton, 1978; Olton et al., 1979, 1980). Recent studies from other laboratories demonstrate possibly similar time-related retention deficits using a t-maze (Hepler et al., 1985), and (post-surgical) acquisition of a multiple-arm, radial maze (Murray and Fibiger, 1985).

The memory impairment caused by NBM lesions in the radial arm maze, reported here, shares a number of operational similarities to the recent memory loss reported in aged rats, mice, New World and Old World monkeys, humans and early-stage Alzheimer patients (Bartus, 1979; Bartus et al., 1978, 1980a,b, 1983a; Davis, 1978; Flicker et al., 1984; Medin, 1969). Despite certain differences among the various paradigms used to test these different species, each exhibits a deficit in memory primarily characterized by: (a) a somewhat preferential inability to remember brief, discrete events; (b) greatest deficits in situations where there is little or no repetition or opportunity to practice or rehearse the information to be remembered; and (c) a time-related decline in retention, which occurs relatively rapidly (usually within minutes or hours) (Bartus et al., 1983a). The operational and conceptual similarities that exist between the deficits produced by nucleus basalis lesions in rats and those reported in early-phase Alzheimer patients and other dementing diseases is consistent with a role for this brain region in the memory loss seen in those neurodegenerative diseases.

However, further work with these same animals cautioned that no simple relationship between this brain region and mediation of memory should be assumed. During the course of several months training on the radial arm maze task, the performance of the lesioned rats on the delay conditions gradually improved. By 6 months after surgery, the previously robust deficit in recent memory had apparently recovered, and retention of the lesioned rats on the task was no longer different from that of the sham controls (Fig. 6).

Following the occurrence of this functional recovery, the rats were trained and tested on the same passive avoidance task which had previously revealed a profound effect of NBM lesions in previous experiments (Flicker et al., 1983). Two additional groups of rats were added to the experimental design. As before, one received a sham lesion while the other was subjected to ibotenic acid infusions into the NBM. However, for these two groups, surgery was conducted only 3.5 weeks prior to behavioral testing. Thus, these two additional groups served as controls to permit comparisons between the effects of recent lesions and longer-term lesions of the NBM.

As reported in previous publications, the recently lesioned rats exhibited a profound retention deficit on the passive avoidance task (Fig. 7). In sharp contrast, however, the rats that had previously recovered recent memory ability of the radial arm maze exhibited no retention deficit on the passive avoidance task. Thus, the recovery of recent memory, which occurred over a period of several months of training and testing on a radial arm maze, apparently generalized to the passive avoidance task, on which no post-lesion practice had been received.

Upon completion of behavioral testing, all rats were sacrificed, their brains removed, and tissue samples dissected from the frontal cortex, temporal/parietal cortex, hippocampus and olfactory bulbs. Determinations of choline acetyltransferase

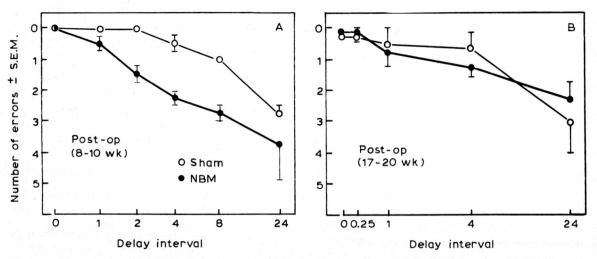

Fig. 6. Time-dependent retention gradients: (A) 8–10 weeks post lesion, showing persistence of NBM deficits, but with possible hint of recovery: and (B) 17–30 weeks post lesion, showing complete behavioral recovery of lesioned rats. (From Bartus et al., 1985c)

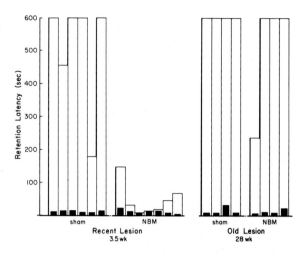

activity (CAT) (Fonnum, 1975), high-affinity choline uptake (HACU) (Simon et al., 1976), and muscarinic receptor binding (Yamamura and Snyder, 1974) were performed. As shown in Table I, these biochemical tests demonstrated that destruction of the nucleus basalis significantly reduced CAT activity and HACU in the cortex, while leaving muscarinic receptor binding intact, as reported by others previously (Johnston et al., 1979, 1981; Kelly and Moore, 1978; Lehmann et

TABLE I

Cholinergic markers determined 2 weeks (recent lesion) or 6 months (longer-term lesion) following destruction of nucleus basalis magnocellularis in rats

			CAT activity[a]	HACU	QNB
Frontal cortex	recent lesion	(a) sham	1.27 ± 0.02	8.59 ± 0.34	0.532 ± 0.09
		(b) NBM	0.69 ± 0.07	5.89 ± 0.25	0.581 ± 0.05
	longer-term lesion	(a) sham	1.42 ± 0.01	9.34 ± 0.74	0.520 ± 0.10
		(b) NBM	0.82 ± 0.07	6.28 ± 0.36	0.487 ± 0.08
Parietal/temporal cortex	recent lesion	(a) sham	1.09 ± 0.07	n.d.	0.747 ± 0.03
		(b) NBM	0.70 ± 0.06	n.d.	0.788 ± 0.03
	longer-term lesion	(a) sham	1.19 ± 0.04	n.d.	0.833 ± 0.02
		(b) NBM	0.88 ± 0.08	n.d.	0.751 ± 0.01
Hippocampus	recent lesion	(a) sham	1.38 ± 0.04	10.42 ± 0.41	0.666 ± 0.01
		(b) NBM	1.39 ± 0.06	9.38 ± 0.50	0.646 ± 0.02
	longer-term lesion	(a) sham	1.42 ± 0.06	10.45 ± 0.41	0.568 ± 0.04
		(b) NBM	1.34 ± 0.09	10.67 ± 0.84	0.646 ± 0.02
Olfactory bulbs	recent lesion	(a) sham	0.77 ± 0.03	n.d.	0.477 ± 0.01
		(b) NBM	0.80 ± 0.03	n.d.	0.457 ± 0.01
	longer-term lesion	(a) sham	0.72 ± 0.03	n.d.	0.522 ± 0.01
		(b) NBM	0.71 ± 0.03	n.d.	0.523 ± 0.01

Values expressed are mean $\pm$ SEM, $n = 4$–7; for analyses of variance tests, see text.
[a]Abbreviations: CAT, choline acetyltransferase (nmol/mg protein/min); HACU, high affinity choline uptake (pmol/mg protein/min); QNB, specific binding of the ^{3}H-labeled, muscarinic antagonist, quinuclidinyl benzilate (pmol/mg protein); n.d., not determined. (From Bartus et al., 1985c)

al., 1980; Pedata et al., 1982; Wenk et al., 1980). Moreover, comparisons between the recent and old lesion revealed that neither cortical CAT activity nor high affinity choline uptake recovered measurably in rats exhibiting the behavioral recovery, nor was there any hint of compensatory changes in the hippocampus or olfactory bulbs (terminal fields for parallel cholinergic pathways). These lasting neurochemical effects of bilateral lesions, therefore, contrast with reports of recovery of cortical CAT activity and high affinity choline uptake following unilateral lesions (Wenk and Olton, 1984). In addition, no changes in muscarinic receptor density were observed in any brain region studied. Finally, histological examination of the lesion site, using standard Nissl staining techniques, revealed no consistent differences in the severity or extent of neurodegeneration in the two groups (Fig. 8). In summary, although severe and selective deficits in recent memory were observed following destruction of basal forebrain cholinergic neurons, complete recovery of the memory loss gradually occurred over the next several months, while no neurochemical or neuroanatomical correlate of this recovery could be identified. Somewhat similar evidence of functional recovery of basal forebrain lesions has been recently reported for rats tested in a t-maze (Hepler et al., 1985) and for monkeys trained on a delayed, non-matching task (Mishkin et al., 1985).

In the present studies, several clear differences in task parameters between the radial arm maze and passive avoidance procedures allow one to exclude a number of salient variables from consideration as relevant to the recovery of function. These include the type of reinforcement used (food vs. shock), response requirement (active discriminatory response vs. inhibitory avoidance), and specific post-lesion task experience (several months on the radial arm maze vs. none on the passive avoidance task). What clearly remained unanswered was whether the dramatic recovery of function could occur spontaneously over a period of time, or alternatively, was dependent upon general stimulation and/or activation of memory-related neurological systems, as occurred during the course of handling the animals

and routinely testing them on the radial arm maze for 6 months following NBM destruction.

To help answer this question two additional groups of rats were given either sham lesions or NBM lesions. Following surgery, they were returned to their home cages for a period of 6 months (i.e., the same time period during which the rats in the preceding experiment received post-lesion training). Contrary to the preceding experiment, however, in this study, no training or task experience was given to the rats between surgery and testing, and except for weekly cleaning and daily feeding, little experimenter interaction occurred with the rats during this time.

The results of this study are illustrated in Fig. 9, demonstrating that when the rats were passively retained for 6 months following NBM destruction, the deficit in the passive avoidance task clearly persisted, relative to sham-operated controls. Thus, the dramatic functional recovery that occurred on both the radial arm maze and passive avoidance paradigms in the prior study apparently did not occur spontaneously, but rather was dependent upon the stimulation and/or experience gained from the routine, post-surgical training and testing on the radial arm maze.

Summary and conclusions

Our data from this series of studies address several separate, but inter-related issues. The first involves the question of the functional role of the NBM (and its cortical cholinergic projections) in mediating memory. Destruction of this brain region produced a profound loss of memory for recent events, while leaving memory for more immediate events and reference memory relatively unimpaired on this task. Thus, these data clearly support the idea that this group of neurons (and their cortical cholinergic efferents) play an important and potentially quantifiable role in mediating recent memory. Certainly, the observation of a gradual recovery after 6 months of regular testing by no means invalidates the functional implications of the lesion effects initially observed. Indeed, there

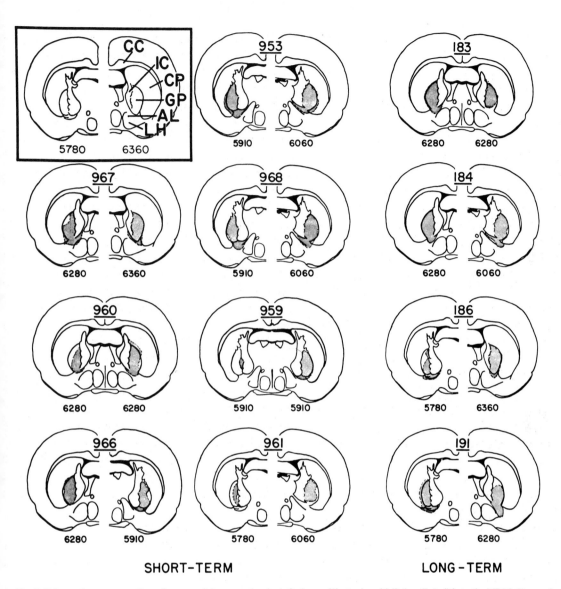

Fig. 8. Schematic representation of neuronal degeneration by infusions of ibotenic acid (2.4 μg/0.4 μl) into the NBM. For each of the 22 lesions in the 11 lesioned rats, the coronal section illustrates the rostro-caudal level at which the lesion (stippled area) reached its maximal extent. The section diagrams were modified from Konig and Klippel (1963). Numbers in the bottom of each section refer to the distance (microns) anterior to the interaural line. Numbers at the top of each pair of sections refer to the individual subject numbers. Sections in the left-hand and middle columns are from the short-term lesion group, whereas sections in the right hand column are from the long-term lesion group. Neuroanatomical structures from the two most extreme rostro-caudal levels are labeled in the diagram on the upper left. Abbreviations: AL, ansa lenticularis; CC, corpus callosum; CP, caudate putamen; GP, globus pallidus; IC, internal capsule; LH, lateral hypothalamus. (From Bartus et al., 1985c)

exist numerous examples of comparable recovery of function following brain lesions (Finger and Stein, 1982; Lashley, 1921; LeVere, 1980). In the present situation, the specificity and severity of the

memory loss initially inflicted by the lesion strongly implicates some role for this nucleus and its pathway in mediating recent memory. This conclusion remains valid in spite of the eventual

356

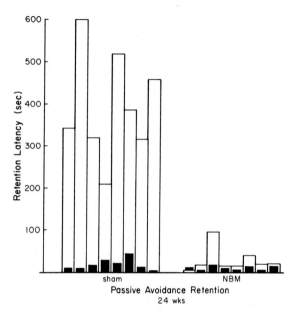

Fig. 9. 24-h retention of passive avoidance task 6 months following sham or NBM lesion. Contrary to the 'old lesion' rats depicted in Fig. 7, which were given 6 months of training post-operationally, and consequently exhibited no passive avoidance deficit, these rats were retained in their home cages for 6 months and exhibited persistence of a clear deficit on the task. The open portion of the bars depicts retention latencies, whereas the solid black bars depict training latencies. (From Bartus et al., 1986)

recovery of the long-term trained rats, and independent of whether or not any neural compensatory changes might ever be found.

The second issue concerns the role that cell loss in the nucleus basalis (and its presumed relation to decreased cortical CAT activity) may play in the early symptoms of Alzheimer's and other neurodegenerative diseases. Certainly, the profound and specific loss of memory following damage to the basal forebrain-cortical cholinergic system provides a strong argument for a possible role. Moreover, the operational similarities between the artificially induced deficit and the memory loss found to occur spontaneously in aged rodents, primates, humans and early-stage Alzheimer patients, make the argument for an important role even more compelling. At the same time, however, complete recovery of the memory deficit did occur, which is certainly contrary to the prognosis given for patients with

Alzheimer's disease, or any of the degenerative diseases in question (who presumably continue to attempt to perform tasks on which they become functionally impaired). A major question which presents itself is whether recovery in the continuously-trained animals would have occurred if the lesion had been given to older animals which suffer certain age-related neurofunctional disturbances (Bartus, 1979; Bartus et al., 1982; Bartus and Dean, 1985; Kubanis and Zornetzer, 1981), possibly including a reduced capacity to recover lost neurobehavioral function (Mufson and Stein, 1980; Stein, 1974; Stein and Firl, 1976). Also of interest would be the effects of combining lesions of the basal forebrain with other areas also implicated in Alzheimer's disease (such as the hippocampus or locus ceruleus). Clearly pertinent to this point are recent preliminary findings in monkeys which suggest that, although more robust and reliable effects are obtained with combined septum/NBM lesions, recovery of the deficit still occurs after several months of training (Mishkin et al., 1985). From a similar perspective, the question of the functional significance of the classic neuropathology of Alzheimer's disease (i.e., neurofibrillary tangles and amyloid plaques) must be considered; perhaps this neuropathology must coexist with the neurodegeneration to cause the severe and permanent loss of cognitive function characteristic of diseases such as Alzheimer's. In other words, given the apparent complexity of these diseases and their clinical manifestations, it seems reasonable to consider that simultaneous degeneration of a number of brain regions, or the existence of a number of different pathologies, may be required to produce not only the profound and permanent loss of memory and related cognitive skills, but also the insidious progression of the symptoms seen in these diseases. Finally, from a different perspective, might it be possible to significantly reduce the functional loss associated with Alzheimer's disease by providing intense, routine practice and remedial training of daily living skills? Clearly, attention to these many issues must be a concern for future research.

The question of species suitability for these

studies is another issue deserving some comment. Although the ventromedial lateral globus pallidus is commonly agreed to represent an area homologous to the primate nucleus basalis of Meynert, the region is poorly defined in rodents and there are differences in its cellular distribution and topographical projections. Further, the nature of the specific memory loss impaired with age and dementia continues to present problems when studied in rodents (see Bartus and Dean, 1985). Alternatively, the similarity of structure and organization of the basal forebrain nuclei in human and non-human primates, combined with the relative similarity of behavioral repertoire and cognitive test capabilities in these species, reduces the assumptions necessary to extrapolate from the effects of lesions in monkeys to the functional consequences of degeneration of the basal forebrain nuclei in aged, demented humans. Thus, a number of advantages argue for the use of non-human primates in these studies.

Nonetheless, future experimental work in both primates and rodents, as well as with post-mortem tissue from various demented and non-demented patient populations, is clearly needed, and should help clarify the role of this brain region in mediating behavior and its relationship to the cognitive loss associated with aging and dementia. Although it is unreasonable to expect studies with animals to unravel single-handedly, the complex mysteries of human Alzheimer's and other dementing diseases, information gained from such studies, and new thinking generated by the questions raised, should ultimately contribute to a more complete understanding.

Acknowledgements

The authors thank Jean Tomara and Kathy Schill for technical assistance and Rhonda Sheppard for help in preparing the manuscript.

References

Altman, H. J., Crosland, R. D., Jenden, D. J. and Berman, R. F. (1985) Further characterizations of the nature of the behavioral and neurochemical effects of lesions to the nucleus basalis of Meynert in the rat. Neurobiol. Aging, 6: 125–130.

Arai, H., Kosaka, K. and Iizuka, R. (1984) Changes of biogenic amines and their metabolites in postmortem brains from patients with Alzheimer-type dementia. J. Neurochem., 43: 388–393.

Arendt, T., Bigl, V., Tennstedt, A. and Arendt, A. (1984) Correlation between cortical plaque count and neuronal loss in the nucleus basalis in Alzheimer's disease. Neurosci. Lett., 48: 81–85.

Bartus, R. T. (1979) Effects of aging on visual memory, sensory processing and discrimination learning in the non-human primate. In J. M. Ordy and K. Brizzee (Eds.), Aging, Sensory Systems and Communication in the Elderly, Vol. 10, Raven Press, New York, pp. 85–114.

Bartus, R. T. and Dean, R. L. (1981) Age related memory loss and drug therapy: possible directions based on animal models. In S. J. Enna, T. Samorajski and B. Beer (Eds.), Brain Neurotransmitters and Receptors in Aging and Age-related Disorders, Raven Press, New York, pp. 209–223.

Bartus, R. T. and Dean, R. L. (1985) Developing and utilizing animal models in the search for an effective treatment for age-related memory disturbances. In C. G. Gottfries (Ed.),

Physiological Aging, Dementia of Alzheimer Type (AD) and Senile Dementia (SD), Press of the Free University of Brussels, Brussels, pp. 231–267.

Bartus, R. T. and Johnson, H. R. (1976) Short term memory in the rhesus monkey: disruption from the anticholinergic scopolamine. Pharmacol. Biochem. Behav., 5: 39–40.

Bartus, R. T., Fleming, D. and Johnson, H. R. (1978) Aging in the rhesus monkey: debilitating effects on short-term memory. J. Gerontol., 33: 858–871.

Bartus, R. T., Dean, R. L. and Beer, B. (1980a) Memory deficits in aged Cebus monkeys and facilitation with central cholinomimetics. Neurobiol. Aging, 1: 145–152.

Bartus, R. T., Dean, R. L., Goas, J. A. and Lippa, A. S. (1980b) Age-related changes in passive avoidance retention: modulation with dietary choline. Science, 209: 301–303.

Bartus, R. T., Dean, R. L., Beer, B. and Lippa, A. S. (1982) The cholinergic hypothesis of geriatric memory dysfunction. Science, 217: 408–417.

Bartus, R. T., Flicker, C. and Dean, R. L. (1983a) Logical principles for the development of animal models of age-related memory impairments. In T. Crook, S. Ferris, and R. T. Bartus (Eds.), Assessment for Geriatric Psychopharmacology, Powley Associates, New Haven, CT, pp. 263–299.

Bartus, R. T., Dean, R. L., Flicker, C. and Beer, B. (1983b) Behavioral and pharmacological studies using animal models of aging: implications for studying and treating dementia of Alzheimer's type. In Banbury Report, Vol. 15, Biological

358

Aspect of Alzheimer's Disease, Cold Spring Harbor Laboratory, New York, pp. 207–218.

Bartus, R. T., Dean, R. L. and Beer, B. (1983c) An evaluation of drugs for improving memory in aged monkeys: implications for clinical trials in humans. *Psychopharmacol. Bull.*, 19: 168–184.

Bartus, R. T., Dean, R. L., Pontecorvo, M. J. and Flicker, C. (1985b) The cholinergic hypothesis: A historical overview, current perspective and future directions. In D. Olton, E. Gamzu and S. Corkin (Eds.), *Memory Dysfunctions, Integration of Animal and Human Research from Clinical and Preclinical Perspectives*, New York Academy of Science, pp. 332–358.

Bartus, R. T., Flicker, C., Dean, R.L., Pontecorvo, M., Figueiredo, J. C. and Fisher, S. K. (1985c) Selective memory loss following nucleus basalis lesions: long term behavioral recovery despite persistent cholinergic deficiencies. *Pharmacol. Biochem. Behav.*, 23: 125–135.

Bartus, R. T., Pontecorvo, M., Flicker, C., Dean, R. L. and Figueiredo, J. C. (1986) Behavioral recovery following bilateral lesions of the nucleus basalis does not occur spontaneously. *Pharmacol. Biochem. Behav.*, 24: 1287–1292.

Benton, J. S., Bowen, D. M., Allen, S. J., Haan, E. A., Davison, A. N., Neary, D., Murphy, R. P. and Snowden, J. S. (1982) Alzheimer's disease as a disorder of isodendritic core. *Lancet*, 1: 456.

Bondareff, W., Mountjoy, C. Q. and Roth, M. (1981) Selective loss of neurons of origin of adrenergic projection to cerebral cortex (nucleus locus coeruleus) in senile dementia. *Lancet*, 1: 783–784.

Bowen, D. M., Smith, C. B., White, P. and Davison, A. N. (1976) Neurotransmitter-related enzymes and indices of hypoxia in senile dementia and other abiotrophies. *Brain*, 99: 459–496.

Bowen, D. M., Allen, S. S. and Benton, J. S. (1983) Biochemical assessment of serotonergic and cholinergic dysfunction and cerebral atrophy in Alzheimer's disease. *J. Neurochem.*, 41: 266–272.

Christie, J. E., Shering, A., Ferguson, J. and Glen, A. I. M. (1981) Physostigmine and arecoline: effects of intravenous infusions in Alzheimer's presenile dementia. *Br. J. Psychiat.*, 128: 46–50.

Coyle, J. T., Price, D. L. and DeLong, M. R. (1983) Alzheimer's disease: A disorder of cortical cholinergic innervation. *Science*, 219: 1184–1190.

Craik, F. I. M. (1977) Age related differences in human memory. In J. E. Birren and K. W. Schaie (Eds.), *Handbook of the Psychology of Aging*, Van Nostrand Reinhold, New York, pp. 384–420.

Crapper, D. R. and Dalton, A. J. (1972) Alterations in short-term retention, conditioned avoidance response acquisition and motivation following aluminum induced neurofibrillary degeneration. *Physiol. Behav.*, 10: 925–932.

Crapper, D. R. and Dalton, A.J. (1973) Aluminum induced

neurofibrillary degeneration, brain electrical activity and alteration in acquisition and retention. *Physiol. Behav.*, 10: 935–945.

Das, G. D. (1971) Projection of the interstitial nerve cells surrounding the globus pallidus: a study of retrograde changes following cortical ablations in rabbits. *Z. Anat. Entwickl. Gesch.*, 133: 135–160.

Davies, P. and Maloney, A. J. F. (1976) Selective loss of central cholinergic neurons in Alzheimer's disease. *Lancet*, 2: 1403.

Davies, P. and Terry, R. D. (1981) Cortical somatostatin-like immunoreactivity in cases of Alzheimer's disease and senile dementia of the Alzheimer type. *Neurobiol. Aging*, 2: 9–14.

Davis, K. L., Mohs, R. C., Davis, B. M., Levy, M. I., Horvath, T. B., Ronsberg, G. S., Ross, A., Rothpearl, A. and Rosen, W. (1982) Cholinergic treatment in Alzheimer's disease: implications for future research. In S. Corkin, K. L. Davis, J. H. Growdon, E. Usdin and R. J. Wurtman (Eds.), *Aging, Alzheimer's Disease, A Report of Progress in Research, Vol. 19*, Plenum Press, New York, pp. 483–494.

Davis, R. T. (1978) Old monkey behavior. *Exp. Gerontol.*, 13: 237–250.

Drachman, D. A. and Leavitt, J. (1974) Human memory and the cholinergic system: a relationship to aging. *Arch. Neurol.*, 30: 113–121.

Drachman, D. A. and Sahakian, B. J. (1980) Memory and cognitive function in the elderly: a preliminary trial of physostigmine. *Arch. Neurol.*, 37: 674–675.

Dubois, B., Mayo, W., Agid, Y., LeMoal, M. and Simon, H. (1985) Profound disturbances of spontaneous and learned behaviors following lesions of the nucleus basalis magnocellularis in the rat. *Brain Res.*, 338: 249–258.

Edstrom, J. P. and Phillis, J. W. (1980) A cholinergic projection from the globus pallidus to cerebral cortex. *Brain Res.*, 189: 524–529.

Fibiger, H. C. (1982) The organization and some projections of cholinergic neurons of the mammalian forebrain. *Brain Res. Rev.*, 4: 327–388.

Finger, S. and Stein, D. G. (1982) *Brain Damage and Recovery: Research and Clinical Perspectives*, Academic Press, New York.

Flicker, C., Dean, R. L., Watkins, D. L., Fisher, S. K. and Bartus, R. T. (1983) Behavioral and neurochemical effect following neurotoxic lesions of a major cholinergic input to the cerebral cortex in the rat. *Pharmacol. Biochem. Behav.*, 18: 973–981.

Flicker, C., Bartus, R. T., Crook, T. and Ferris, S. H. (1984) Effects of aging and dementia upon recent visuospatial memory. *Neurobiol. Aging*, 5: 275–283.

Fonnum, F. (1975) A rapid radiochemical method for the determination of choline acetyltransferase. *J. Neurochem.*, 24: 407–409.

Friedman, E., Lerer, B. and Kuster, J. (1983) Loss of cholinergic neurons in rat neocortex produces deficits in passive avoidance learning. *Pharmacol. Biochem. Behav.*, 19: 309–312.

Gold, P. E. and McGaugh, J. L. (1975) Changes in learning and memory during aging. In J. M. Ordy and K. M. Brizzee (Eds.), *Neurobiology of Aging*, Plenum Press, New York, pp. 145–158.

Gottfries, C. G. (1982) The metabolism of some neurotransmitters in aging and dementia disorders. *Gerontology*, 28 (2): 11–19.

Gray, J. A. and McNaughton, N. (1983) Comparison between the behavioral effects of septal and hippocampal lesions: a review. *Neurosci. Biobehav. Rev.*, 7: 119–188.

Heise, G. A. (1981) Learning and memory facilitators: Experimental definition and current status. *Trends Pharmacol. Sci.*, 2: 158–160.

Heise, G. A. (1984) Behavioral methods for measuring effects of drugs on learning and memory in animals. *Med. Res. Rev.*, 4: 535–558.

Hepler, D. J., Olton, D. S., Wenk, G. L. and Coyle, J. T. (1985) Lesions in nucleus basalis magnocellularis and medial septal area of rats produce qualitatively similar memory impairments. *J. Neurosci.*, 5: 866–873.

Honig, W. K. (1978) Studies of working memory in the pigeon. In S. H. Hulse, H. Fowler and W. K. Honig (Eds.), *Cognitive Processes in Animal Behavior*, Erlbaum, Hillsdale, NJ, pp. 211–248.

Iversen, L. L., Rossor, M. N., Reynolds, G. P., Hills, R., Roth, M., Mountjoy, C. Q., Foote, S. L., Morrison, J. H. and Bloom, F. E. (1983) Loss of pigmented dopamine-β-hydroxylase positive cells from locus coeruleus in senile dementia of Alzheimer's type. *Neurosci. Lett.*, 39: 95–100.

Johnston, M. V., McKinney, M. and Coyle, J. T. (1979) Evidence for a cholinergic projection from neurons in basal forebrain. *Proc. Natl. Acad. Sci. USA*, 76: 5392–5396.

Johnston, M. V., McKinney, M. and Coyle, J. T. (1981) Neocortical cholinergic innervation: a description of extrinsic and intrinsic components on the rat. *Exp. Brain Res.*, 43: 150–172.

Kelly, P. H. and Moore, K. E. (1978) Decrease of neocortical choline acetyltransferase after lesion of the globus pallidus in the rat. *Exp. Neurol.*, 61: 479–484.

Klatzo, I., Wisniewski, H. and Streicher, E. (1965) Experimental production of neurofibrillary degeneration. *J. Neuropathol. Exp. Neurol.*, 24: 187–199.

Konig, J. F. and Klippel, R. (1963) *The Rat Brain: A Stereotaxic Atlas*, Williams and Wilkins, Baltimore, MD.

Kubanis, P. and Zornetzer, S. F. (1981) Age related behavioral and neurobiological changes: A review with emphasis on memory. *Behav. Neur. Biol.*, 31: 115–172.

Kuhar, M. H. (1976) The anatomy of cholinergic neurons. In A. Goldberg and I. Hannin (Eds.), *The Biology of Cholinergic Function*, Raven Press, New York, pp. 3–28.

Lamour, Y., Dutar, P. and Jobert, A. (1982) Spread of acetylcholine sensitivity in the neocortex following lesion of the nucleus basalis. *Brain Res.*, 252: 377–381.

Lashley, K. S. (1929) *Brain Mechanisms and Intelligence: A Quantitative Study of Injuries to the Brain*, University of Chicago Press, Chicago, IL.

Lehmann, J., Nagy, J. I., Atmadja, S. and Fibiger, H. C. (1980) The nucleus basalis magnocellularis: The origin of a cholinergic projection to the neocortex of the rat. *Neuroscience*, 5: 1161–1174.

Lerer, B., Warner, J., Friedman, E., Vincent, G. and Gamzu, E. (1985) Cortical cholinergic impairment and behavioral deficits produced by kainic acid lesions of rat magnocellular basal forebrain. *Behav. Neurosci.*, 99: 661–667.

LeVere, T. E. (1980) Recovery of function after brain damage: a theory of the behavioral deficit. *Physiol. Psychol.*, 8: 297–308.

Lippa, A. S., Pelham, R. W., Beer, B., Critchett, D. J., Dean, R. L. and Bartus, R. T. (1980) Brain cholinergic dysfunction and memory in aged rats. *Neurobiol. Aging*, 1: 13–19.

LoConte, G., Bartolini, L., Casamenti, F., Marconcini-Pepeu, I. and Pepeu, G. (1982) Lesions of cholinergic forebrain nuclei: changes in avoidance behavior and scopolamine actions. *Pharmacol. Biochem. Behav.*, 17: 933–937.

Mann, D. M. A., Yates, P. O. and Marcyniuk, B. (1985) Correlation between senile plaques and neurofibrillary tangle counts in cerebral cortex and neuronal counts in cortex and subcortical structures in Alzheimer's disease. *Neurosci. Lett.*, 56: 51–55.

Medin, D. L. (1969) Form perception and pattern reproduction by monkeys. *J. Comp. Physiol. Psychol.*, 68: 412–419.

Mesulam, M. M. and Van Hoesen, G. W. (1976) Acetylcholinesterase rich projections from the basal forebrain of rhesus monkey to neocortex. *Brain Res.*, 109: 152–157.

Mesulam, M. M., Mufson, E. J., Levey, A. I. and Wainer, B. (1983) Cholinergic innervation of cortex by the basal forebrain: cytochemistry and cortical connections of the septal area, diagonal band nuclei, nucleus basalis (substantia innominata) and hypothalamus in the rhesus monkey. *J. Comp. Neurol.*, 214: 170–197.

Mishkin, M., Aigner, T. G. and Aggleton, J. (1985) Neurobiology of memory in primate brain. *Thirteenth International Congress of Gerontology Abstracts*, p. 20.

Miyamoto, M., Shintani, M., Nagaoba, A. and Nagawa, Y. (1985) Lesioning of the rat basal forebrain leads to memory impairments in passive and active avoidance tasks. *Brain Res.*, 328: 97–104.

Mufson, E. J. and Stein, D. G. (1980) Behavioral and morphological aspects of aging: an analysis of rat frontal cortex. In D. G. Stein (Ed.), *The Psychobiology of Aging: Problems and Perspectives*, Elsevier, New York, pp. 99–125.

Murray, C. L. and Fibiger, H. C. (1985) Learning and memory deficits after lesions of the nucleus basalis magnocellularis: reversal by physostigmine. *Neuroscience*, 14: 1025–1032.

Olton, D. S. (1978) Characteristics of spatial memory. In S. H. Hulse, H. F. Fowler and W. K. Honig (Eds.), *Cognitive Processes in Animal Behavior*, Erlbaum, Hillsdale, NJ, pp. 341–373.

Olton, D. S. and Samuelson, R. J. (1976) Remembrance of places passed: spatial memory in rats. *J. Exp. Psychol. Animal Behav.*, 2: 97–116.

Olton, D. S., Becker, J. T. and Handelmann, G. E. (1979) Hippocampus, space and memory. *Behav. Brain Sci.*, 2: 313–365.

Olton, D. S., Becker, J. T. and Handelmann, G. E. (1980) Hippocampal function: working memory on cognitive mapping. *Physiol. Psychol.*, 8: 239–246.

Pedata, F., LoConte, G., Sorbi, S., Marconcini-Pepeu, I. and Pepeu, G. (1982) Changes in high affinity choline uptake in rat cortex following lesions of the magnocellular forebrain nuclei. *Brain Res.*, 233: 359–367.

Perry, E. K., Tomlinson, B. E., Blessed, G., Bergmann, K., Gibson, P. H. and Perry, R. H. (1978) Correlation of cholinergic abnormalities with senile plaques and mental test scores in senile dementia. *Br. Med. J.*, 2: 1457–1459.

Reisberg, B., Ferris, S. H. and Crook, T. (1982) Signs, symptoms and course of age-associated cognitive decline. In S. Corkin, K. L. Davis, J. H. Growdon, E. Usdin and R. J. Wurtman (Eds.), *Aging, Alzheimer's Disease: A Report of Progress in Research, Vol. 19*, Raven Press, New York, pp. 177–182.

Rogers, J. D., Brogan, D. and Mirra, S. S. (1985) The nucleus basalis of Meynert in neurological disease: a quantitative morphological study. *Ann. Neurol.*, 17: 163–170.

Shute, C. C. D. and Lewis, P. R. (1967) The ascending cholinergic reticular system: neocortical olfactory and subcortical projections. *Brain*, 90: 497–521.

Simon, J. R., Atweh, S. and Kuhar, M. J. (1976) Sodium-dependent high affinity choline uptake: a regulatory step in the synthesis of acetylcholine. *J. Neurochem.*, 26: 909–922.

Stein, D. G. (1974) Some variables influencing recovery of function after central nervous system lesions in the rat. In S. G. Stein, J. J. Rosen and N. Butters (Eds.), *Plasticity and Recovery of Function in the Central Nervous System*, Academic Press, New York, pp. 373–427.

Stein, D. G. and Firl, A. C. (1976) Brain damage and reorganization of function in old age. *Exp. Neurol.*, 52: 157–167.

Strong, R., Hicks, P., Hsu, L., Bartus, R. T. and Enna, S.J. (1980) Age-related alternations in the brain cholinergic system and behavior. *Neurobiol. Aging*, 1: 59–63.

Thomas, J. B. (1972) Nonappetitive passive avoidance in rats with septal lesions. *Physiol. Behav.*, 8: 1087–1092.

Wenk, G. L. and Olton, D. S. (1984) Recovery of neocortical choline acetyltransferase activity following ibotenic acid injection into the nucleus basalis of Meynert in rats. *Brain Res.*, 293: 184–186.

Wenk, H., Volker, B., Meyer, U. (1980) Cholinergic projections from magnocellular nuclei of the basal forebrain to cortical areas in rats. *Brain Res. Rev.*, 2: 295–316.

Whitehouse, P. J., Price, D. L., Clark, A. W., Coyle, J. T. and Delong, M. R. (1981) Alzheimer's disease: evidence for selective loss of cholinergic neurons in the nucleus basalis. *Ann. Neurol.*, 10: 122–126.

Whitehouse, P. L., Price, D. L., Struble, R. G., Clark, A. W., Coyle, J. T. and DeLong, M. R. (1982) Alzheimer's disease and senile dementia: loss of neurons in the basal forebrain. *Science*, 215: 1237–1239.

Wilcock, G. K., Esiri, M. M., Bowen, D. M. and Smith, C. C. T. (1983) The nucleus basalis in Alzheimer's disease: cell counts and cortical biochemistry. *Neuropathol. Appl. Neurobiol.*, 9: 175–179.

Wisniewski, H. M., Bruce, M. E. and Fraser, H. (1975) Infection etiology of neuritic (senile) plaques in mice. *Science*, 190: 1108–1110.

Yamamura, H. I. and Snyder, S. H. (1974) Muscarinic cholinergic binding in rat brain. *Proc. Natl. Acad. Sci. USA*, 711: 725–1729.

Discussion

J. M. PALACIOS: Have you been able to reverse the behavioral deficits seen in the nucleus basalis of Meynert (NBM) lesioned animals with any pharmacological treatment?

ANSWER: The gradual, but eventually complete recovery of the lesioned rats in the radial arm maze prevented controlled studies of drug treatments.

J. HAGAN: Should passive avoidance deficits be interpreted as memory losses? When run as a choice rather than latency paradigm, putative amnesic and facilitatory effects on passive avoidance may no longer appear (Van Haaren and Van de Poll, 1984).

ANSWER: The passive avoidance procedure is a rather crude behavioral paradigm, which, when run in a certain way is very sensitive to the effects of age and cholinergic defects. Several important control groups must be used in order to ultimately conclude that the age-related deficits are related to a loss of memory ability. Many of us in this area of research have included such control groups in our studies and can therefore rule out a number of non-mnemonic variables as being responsible for the behavioral deficit and at the same time suggest a time-related decline in retention of the learned event. Thus, although the passive avoidance paradigm is crude, offers only an approximation of the degree of memory loss, and must employ many control groups to allow one to conclude that memory is primarily being affected, it still can be a useful procedure if carefully and correctly utilized.

A. BJÖRKLUND: Studies on the nigrostriatal dopamine system have shown that lesions of up to 90% of the system are followed by a complete behavioral recovery. Your lesions of the NBM produced a 40% drop in cortical ChAT. Thus, the behavioral recovery you described would be expected on the basis of a partial lesion.

ANSWER: I agree that may be one explanation of the behavioral recovery, but, of course a number of other possibilities also exist.

G. W. VAN HOESEN: The location of your lesions would not seem to destroy the cholinergic input to the hippocampus, but instead that to the somatomotor cortices. These parts of the cortex survive well in Alzheimer's disease and one usually does not associate this cortex with the more cognitive-related aspects of memory. Would you comment on this?

ANSWER: The lesions were indeed intended to spare the hippocampus, but to destroy the cholinergic nucleus of the basal forebrain which projects to the frontal and temporal-parietal cortex. Of course, this area in the rat is believed by many to be homologous to the nucleus basalis of Meynert in the human, which is degenerated in AD; its projection areas in the cortex suffer severe CAT loss, plaques and tangles in AD.

P. W. M. RAAYMAKERS: (1) Do you have any idea on the reason for the discrepancy between your results and our preliminary results which were presented in a poster, with regard to recovery of ChAT activity 4 months after lesions in younger but not in older rats?

(2) Could you discuss in more detail the problem cq. value of rehearsal in an animal model of memory disorders?

ANSWER: (1) No, although our data agree with several other papers demonstrating persistent loss of cholinergic markers with bilateral NBM lesions.

(2) One of the primary types of memory loss that occurs with advanced age in humans and early-stage Alzheimer patients involves an inability to recall information from situations that do not permit practice or the opportunity of rehearsal or repetition of the information. Aged animals typically exhibit similar memory deficits under the same conditions. Logically, if an animal model portends to provide information predictive of this memory loss, it should be attempted to optimize and incorporate these facts.

References

Van Haaren, F. and Van de Poll, N. E. (1984) The effects of a choice alternative on passive avoidance behavior of male and female Wistar rats. *Physiol. Behav.*, 32: 211–215.

D. F. Swaab, E. Fliers, M. Mirmiran, W. A. Van Gool and F. Van Haaren (Eds.)
Progress in Brain Research, Vol. 70.
© 1986 Elsevier Science Publishers B.V. (Biomedical Division)

CHAPTER 23

Experimental studies on the induction and prevention of retrograde degeneration of basal forebrain cholinergic neurons

M. V. Sofroniew[a],*, R. C. A. Pearson[b], O. Isacson[c] and A. Björklund[c]

[a]*Department of Neurosurgery, Johns Hopkins Hospital, Johns Hopkins University, Baltimore, MD, USA*, [b]*Department of Human Anatomy, University of Oxford, Oxford, UK and *[c]*Department of Histology, University of Lund, Lund, Sweden*

Introduction

The substantia innominata of the human basal forebrain (Brissaud, 1893; Forel, 1907) is characterized by distinct aggregations of large neurons originally termed the nucleus of the ansa peduncularis 'Kern der Hirnschenkelschlinge' (Meynert, 1872). These aggregations of neurons were first referred to collectively as the basal nucleus, or basal nucleus of Meynert (Meynertsches Basalganglion) by Koelliker (1896). Equivalent neurons are identifiable in Nissl-stained sections of the basal forebrains of other primates and lower mammals as clusters of large, deeply stained neurons, but their precise location within the basal forebrain shows considerable species variation. Based on a comparative study, Brockhaus (1942) divided Koelliker's extensive basal nucleus into three principal groups: (1) the medial septum and nuclear groups of the diagonal band of Broca, (2) the large neurons in the tuberculum olfactorium and (3) the basal nucleus proper. This latter nucleus was described as comprising clusters of large darkly stained (in Nissl preparations) neurons in the substantia innominata of humans and primates, which in lower mammals to a much greater extent lie dorsally, medial to the pallidum, in accordance with the previous description of Grunthal (1932). These basic subdivisions are still recognized today.

The neurons in these three groups are often referred to collectively as the complex of cholinergic neurons of the basal forebrain, since they stain positively for the cholinergic enzymes acetylcholinesterase (AChE) (Koelle, 1954; Shute and Lewis, 1967; Mesulam and Van Hoesen, 1976; Perry et al., 1982; Rossor et al., 1982b; Henke and Lang, 1983) or choline acetyltransferase (ChAT, Sofroniew et al., 1982, 1985; Armstrong et al., 1983; Houser et al., 1983; Mesulam et al., 1983; Nagai et al., 1983), and most contain both enzymes (Eckenstein and Sofroniew, 1983; Levey et al., 1983). The neurons in the various groups do, however, have differing projections. Neurons in the medial septum and vertical limb of the nucleus of the diagonal band project to the hippocampus (Diatz and Powell, 1954; Swanson and Cowan, 1979), neurons in the horizontal nucleus of the diagonal band project to the olfactory bulb (Price and Powell, 1970), and neurons of the basal nucleus project to the neocortex (Divac, 1975; Kievit and Kuypers, 1975; Jones et al., 1976; Bigl et al., 1982; Mesulam et al., 1983; Pearson et al., 1983a) and amygdala (Woolf and Butcher, 1982). Thus, these three major groups of neurons provide cholinergic afferents to the

---

*Present address: Anatomy School, Downing Street, Cambridge CB2 3DY, UK.

entire mantel of allo- and neocortex in a topo-graphically organized manner (Pearson et al., 1983c). It is also clear that the basal nucleus is the principal source of extrinsic cholinergic afferents to the cortex, such that lesions in the basal nucleus in the rat cause a fall of up to 70% in ChAT activity in the cortex (Johnston et al., 1981). In the rat, the nucleus is less well demarcated than in primates, but it is identifiable as a band of large cholinergic neurons lying principally adjacent to and inter-mingling with the medial border of the internal capsule along its entire rostro-caudal extent (Grun-thal, 1932; Bigl et al., 1982; Sofroniew et al., 1982). Fig. 1 shows the general topography and appear-

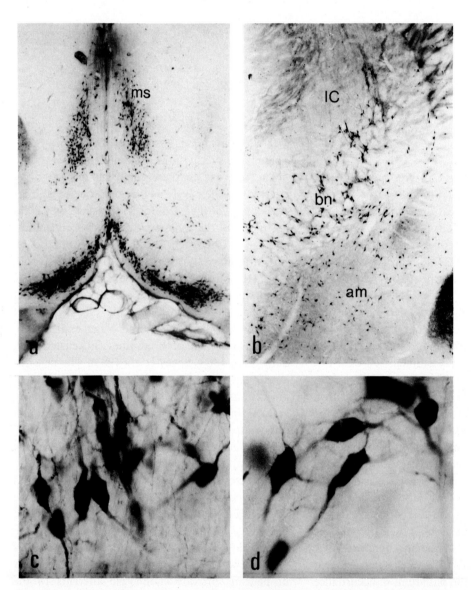

Fig. 1 (a–d). ChAT-positive neurons in frontal section of the rat basal forebrain. (a) Survey of the medial septal nucleus (ms) and nucleus of the diagonal band of Broca. (b) Survey of the basal nucleus (bn) and amygdala (am). (c) Detail of (a) showing cholinergic neurons in the medial septum. (d) Detail of (b) showing cholinergic neurons in the basal nucleus. IC, internal capsule.

ance of cholinergic neurons identified by immuno-histochemical staining for ChAT in the rat medial septum and basal nucleus. Fig. 2 summarizes in schematic form on a sagittal view of the rat brain some of the major identified projections of various central cholinergic neurons, including those from neurons in the basal forebrain complex located in the medial septum, diagonal band, and basal nucleus to different allo- and neocortical areas.

Neurochemical and pathological-anatomical changes in the basal nucleus and other forebrain regions in Alzheimer's disease (AD)

The large cholinergic neurons of the basal fore-brain have recently received much attention because of their reported degeneration during the senile and presenile dementias (Whitehouse et al., 1982; Arendt et al., 1985) as well as during a variety of other diseases such as schizophrenia (von Buttlar-Brentano, 1952), Korsakoff's disease

(Arendt et al., 1983), Parkinson's disease (Arendt et al., 1983; Nakano and Hirano, 1983), and progressive supranuclear palsy (Tagliavini et al., 1983). In addition, experimental evidence suggests that these neurons are involved in cognitive functions (Hepler et al., 1985; Miyamoto et al., 1985). The degeneration of these neurons and the accompanying loss of cholinergic input to various cortical areas may thus be directly related to the loss of such functions which accompany these diseases, and might represent the primary event in some of these diseases. This has been suggested for AD, where there is a marked reduction of ChAT activity in both the cerebral cortex and substantia innominata of the basal forebrain (Bowen et al., 1976; Davies and Maloney, 1976; Perry et al., 1977; Perry et al., 1982; Rossor et al., 1982a,b; Henke and Lang, 1983; Sims et al., 1983). These losses of ChAT activity are accompanied by histopathologic changes affecting the large (mean diameter 30 μm) cells of the basal nucleus and basal forebrain

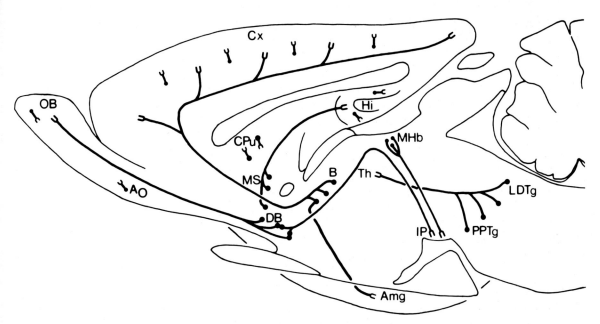

Fig. 2. Schematic sagittal drawing of the rat brain showing major cholinergic pathways based on experimental evidence. Amg, amygdala; AO, anterior olfactory nucleus; B, basal nucleus of Meynert; Cx, cortex; DB, nuclei of the diagonal band; Hi, hippocampus; IP, interpeduncular nucleus; LDTg, laterodorsal tegmental nucleus; MHb, medial habenula nucleus; MS, medial septum; OB, olfactory bulb; PPTg, pedunculopontine tegmental nucleus; Th, thalamus. (From Sofroniew et al., 1985)

complex, the principal source of afferent cholinergic fibers to the cortex, principally a striking loss of the cells (Whitehouse et al., 1982; Arendt et al., 1985) as well as the hypertrophy of some cells (Arendt et al., 1985) as seen in Nissl-stained sections. The severity of these histopathologic changes within the basal forebrain has recently been shown to follow a regional distribution which correlates with the severity of the changes noted in the corresponding target allo- or neocortex (Arendt et al., 1985).

Retrograde effects of cortical ablation on basal forebrain cholinergic neurons

It is not known whether the loss of cells with a mean diameter greater than 30 μm in neuropathological sections of brains with AD as described above represents cell shrinkage or cell death. A similar disappearance of the large cells from the basal nucleus is seen in human and monkey brains after surgical lesions of the cortex (Pearson et al., 1983b) indicating that such changes can be induced retrogradely, so that it is not yet certain if the changes observed in the basal nucleus in AD represent the primary pathology or are secondary to the various processes known to affect the cortex in these diseases. We addressed this question further in experimental studies by examining the effects of different forms of mechanical or chemical damage to the allo- or neocortex on immunohistochemically identified cholinergic neurons in the basal forebrain of the rat.

The details of all surgical and immunohistochemical procedures used in these studies have been described (Sofroniew, 1983; Sofroniew et al., 1983, 1986a). The staining of cholinergic neurons was achieved with immunohistochemical detection of ChAT using a specific monoclonal antibody and the peroxidase-antiperoxidase procedure (Eckenstein and Thoenen, 1982; Sofroniew et al., 1983). In all experimental and control animals, 50 ChAT-containing neurons selected from the different nuclei studied were drawn at a magnification of ×600 and their cross-sectional areas measured

using a semi-automatic image analysis apparatus. The neurons to be drawn were always taken from approximately the same standardized location within each nucleus in different animals. In selected animals, five representative sections at carefully matched levels through the relevant nucleus were drawn with a drawing apparatus, and all the ChAT-positive neurons were plotted. The number of cells on each side was counted, corrected for differences in cell size using the Abercrombie (1946) correction, and compared with the numbers at carefully matched levels of the relevant nucleus in age- and sex-matched normal animals. The significance of the differences observed between animals was confirmed statistically (Sofroniew et al., 1983; Pearson et al., 1984).

For these studies, a large area of cerebral neocortex was mechanically devascularized with a surgical needle on one or both sides, and in other rats the hippocampus was removed on one side by suction as well. The rats were perfused after survival times ranging from 7–495 days. Findings in these rats were compared with those in age- and sex-matched controls.

Normal animals showed little variation with age and sex in the size of the cholinergic cells in the basal nucleus or septum. This was confirmed statistically using Bartlett's test (Bailey, 1959) for the homogeneity of several variances which showed no significant differences. The means of all the normal observations in each nucleus were therefore used for subsequent analysis of the experimental data with Student's t test using a standard deviation derived from the pooled variances of all the normal sides (Pearson et al., 1984).

In animals with unilateral mechanical lesions, following short post-operative survival times (7–14 days), most of the cholinergic cells within the affected part of the basal nucleus on the same side as the lesion appeared swollen, with their nuclei eccentric and sometimes displacing the plasma membrane (Sofroniew et al., 1983). At 19–21 days, fewer cells showed these changes, the majority having shrunken somata and dendrites. By 28 days, the acute changes were no longer visible, and

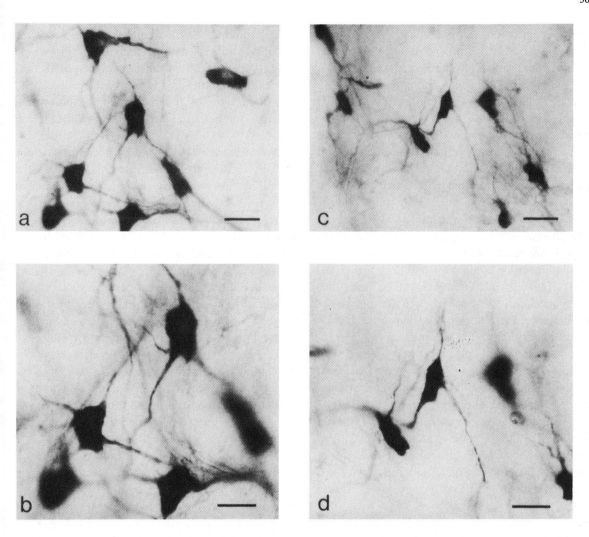

Fig. 3 (a–d). ChAT-positive neurons in a rat with a large unilateral cortical ablation and a post-operative survival time of 28 days. (a) Group of cholinergic neurons from the basal nucleus of the unoperated side. Scale bar = 30 μm. (b) Higher magnification photomicrograph of cells in (a). Scale bar = 20 μm. (c) Group of shrunken cholinergic neurons from the basal nucleus of the operated side at precisely the same level as in (a). Note the shrunken cell bodies. Scale bar = 30 μm. (d) Higher magnification photomicrograph of cells in (c). Note the marked shrinkage of the dendrites compared with the cells in the unoperated side (b). Scale bar = 20 μm. (From Sofroniew et al., 1983)

all the affected cells appeared shrunken (Fig. 3). In any one animal, not all of the cells on the side of the lesion showed these changes, a few apparently normal cells being present at all levels. The site and extent of the degeneration within the nucleus varied with the size and position of the cortical lesion, anterior lesions causing the most severe degeneration anteriorly in the nucleus and pos-

terior lesions affecting the posterior part. At survival times greater than 25 days (32–495 days) the appearance of degenerate cells within the nucleus did not appreciably alter. These qualitative observations were confirmed quantitatively by the measurement of cell sizes in all animals. The values of mean cell area in each experimental animal were compared individually with the mean for the normal population using Student's *t* test, and showed significant shrinkage after all survival times greater than 19 days (Sofroniew et al., 1983; Pearson et al., 1984). Fig. 4 compares cell sizes in animals with different post-operative survival times.

An unexpected observation in animals with unilateral mechanical lesions was that at all survival times examined, the cholinergic neurons of the basal nucleus on the unoperated side were significantly larger than those in the same nucleus in normal animals, as determined by comparing the values of mean cell area in each experimental animal individually with the mean for the normal population using Student's *t* test (Pearson et al., 1984). The cells measured were taken from that part of the nucleus which showed the maximum shrinkage on the lesioned side. This hypertrophy had begun at 7 days and persisted up to 300 days post-operatively (Fig. 4), the longest survival time examined.

Two animals with unilateral lesions of the cortex and post-operative survival times of 120 and 84 days were age- and sex-matched with two normal animals. The number of cells stained for AChE in one pair, and ChAT in the other pair, were counted at five carefully matched levels of the basal nucleus. These counts, and their values corrected

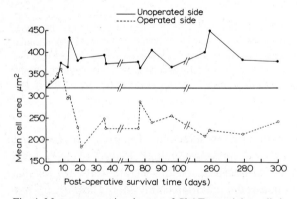

Fig. 4. Mean cross-sectional areas of ChAT-containing cells in the basal nucleus following different survival times after damage to the cerebral cortex of one side. The solid line represents the mean for the normal animals (319 μm²). (From Pearson et al., 1984)

(Abercrombie, 1946) to take account of the difference in cell size on each side, showed no significant side-to-side difference between the left sides of the control and experimental animals and the right sides of the control and experimental animals for both staining methods (Sofroniew et al., 1983).

Following removal of the hippocampus of one side by suction, the cholinergic cells in the medial septal nucleus show marked changes. In contrast to the basal nucleus after unilateral cortical damage, the most striking feature of the changes in this nucleus was a dramatic reduction in the numbers of ChAT-positive cells (Fig. 14a,b). The disappearance of cholinergic neurons is already apparent after a 7-day post-operative survival, and reaches maximum (75%) 14 days after operation, beyond which there is no further detectable loss. The cells in the 7-day survival animal are of normal size, but by the 14th post-operative day, the remaining neurons in the nucleus ipsilateral to the lesion are significantly shrunken, and this decrease remains fairly constant at all survival times up to 245 days, the longest post-operative time examined (Sofroniew et al., 1986a).

These findings indicate that both cell shrinkage and cell loss can be induced retrogradely in cholinergic neurons of the basal forebrain following damage to their terminals in target neo- or allocortex. The degeneration observed here is similar in many ways to the retrograde changes classically described following axotomy of peripheral nerves, with a stage of 'primäre Reizung' (Nissl, 1892) in which the cells swell, followed by 'retrograde atrophy', during which the cells shrink and some die (see Brodal, 1981). The findings further demonstrate that cells located in different portions of the basal forebrain complex of cholinergic neurons react differently to this type of insult depending on the projection system involved, such that neurons projecting to neocortex shrink and persist, while neurons projecting to hippocampal allocortex shrink and die. The reasons for this difference in reaction is at present unclear, but may be related to differences in the number of distant and local collaterals present which may sustain a neuron after axotomy of one of its principal axons. These findings may be of interest when considering the recent report by Arendt et al. (1985) of regional differences in the distribution of pathological findings in the basal nucleus in AD which correlate with differences in the severity of the pathology of the appropriate target cortex. In addition, hypertrophy of certain cholinergic forebrain neurons occurred in the experimental animals on the side opposite to the unilateral cortical lesions. While the mechanism of this hypertrophy is at present unclear, it is also of interest to note that hypertrophied neurons have been reported as part of the histopathologic changes found in the basal forebrain in AD (Arendt et al., 1985).

Observations on immunohistochemically stained cholinergic neurons in human brains with Alzheimer's disease

In order to study the appearance and number of cholinergic cells in basal forebrains suffering from AD and to compare these with the results of our experimental studies in animals, we applied the same histological procedures just described to human brains, in one case of AD and in two age- and sex-matched normal brains (Pearson et al., 1983d).

Case HA1 was a 72-years-old man with a 3.5-year clinical history of dementia which began with a gradual deterioration of memory over 2 years. An examination of his mental state 14 months before death showed him to be grossly disorientated with a very poor memory. The last year of his life was spent in hospital where he died of carcinoma of the bronchus. The appearance of the basal nucleus was compared with that in the brains of two known undemented men, HN1 aged 76 and HN2 aged 82, who died of cardiac related events. The brains were removed at autopsy and processed for immunohistochemical staining of ChAT., histochemical staining of AChE and neuropathological examination. Neuropathological examination of the cortex showed numerous argyrophilic

plaques and neurofibrillary tangles in HA1 and the absence of such features typical of AD in cases HN1 and HN2. In three AChE- and three ChAT-stained sections taken from these brains at carefully matched levels, the stained cells in six fields (each 600×900 μm) within the basal nucleus were plotted and counted, and 100 randomly selected ChAT-stained cells were drawn and their cross-sectional areas measured.

All findings were essentially identical in the two control brains. With the AChE method both the cell bodies and the neuropil of the basal nucleus in the normal brains were very heavily stained, whereas in the AD brain there was a marked reduction in the staining of the neuropil, even though numerous smaller and sometimes paler AChE neurons were still present. The immunohistochemical detection of ChAT clearly showed the large cholinergic cells in the nucleus of the normal brains, while in the AD brain the ChAT-positive cells, though still numerous, appeared smaller (Pearson et al., 1983d). This qualitative impression was confirmed quantitatively using cell area measurements, and the change in cell size appeared to involve the whole population of cells. The histogram in Fig. 5 shows that the majority of the cholinergic cells in the AD brain is smaller than the mean of the cell areas in the control brain.

Comparison of the counts in individual matched fields between the control and AD brains for each staining method using a paired t test showed no significant difference, suggesting that no significant loss of cells in the AD brain was found using either staining procedure. Other authors have also reported on the appearance of cholinergic neurons in the basal forebrain in AD using histochemical stains for AChE or immunohistochemical staining of ChAT. These studies include reports showing no significant reduction in the number of cells as we do (Perry et al., 1982), as well as reports of substantial reductions in the number of cells (Nagai et al., 1983). Differences such as these are perhaps reconcilable. Basal forebrain neurons may be affected differently in different cases of the disease, varying with the age at onset of the disease

370

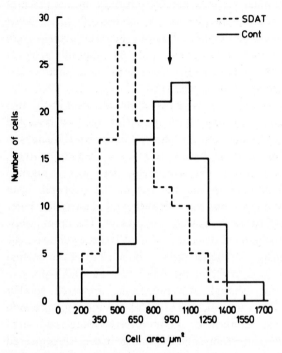

Choline acetyltransferase positive cells

Fig. 5. Histogram to show difference in cross-sectional areas of ChAT-positive neurons in the basal nucleus between the control and Alzheimer (SDAT) brains. Arrow indicates mean of cell areas in control brain and it can be seen that the majority of the cells in the SDAT brain, are smaller than this mean. (From Pearson et al., 1983d)

and with its duration. Such variations could also be accounted for by differences in sampling techniques in view of the striking regional differences in the severity of the pathology in different regions within the basal forebrains as reported by Arendt et al. (1985).

Thus, to summarize briefly, some of the basic changes affecting cholinergic neurons within the basal forebrain in AD include (1) loss of cells, (2) shrinkage of cells, (3) hypertrophy of some cells, and all of these changes appear to show regional differences of severity within the basal forebrain correlating with the severity of the pathology found in the corresponding target cortex. All of these changes can be induced retrogradely in

cholinergic basal forebrain neurons in experimental animals by damaging allo- or neocortex, and these changes within the basal forebrain are also regionally specific, related to the area of cortex damaged.

Chemical lesions with excitotoxic amino acids or colchicine

The animal experiments described thus far have examined the retrograde effect of mechanical damage to the target cortex on basal forebrain cholinergic neurons. However, mechanical lesions of this nature directly damage and destroy the terminals of the cholinergic neurons within the cortex, and such a direct destruction of these terminals within the cortex is not known to occur in AD. The histopathology of the cortex in AD is characterized by the presence of plaques and tangles, and by the loss of cortical neurons (Corsellis, 1976; Wilcock and Esiri, 1982). Tangles have been shown to share antigenic determinants with neurofilaments (Anderton et al., 1982; Dahl et al., 1982) and disturbances in neurofilaments and axonal transport have been proposed as a possible basic mechanism underlying certain diseases of the central nervous system including AD (Gajdusek, 1985). We therefore undertook studies to examine the effect upon cholinergic neurons in the basal forebrain of depleting different cortical areas of neurons using excitotoxic amino acids, or of disrupting neurofilaments and microtubules in the axons of the cholinergic neurons with colchicine.

Excitotoxin experiments

In these experiments, the excitotoxic amino acids kainic acid (KA), N-methyl-D-aspartic acid (NMAA), or ibotenic acid (IBO), were spread evenly over the exposed surface of an area of dura overlying the cortex on one side (Guldin and Markowitsch, 1982). These excitotoxic amino acids are known to selectively deplete an area of local neuronal perikarya, while sparing axons of passage or local terminals (Coyle and Schwarcz,

1983). As controls, two rats were sham-operated in which the dura was exposed but no toxin applied, and in one rat each, glutamic acid (GLU) or ascorbic acid (ASC) were applied to the dura instead of excitotoxin. In several rats, KA was applied directly to the exposed surface of the hippocampus after removal of the cortex. The rats were perfused after survival times ranging from 49–133 days. The findings are described in detail elsewhere (Sofroniew and Pearson, 1985; Sofroniew et al., 1986a).

Appearance of the cerebral cortex and hippocampus

In both sham-operated animals surviving for 56 or 63 days post-operatively and in the rats receiving GLU or ASC onto the dura, the cerebral cortex underlying the area of exposed dura showed a normal cytoarchitecture (Fig. 6) compared with that seen on the unoperated side and in unoperated animals. In contrast, the cortex underlying the dura onto which KA, NMAA or IBO had been applied showed characteristic changes after all survival times, ranging from 49–133 days. There

was a severe loss of neurons in all layers, a disruption of the typical lamination and cytoarchitecture, and a shrinkage in the thickness of the cortex (Fig. 6). All of these effects were more severe following application of KA, which caused about a 75% reduction in cortical thickness, as compared with NMAA or IBO which caused about 50% and 25% reductions, respectively. In all cases, a rim of cortical tissue containing neurons and ranging from 25–75% of its original thickness (Fig. 6), remained over the surface of the hemisphere underlying the treated dura, and there was no discernible damage to the white matter under the cortex or to structures deep to this. In a similar manner, after application of excitotoxins to the ventricular surface of the hippocampus, this structure was also severely depleted of neurons and was reduced to about 25–30% of its normal surface area on tissue sections.

Appearance of cells in the basal nucleus

In sham-operated and GLU or ASC control animals, cholinergic neurons in the basal nucleus

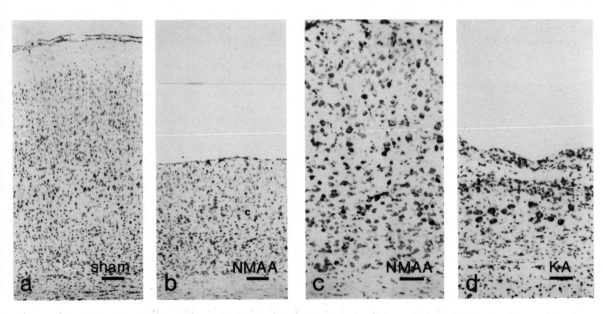

Fig. 6 (a–d). Thionin-stained sections of the cerebral cortex after various experimental procedures. (a) Exposure of the overlying dura without application of a toxin (sham). Scale bar = 100 μm. (b) Application of *N*-methyl-D-aspartic acid (NMAA) to the overlying dura. Scale bar = 100 μm. (c) Detail of (b). Scale bar = 50 μm. (d) Application of kainic acid (KA) to the overlying dura. Scale bar = 50 μm. (From Sofroniew and Pearson, 1985)

on both sides were normal in appearance and the measured mean cross-sectional areas were in the normal range. In contrast, in the KA, NMAA and IBO animals, cholinergic neurons in the basal nucleus on the side ipsilateral to the treated cortex were significantly smaller than neurons in the basal nucleus on the contralateral side (Fig. 7) and of those in normal animals. The mean size of neurons in the basal nucleus contralateral to the excitotoxin-treated cortex remained within the normal range in contrast to the hypertrophy of such neurons seen after a unilateral mechanical lesion of the cortex (Fig. 8).

Medial septal nucleus

In animals in which solid KA was applied to the ventricular surface of the hippocampus of one side following removal of the overlying cortex, the hippocampus was reduced to less than a third of its normal cross-sectional area, with marked cell loss in all subdivisions, although the dentate gyrus was least affected. The ChAT-positive cells of the ipsilateral medial septum were significantly shrunken, but in contrast to the animals with removal of the hippocampus, there is little if any cell loss (Sofroniew et al., 1986a).

These findings show that cholinergic basal forebrain neurons undergo a severe shrinkage in response to lesion of their target cortex with excitotoxic amino acids, indicating that they can undergo retrograde degeneration transneuronally, i.e. secondary to a loss of their target cortical neurons. The normal appearance of these neurons in the sham-operated animals shows that the changes observed following application of the excitotoxins were not due to a mechanical or vascular disturbance of the cortex. The toxicity of these amino acids is thought to be related to their excitatory effects and their ability to bind irreversibly to specific receptors (Coyle and Schwarcz, 1983). They have been shown to kill neurons with cell bodies in the region of application while sparing axons of passage and their neurons of origin (Coyle and Schwarcz, 1983). It seems unlikely that the toxins directly affected the terminals of cholinergic neurons, since approximately 70% of the ChAT activity present in the cortex is thought to derive from neurons outside the cortex (Johnston et al., 1981), and it has been reported that the injection of KA into the cortex causes no appreciable loss of ChAT activity from treated cortex following survival times after which

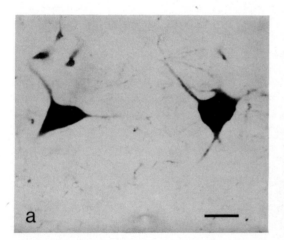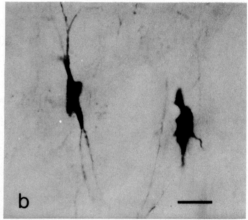

Fig. 7 (a and b). ChAT-positive neurons in a rat treated with kainic acid extradurally over the cerebral cortex of one side. (a) Cholinergic neurons from the dorsal central portion of the basal nucleus on the side opposite the treated cortex. Scale bar = 20 μm. (b) Shrunken cholinergic neurons from the equivalent region of the dorsal central portion of the basal nucleus on the same side as the treated cortex. Scale bar = 20 μm. (From Sofroniew and Pearson, 1985)

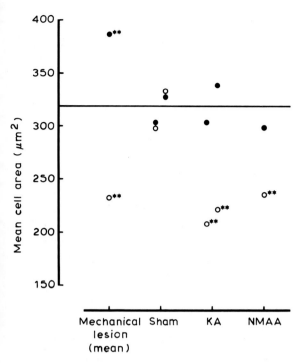

Fig. 8. Mean cross-sectional areas of cholinergic neurons in the basal nucleus of both sides following different experimental procedures involving the cerebral cortex of one side: mechanical lesion, sham operation (i.e. exposure of the dura), or application of kainic (KA) or N-methyl-D-aspartic acid (NMAA) to the dura overlying the cortex. The bar at 319 μm^2 indicates the mean size of basal nucleus neurons in normal animals. The solid circles indicate the mean size of neurons on the side opposite, and the open circles that of the neurons on the same side as the treated cortex. The value for the mechanical lesion represents the mean of 10 animals whereas the other values represent individual animals. **, $p < 0.001$ versus the normal mean. (From Sofroniew and Pearson, 1985)

there was severe loss of cortical neurons (Lehmann et al., 1980). Kainic acid, therefore, appears to cause little or no direct initial damage to cholinergic terminals in the cortex. In addition, ultrastructural analysis of the KA-treated cerebellar cortex showed persistence of presynaptic elements with attached post-synaptic fragments deriving from degenerated neurons long after those neurons had died and their remaining debris cleared from the tissue (Herndon et al., 1980). Thus it seems likely that the basal forebrain neurons degenerated

secondary to a loss of cortical neurons, rather than to a direct effect upon the neurons themselves.

Unilateral intraventricular injection of colchicine

In three young adult animals 100 $\mu g/20$ μl of colchicine (in distilled water) was injected into the lateral ventricle at a point adjacent to the fimbria and the ascending fibers of basal nucleus neurons and the animals were allowed to survive for 24 or 48 h. Colchicine is known to disrupt neurofilaments and microtubules (Dahlstrom, 1968; Kreutzberg, 1969), blocking axonal transport.

In the ipsilateral basal nucleus (Fig. 9) and medial septum, the ChAT-positive cells were

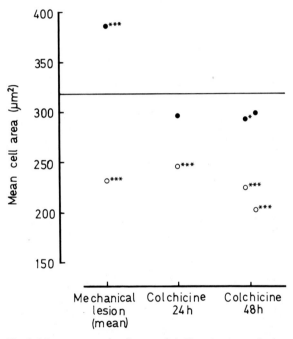

Fig. 9. Mean cross-sectional areas of cholinergic neurons in the basal nucleus of both sides following administration of colchicine into the left lateral cerebral ventricle near the axons of forebrain cholinergic neurons passing to the cortex. The bar at 319 μm^2 indicates the mean size of basal nucleus neurons in normal animals. The solid circles indicate the mean size of neurons on the side opposite, and the open circles that of the neurons on the same side as the injection was made. The value for the mechanical lesion represents the mean of 10 animals whereas the other values represent individual animals. *, $p < 0.05$; ***, $p < 0.001$ versus the normal mean.

significantly smaller both than those in the contra-lateral nuclei and the pool of normal animals (Sofroniew et al., 1986a). This shrinkage was similar in degree to that seen following cortical or hippocampal damage. The change was not accompanied by any cell loss.

These findings suggest that basal forebrain cholinergic neurons will undergo retrograde degeneration secondary to a disruption of axonal neurofilaments and microtubules, although another toxic effect of the colchicine cannot be excluded. This disruption blocks axonal transport between the perikaryon and its target and would prevent the retrograde transport of any trophic factors, as have been described in other neuronal systems (Thoenen and Barde, 1980).

Thus, to summarize briefly, the findings of these two sets of experiments suggest that basal forebrain cholinergic neurons will not only undergo retrograde degeneration following mechanical lesion of their target cortex which damages their terminals directly, but will undergo a similar retrograde degeneration transneuronally, i.e. secondary to a loss of cortical neurons without an initial direct insult to the terminals. Furthermore, they will also shrink and degenerate secondary to a blockade of transport between the neuronal cell body and its target neurons caused by disruption of axonal neurofilaments. These findings are compatible with the possibility that the degeneration of basal forebrain neurons observed in AD is retrogradely induced, i.e. secondary to the pathological processes known to affect the cortex in this disease.

Hypertrophy of cholinergic basal nucleus neurons after section of the corpus callosum

As described above, previous studies have shown that while basal forebrain cholinergic neurons ipsilateral to the lesion shrink following unilateral damage of the cerebral cortex, neurons on the contralateral side hypertrophy. The mechanism of this hypertrophy is at present unknown, but it occurs in all ages of animals and persists for up to 300 days, the longest survival time thus far

examined. Hypertrophy of some neurons in the basal forebrain in AD has been reported (Arendt et al., 1985), and it was of interest to further examine the possible factors involved in the hypertrophy observed in experimental animals. The hypertrophy within the basal nucleus seen after unilateral cortical damage in experimental animals is regionally specific, localized to the area of the nucleus which corresponds to that showing retrograde degeneration on the opposite side; therefore, it is unlikely that the stimulus is a diffusible trophic substance. It is possible that denervation of the undamaged cortex may lead to the enlargement of these cholinergic neurons on the unoperated side, and this was examined by section of the corpus callosum (Pearson et al., 1985a, 1986).

At various ages (1–56 days), the midline of the cerebral hemisphere was exposed under ether anesthesia, and the corpus callosum was sectioned over most of its length using an iridectomy knife inserted to a depth of about 4 or 5 mm immediately to one side of the sagittal sinus. Following different survival periods, the animals were perfused and their brains processed for immunohistochemical detection of ChAT as described above, and ChAT-containing cells within the basal nucleus of each side at a standard site within the central dorsal portion of the nucleus, were drawn at a magnification of ×600, and their cross-sectional areas were measured using a semi-automatic image analysis apparatus. These were compared with the already available pool of data obtained in the same way in normal animals from the same breeding colony using Student's t test as in the studies described above.

In all cases, the corpus callosum could be seen to be divided over most of its anteroposterior extent (Fig. 10). The damage to cingulate cortex through which the iridectomy knife had been passed, varied and was greater in animals operated upon as adults than as infants, but involved only a small portion of this. The underlying hippocampus was sometimes involved in the lesion, but deeper structures and the cortex of the lateral surface were always intact.

In all experimental animals, the mean cross-

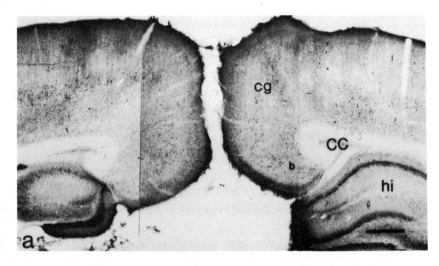
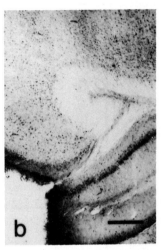

Fig. 10 (a and b). (a) Photomicrograph of a section processed for the immunohistochemical detection of choline acetyltransferase and counterstained with thionin in a rat operated upon the first postnatal day. Note the complete division of the corpus callosum. cg, cingulate cortex; CC, corpus callosum; hi, hippocampus. Scale bar = 500 μm. (b) Higher magnification of area (b) shown in (a). Note how the subcortical white matter ends deep to the cingulate cortex. Scale bar = 300 μm. (From Pearson et al., 1985a)

sectional diameter of the ChAT-containing cells of the basal nucleus of both sides was significantly greater than that seen in normal animals. This hypertrophy was present by 21 days and persisted up to 62 days post-operatively, the longest survival time examined. The degree of hypertrophy was greatest when the operation was performed on the first post-natal day, though it occurred at all ages examined, up to fully adult, and the hypertrophy of the cholinergic cells of the basal nucleus following sectioning of the corpus callosum was similar in appearance (Fig. 11) and magnitude (Fig. 12) to that seen following contralateral cortical damage (Pearson et al., 1984, 1986).

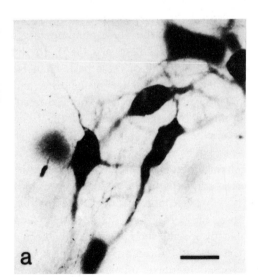
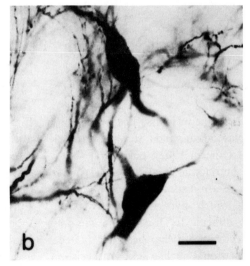

Fig. 11 (a and b). Photomicrographs of choline acetyltransferase containing cells in the basal nucleus. (a) In a normal animal, (b) in an experimental animal following section of the corpus callosum at 56 days of age. Scale bar = 20 μm. (From Pearson et al., 1985a)

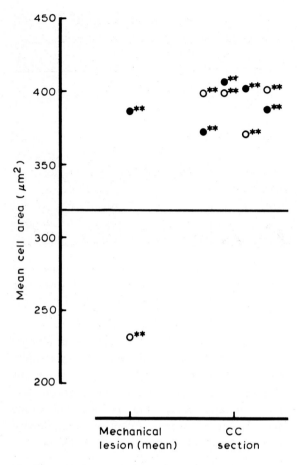

Fig. 12. Mean cross-sectional areas of cholinergic neurons in the basal nucleus of both sides following section of the corpus callosum in adult animals. The bar at 319 μm^2 indicates the mean size of basal nucleus neurons in normal animals. The value following mechanical lesion represents the mean of 10 animals. $\bigcirc$, left side; $\bullet$, right side; ** $p < 0.001$ vs the normal mean. (From Pearson et al., 1985a)

The hypertrophy of neurons has been found in the central (Goldschmidt and Steward, 1980; Hendrickson and Dineen, 1982), peripheral (Nittono, 1923) and autonomic (Gabella, 1984) nervous systems. There are distinct differences in the circumstances in which hypertrophy has been found, and it is difficult to discern the factors determining its occurrence. It has been postulated that increases in neuronal nucleic acid synthesis in relation to contralateral lesions represent a form of compensation for the damage; this has been called 'work hypertrophy' (Watson, 1965, 1968). It is probable that hypertrophy of neurons is a widespread phenomenon. Of particular interest to the present findings are the observations that hypertrophy may represent a cell soma event accompanying distant axonal sprouting (Goldschmidt and Steward, 1980; Hendrickson and Dineen, 1982). Thus, the enlargement of neurons observed in the studies presented here may occur as part of a reactive sprouting response to denervation of the cortex to which they project. Further experiments will be required to test this possibility.

Comparison of changes in cholinergic forebrain neurons in Alzheimer's disease with changes observed in experimental animals

As described above, the basic changes observed in cholinergic forebrain neurons in AD using histochemical or immunohistochemical staining techniques are loss of neurons and shrinkage of neurons. From histopathologic studies it is also likely that some of these neurons undergo hypertrophy and that the various changes observed exhibit a regional variation within the basal forebrain in degree of severity (Arendt et al., 1985). Furthermore, this regional variation in degree of severity appears to correlate with the severity of the pathology seen in the corresponding target allo- or neocortex (Arendt et al., 1985). In the studies described here, all of these basic changes, i.e. loss of neurons, shrinkage of neurons and hypertrophy of neurons, have been induced retrogradely in the cholinergic neurons of the basal forebrains of experimental animals. Cell shrinkage and cell loss have been induced retrogradely by direct mechanical damage to the terminals and the target cortex and cells in the acute phase of this degeneration hypertrophy prior to degeneration. Furthermore, these reactions are regionally and topographically specific such that cells are affected in that part of basal forebrain projecting to the area of cortex lesioned. In addition, cells in different parts of the forebrain are affected in differing degrees of severity, such that cells in the basal nucleus shrink and persist while those in the medial septum both shrink and many die. In addition, neurons on the side opposite to a unilateral cortical lesion undergo hypertrophy, perhaps in response to a denervation of their appropriate target cortex. However, direct mechanical or ischemic damage to cholinergic terminals in the cortex are not known to occur in AD. The pathology of the cortex in this disease includes cell loss and possible disturbances of neurofilaments. Additional animal experiments showed that retrograde shrinkage could also be induced in basal forebrain neurons by application of toxins which depleted the target cortex of endogenous neurons while not initially damaging the cholinergic terminals. Disruption of neurofilaments in the axons of these neurons also resulted in shrinkage of the neurons. These findings suggest that these neurons will undergo retrograde degeneration in the absence of their cortical target neurons or if axonal transport between the parent cell soma and its terminals is blocked. Together, these findings indicate that changes observed in cholinergic basal forebrain in AD could be secondary to the pathology known to affect the cortex in this disease (Corsellis, 1976; Wilcock and Esiri, 1982). It has recently been proposed that the pathology in AD spreads along known pathways (Pearson et al., 1985b) and that the basal forebrain may simply be affected by virtue of its allo- or neocortical connections.

Prevention of retrograde changes by parenteral administration of gangliosides or with fetal cortical cell-suspension grafts

In the studies described thus far, degeneration of basal forebrain cholinergic neurons has been induced retrogradely in experimental animals in several ways. Such experimentally induced degeneration, with its quantitative documentation, also provides experimental models in which to test procedures attempting to prevent neuronal degeneration. In this section experiments are presented in which retrograde degeneration of basal fore-

brain cholinergic neurons has been prevented (1) by administration of gangliosides to animals with unilateral mechanical lesions of the cortex or (2) by implantation of fetal cortical cell suspension grafts to animals with excitotoxic amino acid lesions of the cortex.

Ganglioside treatment studies

Gangliosides are sialic acid containing glycosphingolipids located in the outer leaflets of neuronal cell membranes (Zambotti et al., 1972; Ledeen, 1978), which have been shown to exert effects on neuronal growth in various situations, including during regeneration (see Rapport and Gorio, 1981).

Intraperitoneal administration of gangliosides enhances axonal sprouting during peripheral reinnervation (Ceccarelli et al., 1976; Gorio et al., 1980), accelerates the recovery of ChAT and AChE activities in the hippocampus following septal lesions (Wojcik et al., 1982), and promotes the reinnervation of the striatum by dopaminergic fibers following hemitransection of the nigrostriatal pathway (Toffano et al., 1983), possibly by enhancing collateral sprouting (Agnati et al., 1983). Furthermore, it substantially reduces the amount of retrograde degeneration of dopaminergic neurons in the substantia nigra, which normally accompanies such a transection (Toffano et al., 1984). We therefore examined the effect of ganglioside administration on cholinergic neurons in the basal forebrain in rats with extensive unilateral ablation of the cerebral cortex and hippocampus (Sofroniew et al., 1986b).

A large area of cerebral neocortex was devascularized and a large portion of the underlying hippocampus was removed by suction on the left side in one group of rats. Beginning on the day of operation GM_1 ganglioside (monosialoganglioside) was administered to these rats and a group of unoperated controls intraperitoneally daily at a dose of 30 mg/kg per day until after 30 days, when all animals were perfused and sections through the basal nucleus processed for immunohistochemical staining of ChAT. In each animal, 50 cells in the dorsal central portion of the basal nucleus were drawn and their cross-sectional areas measured. The values of mean cell area in each animal were compared with the mean for the normal population available from previous studies as described above.

Control animals

The intraperitoneal administration of GM_1 to normal rats for 30 days significantly altered the mean size of cholinergic neurons in several sides of the basal nucleus and medial septal nucleus in three individual animals. Thus, while a number of individual values were in the large normal range, some values significantly exceeded this, and the overall mean of cholinergic neurons in the basal nucleus was significantly larger than the normal mean.

Animals with unilateral lesions of the neocortex and hippocampus

The mean cell areas of cholinergic neurons in both the medial septal nucleus and basal nucleus (Fig. 13) on the operated side of each rat given GM_1 post-operatively for 30 days were within the normal ranges, as were the means for all three lesioned sides in each nucleus. In contrast, the mean cell areas of cholinergic neurons in both the medial septal nucleus and basal nucleus on the side opposite to the lesions of the cortex in each of these rats were significantly larger than those in normal animals, and this hypertrophy was of a magnitude similar to that seen in lesioned animals which had not been given GM_1. In addition, cell counts showed no significant reduction in the number of cholinergic neurons in the medial septal nucleus in lesioned animals given GM_1 as compared with an average loss of about 75% in lesioned but untreated animals (Fig. 14).

This study showed that chronic GM_1 ganglioside treatment completely prevented not only the retrograde shrinkage of cholinergic neurons in the basal forebrain but also the reduction in cell number in the septum which occurs in animals with

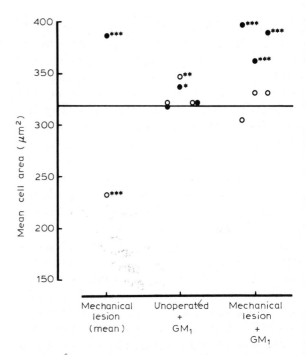

Fig. 13. Mean cross-sectional areas of cholinergic neurons in the basal nucleus of both sides following chronic administration of GM_1 ganglioside to unoperated animals or to animals undergoing mechanical lesion of the cerebral cortex of the left side. The bar at 319 μm^2 indicates the mean size of basal nucleus neurons in normal animals. The solid circles indicate the mean size of neurons on the side opposite, and the open circles that of the neurons on the same side as the lesioned cortex. The value for the mechanical lesion represents the mean of 10 animals whereas the other values represent individual animals. *, $p < 0.05$; **, $p < 0.01$; ***, $p < 0.001$ vs the normal mean.

unilateral ablation of the neocortex and hippocampus. In addition, such treatment resulted in a small but significant increase in the size of some basal forebrain cholinergic neurons in normal (i.e. unoperated) animals. This latter observation is perhaps not surprising, since a characteristic feature of the gangliosides is neuronal hypertrophy (Escourolle and Poirier, 1978). GM_1 treatment has also been reported to have a protective effect in reducing the degeneration of neurons in the substantia nigra following nigrostriatal transection (Toffano et al., 1984), and gangliosides have been shown to promote neurite outgrowth in culture and to facilitate sprouting during regeneration.

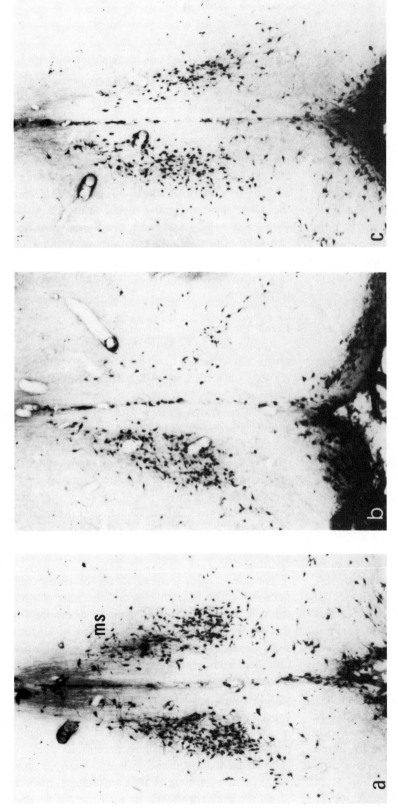

Fig. 14 (a–c). Frontal sections stained for ChAT through the medial septal nuclei of three different rats: (a) normal animal, (b) animal with the hippocampus removed on one side, (c) animal with the hippocampus removed on one side and treated chronically with GM₁ ganglioside. Note that hippocampal removal results in the loss of most of the cholinergic neurons in the ipsilateral medial septum and that this loss is prevented by chronic treatment with GM₁ ganglioside.

379

The possible mechanisms underlying these effects can only be speculated upon at this time. GM_1 is an important structural component of neuronal membranes, and the degenerative process which results in shrinkage may involve the rechanneling of substances into acutely needed metabolic pathways. The ready availability of an excess amount of a particular complex substance, such as the gangliosides, may thus protect the cell from some of the adverse effects of rechanneling available resources. In this context it is important to note that exogenously given GM_1 crosses the blood–brain barrier (Orlando et al., 1979) and can be incorporated into neuronal membranes (Toffano et al., 1984).

Fetal cortical graft studies

As described above, degeneration of cholinergic neurons can be induced retrogradely in the basal forebrain by lesions of the allo- or neocortex by application of excitotoxic amino acids and depleting these structures of intrinsic neurons. We therefore examined the possibility that replacing the neurons lost from cortex previously lesioned with KA with neurons in cell suspension grafts of fetal cortex will prevent the retrograde degeneration of basal forebrain cholinergic neurons, which normally accompanies such a lesion (Sofroniew et al., 1986c).

Three groups of experimental rats were examined in this study, normal controls, rats with KA applied as a powder to the dura overlying the cerebral cortex of one side as described above, and rats receiving cell suspension grafts of fetal cortex 4 days after application of KA to the dura of one side. Cell suspensions of fetal cortex were prepared using 14–16 mm fetuses. Grafts were placed by making several 0.1-μl injections of cell suspension into that portion of the cerebral cortex of one side underlying the dura which had been covered with KA 4 days previously. Rats from these three groups were fixed by perfusion 38–52 days post KA application for histological examination. Rats from these same groups have also been examined

at 10 and 30 days for biochemical determinations of marker enzymes in KA-lesioned and grafted cortex, as well as at 120 days post-operatively for connections made between host and graft using retrograde tracing as described in detail elsewhere (Isacson et al., 1986). Rats were perfused, sections prepared and immunohistochemically stained for ChAT, and neurons were measured in the basal nucleus as described above. The findings from these rats were compared using Student's *t* test with each other, and with previously obtained values from normal rats, from rats with unilateral mechanical lesions of the cerebral cortex, and from rats with application of KA and other substances to the dura.

Cerebral cortex

Application of KA to the dura resulted in a severe depletion of neurons from the underlying cortex with a disruption of cortical lamination as described above. In contrast, rats receiving cortical suspension grafts 4 days after KA application showed a pronounced increase of about 50–75% in local cortical depth (Fig. 15) at all survival times. The areas of grafted cortex did not show recognizable cortical lamination and appeared as large masses of cells. Staining for AChE showed numerous presumptive cholinergic fibers innervating these grafts.

Basal nucleus

The mean cross-sectional areas of cholinergic neurons in the basal nucleus of the four normal sides from the two normal animals examined for this study, as well of the overall mean of all four sides was not significantly different from the value obtained from a previous larger series of normal animals (Pearson et al., 1984). This previous mean was therefore used for comparison with the new experimental results. Extradural application of KA in the present study resulted in a significant reduction in the mean cross-sectional area of cholinergic neurons in the ipsilateral basal nucleus, while the size of those in the contralateral nucleus remained unchanged in a manner similar to that

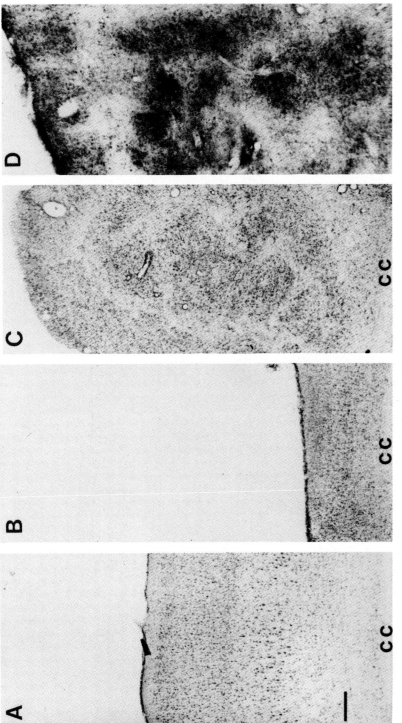

Fig. 15 (A–D). Photomicrographs of representative sections of cortex from an unoperated control side (A), from a KA-lesioned side 52 days after operation (B), and from a KA-lesioned rat that also received a cortical transplant 52 days after KA lesion (C), stained with cresyl-violet. A section from the same transplanted rat as in (C) stained for the acetylcholine-degrading enzyme acetylcholinesterase (D) shows a patchy fiber distribution within the cortical transplant. All photographs are at the same magnification; scale bar = 370 μm. cc, corpus callosum. (From Sofroniew et al., 1986c)

382

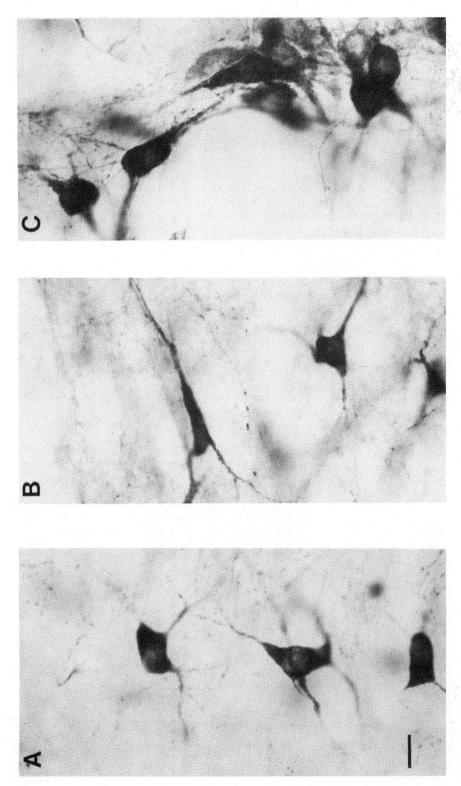

Fig. 16 (A–C). Photomicrographs from the dorsal central portion of the basal nucleus of sections stained with a monoclonal antibody directed against ChAT. Cholinergic neurons shown are from an unoperated control rat (A), a KA-lesioned rat, ipsilateral to the lesion (B), and a KA-lesioned rat that also received a cortical transplant (C). All photographs are of the same magnification; scale bar = 12.4 μm. (From Sofroniew et al., 1986c)

previously described (Sofroniew and Pearson, 1985) (Fig. 16). In all rats receiving cortical cell suspension grafts 4 days after extradural KA application, the mean cross-sectional areas of cholinergic neurons in both the ipsi- and contralateral basal nuclei were not significantly different from the overall mean in normal animals (Fig. 17).

These findings show that cell suspension grafts of fetal cortical cells into cerebral cortex previously lesioned with KA, can prevent the retrograde degeneration of cholinergic neurons in the ipsilateral basal nucleus which normally accompanies such a lesion. It is thought that this degeneration is transneuronal, i.e. secondary to a loss of neurons from the cortex rather than to direct damage of the afferent terminals of the cholinergic neurons in the cortex (Sofroniew and Pearson, 1985). This is

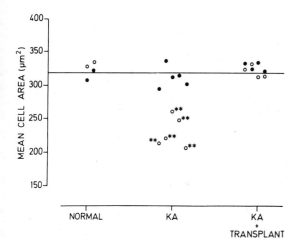

Fig. 17. Comparison of mean cross-sectional cell area of ChAT-positive neurons in the dorsal central portion of the basal nucleus from individual animals in three groups: (a) normal unoperated controls, (b) KA-lesioned rats, and (c) KA-lesioned rats that also received cortical suspension grafts into the cortex. Each symbol represents the mean value of 50 randomly sampled ChAT-positive cell bodies on both sides in each animal. The value for the left side, indicated by open circles, is the operated side in the experimental animals. The value for the contralateral unoperated side for each animal is indicated by solid circles. Corresponding left and right values are above each other. The horizontal line given at 319 μm^2 is the mean cross-sectional area of cholinergic neurons in the basal nucleus. Side differences for each animal, using Student's related t test, are indicated by **, $p < 0.001$. (From Sofroniew et al., 1986c)

further supported by the biochemical determination which showed a decrease in GAD but no decrease in ChAT in the cortical remnants 10 days post KA application. This indicates a severe reduction in the number of endogenous (GAD-producing) neurons with little or no reduction in the ChAT contained in afferent cholinergic fibers and terminals. Thus, the grafts were made into cortical tissue which had been severely depleted of neurons, but which still contained afferent cholinergic fibers, establishing a potential link between basal nucleus neurons and the cortical graft. Further evidence for such connections was obtained from retrograde tracing analysis with horseradish peroxidase, which showed that cholinergic basal forebrain neurons projected into the grafts (Isacson et al., 1986).

Together, these findings support the conclusion that cholinergic neurons of the basal forebrain receive a trophic influence from their target cortical neurons, that they will degenerate in the absence of this influence, and that grafted cortical neurons can substitute for endogenous neurons in providing this influence. The nature of this influence is in this specific case not known, but examples for retrogradely transported trophic factors are well documented in neurobiology (Thoenen and Barde, 1980). Indeed, it has been shown that nerve growth factor, which is normally produced in the cortex (Korsching et al., 1985), can be retrogradely transported from the cortex to the basal nucleus (Seiler and Schwab, 1984).

General discussion, summary and closing remarks

As described above, it is generally accepted that there are marked changes in the basal nucleus in AD brains, with a severe loss of large neurons in Nissl-stained sections and a loss of biochemically measured ChAT activity from the region which contains the nucleus. The studies presented here developed from the observation that cells of the basal nucleus undergo retrograde degeneration following cortical damage in monkey and man which is similar in appearance to that seen in AD.

384

In our initial experimental studies we found that cholinergic cells in the rat basal nucleus shrink following mechanical lesions of the cortex but do not die, while cells in the medial septum died after lesion of the hippocampus. Parallel to these studies we found in a case of AD that ChAT-positive neurons in the basal nucleus were shrunken, but undiminished in number, compared with an age- and sex-matched control brain. These findings do not exclude the possibility that significant cell loss may be present in cases of AD with presenile onset or in cases of AD with longer histories, but they clearly demonstrate that clinical AD can occur without significant cell loss from the basal nucleus. To investigate further whether or not such an effect might be the result of factors initially affecting cortical neurons as opposed to directly disturbing afferent fibers to the cortex, additional experiments were conducted in which lesions were made in the cortex of experimental animals with the excitotoxic amino acids, KA or NMAA. This resulted in a similar shrinkage, suggesting that the cholinergic neurons of the basal nucleus will not only undergo retrograde degeneration following mechanical lesions which damage their terminals directly, but will also undergo a similar retrograde degeneration transneuronally, i.e. secondary to a loss of neurons in the cortex without an initial direct insult to the terminals. Lastly, we examined several means by which such experimentally induced retrograde degeneration might be prevented. In these studies, we found that treatment with GM_1 ganglioside not only prevents the shrinkage of these cholinergic neurons following mechanical damage to the allo- or neocortex, but also prevents the retrograde cell death induced by ablation of the hippocampus, which further supports the growing body of evidence that gangliosides may have a protective influence on injured neurons and may promote repair and regeneration. In addition, we found that cell suspension grafts of fetal cortical neurons into the cerebral cortex of adult animals lesioned with excitotoxic amino acids completely prevented the retrograde degeneration of cholinergic neurons, which normally accompanies such a lesion. This further supported the evidence that basal forebrain cholinergic neurons receive a trophic influence from their target cortical neurons that they will degenerate in the absence of this influence, and indicates that grafted cortical neurons can substitute for endogenous neurons in providing this influence.

In conclusion, although it cannot yet be determined whether or not the observed changes involving cholinergic neurons in the basal nucleus in AD are the primary pathology or are secondary to changes in the cerebral cortex, retrograde cell degeneration can occur in the nucleus in the human brain after cortical damage, and the studies presented here showed marked similarities between the findings in brains with AD and those in the experimental animals with mechanical or chemical lesions in the cortex. The possibility of a retrograde effect upon the basal nucleus in AD can, therefore, not be excluded. It has been proposed that the pathology in AD spreads along known interneuronal connections. The findings presented here clearly raise the possibility that the degeneration of neurons in the basal nucleus observed in AD might be secondary to a process which directly affects the axons of these neurons within the cortex, or might be a consequence of the pathological processes known to affect cortical neurons in this disease.

References

Abercrombie, M. (1946) Estimation of nuclear populations from microtome sections. *Anat. Rec.*, 94: 239–247.

Agnati, L. F., Fuxe, K., Calza, L., Benfenati, F., Cavicchioli, L., Toffano, G. and Goldstein, M. (1983) Gangliosides increase the survival of lesioned nigral dopamine neurons and favour the recovery of dopaminergic synaptic function in striatum of rats by collateral sprouting. *Acta Physiol. Scand.*, 119: 347–363.

Anderton, B. H., Breinburg, D., Downes, M. J., Green, P. J., Tomlinson, B. E., Ulrich, J., Wood, J. N. and Kahn, J. (1982) Monoclonal antibodies show that neurofibrillary tangles and neurofilaments share antigenic determinants. *Nature (Lond.)*, 298: 84–86.

Arendt, T., Bigl, V., Arendt, A. and Tennstadt, A. (1983) Loss of neurons in the nucleus basalis of Meynert in Alzheimer's disease, paralysis agitans and Korsakoff's disease. *Acta Neuropathol. (Berl.)*, 61: 101–108.

Arendt, T., Bigl, V., Tennstadt, A. and Arendt, A. (1985) Neuronal loss in different parts of the nucleus basalis is related to neuritic plaque formation in cortical target areas in Alzheimer's disease. *Neuroscience*, 14: 1–14.

Armstrong, D. M., Saper, C. B., Levey, A. I., Wainer, B. H. and Terry, R. D. (1983) Distribution of cholinergic neurons in rat brain: demonstrated by the immunocytochemical localization of choline acetyltransferase. *J. Comp. Neurol.*, 216: 53–68.

Bailey, N. T. J. (1959) *Statistical Methods in Biology*, Edinburgh University Press, Edinburgh, p. 191.

Bigl, V., Woolf, N. J. and Butcher, L. L. (1982) Cholinergic projections from the basal forebrain to frontal, parietal, temporal, occipital and cingulate cortices: a combined fluorescent tracer and acetylcholinesterase analysis. *Brain Res. Bull.*, 8: 727–749.

Bowen, D. M., Smith, C. B., White, P. and Davison, A. N. (1976) Neurotransmitter-related enzymes and indices of hypoxia in senile dementia and other abiotrophies. *Brain*, 99: 459–496.

Brissaud, E. (1893) *Anatomie du Cerveau de l'Homme, Morphologie des Hemisphères Cérébraux ou Cerveau Proprement Dit*, Masson, Paris.

Brockhaus, H. (1942) Vergleichend-anatomische Untersuchungen über den Basalkernkomplex. *J. Psychol. Neurol.*, 51: 57–95.

Brodall, A. (1981) *Neurological Anatomy in Relation to Clinical Medicine*. Oxford University Press, New York.

Ceccarelli, B., Aporti, F. and Finesso, M. (1976) Effects of brain gangliosides on functional recovery in experimental regeneration and reinnervation. *Adv. Exp. Med. Biol.*, 21: 275–293.

Corsellis, J. A. N. (1976) Ageing and the dementias. In W. Blackwood and J. A. N. Corsellis (Eds.), *Greenfield's Neuropathology*, 3rd Edn. Edward Arnold, London, pp. 796–848.

Coyle, J. T. and Schwarcz, R. (1983) The use of excitatory amino acids as selective neurotoxins. In A. Björklund and T. Hökfelt (Eds.), *Handbook of Chemical Neuroanatomy, Methods in Chemical Neuroanatomy, Vol. 1*, Elsevier, Amsterdam, pp. 508–527.

Dahl, D., Selkoe, D. J., Pero, R. T. and Bignami, A. (1982) Immunostaining of neurofibrillary tangles in Alzheimer's senile dementia with a neurofilament antiserum. *J. Neurosci.*, 2: 113–119.

Dahlstrom, A. (1968) Effect of colchicine on transport of amine storage granules in sympathetic nerves of rat. *Eur. J. Pharmacol.*, 5: 111–112.

Daitz, H. M. and Powell, T. P. S. (1954) Studies on the connexions of the fornix system. *J. Neurol. Neurosurg. Psychiat.*, 17: 75–82.

Davies, P. and Maloney, A. J. F. (1976) Selective loss of central cholinergic neurons in Alzheimer's disease. *Lancet*, 2: 1403.

Divac, I. (1975) Magnocellular nuclei of the basal forebrain project to neocortex, brain stem and olfactory bulb. Review of some functional correlates. *Brain Res.*, 93: 385–398.

Eckenstein, F. and Sofroniew, M. V. (1983) Identification of central cholinergic neurons containing both choline acetyltransferase and acetylcholinesterase and of central neurons containing only acetylcholinesterase. *J. Neurosci.*, 3: 2286–2291.

Eckenstein, F. and Thoenen, H. (1982) Production of specific antisera and monoclonal antibodies to choline acetyltransferase: characterization and use for identification of cholinergic neurons. *EMBO J.*, 1: 363–368.

Escourolle, R. and Poirier, J. (1978) *Manual of Basic Neuropathology*, W. B. Saunders, Philadelphia.

Forel, A. H. (1907) *Gesammelte hirnanatomische Abhandlungen mit einem Aufsatz über die Aufgaben der Neurobiologie*, Reinhardt, Munich.

Gabella, G. (1984) Size of neurons and glial cells in the intramural ganglia of the hypertrophic intestine of the guinea-pig. *J. Neurocytol.*, 13: 73–84.

Gajdusek, D. C. (1985) Hypothesis: interference with axonal transport of neurofilament as a common pathogenetic mechanism in certain diseases of the central nervous system. *N. Engl. J. Med.*, 312: 714–719.

Goldschmidt, R. B. and Steward, O. (1980) Time course of increases in retrograde labeling and increases in cell size of entorhinal cortex neurons sprouting in response to unilateral entorhinal lesions. *J. Comp. Neurol.*, 189: 359–379.

Gorio, A., Carmignoto, G., Facci, L. and Finesso, M. (1980) Motor sprouting induced by ganglioside treatment. Possible implication for gangliosides on neuronal growth. *Brain Res.*, 197: 236–241.

Grunthal, E. (1932) Vergleichend anatomische Untersuchungen über den Zellbau des Globus pallidus und Nucleus basalis der Saüger und des Menschen. *J. Psychol. Neurol.*, 44: 403–428.

Guldin, W. O. and Markowitsch, H. J. (1982) Epidural kainate, but not ibotenate, produces lesions in local and distant regions of the brain. A comparison of the intracerebral actions of kainic acid and ibotenic acid. *J. Neurosci. Meth.*, 5: 83–93.

Hendrickson, A. and Dineen, J. T. (1982) Hypertrophy of neurons in dorsal lateral geniculate nucleus following striate cortex lesions in infant monkeys. *Neurosci. Lett.*, 30: 217–222.

Henke, H. and Lang, W. (1983) Cholinergic enzymes in neocortex, hippocampus and basal forebrain on non-neurological and senile dementia of Alzheimer-type patients. *Brain Res.*, 267: 218–231.

Hepler, D. J., Olton, D. S., Wenk, G. L. and Coyle, J. T. (1985) Lesions in nucleus basalis magnocellularis and medial septal area of rats produce qualitatively similar impairments. *J. Neurosci.*, 5: 866–873.

386

Herndon, R. M., Coyle, J. T. and Addicks, E. (1980) Ultrastructural analysis of kainic acid lesion to cerebellar cortex. *Neuroscience*, 5: 1015–1026.

Houser, C. R., Crawford, G. D., Barber, R. P., Salvaterra, P. M. and Vaughn, J. E. (1983) Organization and morphological characteristics of cholinergic neurons: an immunocytochemical study with a monoclonal antibody to choline acetyltransferase. *Brain Res.*, 266; 97–119.

Isacson, O., Sofroniew, M. V. and Bjorklund, A. (1986) Biochemical and histochemical studies on grafts of fetal cortical neurons to cerebral cortex lesioned with excitotoxic amino acids, in preparation.

Johnston, M. V., McKinney, M. and Coyle, J. T. (1981) Neocortical cholinergic innervation: a description of extrinsic and intrinsic components in the rat. *Exp. Brain Res.*, 43: 159–172.

Jones, E. G., Burton, H., Saper, C. B. and Swanson, L. W. (1976) Midbrain, diencephalic and cortical relationships of the basal nucleus of Meynert and associated structures in primates. *J. Comp. Neurol.*, 167: 385–420.

Kievit, J. and Kuypers, H. G. J. M. (1975) Subcortical afferents to the frontal lobe in the rhesus monkey studied by means of retrograde horseradish peroxidase transport. *Brain Res.*, 85: 261–266.

Koelle, G. B. (1954) The histochemical localization of cholinesterases in the central nervous system of the rat. *J. Comp. Neurol.*, 100: 211–235.

Koelliker, A. (1896) *Handbuch der Gewebelehre des Menschen. Vol. 2.* Leipzig, p. 456.

Korsching, S., Auburger, G., Heumann, R., Scott, J. and Thoenen, H. (1985) Levels of nerve growth factor and its mRNA in the central nervous system of the rat correlate with cholinergic innervation. *EMBO J.*, 4: 1389–1393.

Kreutzberg, G. (1969) Neuronal dynamics and flow. IV. Blockage of intra-axonal enzyme transport by colchicine. *Proc. Natl. Acad. Sci. USA*, 62: 722–728.

Ledeen, R. W. (1978) Ganglioside structure and distribution: are they located at the nerve ending? *J. Supramol. Struct.*, 8: 1–17.

Lehmann, J., Nagy, J. I., Atmadja, S. and Fibiger, H. C. (1980) The nucleus basalis magnocellularis: the origin of a cholinergic projection to the neocortex of the rat. *Neuroscience*, 5: 1161–1174.

Levey, A. I., Wainer, B. H., Mufson, E. J. and Mesulam, M. M. (1983) Co-localization of acetylcholinesterase and choline acetyltransferase in the rat cerebrum. *Neuroscience*, 9: 9–22.

Mesulam, M. M. and Van Hoesen, G. W. (1976) Acetylcholinesterase-rich projections from the basal forebrain of the Rhesus monkey to neocortex. *Brain Res.*, 109: 152–157.

Mesulam, M. M., Mufson, E. J., Levey, A. I. and Wainer, B. H. (1983) Cholinergic innervation of cortex by the basal forebrain: cytochemistry and cortical connections of the septal area, diagonal band nuclei, nucleus basalis (substantia innominata) and hypothalamus in the rhesus monkey. *J. Comp. Neurol.*, 214: 170–197.

Meynert, T. (1872) Vom Gehirn der Säugetiere. *Stricker's Handbuch der Lehre von den Geweben des Menschen und der Thiere, Vol. 2*, Engelmann, Leipzig, pp. 694–838.

Miyamoto, M., Shintani, M., Nagaoka, A. and Nagawa, Y. (1985) Lesioning of the rat basal forebrain leads to memory impairments in passive and active avoidance tasks. *Brain Res.*, 328: 97–104.

Nagai, T., McGeer, P. L., Peng, J. H., McGeer, E. G. and Dolman, C. E. (1983) Choline acetyltransferase immunohistochemistry in brains of Alzheimer's disease patients and controls. *Neurosci. Lett.*, 36: 195–199.

Nakano, I. and Hirano, A. (1983) Neuron loss in the nucleus basalis of Meynert in parkinsonism-dementia complex of Guam. *Ann. Neurol.*, 13: 87–91.

Nissl, F. (1892) Über die Veränderungen der Ganglienzellen am Facialiskern des Kaninchens nach Ausreissung der Nerven. *Allg. Z. Psychiat.*, 48: 197–198.

Nittono, K. (1923) On bilateral effects from the unilateral section of branches of the nervus trigeminus in the albino rat. *J. Comp. Neurol.*, 35: 133–161.

Orlando, P., Cocciante, G., Ippolito, G., Massari, P., Roberti, S. and Tettamanti, G. (1979) The fate of tritium-labelled GM_1 ganglioside injected in mice. *Pharmacol. Res. Commun.*, 11: 759–773.

Pearson, R. C. A., Gatter, K. C., Brodal, P. and Powell, T. P. S. (1983a) The projection of the basal nucleus of Meynert upon the neocortex in the monkey. *Brain Res.*, 259: 132–136.

Pearson, R. C. A., Gatter, K. C. and Powell, T. P. S. (1983b) Retrograde cell degeneration in the basal nucleus in monkey and man. *Brain Res.*, 261: 321–326.

Pearson, R. C. A., Gatter, K. C. and Powell, T. P. S. (1983c) The cortical relationships of certain basal ganglia and the cholinergic basal forebrain nuclei. *Brain Res.*, 261: 327–330.

Pearson, R. C. A., Sofroniew, M. V., Cuello, A. C., Powell, T. P. S., Eckenstein, F., Esiri, M. M. and Wilcock, G. K. (1983d) Persistence of cholinergic neurons in the basal nucleus in a brain with senile dementia of the Alzheimer's type demonstrated by immunohistochemical staining for choline acetyltransferase. *Brain Res.*, 289: 375–379.

Pearson, R. C. A., Sofroniew, M. V. and Powell, T. P. S. (1984) Hypertrophy of immunohistochemically identified cholinergic neurons of the basal nucleus of Meynert following ablation of the contralateral cortex in the rat. *Brain Res.*, 311: 194–198.

Pearson, R. C. A., Sofroniew, M. V. and Powell, T. P. S. (1985a) Hypertrophy of cholinergic neurons of the rat basal nucleus following section of the corpus callosum. *Brain Res.*, 338: 337–340.

Pearson, R. C. A., Esiri, M. M., Hiorns, R. W., Wilcock, G. K. and Powell, T. P. S. (1985b) Anatomical correlates of the distribution of the pathological changes in the neocortex in

Alzheimer's disease. *Proc. Natl. Acad. Sci. USA*, 82: 4531–4535.

Pearson, R. C. A., Sofroniew, M. V. and Powell, T. P. S. (1986) The cholinergic nuclei of the basal forebrain of the rat: hypertrophy following contralateral cortical damage or section of the corpus callosum. *Brain Res.*, in press.

Perry, E. K., Perry, R. H., Blessed, G. and Tomlinson, B. E. (1977) Necropsy evidence of central cholinergic deficits in senile dementia. *Lancet*, 1: 189.

Perry, R. H., Candy, J. M., Perry, E. K., Irving, D., Blessed, G., Fairbairn, A. F. and Tomlinson, B. E. (1982) Extensive loss of choline acetyltransferase activity is not reflected by neuronal loss in the nucleus of Meynert in Alzheimer's disease. *Neurosci. Lett.*, 33: 311–315.

Price, J. L. and Powell, T. P. S. (1970) An experimental study of the origin and the course of the centrifugal fibres to the olfactory bulb in the rat. *J. Anat.*, 107: 215–237.

Rapport, M. M. and Gorio, A. (Eds.) (1981) *Gangliosides in Neurological and Neuromuscular Function, Development and Repair*, Raven Press, New York.

Rossor, M. N., Garrett, N. J., Johnson, A. L., Mountjoy, C. Q., Roth, M. and Iversen, L. L. (1982a) A post-mortem study of the cholinergic and GABA systems in senile dementia. *Brain*, 105: 313–330.

Rossor, M. N., Svendsen, C., Hunt, S. P., Mountjoy, C. Q., Roth, M. and Iversen, L. L. (1982b) The substantia innominata in Alzheimer's disease: an histochemical and biochemical study of cholinergic marker enzymes. *Neurosci. Lett.*, 28: 217–222.

Seiler, M. and Schwab, M. E. (1984) Specific retrograde transport of nerve growth factor (NGF) from neocortex to nucleus basalis in the rat. *Brain Res.*, 300: 33–39.

Shute, C. C. D. and Lewis, P. R. (1967) The ascending cholinergic reticular system: neocortical, olfactory and subcortical projections. *Brain*, 90: 497–520.

Sims, N. R., Bowen, D. M., Allen, S. J., Smith, C. C. T., Neary, D., Thomas, D. J. and Davison, A. N. (1983) Presynaptic cholinergic dysfunction in patients with dementia. *J. Neurochem.*, 40: 503–509.

Sofroniew, M. V. (1983) Golgi-like immunoperoxidase staining of neurons producing specific substances or of neurons transporting exogenous tracer proteins. In A. C. Cuello (Ed.), *Immunohistochemistry*, John Wiley, New York, pp. 431–447.

Sofroniew, M. V. and Pearson, R. C. A. (1985) Degeneration of cholinergic neurons in the basal nucleus following kainic or *N*-methyl-D-aspartic acid application to the cerebral cortex in the rat. *Brain Res.*, 339: 186–190.

Sofroniew, M. V., Eckenstein, F., Thoenen, H. and Cuello, A. C. (1982) Topography of choline acetyltransferase-containing neurons in the forebrain of the rat. *Neurosci. Lett.*, 33: 7–12.

Sofroniew, M. V., Pearson, R. C. A., Eckenstein, F., Cuello, A. C. and Powell, T. P. S. (1983) Retrograde changes in cholinergic neurons in the basal forebrain of the rat following cortical damage. *Brain Res.*, 289: 370–374.

Sofroniew, M. V., Campbell, P., Cuello, A. C. and Eckenstein, F. (1985) Central cholinergic neurons visualized by immunohistochemical detection of choline acetyltransferase. In G. Paxinos and C. Watson (Eds.), *The Rat Nervous System. Vol. 1. Forebrain and Midbrain.*, Academic Press, Sydney, pp. 471–485.

Sofroniew, M. V., Pearson, R. C. A. and Powell, T. P. S. (1986a) The cholinergic nuclei of the basal forebrain of the rat: normal structure, development and experimentally induced degeneration. *Brain Res.*, in press.

Sofroniew, M. V., Pearson, R. C. A., Cuello, A. C., Tagari, P. C. and Stevens, P. H. (1986b) Parenterally administered GM₁ ganglioside prevents retrograde degeneration of cholinergic cells of the rat basal forebrain. *Brain Res.*, in press.

Sofroniew, M. V., Isacson, O. and Bjorklund, A. (1986c) Cortical grafts prevent atrophy of cholinergic basal nucleus neurons induced by excitotoxic cortical damage. *Brain Res.*, 378: 409–415.

Swanson, L. W. and Cowan, W. M. (1979) The connections of the septal region in the rat. *J. Comp. Neurol.*, 186: 621–656.

Tagliavini, F., Pilleri, G., Gemignani, F. and Lechi, A. (1983) Neuronal loss in the basal nucleus of Meynert in progressive supranuclear palsy. *Acta Neuropathol. (Berl.)*, 61: 157–160.

Thoenen, H. and Barde, Y. A. (1980) Physiology of nerve growth factor. *Physiol. Rev.*, 60: 1284–1335.

Toffano, G., Savoini, G. E., Moroni, F., Lombardi, M. G., Calza, L. and Agnati, L. F. (1983) GM₁ ganglioside stimulates the regeneration of dopaminergic neurons in the central nervous system. *Brain Res.*, 261: 163–166.

Toffano, G., Savoini, G. E., Moroni, F., Lombardi, G., Calza, L. and Agnati, L. F. (1984) Chronic GM₁ ganglioside treatment reduces dopamine cell body degeneration in the substantia nigra after unilateral hemitransection in rat. *Brain Res.*, 296: 233–239.

Von Buttlar-Brentano, K. (1952) Pathohistologische Feststellungen am Basalkern Schizophrener. *J. Nerv. Ment. Dis.*, 116: 646–653.

Watson, W. E. (1965) An autoradiographic study of the incorporation of nucleic acid precursors by neurons and glia during nerve regeneration. *J. Physiol. (Lond.)*, 180: 741–753.

Watson, W. E. (1968) Observations on the nucleolar and total cell body nucleic acid of injured nerve cells. *J. Physiol. (Lond.)*, 196: 655–676.

Whitehouse, P. J., Price, D. L., Struble, R. G., Clark, A. W., Coyle, J. T. and DeLong, M. R. (1982) Alzheimer's disease and senile dementia: loss of neurons in the basal forebrain. *Science*, 215: 1237–1239.

Wilcock, G. K. and Esiri, M. M. (1982) Plaques, tangles and dementia, a quantitative study. *J. Neurol. Sci.*, 56: 343–356.

Wojcik, M., Ulas, J. and Oderfeld-Nowak, B. (1982) The stimulating effect of ganglioside injections on the recovery of choline acetyltransferase and acetylcholinesterase activities in the hippocampus of the rat after septal lesions. *Neuroscience*, 7: 495–499.

Woolf, N. J. and Butcher, L. L. (1982) Cholinergic projections to the basolateral amygdala: a combined Evans Blue and acetylcholinesterase analysis. *Brain Res. Bull.*, 8: 751–763.

Zambotti, V., Tettamanti, G. and Arrigoni, M. (1972) *Glycolipids, Glycoproteins, and Mucopolysaccharides of the Nervous System*, Plenum Press, New York.

Discussion

A. BJÖRKLUND: How do you reconcile your observations on cell shrinkage in the basal nucleus of Alzheimer patients with reports from other labs of an actual cell loss?

M. V. SOFRONIEW: There are now several studies by different authors in which cell loss or the absence of cell loss is reported in the basal forebrain in AD using staining procedures for AChE or ChAT. Our own study showed no cell loss, but a generalized cell shrinkage of ChAT-positive cells so that these cells might well have been beneath the size limit for 'large' basal forebrain neurons as identified in Nissl stained pathological sections. They would thus have not been counted and would have contributed to the impression of cell loss if analyzed using a Nissl stain. Thus, one thing to consider when comparing results is the procedure used, i.e. Nissl stains versus histochemical stains. Nevertheless, there are also histochemical studies which report cell loss, and as more information is collected, several important points seem to be emerging. It seems likely that AD may not represent a homogenous pathological entity in that differences may be observed in the basal forebrain in relation to age of the patient at onset of the disease and duration of the disease prior to death. Furthermore, as shown by Arendt et al., (1985) regional differences within the basal forebrain exist as regards the severity of the pathology observed, and these regional differences are correlated with severity of the pathology observed in the corresponding allo- or neocortex to which they project. This brings me to our main point: of consequence is not establishing whether or not cell shrinkage *or* cell death occurs, since it is likely that both occur, but rather determining whether or not these changes in the basal forebrain occur as a primary pathology, or are merely changes which occur secondary to the pathology of the allo- or neocortex to which the cholinergic neurons project.

P. D. COLEMAN: *Comment*: the issue of neuronal death or survival after lesion of terminal fields was studied a number of years ago by Jerzy Rose in thalamo-cortical systems. He described two classes of axonal projections: essential, which were essential to the survival of neurons, and sustaining which were not required for neuronal survival, but did contribute to neuronal resistance to retrograde degeneration after lesion of other portions of its axonal projection. He did not have available the methods to visualize details of terminal field configuration but his basic concepts may well be germane to the present discussion.

K. IQBAL: How long after the surgical lesion was ganglioside GM_1 administered?

M. V. SOFRONIEW: Ganglioside was given beginning with the day of surgery and was given daily thereafter until the animals were perfused.

D. M. GASH: Is it necessary to continue GM_1 ganglioside treatment in lesioned animals to maintain neuronal survival, or do the neurons at risk become stabilized by relatively short-term treatment?

M. V. SOFRONIEW: This is something we have not yet tested. In our initial experiments presented here we examined only the effect of chronic treatment with ganglioside.

D. F. SWAAB: Is cell shrinkage preceding cell loss in time? How is the ratio between these two phenomena changing with time?

M. V. SOFRONIEW: It is of course difficult to answer this with certainty since we cannot follow specific cells in time but can only analyze populations of cells at certain points in time. Given this limitation it seems that yes, in those areas where cell death occurs, it appears to be preceded by cell shrinkage in so far as the size of the population of cells decreases before the number does.

J. M. PALACIOS: Do you think there is a trophic factor in the cortex 'responsible' for the size of the neurons in the basal forebrain? Are you aware of any attempt to isolate this factor or to use cell free extracts to compensate for the effects in basal forebrain neurons?

M. V. SOFRONIEW: It does seem likely that cortical neurons have a trophic influence upon cholinergic neurons in the basal forebrain, in that destruction of cortical neurons or of connections between basal forebrain and cortex leads to the degeneration of the cholinergic neurons whereas this degeneration does not occur if depleted endogenous cortical neurons are replaced by grafts of fetal cortical cells. The nature of this trophic influence is not clear. It may or may not be a chemical factor. In this context it is of interest to note that NGF (nerve growth factor) has been shown to be produced in the cortex (Korsching et al., 1985) and to be retrogradely transported by basal forebrain neurons (Seiler and Schwab, 1984). I also believe a chemical factor has been identified in hippocampal extracts which has a trophic effect on septal neurons.

A. J. CROSS: Have you studied retrograde changes in other neurons projecting to the neocortex such as the locus ceruleus or raphe nuclei? Are these changes specific to the cholinergic system?

M. V. SOFRONIEW: In some of our initial animals with mechanical lesions of neocortex on one side we also looked at neurons in the locus ceruleus stained for tyrosine hydroxylase. In these we also found some cell shrinkage which was bilateral in this nucleus. We have not yet had time to sufficiently analyse all the data we have, but it seems likely that such changes are not confined to the cholinergic system.

J. KORF: What happened with the levels of acetylcholinesterase or choline acetyltransferase in your preparation in which the cortex was exposed to kainic acid? Are the observed changes similar to those seen in the cortex of Alzheimer's disease?

M. V. SOFRONIEW: A study examining this is just being completed (Isacson et al., 1986). Basically there is little initial change in the levels of these enzymes in the cortex at 4 or 10 days post treatment, but there is a decrease in activity after 30 or more days. In AD the cortex shows decreased activities of these enzymes.

For references see list on pp. 384–387.

D. F. Swaab, E. Fliers, M. Mirmiran, W. A. Van Gool and F. Van Haaren (Eds.)
Progress in Brain Research, Vol. 70.
© 1986 Elsevier Science Publishers B.V. (Biomedical Division)

CHAPTER 24

Scrapie and its association with 'amyloid-like' fibrils and glycoproteins encoded by cellular genes: an animal model for human dementia

J. Goudsmit[a] and F. W. Van der Waals

[a]*Virology Department, Academic Medical Center, Meibergdreef 9, 1105 AZ Amsterdam ZO, The Netherlands*

Introduction

Alzheimer's disease (AD) is generally considered the most frequent cause of dementia in the Western world. The discovery by Gajdusek et al. (1966) and Gibbs et al. (1968) that two chronic degenerative diseases of the brain, kuru and Creutzfeldt-Jakob disease (CJD) could be transmitted to non-human primates led the way to a worldwide search for transmissible agents in other chronic diseases of the central nervous system of unknown etiology, like AD.

In 1959, Hadlow brought the similarity between scrapie in sheep and kuru in man to the attention of the scientific community stating that "one might surmise that the pathogenetic mechanisms involved in scrapie — however unusual they may be — are unlikely to be unique in the province of animal pathology".

In this review we will illustrate the similarities and differences between the human dementias, CJD and AD and scrapie. Subsequently, the elegance of the hamster-scrapie model for human dementia will be outlined.

Clinical, pathological and epidemiological similarities between Alzheimer's disease and Creutzfeldt-Jakob disease

CJD closely resembles AD in course and duration of clinical disease (Brown et al., 1979; Masters et al., 1981) and the characteristic EEG changes of CJD may occur in typical AD cases (Ehle and Johnson, 1977). Senile plaques and neurofibrillary tangles, pathological hallmarks of AD, are occasionally seen in CJD (Traub et al., 1977) and spongiform change, a hallmark of CJD, may be present in AD (Flament-Durand and Couck, 1979; Mancardi et al., 1981). Both AD and CJD occur in approximately 10% of the cases within families with an autosomal pattern of inheritance (Masters et al., 1981; Goudsmit et al., 1981). Coexistence of AD and CJD in families has been reported as well as conjugal cases (Masters et al., 1981). Familial CJD can be transmitted to non-human primates as easily as sporadic CJD. Finally, brain suspensions from patients with familial AD contain a factor inducing *in vitro* cell-fusion in almost the same frequency as CJD (Fig. 1) (Moreau-Dubois et al., 1981). These observations indicate a strong similarity between the extremely rare dementia CJD and the most frequent form of dementia of man, AD.

Transmissibility of Creutzfeldt-Jakob disease, Alzheimer's disease and scrapie to laboratory animals

Transmission of CJD to non-human primates has been accomplished repeatedly by inoculating animals intracerebrally with suspensions of brain tissue (Goudsmit et al., 1980) with the same success

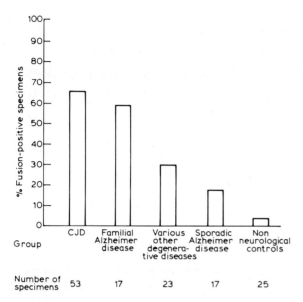

Fig. 1. Frequency of in vitro cell fusion induced by brain suspensions from patients with CJD, AD and various other neurological and non-neurological diseases. (From Moreau-Dubois et al., 1981)

TABLE I

Attempts to transmit Alzheimer's disease to non-human primates[a]

	Familial Alzheimer's disease	Sporadic Alzheimer's disease
Positives (unrepeated)	2	0
Negatives	12	45

[a]Results through June 1982. Except as noted, all inocula were supernatants from 2 000-rpm centrifuged 1–20% ground brain suspensions, given as 0.1–0.3 ml intracerebral inoculations. Most specimens were inoculated into at least two animals. (From Brown et al., 1982)

rate as primary transmissions of kuru to primates and of scrapie to sheep, mice and hamsters. In all of these cases the clinical and pathological features of the inoculated animals closely resembled the disease in the natural host from which the inoculum was taken. In addition, experimental kuru and CJD is almost indistinguishable from experimental scrapie in the same host. Unfortunately, the transmissibility of AD to laboratory animals has been shown to be unsuccessful (Goudsmit et al., 1980; Brown et al., 1982). Table I shows the attempts to transmit AD to non-human primates. Of the 45 attempts to transmit sporadic AD to chimpanzees none of the inoculated animals showed signs of AD after a duration exceeding more than two standard deviations of the mean incubation period of experimental CJD in the same species. Of the 14 attempts to transmit familial AD 12 were negative according to the criteria mentioned before, while two brain suspensions of familial AD cases induced a spongiform encephalopathy in the inoculated animal, but not AD (Goudsmit et al., 1980). These two transmissions

could not be repeated. Table II shows the details of the confusing transmission experiments with tissues of the latter two AD cases.

These data indicate that AD cannot be induced in non-human primates like CJD, although some similarities between the two dementias exist. This leaves CJD as the only dementia that is transmissible to laboratory animals. Only if the changes in the brain of CJD- and scrapie-inoculated animals are in any respect comparable to the changes in the brain of AD patients, these animal models are of any value for the understanding of AD.

Host range and clinical signs of experimental scrapie and Creutzfeldt-Jakob disease

Both CJD and scrapie can be transmitted to Old- and New-World monkeys, to goats, guinea pigs, hamsters and mice (Gibbs et al., 1979). However, strain variation occurs, resulting in significant differences in incubation period, host range, duration and type of clinical disease. In addition, these parameters may change during passage. On the other hand, one has to realize that the neuropathological findings resulting from either scrapie or CJD inoculation are virtually indistinguishable. Spongiform encephalopathy remains the hallmark of both scrapie and CJD in the natural and

TABLE II

Cases of Alzheimer's disease inoculated into non-human primates with transmission of a spongiform encephalopathy[a]

Patient	Inoculum source[b]	Primate host	Route of inoculation[c]	Date of inoculation	Duration (months)	Neuro-pathology
A.Yo.	Brain + LSHK	Chimpanzee	ic,iv,sc[d]	1968	166	
	Brain + LSHK	Squirrel	ic,iv,sc[d]	1968	23 (died)	Pos
	Brain + LSHK	Cynomolgous	ic,iv,sc[d]	1968	30 (died)[e]	Neg
	Brain	Squirrel	ic,iv	1973	46 (died)[e]	Neg
	Brain	Squirrel	ic,iv	1973	52 (died)[e]	Neg
	Brain	Chimpanzee	ic,iv	1975	84	
	Brain	Afr. Green	ic,iv	1975	88	
	Brain	Afr. Green	ic,iv	1975	88	
	Brain	Cynomolgous	ic,iv	1975	88	
	Brain	Cynomolgous	ic,iv	1975	88	
	Brain	Rhesus	ic,iv	1975	88	
	Brain	Capuchin	ic,iv	1975	88	
	Brain	Capuchin	ic,iv	1975	88	
	Brain	Spider	ic,iv	1975	61 (died)[e]	Neg
	Brain	Spider	ic,iv	1975	88	
	Brain	Squirrel	ic,iv	1975	88	
B.Ha.	Brain bx	Squirrel	ic,iv	1972	29 (died)	Pos
	Brain bx	Capuchin	ic,iv	1972	40 (died)	Pos
	Brain bx	Chimpanzee	ic,iv	1975	61 (died)[e]	Neg
	Brain bx	Capuchin	ic	1975	33 (died)[e]	Neg
	Brain bx	Squirrel	ic	1975	83	
	Urine	Capuchin	ic	1976	42 (died)[e]	Neg
	Urine	Squirrel	ic	1976	70	
	Feces	Squirrel	ic	1976	70	
	Saliva	Squirrel	ic	1976	70	

[a]Five animals dying of non-neurologic intercurrent illnesses less than 1 year after inoculation are not included in the Table.
[b]LSHK, liver, spleen, heart, kidney.
[c]ic, intracerebral; iv, intravenous; sc, subcutaneous. All inocula were supernates from 2 000 rpm centrifuged 10% ground tissue suspensions.
[d]Inoculated ic and iv with brain suspension and sc with a pool of the visceral suspensions.
[e]Non-neurologic illness.
(From Brown et al., 1982)

experimental host. Variation occurs in distribution of the lesions and, for instance, amyloid plaque formation, like in kuru. Clinically, experimental scrapie mimics experimental CJD (Manuelidis and Manuelidis, 1979).

For all these reasons and to avoid, for safety sake, to work with human agents, the best animal model for CJD appears to be the scrapie-infected hamster. For practical purposes one likes to take a strain of agents with high infectivity and short incubation time. The scrapie strain 263K, isolated by Kimberlin and Walker, with a very short incubation time (± 50–70 days) and over 1 000 times more infectivity than any typical CJD isolate (Kimberlin and Walker, 1978), serves this goal best. Clinically, scrapie induced by the 263K strain in hamsters can be diagnosed without difficulty, based on locomotor symptoms (jerks and ataxia) and differences in behaviour (activity and rearing) (Goudsmit et al., 1983) (Fig. 2).

394

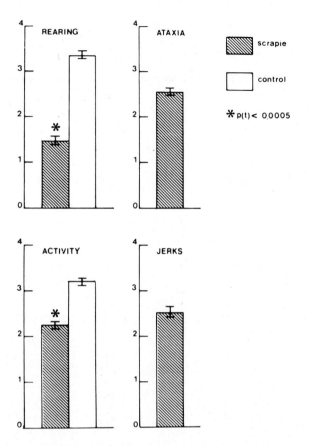

Fig. 2. Locomotor symptoms (jerks and ataxia) of scrapie-infected hamster and differences in behaviour (activity and rearing) between scrapie-infected and control animals at 60–70 days after inoculation. *, $p(t) = 0.0005$; error bars: SE of the means. (From Goudsmit et al., 1983)

Nature of the scrapie agent

Scrapie infectivity is dependent on protein (Prusiner et al., 1981), ruling out the possibility that the scrapie agent is a viroid composed exclusively of nucleic acid. Radiosensitivity of viruses is a function of both nucleic acid mass and strandedness, but not exclusively as is suggested in the 'target' theory. The 'target' theory assumes a direct relationship between virus size and radiosensitivity (Rohwer, 1984). Comparison of the radiosensitivity of viruses of known nucleic acid size and the radiosensitivity of the scrapie agent places scrapie

with the smaller viruses not requiring a sub-viral size to plot the data (Rohwer, 1984) (Fig. 3). In accord with these findings the ability of the scrapie agent to penetrate a gel is shared by conventional viruses (Rohwer, 1984). Recently, a unique RNA species of approximately 100 bases (4.3S) has been reported to be associated with scrapie infectivity (Dees et al., 1985). These findings are compatible with a virus-like agent composed of protein and nucleic acid either replicating by virally or host-encoded enzymes (Dickinson and Outram, 1979; Eklund et al., 1963; Merz et al., 1983). On the other hand it rules out that the scrapie agent is a proteinaceous infectious particle (prion) composed of protein alone and replicating by reverse translation or protein-directed protein synthesis (Prusiner, 1982).

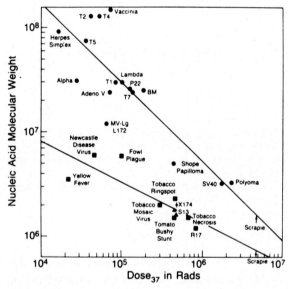

Fig. 3. Radiosensitivity of viruses as a function of the molecular weight of nucleic acids. The reciprocals of the inactivation rate constant are plotted against the molucular weight of the nucleic acid component of the virus, obtained where possible from sequence or restriction enzyme data. ●, Double-stranded DNA viruses; ■, single-stranded RNA viruses; ▲, single-stranded DAN viruses. Separate regression lines have been drawn through the double-stranded and single-stranded virus data. (From Rohwer, 1984)

Filamentous structures associated with Creutzfeldt-Jakob disease and scrapie in natural and experimental hosts

Scrapie-associated fibrils (SAF) are first observed in scrapie-infected mouse brains by negative stain electron microscopy (Merz et al., 1981). Subsequently, SAF has been shown to be present in human CJD and sheep scrapie as well as in experimental CJD, kuru and scrapie in primates, and experimental scrapie in mice and hamsters (Merz et al., 1984). SAF are absent from brains of ALS and AD patients, although amyloid and paired helical filaments, the hallmarks of AD show a striking similarity with SAF (Fig. 4). Recently it has been shown that a polyclonal antibody to SAF identifies 70% of CJD specimens by immunoblot analysis, while a specific ELISA for SAF could be developed based on the same polyclonal antibody (Brown et al., 1986). It is also possible to identify SAF in tissue slides by immunocytochemistry following proteinase K treatment (Merz, personal communication).

A proteinase K-resistant glycoprotein with M_r 27 000–30 000 is a major component of SAF in CJD and scrapie

Bolton et al. (1982) reported that a diffuse protein band in polyacrylamide gel of relative molecular

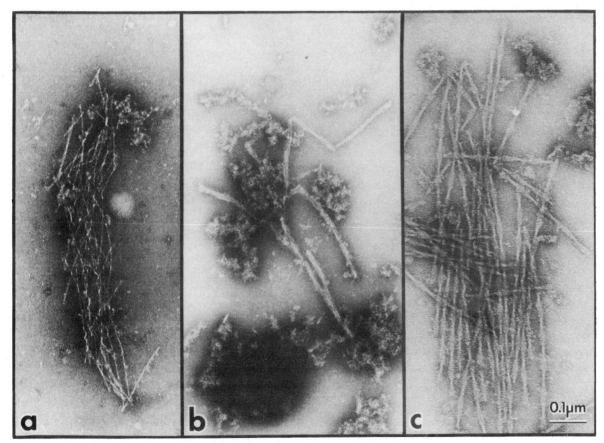

Fig. 4. Amyloid (a), scrapie-associated fibrils (b) and paired helical filaments (c) after negative staining and electron microscopy (×86 000). (From Van der Waals and Goudsmit, 1985)

mass (M_r) 27 000–30 000 was present in scrapie brain preparations and not in control preparations. This protein was shown to be proteinase K resistant. A protein with a similar M_r (26 000–30 000) was subsequently shown to be present in preparations of purified hamster scrapie (Diringer et al., 1983) and associated with infectivity. An antigenically related protein with similar M_r is present in brain preparations of CJD in man and experimental CJD in laboratory animals

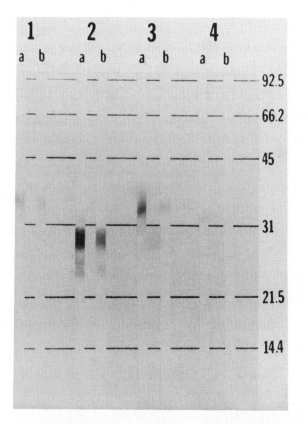

Fig. 5. Immunoblots of control and scrapie-infected hamster brain preparations. Proteins were extracted with 0.1% sarkosyl and aliquots were electrophoreses into SDS 12% polyacrylamide gels, transferred on to nitrocellulose paper, immunoblotted with rabbit anti-PrP 27–30, followed by horseradish peroxidase conjugated goat anti-rabbit IgG. Extracts from scrapie-infected brain (lanes 1 and 2) and normal brain (lanes 3 and 4) are shown. Proteinase K digested samples are shown in lanes 2 and 4. Western blots were performed with PrP 27–30 antisera (lanes denoted (a)) and affinity-purified PrP 27–30 antibodies (lanes denoted (b)). (From Oesch et al., 1985)

(Bendheim et al., 1985; Manuelidis et al., 1985; Brown et al., 1986). Fig. 5 (Oesch et al., 1985) shows clearly that before proteinase K treatment antigenically related proteins of M_r 33 000–35 000 are present in both infected and control brain preparations. After treatment of the brain preparation with proteinase K, the proteins of normal brain are completely digested while in scrapie brain preparations partially degraded proteins of M_r 27 000–30 000 and 23 000–26 000 are still present. The deduced amino acid sequence of this protein has a hydrophobic C terminus and a strech of hydrophobic animo acids near the N terminus confining a region with potentially beta structure (Oesch et al., 1985). SAF, similar to cerebral amyloid, shows green-red birefringence after staining with Congo red (Glenner et al., 1974), a property attributed to domains with a high degree of beta structure (Glenner et al., 1972). This has led (Prusiner et al., 1983) to the hypothesis that amyloid in scrapie, CJD and even in AD is infectious. However, no evidence for this far-reaching conclusion is available (Goudsmit et al., 1980).

The question remains of what distinguishes these proteins in scrapie-infected brain from a similar protein in normal brain. In scrapie-infected brain these proteins undergo most likely some kind of post-translational change, that makes them partially resistant to proteinase K, for instance glycosylation. This accords very well with the recent finding that p27–30 is a sialoglyco protein (Bolton et al., 1985).

Scrapie-associated glycoprotein is encoded by a cellular gene present in normal brain

Oesch et al. (1985) have succeeded in selecting a DNA clone encoding p27–30 from a scrapie-infected hamster brain cDNA library by oligonucleotide probes corresponding to the N terminus of the protein. Using this DNA as probe, normal as well as infected brain DNA showed specific hybridisation in hamsters, mice and man. p27–30-related mRNA was also found at the same level in normal and scrapie-infected brain.

No p27–30 nucleic acids were found in purified preparations of scrapie agent, suggesting that p27–30 is not encoded by a particle-associated nucleic acid.

The presence of SAF and proteinase K resistant protein p27–30 in the brain appears to be a common pathological feature of CJD and scrapie, and most likely reflects enhanced and aberrant expression of cellular genes present in normal tissues like brain, heart, lung, spleen and kidney (Oesch et al., 1985).

Summary and conclusions

CJD in humans can be considered a cerebral amyloidosis with SAF as ultrastructural hallmark. As such, the similarity of CJD and AD, with PHF as ultrastructural characteristic, is obvious. CJD is transmissible to laboratory animals and AD is not.

Scrapie and CJD induce apparently enhanced expression of cellular genes and aberrant post-translational processes resulting in deposits of SAF in the brain. Although the disease-inducing factors may differ between AD and CJD, similar pathogenetic processes to CJD can easily be envisioned for AD, leading to formation and deposition of amyloid and neurofibrillary tangles. In a recent paper, Gajdusek (1985) suggested that the common pathogenetic mechanism in AD and CJD may be the interference with axonal transport of neurofilament.

Future studies should be aimed at establishing the antigenic relatedness between amyloid, paired helical filaments, SAF and neurofilaments. In addition the pathogenesis of these beta structure proteins, for instance with respect to interference with axonal transport of neurofilament, should be a priority in dementia studies.

Scrapie, so easily transmissible to small rodents, serves as a good model for CJD, while, in addition, it may shed new light on the development of amyloid and neurofibrillary tangles in AD/SDAT.

References

Bendheim, P. E., Bockman, J. M., McKinley, M. P., Kingsbury, D. T. and Prusiner, S. B. (1985) Scrapie and Creutzfeldt-Jakob disease prion proteins share physical properties and antigenic determinants. *Proc. Natl. Acad. Sci. USA*, 82: 997–1001.

Bolton, D. C., McKinley, M. P. and Prusiner, S. B. (1982) Identification of a protein that purifies with the scrapie prion. *Science*, 218: 1309–1311.

Bolton, D. C., Meyer, R. K. and Prusiner, S. B. (1985) Scrapie PrP 27–30 is a sialoglycoprotein. *J. Virol.*, 53: 596–606.

Brown, P., Cathala, F., Sadowsky, D. and Gajdusek, D. C. (1979) Creutzfeldt-Jakob disease in France. II. Clinical characteristics of 124 consecutive verified cases during the decade 1968–1977. *Ann. Neurol.*, 6: 5, 430–437.

Brown, P., Salazas, A. M., Gibbs, Jr, C. J. and Gajdusek, D. C. (1982) Alzheimer disease and transmissible virus dementia. *Ann. NY Acad. Sci.*, 396: 131–143.

Brown, P., Coker-Vann, M., Pomeroy, K., Asher, D. M., Gibbs, C. J. and Gajdusek, D. C. (1986) Immunological diagnosis of Creutzfeldt-Jakob disease. *N. Engl. J. Med.*, in press.

Dees, C., McMillan, B. C., Wade, W. F., German, T. L. and Marsh, R. F. (1985) Characterization of nucleic acids in membrane vesicles from scrapie-infected hamster brain. *J. Virol.*, 55: 126–132.

Dickinson, A. G. and Outram, G. (1979) The scrapie replication-site hypothesis and its implications for pathogenesis. In S. B. Prusiner and W. J. Hadlow (Eds.), *Slow Transmissible Diseases of the Nervous System, Vol. 2*, Academic Press, New York, pp. 13–31.

Diringer, H., Gelderblom, H., Hilmert, H., Ozel, M., Edelbluth, C. and Kimberlin, R. H. (1983) Scrapie infectivity, fibrils and low molucular weight protein. *Nature*, 306: 476–478.

Ehle, A. L. and Johnson, P. C. (1977) Rapidly evolving EEG changes in a case of Alzheimer's disease. *Ann. Neurol.*, 1: 593–595.

Eklund, C. M., Hadlow, W. J. and Kennedy, R. C. (1963) Some properties of the scrapie agent and its behavior in mice. *Proc. Soc. Exp. Biol. Med.*, 112: 974–979.

Flament-Durand, J. and Couck, A. M. (1979) Spongiform alterations in brain biopsies of presenile dementia. *Acta Neuropathol. (Berl.)*, 46: 159–162.

Gajdusek, D. C. (1985) Hypothesis: interference with axonal transport of neurofilament as a common pathogenic mechanism in certain diseases of the central nervous system. *N. Engl. J. Med.*, 312: 714–719.

Gajdusek, D. C., Gibbs, C. J. Jr. and Alpers, M. (1966) Experimental transmission of a kuru-like syndrome to chimpanzees. *Nature*, 209: 5025, 794–796.

Gibbs, C. J. Jr., Gajdusek, D. C., Asher, D. M., Alpers, M. P., Beck, E., Daniel, P. M. and Mathews, W. B. (1968) Creutzfeldt-Jakob disease (subacute spongiform encephalo-

398

pathy): transmission to the chimpanzee. *Science*, 161: 3839, 388–389.

Gibbs, C. J. Jr., Gajdusek, D. C. and Amyx, H. (1979) Strain variation in the viruses of Creutzfeldt-Jakob disease and kuru. In S. B. Prusiner and W. J. Hadlow (Eds.), *Slow Transmissible Diseases of the Nervous System, Vol. 2*, Academic Press, New York, pp. 87–110.

Glenner, G. G., Eanes, E. D. and Page, D. L. (1972) The relation of the properties of Congo red-stained amyloid fibrils to the β-conformation. *J. Histochem. Cytochem.*, 20: 821–826.

Glenner, G. G., Eanes, E. D., Bladen, H. A., Linke, R. P. and Termine, J. D. (1974) β-plated sheet fibrils. A comparison of native amyloid with synthetic protein fibrils. *J. Histochem. Cytochem.*, 22: 1141–1158.

Goudsmit, J., Morrow, C. H., Asher, D. M., Yanagihara, R. T., Masters, C. L., Gibbs, C. J. Jr. and Gajdusek, D. C. (1980) Evidence for and against the transmissibility of Alzheimer's disease. *Neurology*, 30: 9, 945–950.

Goudsmit, J., White, B. J., Weitkamp, L. R., Keats, B. J., Morrow, C. H. and Gajdusek, D. C. (1981) Familial Alzheimer's disease in two kindreds of the same geographic and ethnic origin: a clinical and genetic study. *J. Neurol. Sci.*, 49: 1, 79–89.

Goudsmit, J., Rohwer, R. G., Silbergeld, E. K., Neckers, L. M. and Gajdusek, D. C. (1983) Scrapie in hamsters: clinical disease and disturbances in the serotonergic pathway. In Court and F. Cathala (Eds.), *Virus Non-conventionnels et Affections du Système Nerveux Central*, Masson, Paris, pp. 453–476.

Hadlow, W. J. (1959) Scrapie and kuru. Lancet, ii: 289–290.

Kimberlin, R. H. and Walker, C. (1978) Evidence that the transmission of one source of scrapie agent to hamsters involves separation of agent strains from a mixture. *J. Gen. Virol.*, 39: 487–496.

Mancardi, G. L., Mandybur, T. I. and Liwncz, B. H. (1981) Ultrastructural study of the spongiform-like abnormalities in Alzheimer's disease. *J. Neuropathol. Exp. Neurol.*, 40: 360.

Manuelidis, E. E. and Manuelidis, L. (1979) In S. B. Prusiner and W. J. Hadlow (Eds.), *Slow Transmissible Diseases of the Nervous System, Vol. 2*, Academic Press, New York, pp. 147–173.

Manuelidis, L., Velley, S. and Manuelidis, E. E. (1985) Specific proteins associated with Creutzfeldt-Jakob disease and

scrapie share antigenic and carbohydrate determinants. *Proc. Natl. Acad. Sci. USA*, 82: 4263–4267.

Masters, C. L., Gajdusek, D. C. and Gibbs, C. J. Jr. (1981) The familial occurrence of Creutzfeldt-Jakob disease and Alzheimer's disease. *Brain*, 104: 3, 535–558.

Merz, P. A., Somerville, R. A., Wisniewski, H. M. and Iqbal, K. (1981) Abnormal fibrils from scrapie-infected brains. *Acta Neuropathol.*, 54: 63–74.

Merz, P. A., Somerville, R. A., Wisniewski, H. M. and Manuelidis, E. E. (1983) Scrapie-associated fibrils in Creutzfeldt-Jakob disease. *Nature (Lond.)*, 306: 474–476.

Merz, P. A., Rohwer, R. G., Wisniewski, H. M., Somerville, R. A., Gibbs, C. J. Jr. and Gajdusek, D. C. (1984) Infection specific particle from the unconventional slow virus diseases. *Science*, 225: 437–440.

Moreau-Dubois, M. C., Brown, P., Goudsmit, J., Cathala, F. and Gajdusek, D. C. (1981) Biological distinction between sporadic and familial Alzheimer disease by an in vitro cell fusion test. *Neurology*, 31: 3, 323–326.

Oesch, B., Westaway, D., Wälchli, M., McKinley, M. P., Kent, S. B., Aebersold, R., Barry, R. A., Tempst, P., Teplow, D. B., Hood, L. E., Prusiner, S. B. and Weissmann, C. (1985) A cellular gene encodes scrapie PrP 27-30 protein. *Cell*, 40: 735–746.

Prusiner, S. B. (1982) Novel proteinaceous infectious particles cause scrapie. *Science*, 216: 136–144.

Prusiner, S. B., McKinley, M. P., Groth, D. F., Bowman, K. A., Mock, N. I., Cochran, S. P. and Mariarz, F. R. (1981) Scrapie agent contains a hydrophobic protein. *Proc. Natl. Acad. Sci. USA*, 78: 6675–6679.

Prusiner, S. B., McKinley, M. P., Bowman, K. A., Bolton, D. C., Bendheim, P. E., Groth, D. F. and Glenner, G. G. (1983) Scrapie prions aggregate to form amyloid-like birefringent rods. *Cell*, 35: 349–358.

Rohwer, R. G. (1984) Scrapie infectious agent is virus-like in size and susceptibility to inactivation. *Nature (Lond.)*, 308: 658–662.

Traub, R., Gajdusek, D. C. and Gibbs, C. J. Jr. (1977) Transmissible virus dementia: The relation of transmissible spongiform encephalopathy to Creutzfeldt-Jakob disease. In M. Kinsbourne and L. Smith (Eds.), *Aging and Dementia*, Spectrum Publ. Flushing, New York, pp. 91–172.

Van der Waals, F. W. and Goudsmit, J. (1985) Characteristics of the CJD agent: new perspectives of the pathogenesis of dementia. *Ned. Tijdschr. Gen.*, 129: 1275–1280, in Dutch.

D. F. Swaab, E. Fliers, M. Mirmiran, W. A. Van Gool and F. Van Haaren (Eds.)
Progress in Brain Research, Vol. 70.
© 1986 Elsevier Science Publishers B.V. (Biomedical Division)

CHAPTER 25

Aluminum: a role in degenerative brain disease associated with neurofibrillary degeneration

D. R. Crapper McLachlan and M. F. A. Van Berkum

Departments of Physiology and Medicine, Faculty of Medicine, University of Toronto, Toronto, Ontario, Canada

Introduction

Concentrations of aluminum which are toxic to many biochemical processes are found in at least 10 human neurological conditions (Crapper McLachlan and DeBoni, 1980). However, four primary neurodegenerative conditions of late adult life are of particular interest: senile and presenile dementia of the Alzheimer type, Down syndrome with Alzheimer disease, the Guam parkinsonism-dementia complex (PD) and Guam amyotrophic lateral sclerosis (ALS). Each of these diseases is linked by two important markers: (1) neurons exhibit neurofibrillary degeneration composed of aggregates of 10 nm paired helical filaments; (2) neurons with neurofibrillary degeneration contain elevated concentrations of aluminum.

A number of independent studies have demonstrated aluminum to occur in high concentration in the presence of neurofibrillary degeneration of the Alzheimer type (Crapper et al., 1973, 1976, 1980; Trapp et al., 1978; Perl and Brody, 1980; Perl et al., 1982; Garruto et al., 1984; Masters et al., 1985; Yoshimasu et al., 1985). Aluminum has also been detected in the amyloid cores of senile plaques by Duckett and Galle (1976), Candy et al., (1986) and Masters et al. (1985). The latter two groups report that aluminum complexed with silicon and aluminum silicate appears to form the insoluble residue of both amyloid of senile plaques and the neurofibrillary tangle. The contribution of aluminum to the pathogenesis of these diseases has remained uncertain. One interpretation attributes the accumulation of aluminum in neurons with neurofibrillary degeneration to an increase in cation binding sites within degenerating neurons and therefore of trivial significance. An alternative interpretation postulates that aluminum may play an active role in the pathogenesis of the disease and contribute to the molecular disorders which eventually result in altered function and cell death. The weight of evidence now favors the latter possibility.

A satisfactory hypothesis explaining the etiology or pathogenesis of any of the diseases associated with neurofibrillary degeneration has not yet been advanced. Several observations, however, suggest that environmental factors may contribute to the degenerative process. Head injury has been implicated as a risk factor for Alzheimer disease (Mortimer et al., 1985; Heyman et al., 1984) and a factor in the neurofibrillary associated condition, dementia pugilistica (Corsellis, 1978). Alzheimer type neurofibrillary degeneration may also occur in a number of other diseases, many of which are

---

Correspondence to: D. R. McLachlan, Department of Physiology, Room 3318, Medical Sciences Building, University of Toronto, Toronto, Ontario, Canada M5S 1A8.

related to environmental or infectious agents (Wisniewski et al., 1979).

The strongest evidence in support of an environmental factor in the pathogenesis of neurofibrillary diseases arises from the epidemiological studies of Guam PD/ALS syndromes. An initial working hypothesis of one investigative team (Reed et al., 1966) was that the world-wide distribution of PD/ALS was due to rare genetic traits or mutations and that the exceptionally high occurrence in Guam was due to a highly penetrant form in an isolated population. However, several epidemiological studies have failed to support either a genetic or an infectious etiology for these diseases (Reed et al., 1966; Reed and Brody, 1975). The unusual geographic distribution of the diseases in Guam strongly implicated environmental factors as the cause. Two additional geographic loci of high incidence of similar neurodegenerative illness have also been described: the Auyu and Jakai people of Irian New Guinea (Gajdusek and Salazar, 1982) and certain regions of the Kii peninsula of Japan (Yase, 1977). Epidemiological studies in these loci also support environmental determinants, perhaps through the food chain.

The possibility that trace elements might be important in the etiology of the Guam and Kii peninsula cases was suggested by Yase and his co-workers (Yase, 1977, 1980). These workers postulated that a low intake of calcium induces a secondary hyperparathyroidism with calcium deposition in vulnerable central nervous system tissues along with the deposition of manganese, lead and aluminum. The combined insult of calcium deprivation and environmental exposure to toxic trace metals was postulated to result in neural degeneration. Recent general support for this hypothesis has been advanced by Yanagihara et al. (1984). These hypotheses regard the neurodegenerative process to result from an interaction of several processes and do not assign a specific role to aluminum. The evidence outlined below, however, indicates that aluminum may have a central role in the pathogenesis of the degenerative process.

Aluminum bioavailability

Aluminum is a highly reactive trivalent cation existing in a number of hydrated species and organic and inorganic complexes. Consideration of atomic properties and metal ion solution chemistry led Nieboer and Richardson (1980) to classify aluminum and calcium in the same category. These ions prefer similar ligands and are 'oxygen seeking'. Blaustein and Goldman (1968) found the aluminum effects upon sodium and potassium voltage sensitive conductance in excitable neuronal membranes under voltage clamp conditions to resemble calcium at physiological concentrations. Indeed aluminum acted as 'super calcium'. The high charge density of Al(III) ($e/r = 5.88$) gives aluminum ionic bonds greater covalent characteristics resulting in slow dissociation rates for bound aluminum. Furthermore, precise determination of aluminum bioavailability, especially in a physiological environment where numerous natural aluminum ligands exist, is complex and difficult to achieve (Haug, 1984). Both silicon and fluorine form insoluble complexes with aluminum and influence the availability of aluminum in water supplies and biological fluids (Iler, 1979). Plant ligands such as the flavinoids, organic acids, food additives and medicinal preparations are important sources of aluminum (Lione, 1983).

Aluminum absorption is dependent on pH (Kaehny et al., 1977), and the solubility of aluminum compounds (Litman, 1967; Cam et al., 1976). In rat inverted jejunum preparations, aluminum absorption also depends on oxidative phosphorylation, glucose and temperature, suggesting an energy-dependent, carrier-mediated mechanism with maximal aluminum absorption in the absence of calcium (Feinroth et al., 1982). This supports an earlier report of increased aluminum absorption in Ca/Mg deficient diets (Yase, 1980).

Further, aluminum absorption and retention is increased in rats treated with parathyroid hormone (PTH) (Mayor et al., 1980a,b), while in chickens, treatment with 1,25-$(OH)_2$ D_3, the active metabolite of vitamin D, increases brain aluminum content

(Long et al., 1980). Dietary zinc deficiency also increases aluminum absorption in the gut (Wenk and Stemmer, 1983) while fluoride decreases aluminum absorption (Still and Kelley, 1980).

In dogs, 60–70% of plasma aluminum is carried by transferrin (Trapp, 1983), 10% to 20% by albumin and the remaining 20% is ultrafiltrable (Kovalchik et al., 1980). The half-life of a single injection of aluminum was 276 min with 10–20% of serum aluminum removed in the first 150 min by renal excretion (Henry et al., 1984). Serum calcium levels increased 15% after 2 weeks of injections (1 mg/kg) but serum immunoreactive PTH content and PTH response to an EDTA-induced hypocalcemia remained unaltered (Henry et al., 1984).

The brain, therefore, is well protected from aluminum by: (1) environmental bioavailability; (2) selective absorption in the gut; (3) rapid binding to plasma proteins, especially transferrin and albumin; and (4) renal and probably bile excretion of plasma aluminum.

To be absorbed by neurons, aluminum must first penetrate the blood–brain barrier (Bradbury, 1984), and several lines of evidence suggest that competence of this barrier varies widely among mammalian species. Compared to cats or rabbits, rodents and primates are relatively resistant to the encephalopathic effects of either intravenous or intracranial injections of aluminum (King et al., 1975). Rodents also have a greater capacity to rapidly remove aluminum from the brain. It is hypothesized that normal human, and probably rodent brain, contain either a natural barrier or a physiological ligand of high capacity capable of protecting both the glial and neuronal compartments from aluminum toxicity. We postulate defects in these protective mechanisms in neurodegenerative diseases associated with neurofibrillary degeneration, perhaps genetic or possibly acquired with aging, which result in the release of the toxic properties of aluminum.

Aluminum neurotoxicity

Aluminum affects a remarkably large number of nuclear, cytoplasmic, membrane and synaptic functions. An up-to-date review of the several mechanisms of aluminum neurotoxicity appears elsewhere (Crapper et al., 1985). Of the many disturbances in cellular function known to result from aluminum intoxication, the effects upon calcium homeostasis and neurofilament transport appear to be particularly important to the neurodegenerative diseases associated with neurofibrillary degeneration.

Aluminum effects on calcium homeostasis

Tissue calcium content

Yoshimasu and co-workers (1976) and Yase (1977, 1980), employing neutron activation, reported an increase in both calcium and aluminum in the spinal cord from cases of ALS from Guam and the Kii peninsula of Japan. These workers speculated that metallic ions such as aluminum may alter calcium transport. X-ray emission studies by Perl and Brody (1980), Perl et al. (1982) and Garruto et al. (1984) demonstrated that aluminum and calcium were markedly elevated in both the nucleus and cytoplasm of neurons with neurofibrillary degeneration but manganese, magnesium, silicon and iron were not elevated. Since calcium accumulation occurs in injured and degenerating tissues in all body organs, the occurrence of increased concentrations of aluminum and calcium in neurons with neurofibrillary degeneration might be considered non-specific. However, in healthy brain tissues of rabbits a single intracranial injection of aluminum results in a delayed, progressive, rise in total brain calcium content (Farnell et al., 1985). The rise in tissue calcium correlates well with the progressive behavioral and motor abnormalities of the encephalopathy (Farnell et al., 1985).

Total tissue calcium content of control, age-matched, rabbit prosencephalon is 263 μg/g dry weight as measured by atomic absorption or inductively coupled plasma emission spectroscopy. About 7 to 10 days after aluminum injection, or at the end of the early, asymptomatic stage of the encephalopathy the content had risen to 294 μg/g.

At the end of the second stage, characterized by learning-memory deficits and the appearance of minor motor control difficulties, the calcium content was 340 $\mu g/g$. When animals reach the third, or terminal, stage of the encephalopathy they exhibit major motor dysfunction and the average total tissue calcium content was found to be 550 $\mu g/g$. While the total sodium and magnesium content in the same tissue is not altered as the calcium rises, potassium concentration increased by 16% in the last stage of the encephalopathy (Van Berkum et al., in preparation).

The aluminum-induced changes in calcium content correlate strongly with alterations in neuronal electrical activity and the appearance of behavioral and neurological motor signs of the encephalopathy. In hippocampal slices removed from control and aluminum-injected rabbits at various stages of the encephalopathy, the normal relation between the population EPSP and the population CA 1 spike output potential was altered, indicating an increase in spike-generating threshold. The changes were partially reversed by increasing the calcium concentration in the bathing medium. Long-term potentiation was also affected in the encephalopathy. Long-lasting potentiation of electrical activity within the hippocampus has been postulated as the mechanism responsible for electrical changes observed in the hippocampus during classical conditioning (Berger et al., 1976, 1978). Calcium-dependent steps appear to be involved in the alterations in membrane properties which modify synaptic efficacy at presynaptic (Turner et al., 1982) and postsynaptic sites (Baudry and Lynch, 1980). A reduction in long-term potentiation occurs in the aluminum encephalopathy (Farnell et al., 1982) and is temporally related to the learning-memory changes which develop in the early middle stage of the encephalopathy (Crapper and Dalton, 1973; Petit et al., 1980; Rabe et al., 1982; Yokel, 1983). Farnell et al. (1985) demonstrated that modest depressions in long-term potentiation could be restored to control values when the concentration of calcium was increased in the bathing medium. Thus, aluminum disturbs not only the intracellular regulation of calcium but important calcium-dependent electrophysiological functions. Therefore, it is reasonable to consider aluminum causing the increase in calcium content found in human neurons with neurofibrillary degeneration. Furthermore, the aluminum-induced disorder in calcium metabolism may be partly responsible for the alterations in neuron functions underlying clinical dementia and neuron survival.

At present, two principal molecular mechanisms regulating intracellular calcium content are known to be disturbed in the brain by aluminum: one involves the important intracellular messenger, calmodulin; the other involves voltage-dependent calcium permeability in synaptic terminals.

Calmodulin and aluminum

Calmodulin (CaM) is a highly conserved ubiquitous protein with four high-affinity calcium-binding sites (Babu et al., 1985; Means et al., 1982). It has been implicated in a number of cellular functions including cyclic AMP regulation via both adenylate cyclase (Brontium et al., 1975) and 3',5'-cyclic nucleotide phosphodiesterase (Lin et al., 1974), regulation of calmodulin-dependent kinase activity (Schulman and Greengard, 1978) and interactions with both tubulin (Deerly et al., 1984) and actin (Weeds, 1982) to regulate the cytoskeleton.

Aluminum binds to CaM with 10 times higher affinity than calcium and induces a conformational change that reduces the alpha helical content by 30% and increases the total hydrophobic surface area 20-fold (Seigle and Haug, 1983a). This may alter CaM's ability to bind substrate proteins and disturb the equilibrium between cytosolic and membrane bound CaM. Both these conformational changes are quenched by EGTA or by pretreatment of CaM with citric acid. However, once aluminum binds to CaM, citric acid can only partially restore CaM to its native structure (Suhayda and Haug, 1984). It is doubtful that CaM, freed from aluminum, remains fully active because a net reduction in the alpha helical content prevails. Nevertheless in vivo, CaM may be partially protected from aluminum toxicity by endogenous citrate.

When aluminum binds to CaM at a 3:1 mole ratio (A1/CaM), CaM is unable to stimulate phosphodiesterase in vitro (Seigle and Haug, 1983a). Aluminum also inhibits CaM stimulation of Ca-Mg ATPase activity in barley root membranes at an A1/CaM mole ratio of 3:1 (Seigle and Haug, 1983b). This latter effect would result in an in vivo accumulation of intracellular Ca (Hincke and Demaille, 1984). Indeed, the activity of calmodulin as a calcium-calmodulin activator of the enzyme $3',5'$-cyclic nucleotide phosphodiesterase declined progressively in the rabbit brain as the aluminum encephalopathy developed (Farnell et al., 1985). For hippocampal extracts, the K_m for control tissue was 0.019 pM calmodulin, expressed in terms of calmodulin measured by radioimmune assay, and 0.038 pM in the middle stages of the encephalopathy. In the late stage, rabbit hippocampus required almost three times as much calmodulin to achieve the same rate of release of phosphorus as calmodulin extracted from control hippocampus, at a K_m value of 0.053 pM. Since calmodulin is a major intracellular receptor of calcium and mediator of many calcium effects in eukaryotes, the known effects of aluminum upon this pivotal molecule predict that the activity of calmodulin would no longer be regulated by calcium flux and other biochemical mechanisms would be altered in addition to the failure to maintain normal intracellular calcium concentration.

Aluminum and calmodulin gene expression

Following direct intracranial injection of a soluble aluminum salt, the metal rapidly associates with DNA containing nuclear structures (Crapper et al., 1980). In the human diseases with neurofibrillary degeneration, aluminum is also found in high concentration within the nucleus (Crapper et al, 1980; Perl and Brody, 1980; Perl et al., 1982; Garruto et al., 1984). Karlik et al. (1980) demonstrated an interaction of aluminum species with DNA, in vitro, supporting the hypothesis that intranuclear aluminum could alter, in vivo, gene expression directly as well as indirectly through the calcium-calmodulin pathway (Cheung, 1984).

Sarkander et al. (1983) and Matsumoto and Morimura (1980) studied the effects of aluminum on 'run-on' transcription of isolated chromatin spreads and observed a significant 50% decrease in template activity. The effect of aluminum upon transcription processes in the intact brain are complex. Van Berkum et al. (in preparation) using a quantitative dot blot hybridization assay have observed a 40% reduction in yield of calmodulin messenger RNA within 24 h of aluminum exposure. The reduction is observed when the data are expressed as the amount of CaM messenger (in intensity units) per g of tissue or as a percentage of total poly(A)+mRNA. Poly(A)+ messenger RNA content was measured in total iRNA extracts by a modification of the ^{3}H-poly(U) assay of Bantle and Hahn (1976). The calmodulin cDNA probe was generously provided by A. R. Means (Baylar College of Medicine, Houston, TX) in a collaborative study. Table I is based upon the analysis of 448 data points from 13 control and 18 aluminum-treated rabbits and indicates that the percentage of calmodulin message in the poly(A)+ population is markedly reduced 24 h after aluminum injection and remains low throughout the encephalopathy. There is partial escape from the inhibitory effect toward the late stages of the encephalopathy. We interpret the data to indicate that calmodulin gene expression is directly inhibited by aluminum.

The mechanism by which aluminum influences calmodulin gene expression has not yet been experimentally examined. However, considering the affinity of aluminum for intranuclear binding sites in both native DNA (Karlik et al., 1980) and chromatin (Crapper et al., 1980), aluminum may bind directly to: (1) the promoter/repressor regions of the calmodulin gene; (2) promoter/repressor signal proteins; or (3) interfere with the interaction of the promoter/repressor protein and the DNA binding site. Interestingly, in the 5' flanking regions

TABLE I

Day post injection	Intensity CaM/ng(A)						
	control	n	number of assays	Al-treated	n	number of assays	p $<$
1	0.32 ± 0.03^a	2	24	0.18 ± 0.01	2	24	p 0.007; ANOVA
3	0.27 ± 0.01	2	30	0.21 ± 0.01	4	60	p 0.007; ANOVA
7	0.29 ± 0.02	3	44	0.21 ± 0.01	5	76	p 0.007; ANOVA
10	0.26 ± 0.01	3	44	0.24 ± 0.01	4	54	0.08 p 0.09
12	0.27 ± 0.01	3	44	0.25 ± 0.01	3	43	0.08 p 0.09

Calmodulin messenger RNA measured in dot blot hybridization assay of iRNA prepared from rabbit cerebral tissue. Each dot was photometrically scanned, digitized and normalized to the absolute absorption of the filter. Poly(A) content ng(A) was measured by a ^{3}H-poly(U) assay.
[a]Standard error of the mean.

of the chicken calmodulin gene, between -69 and -58, a sequence having 67% homology with the metalothionine metal induction sequence, CNTTTGCNCNCG, has been observed (Searle et al., 1984; Simmen et al., 1985). This site potentially provides a locus for competitive interaction between calcium and aluminum.

Although the mechanism of escape from aluminum inhibition of CaM messenger production is also not understood, the escape occurs late in the encephalopathy when the tissue calcium content has risen to approximately 130% above control concentrations. One hypothesis of escape is that the depression of CaM message production results eventually in a reduction in the translation product. A reduction in cytoplasmic calmodulin would predict reduced calcium extrusion which in turn would increase intranuclear calcium. A rise in intranuclear calcium would tend to displace aluminum from the gene locus of inhibition. Displacement of aluminum from nuclear to cytoplasmic compartments, in the middle stages of the encephalopathy, is also consistent with the observation that during the middle and latter stages of the encephalopathy, extracted calmodulin becomes progressively less efficacious as a stimulator of phosphodiesterase in vitro (Farnell et al., 1985). Hence, the 'toxicity' of aluminum may become manifest only when the cytoplasmic levels begin to rise because the metal has a high affinity and profound effect upon the gene product, calmodulin.

Aluminum and synaptosome calcium conductance

Late in the encephalopathy, isolated synaptosome membrane preparations demonstrate a decrease in the voltage-induced calcium conductance mechanism. While the change has been observed late in the encephalopathy when intracellular calcium is elevated, the change is of such a magnitude that it is most probably related to a direct membrane effect rather than a secondary effect due to reduced electrochemical gradient for calcium or potassium.

Synaptosomes were isolated from age-matched control rabbit brains and from various stages of the encephalopathy by the methods of Kreuger et al. (1979) and Hajos (1975). In the presence of 5 mM potassium, the uptake of calcium for rabbit synaptosomes was 0.0455 nM/mg protein per min for control and 0.0401 nM/mg protein per min for the aluminum-treated preparations from the third stage of the encephalopathy ($p > 0.2$). Following depolarization in 75 mM potassium, the synaptosome membranes extracted from aluminum-treated animals demonstrated a 33% reduction in calcium uptake which was significant at the $p < 0.02$ level: control = 0.1355, ($n = 13$); aluminum 0.0897 nM/mg protein per min, ($n = 8$). Assuming that the in vitro synaptosomes had 210% higher ionic calcium content than control (Farnell et al., 1985), the reduction in the electrochemical gradient would reduce the influx of calcium by only 7%. While the intraneuronal calcium ion concentration in the aluminum encephalopathy has not yet been measured, the 33% reduction in voltage-dependent calcium influx is probably related to membrane calcium channel occlusion. Occlusion of voltage-dependent calcium channels could perform a homeostatic protective function and prevent further calcium influx. The molecular mechanisms responsible for the reduction in voltage-sensitive calcium channels may be the result of either a local membrane effect, for example: channel block, or an intranuclear effect of aluminum upon the genes responsible for voltage-dependent calcium channels, analogous to inhibition of the calmodulin gene. If future work supports the latter hypothesis, a specific effect upon electrically excitable neuron-specific genes would help explain why certain cells within the central nervous system exhibit such a high sensitivity to aluminum toxicity compared to other body organs, (Doellken, 1897).

Aluminum and the cytoskeleton

The alterations in calcium homeostasis occur in cells such as the hippocampal CA1 pyramidal-shaped neuron without concomitant morphological change (Farnell et al., 1982). However, there are several classes of neurons including pyramidally shaped neurons of the pyriform and neocortex and motor neurons which exhibit neurofibrillary degeneration. The neurofibrillary material is composed of 10-nm neurofilaments which exhibit evidence of hyperphosphorylation (Troncoso et al., 1985). However, the alterations which result in paired helical filament formation characteristic of the Alzheimer neurofibrillary tangle are not induced by aluminum in human neurons in tissue culture (Crapper et al., 1978). Recent evidence suggests that the accumulation of neurofilaments in the aluminum encephalopathy in the soma and proximal processes is related to a failure of anterograde movement into axons (Bizzi et al., 1984), possibly because hyperphosphorylation may have altered the mechanisms responsible for the transport of the neurofilaments (Sternberger et al., 1985). Recent evidence now favors the hypothesis that Alzheimer neurofibrillary tangles are composed of modified neurofilaments, although the exact mechanisms resulting in PHF formation remain unknown. The Alzheimer PHFs are also hyperphosphorylated, but the sites appear to differ somewhat from the sites phosphorylated in the aluminum encephalopathy (Sternberger et al., 1985). The role of the calcium-calmodulin system in the regulation of phosphorylation is widely recognized (Means et al., 1982). The role aluminum may play in the control of phosphorylation, either directly or through an effect on gene regulation, will be a fruitful area for future investigation.

This hypothesis argues that a selective defect in the blood–brain barrier permits aluminum to gain access in high concentration to certain neurons in Alzheimer's disease. Aluminum in solution has a number of nuclear, cytoplasmic and membrane toxic effects including deregulation of calcium homeostasis and neurofilament hyperphosphorylation. These toxic effects together with other yet to be defined disorders in AD are postulated to change the intraneuronal environment sufficiently to induce the formation of both neurofibrillary tangles and aluminum silicate. If, as speculated by Masters et al., the aluminum silicates assumed the structure of Montmorillonite clays, this inorganic matrix could exert an organization influence upon proteins and influence the structure of both amyloid and paired helical filaments.

Conclusion

The weight of evidence indicating that aluminum influences both genetic and cytoplasmic processes strengthens the hypothesis that aluminum may be actively involved in the promotion of neurofibrillary degeneration in human disease. The hypothesis is still incomplete, however, since many additional factors are undoubtedly operative in the induction of the paired helical conformation (De Boni and McLachlan, 1985) and initiation of the entire process. Application of recombinant DNA technology holds promise for the rapid identification of the alterations in gene expression which are driven by aluminum, those which are the result of yet to be identified environmental factors and those which are genetic.

Acknowledgements

This study was supported by the Ontario Mental Health Foundation and the Scottish Rite Charitable Foundation.

References

Babu, Y. S., Sack, J. S., Greenhough, T. J., Bugg, C. C., Means, A. R. and Cook, W. J. (1985) Three-dimensional structure of calmodulin. *Nature*, 315: 37–40.

Bantle, J. A. and Hahn, W. E. (1976) Complexity and characterization of polyadenylated RNA in the mouse brain. *Cell*, 8: 139–150.

Baudry, M. and Lynch, G. (1980) Hypothesis regarding the cellular mechanisms responsible for long-term synaptic potentiation in the hippocampus. *Exp. Neurol.*, 68: 202–204.

Berger, T. W. and Thompson, R. F. (1978) Neuronal plasticity in the limbic system during classical conditioning of the rabbit nictitating membrane response. I. The hippocampus. *Brain Res.*, 145: 323–346.

Berger, T. W., Alger, B. and Thompson, R. F. (1976) Neuronal substrate of classical conditioning in the hippocampus. *Science*, 192: 483–485.

Bizzi, A., Crane, R. C., Autilio-Gambetti and Gambetti, P. (1984) Aluminum effect on slow axonal transport; a novel impairment of neurofilament transport. *J. Neurol. Sci.*, 4: 722–731.

Blaustein, M. P. and Goldman, D. F. (1968) The action of polyvalent cations on the voltage-clamped lobster axon. *J. Gen. Physiol.*, 51: 279–291.

Bradbury, M. W. B. (1984) The structure and function of the blood-brain-barrier. *Fed. Proc.*, 43: 186–190.

Brontium, C. O., Huang, Y. C., Breckenridge, B. McL. and Wolff, D. J. (1975) Identification of a calcium-binding protein as a calcium-dependent regulation of brain adenyl cyclase. *Proc. Natl. Acad. Sci. USA*, 72: 64–68.

Cam, J. M., Luck, V. A., Eastwood, J. B. and De Wardener, H. E. (1976) The effects of aluminum hydroxide orally on calcium, phosphorus and aluminum metabolism in normal subjects. *Clin. Sci. Mol. Med.*, 51: 407–414.

Candy, J. M., Klinowski, J., Perry, R. H., Perry, E. K., Fairbairn, A., Oakley, A. E., Carpenter, T. A., Atack, J. R., Blessed, G. and Edwardson, J. A. (1986) Alumino-silicates and senile plaque formation in Alzheimer's disease. *Lancet*, 354–357.

Cheung, W. Y. (1984) Calmodulin: its potential role in cell proliferation and heavy metal toxicity. *Fed. Proc.*, 43: 2995–2999.

Corsellis, J. (1978) Post traumatic dementia. In R. Katzman, R. D. Terry and K. L. Bick (Eds.), *Alzheimer's Disease and Related Disorders, Aging, Vol. 7*, Raven Press, New York, pp. 125–133.

Crapper, D. R. and Dalton, A. J. (1973) Alterations in short-term retention, conditioned avoidance response acquisition and motivation following aluminum induced neurofibrillary degeneration. *Physiol. Behav.*, 10: 925–933.

Crapper-McLachlan, D. R. and De Boni, U. (1980) Aluminum in human brain disease — An overview. *Neurotoxicology*, 1: 3–16.

Crapper, D. R., Krishnan, S. S. and Dalton, A. J. (1973) Brain aluminum distribution in Alzheimer's disease and experimental neurofibrillary degeneration. *Science (Wash.)*, 180: 511–513.

Crapper, D. R., Krishnan, S. S. and Quittkat, S. (1976) Aluminum, neurofibrillary degeneration and Alzheimer's disease. *Brain*, 99: 67–79.

Crapper, D. R., Karlik, S. and De Boni, U. (1978) Aluminum and other metals in senile (Alzheimer) dementia. In R. Katzman, R. D. Terry and K. L. Bick (Eds.), *Alzheimer's Disease, Senile Dementia and Related Disorders, Aging, Vol. 7*, Raven Press, New York, pp. 471–485.

Crapper, D. R., Quittkat, S., Krishnan, S. S., Dalton, A. J. and De Boni, U. (1980) Intranuclear aluminum content in Alzheimer's disease, dialysis encephalopathy and experimental aluminum encephalopathy. *Acta Neuropathol. (Berl.)*, 50: 19–24.

Crapper, D. R., Kruck, T. and Van Berkum, M. F. A. (1985) Aluminum and neurodegenerative disease: therapeutic implications. *Am. J. Kidn. Dis.*, 6: 322–329.

De Boni, U. and McLachlan Crapper, D. R. (1985) Controlled induction of paired helical filaments of the Alzheimer type in cultured neurons, by glutamate and aspartate. *J. Neurol. Sci.*, 68: 105–118.

Deerly, W. J., Means, A. R. and Brinkley, B. R. (1984) Calmodulin-microtubule association in cultured mammalian cells. *J. Cell. Biol.*, 98: 904–910.

Doellken, V. (1897) Ueber die Wirkung des Aluminium mit besonderer Berücksichtigung der durch das Aluminium verursachten Läsionen im Zentralnervensystem. *Naunyn-Schmiedeb. Arch. Exp. Pathol. Pharmakol.*, 40: 58–120.

Duckett, S. and Galle, P. (1976) Mise en évidence de l'aluminium dans les plaques de la maladie d'Alzheimer:

étudiée à la microsonde de Castaing. *C. R. Acad. Sci. Paris*, 282: 393–395.

Farnell, B. J., De Boni, U. and Crapper McLachlan, D. R. (1982) Aluminum neurotoxicity in the absence of neurofibrillary degeneration in CA1 hippocampal pyramidal neurons in vitro. *Exp. Neurol.*, 78: 241–258.

Farnell, B. J., Crapper-McLachlan, D. R., Baimbridge, K., De Boni, U., Wong, L. and Wood, P. L. (1985) Calcium metabolism in aluminum encephalopathy. *Exp. Neurol.*, 88: 68–83.

Feinroth, M., Feinroth, M. V. and Berlyne, G. M. (1982) Aluminum absorption in the rat everted gut sac. *Min. Electr. Metab.*, 8: 29–35.

Gajdusek, C. D. and Salazar, A. M. (1982) Amyotrophic lateral sclerosis and parkinsonian syndromes in high incidence among the Auya and Jakai people of West New Guinea. *Neurology*, 32: 107–126.

Garruto, R. M., Fukaton, R., Yanagihara, R., Gajdusek, C. D., Hook, G. and Fiori, C. (1984) Imaging of calcium and aluminum in neurofibrillary tanglebearing neurons in Parkinsonism dementia of Guam. *Proc. Natl. Acad. Sci. USA*, 81: 1875–1879.

Hajos, F. (1975) An important method for the preparation of synaptosomal fractions in high purity. *Brain Res.*, 93: 485–489.

Haug, A. (1984) Molecular aspects of aluminum neurotoxicity. *CRC Crit. Rev. Plant Sci.*, 1: 345–373.

Henry, D. A., Goodman, W. G., Nadelman, R. K., Di Domenico, N. C., Alfrey, A. C., Slatopolsky, E., Stanley, T. M. and Coburn, J. W. (1984) Parenteral aluminum administration in the dog: I. Plasma kinetics, tissue levels, calcium metabolism, and parathyroid hormone. *Kidney Int.*, 25: 362–369.

Heyman, A., Wilkinson, W. E., Stafford, J. A., Helms, M. S., Sigmon, A. H. and Weinberg, T. (1984) Alzheimer's disease: a study of epidemiologic aspects. *Ann. Neurol.*, 15: 335–341.

Hincke, M. T. and Demaille, J. G. (1984) Calmodulin regulation of the ATP dependent calcium uptake by inverted vesicles prepared from rabbit synaptosomal plasma membranes. *Biochim. Biophys. Acta*, 771: 188–194.

Iler, R. K. (1979) *The Chemistry of Silica*. J. Wiley and Sons, New York, pp. 756.

Kaehny, W. D., Alfrey, A. C., Halman, R. E. and Shorr, W. J. (1977) Aluminum transfer during hemodialysis. *Kidney Int.*, 12: 361–365.

Karlik, S. J., Eichhorn, G. L., Lewis, P. N. and Crapper, D. R. (1980) Interaction of aluminum species with deoxyribonucleic acid. *Biochemistry*, 19: 5991–5998.

King, G., De Boni, U. and Crapper, D. R. (1975) Effect of aluminum on conditioned avoidance response aquisition in the absence of neurofibrillary degeneration. *Pharmacol. Biochem. Behav.*, 3: 1003–1009.

Kovalchik, M. T., Kaehny, W. D., Hegg, A. P., Jackson, F. T. and Alfrey, A. C. (1980) Aluminum kinetics during hemodialysis. *J. Lab. Clin. Med.*, 92: 712–720.

Kreuger, B. K., Ratzlaff, R. W., Strichary, G. G. and Blaustein, M. P. (1979) Saxitoxin binding to synaptosomal membranes and solubilized binding sites from rat brain. *J. Membr. Biol.*, 50: 287–340.

Lin, Y. M., Lui, Y. R. and Cheung, W. Y. (1974) Cyclic 3',5'-nucleotide phosphodiesterase: purification, characterization and active form of the protein activator from bovine brain. *J. Biol. Chem.*, 249: 4943–4954.

Lione, A. (1983) The prophylactic reduction of aluminum intake. *Fed. Chem. Toxicol.*, 21: 103–109.

Litman, A. (1967) Reactive and nonreactive aluminum hydroxide gels: dose response relationships in vivo. *Gastroenterology*, 52: 948–951.

Long, J. F., Nagode, L. A., Kendig, A. and Liss, L. (1980) Axonal swelling of Purkinje cells in chickens associated with high intake of 1,25 $(OH)_2D_3$ including microanalysis. *Neurotoxicology*, 1: 111–120.

Masters, C. L., Multhaup, G., Simms, G., Pottycisser, J., Martins, R. N. and Beyreuther, K. (1985) Neuronal origin of a cerebral amyloid: neurofibrillary tangles of Alzheimer's disease contain the same protein as the amyloid of plaque cores and blood vessels. *EMBO*, 4: 2757–2763.

Matsumoto, H. and Morimura, S. (1980) Repressed template activity of chromatin of pea roots treated by aluminum. *Plant Cell Physiol.*, 21: 951–959.

Mayor, G. H., Remedi, R. F., Sprague, S. M. and Lowell, K. L. (1980a) Central nervous system manifestations of oral aluminum: effect of parathyroid hormone. *Neurotoxicology*, 1: 33–42.

Mayor, G. H., Sprague, S. M., Haurani, M. R. and Sanchez, T. V. (1980b) Parathyroid hormone mediated aluminum deposition and egress in the rat. *Kidney Int.*, 17: 40–44.

Means, A. R., Tash, J. S. and Chafauleas, J. G. (1982) Physiological implications of the presence, distribution and regulation of calmodulin in eukaryotic cells. *Physiol. Rev.*, 62: 1–39.

Mortimer, J. A., French, L. R., Hutton, J. T. and Schuman, L. M. (1985) Head injury as a risk factor for Alzheimer's disease. *Neurology*, 35: 264–267.

Nieboer, E. and Richardson, D. H. S. (1980) The replacement of the nondescript term "Heavy Metals" by a biologically and chemically significant classification of metal ions. *Environm. Pol. (Series B)*, 3–26.

Perl, D. P. and Brody, A. R. (1980) Alzheimer's disease: x-ray spectrometric evidence of aluminum accumulation in neurofibrillary tangle-bearing neurons. *Science*, 208: 297–299.

Perl, D. P., Gajdusek, D. C., Garruto, R. W., Yanazihara, R. T. and Gibbs, C. J. (1982) Intraneuronal aluminum accumulation in amyotrophic lateral sclerosis and Guam parkinsonism — dementia of Guam. *Science (Wash.)*, 217: 1053–1055.

Petit, T. L., Biederman, G. B. and McMullen, P. A. (1980) Neurofibrillary degeneration, dendritic dying back and learning-memory deficits after aluminum administration: implications for brain aging. *Exp. Neurol.*, 67: 152–162.

Rabe, A., Lei, M., Shek, J. and Wisniewski, H. (1982) Learning deficit in immature rabbits with aluminum-induced neurofibrillary degeneration. *Exp. Neurol.*, 76: 441–446.

Reed, D., Plato, C., Elizan, T. and Kurland, L. T. (1966) The amyotrophic lateral sclerosis, parkinsonism-dementia complex: a ten-year follow up in Guam. Part 1. Epidemiological studies. *Am. J. Epidemiol.*, 83: 54–73.

Reed, D. M. and Brody, J. A. (1975) Amyotrophic lateral sclerosis and parkinsonism-dementia of Guam, 1947–1972. *Am. J. Epidemiol.*, 101: 287–301.

Sarkander, H. I., Balb, G., Schlosser, R., Stoltenburg, G. and Lux, R. M. (1983) Blockade of neuronal brain RNA initiation sites by aluminum: a primary molecular mechanism of aluminum induced neurofibrillary changes. In J. Cervos-Navarro and H. I. Sarkander (Eds.), *Brain Aging, Aging, Vol. 21*, Raven Press, New York, pp. 259–274.

Schulman, H. and Greengard, P. (1978) Stimulation of brain membrane protein phosphorylation by calcium and an endogenous heat-stable protein. *Nature*, 271: 478–479.

Searle, P. F., Davison, B. L., Stuart, G. W., Wilkie, T. M., Norstedt, G. and Palmiter, R. D. (1984) Regulation, linkage and sequence of mouse metallothionein I and II genes. *Mol. Cell. Biol.*, 4: 1221–1230.

Seigle, N. and Haug, A. (1983a) Aluminum interactions with calmodulin. Evidence for altered structure and function from optical and enzymatic studies. *Biochim. Biophys. Acta*, 744: 36–45.

Seigle, N. and Haug, A. (1983b) Calmodulin-dependent formation of membrane potential in barley root plasma membrane vesicles: a biochemical model of aluminum toxicity in plants. *Physiol. Plant*, 59: 285–291.

Simmen, R., Tanaka, T., Fang, Ts'ui K., Putkey, W., Scott, M., Lai, E. and Means, A. R. (1985) The structural organization of the chicken calmodulin gene. *J. Biol. Chem.*, 260: 907–912.

Sternberger, N. H., Sternberger, L. A. and Ulrich, J. (1985) Aberrant neurofilament phosphorylation in Alzheimer's disease. *Proc. Natl. Acad. Sci. USA*, 82: 4274–4276.

Still, C. N. and Kelley, P. (1980) On the incidence of primary degenerative dementia vs. water fluoride content in South Carolina. *Neurotoxicology*, 1: 125–131.

Suhayda, C. G. and Haug, A. (1984) Organic acids prevent aluminum-induced conformational changes in calmodulin. *Biochem. Biophys. Res. Commun.*, 119: 376–381.

Trapp, G. A. (1983) Plasma aluminum is bound to transferrin. *Life Sci.*, 33: 31–316.

Trapp, G. A., Miner, G. D., Zimmerman, R. L., Master, A. R.

and Heston, L. L. (1978) Aluminum levels in brain in Alzheimer's disease. *Biol. Psychol.*, 13: 709–718.

Troncoso, V. C., Sternberger, L. A., Sternberger, N. H., Hoffman, P. N. and Price, D. L. (1985) Immunocytochemical studies of neurofilament antigens in the neurofibrillary pathology induced by aluminum. *J. Neuropathol. Exp. Neurol.*, 44: 332.

Turner, R. W., Baimbridge, K. G. and Miller, J. J. (1982) Calcium-induced long-term potentiation in the hippocampus. *Neuroscience*, 7: 1411–1416.

Van Berkum, M. F. A., Means, A. R. and Crapper McLachlan, D. R. (1986) Calmodulin, α-tubulin, β-actin and neurofilament (68 000 m.w.) messenger RNA concentrations in rabbit forebrain during aluminum-induced encephalopathy, under editorial review.

Weeds, A. (1982) Actin-binding proteins — regulators of cell architecture and motility. *Nature*, 296: 811–816.

Wenk, G. L. and Stemmer, K. L. (1983) Suboptimal dietary Zn intake increases aluminum accumulation with the rat brain. *Brain Res.*, 288: 393–395.

Wisniewski, K., Jervis, G. A., Moretz, R. C. and Wisniewski, H. M. (1979) Alzheimer neurofibrillary tangles in diseases other than senile and presenile dementia. *Ann. Neurol.*, 5: 288–294.

Yanagihara, R., Garruto, R. M., Gajdusek, C. D., Tomita, A., Uchikawa, T., Konagaya, Y., Chen, K.-M., Sohue, I., Plato, C. and Gibbs, C. J. (1984) Calcium and vitamin D metabolism in Guamanian chamorros with amyotrophic lateral sclerosis and parkinsonism dementia. *Ann. Neurol.*, 15: 42–48.

Yase, Y. (1977) The basic process of amyotrophic lateral sclerosis as reflected in Kii peninsula and Guam. *Excerpta Medica International Congress I Series 434, Neurology*, 43: 1.

Yase, Y. (1980) The role of aluminum in CNS degeneration with interactions of calcium. *Neurotoxicology*, 1: 101–110.

Yokel, R. A. (1983) Repeated systemic aluminum exposure effects on classical conditioning of the rabbit. *Neurobehav. Toxicol. Teratol.*, 5: 41–46.

Yoshimasu, F., Nebayashi, Y., Yase, Y., Iwata, W. and Sasajima, K. (1976) Studies on amyotrophic lateral sclerosis by neutron activation and analysis. *Folia Psychiat. Neurol. Jap.*, 30: 49–55.

Yoshimasu, F., Yasui, M., Yoshida, H., Yoshida, S., Lebayashi, Y., Yase, Y., Gajdusek, D. C. and Chen, K. M. (1985) Aluminum in Alzheimer's disease in Japan and Parkinsonism-dementia in Guam. *XIIIth World Congress of Neurology, Hamburg*, Abstract 15.07.02.

Discussion

R. T. BARTUS: Would you care to comment or speculate on the source of aluminum in the brains of AD patients? Assuming the role of aluminum in the neurodegenerative dysfunctions of AD, do you feel any danger from daily, life-long consumptions of aluminum from antiacids, antiperspirants, etc.?

ANSWER: The source of aluminum is both through the respiratory system and through the food chain. Approximately 10–50 mg of aluminum is ingested daily in the average North-American diet. The question of whether life-long consumption of aluminum in various forms constitutes a risk for Alzheimer's disease cannot be answered at this time. It will be necessary to more precisely evaluate the role of aluminum in the pathogenesis of the disease and in the assembly of paired helical filaments of neurofibrillary degeneration and amyloid of neuritic plaques.

Certainly the normal mammal has extremely effective barriers to aluminum, and these include the intestinal transport systems, the blood transport and urinary excretion, as well as the blood–brain barrier. What is not known at the present time is the effect of aluminum speciation upon penetration of the blood–brain barrier, and various ligands which may facilitate transcellular transport of aluminum.

D. F. SWAAB: You mentioned alcohol dementia as a condition in which Al was accumulated. Does this mean that Al accumulation is secondary to brain damage?

ANSWER: The presence of aluminum deposits in the brain of a patient with alcohol-associated dementia was reported by LaPresle et al. (1975). I believe this case is of importance because extensive damage to the basal ganglia had occurred, and mineralization of the blood vessels in the damaged area had occured. This is the first report of a trace metal analysis of the striatal nigral syndrome, and the presence of aluminum and calcium suggest that this may play a pathogenic role in this particular individual. A number of studies have shown that aluminum does not occur in such conditions as Jakob-Creutzfeldt disease, where there is extensive damage to neurons and glia. However, the accumulation of aluminum as secondary damage in certain degenerative conditions cannot be excluded. It is the marked similarity between the neurotoxicity of aluminum in experimental animals, and the presence of aluminum in similar neurodegenerative conditions in man, which have prompted an investigation of the possible relationship of aluminum to human diseases.

R. D. TERRY: What is the state of calmodulin in native Alzheimer's disease?

ANSWER: We have previously shown that Alzheimer's disease is associated with a 30–40% reduction in calmodulin as measured by the radioimmune assay. We have also shown that the Line-Weaver-Burke plots for calmodulin extracted from Alzheimer affected neocortex exhibits a disturbance in kinetics similar to that which is seen in the aluminum encephalopathy. We are currently measuring the yield of messenger RNA for calmodulin in Alzheimer's disease.

J. M. CANDY: Calcium activated protease has a calmodulin-like calcium binding site and I wonder if an interaction of aluminum with this site may be responsible for accumulation of neurofilaments.

ANSWER: A very excellent idea worthy of further testing.

J. KORF: (1) How can you explain cell specific changes in Alzheimer's disease by a rather general influence in calmodulin,

a universally occurring compound. So why are not all cells affected?

(2) Can you indicate the possible role of mitochondria in the action of A1 as far as Calcium-mediaton is implied. Mitochondria have a great capacity to buffer the cytoplasmic levels of calcium.

ANSWER: Both of these questions are thought-provoking. It is difficult to explain the specific cell loss which occurs in Alzheimer's disease only by an affect upon a ubiquitous intracellular messenger such as calmodulin.

Perhaps, the most important question for us to address is what other unique neuronal markers are affected by aluminum. It is possible that the genetic expression of a unique neuronal marker, possibly associated with a voltage dependent calcium conductance system, might more adequately account for the selective vulnerability to aluminum toxicity.

The question of an effect of aluminum upon the mitochondrial system cannot be excluded. The only observations we have at present are that total tissue calcium increases in a delayed fashion after the application of aluminum to the nervous system, but we have not done subcellular fractionations to localize where the increased calcium is. This work remains to be done.

J. M. B. V. DE JONG: Have you studied metallothiamin?

ANSWER: Metallothiamines have been examined in Alzheimer's disease, and we were unable to detect a difference in content between Alzheimer and controls. We have no evidence that the metallothiamines are disordered in Alzheimer's disease.

R. T. BARTUS: Assuming a role for aluminum in the neurodegenerative dysfunction of AD, do you believe that calmodulin-activating agents might be able to circumvent the neuropathology characteristic of the disease?

ANSWER: The issue of whether a calmodulin activating agent might be of benefit in Alzheimer's disease is intriguing. Such agents would be worth trying in the experimentally induced aluminum encephalopathy before embarking upon studies in man. This would be a worthy investigation.

D. M. GASH: Would you comment further on your clinical trials using Al chelating agents? At what stage of AD do you begin treatment and what are your criteria for selecting patients?

ANSWER: We are carrying on a clinical trial with a trivalent metal chelating agent, Desferrioxamine. While the stability constant, in vitro, is higher for iron than for aluminum, the stability constant for aluminum is still many orders of magnitude higher than for the divalent and monovalent metals. The study is in progress and a firm conclusion cannot as yet be drawn from this study. The patients included in this study are those that have been recently diagnosed, and can be considered to be in the first third of the illness. It is conceivable that because aluminum binds to DNA and has a number of nuclear affects, removal of aluminum may not stop the progress of the disease. Aluminum may be important in initiating some pathogenic mechanism early in the disorder. However, should the outcome of the clinical trial indicate that removal of aluminum results in altered clinical course, then reduction in exposure of aluminum to those at risk for Alzheimer's disease might be worthy of further study.

References

LaPresle, J., Duckett, S., Galle, P. and Cartier, L. (1975) Documents cliniques, anatomiques et biophysiques dans une encéphalopathie avec présence de dépôts d'aluminium. *C. R. Soc. Biol.*, 169: 282–285.

SECTION IV

Therapeutic strategies

D. F. Swaab, E. Fliers, M. Mirmiran, W. A. Van Gool and F. Van Haaren (Eds.)
Progress in Brain Research, Vol. 70.
© 1986 Elsevier Science Publishers B.V. (Biomedical Division)

CHAPTER 26

Clinical strategies in the treatment of Alzheimer's disease

D. F. Swaab and E. Fliers

Netherlands Institute for Brain Research, Meibergdreef 33, 1105 AZ Amsterdam Zuidoost, The Netherlands

Introduction

Every culture has tried to obtain life extension. A 2400-years-old example is the Babylonian-Assyrian epos of Gilgamesh, who tried in vain to escape the aging process by bathing in the fountain of youth and by eating the herb of life. The latter endeavor makes clear that 'research' in the pharmacological prevention of the symptoms of aging has a long history. From the pharmacological literature of the last century it is evident that hypotheses concerning the causal factors of aging and Alzheimer's disease as well as the therapies for treating them were often changing parallel to neurobiological interests and fashions. Clinical strategies were not specific for Alzheimer's disease, but passively followed new developments in medicine and research by trying out nearly every new compound or idea relevant to this condition. This may also explain why therapies that were considered to be 'rational' in the light of a new development, appeared nonsensical as soon as new insights developed.

The approach of trying out everything that is new in neurobiology on Alzheimer patients does not preclude of course the possibility either that an effective substance will be found, or that its proposed mechanism of action will indeed turn out to be correct. However, the chance of success of this strategy is very small. Repeatedly, ideas about the etiology of Alzheimer's disease have been adapted immediately to new disciplines or insights that developed in neurosciences. Thus changes in

hormone levels, blood supply, metabolism, and transmitters have been pinpointed as possible causes of brain aging and Alzheimer's disease. Subsequently, a 'new and promising' therapy was claimed to have a 'rational' basis and was tried out on Alzheimer patients. This history might make us less optimistic about all the ongoing clinical trials, and even more convinced about the necessity of fundamental research in Alzheimer's disease before a therapy with a reasonable chance of success will ever succeed in being developed.

Experimental endocrinology started in 1848 when Berthold, professor of medicine at the University of Göttingen, showed that the atrophy of the comb and the changes in behavior following castration of cockerels, could be prevented by transplantation of testis (cf. Tausk, 1976). Endocrine experiments in animals were followed by series of observations on the possible effects of gonadal hormones on the process of aging and dementia in man. Brown-Séquard (1889), at the age of 72, injected himself with extracts prepared from crushed testicles of guinea-pigs or dogs. We may wonder now how little of the active steroids these aqueous extracts must have contained. Yet he claimed that both his physical and intellectual powers increased. Lorand (1913) reviewed the 'marvelous effects' of ovarian extracts, thyroid extracts and extracts of testicles on the prevention and treatment of the symptoms of old age. Lorand too ('for experimental purposes', as he explained, apparently being in need of an apology) subsequently tried out testicular extracts from the pig on himself and confirmed the increase in 'muscular and mental' powers. In the line of thought of that period, transplantation of animal testicular tissue to the testis of aged men was quite logical. This treatment, with monkeys as donors was indeed reported to be very successful in old animals including man (Voronoff, 1925).

In the same period an indirect way of increasing gonadal hormone levels was proposed by Steinach. He claimed to have experimental evidence for 'hormone accumulation' by ligation of the vas deferens, an operation that would result in 'reactivation'. He subsequently asked the Viennese surgeon and urologist Dr. Robert Lichtenstern "to perform vasoligature on suitable patients for reactivation purposes". Lichtenstern carried out the first 'Steinach' operation on November 1, 1918 on the vas deferens of an 'exhausted and prematurely old man'. This operation was followed by 'many thousands — perhaps even tens of thousands — of successful repetitions'. Steinach called the operation "a means of enriching our stock of remedies against pre-senility, inasmuch it removes disturbances of the central nervous system" (Steinach and Loebel, 1940). Reading through their case histories labelled as 'premature senility', 'moods of depression' are mentioned remarkably often. In those days, the differential diagnosis between depression and dementia will already have been a difficult one, and a beneficial effect of this operation upon depression might be the explanation of the astonishing high success rate of some 80%. It is a pity that Steinach's misconception may have contributed to preventing serious study on the effects of testosterone treatment on aging subjects, since, at present, we know that testosterone levels are indeed decreasing during senescence (Deslypere and Vermeulen, 1984; Warner et al., 1985). Although we do not have any data on testosterone levels in dementia, changes would probably have strong effects on several transmitter systems in the brain. In the old rat, decreased testosterone levels seem to be the most probable explanation for the diminishment of vasopressin-containing fibers originating, e.g., from the bed nucleus of the stria terminalis (Fliers et al., 1985a), although experimental confirmation has still to be performed. Whether or not similar testosterone-dependent fiber systems do also exist in the human brain is not known.

In the subsequent period in our story, the condition of the blood vessels was put central, as appears from the slogan 'a man is as old as his blood vessels' (e.g. Foley, 1956). The idea that dementia was caused by arteriosclerosis of the cerebral vessels led to the development of 'vasodilatators' (see below). Hyperbaric and normobaric oxygen therapy also fit into the vascular hypothesis of aging (McFarland, 1963) and dementia. The initially reported improvements obtained with the use of these therapies were not confirmed in later studies (Wittenborn, 1981; White et al., 1975).

In the meantime, psychotropic drugs had been developed that appeared to be effective, e.g., in treating schizophrenia and depression. They were subsequently applied, without any beneficial effects, in dementia. Such medicines were followed by the 'geronto-psychiatric drugs' that would be 'specifically' beneficial for the elderly patient with mental impairments, again without great success, however.

The recent boom in our knowledge concerning neurotransmitters has resulted in a new direction in gerontological treatments viz. transmitter substitution therapies. In addition, possibly under the influence of social sciences on medicine, increasing attention is currently being paid to non-pharmacological therapies, such as the effects of food or environment (Lieberman and Abou-Nader, 1986; Roth et al., 1986). However, in spite of all these efforts, we still have no effective therapy for

---

Fig. 1. (a) Old ram (No. 14) in 1918, before transplantation. (b) The same old ram (No. 14) in 1923, five and a half years after transplantation. (c) Operation on a human: one of the grafts, obtained from a monkey testicle, is fixed by four sutures of catgut in the left sinus, the glandular side facing the tunica vaginalis. (d) M.T. 74 years old in 1923, before transplantation. (e) M.T. 76 years old in 1925, two and a half years after transplantation. (From Voronoff, 1925)

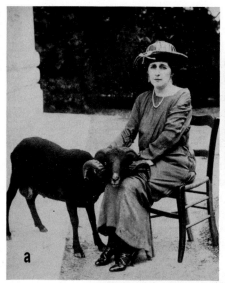

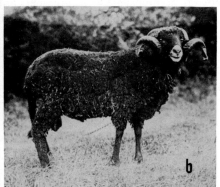

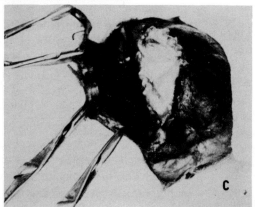

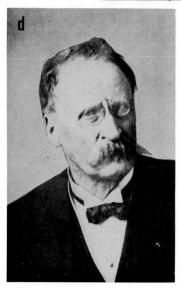

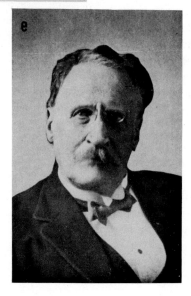

Fig. 1.

Alzheimer's disease, which is perhaps not surprising, since its etiology has not yet been elucidated. There may in fact not even exist any such thing, in view of the possibility that Alzheimer's disease may represent an accelerated form of the normal aging process. Such ignorance merely stresses the importance of more fundamental research into the process underlying normal aging of the brain, and Alzheimer's disease in particular. The modest beneficial effects that have been reported for various pharmacological and non-pharmacological therapies and that are reviewed in the present paper might provide some clues for effective further research.

Cerebral vasodilatators

The use of cerebral vasodilatators was based upon the assumption that dementia was largely caused by cerebral arteriosclerosis. The justification for the use of such drugs in Alzheimer's disease is at present weak. Moreover, even if AD were to have a vascular cause and vasodilatators were effective, one could wonder how arteriosclerotic arteries would be able to dilate (Branconnier and Cole, 1977; Yesavage et al., 1979).

Carbon dioxide and *carbonic anhydrase inhibitors* (e.g., acetazolamide) have been used in dementia without effective therapeutic consequences (Ban, 1978; Cole and Liptzin, 1984).

Papaverine, an ancient drug found in opium and having morphine-like analgesic activity, and the related drug *cyclandelate* have been among the most widely prescribed categories of agents in the treatment of 'arteriosclerotic' dementias. It is questionable, whether the reported therapeutic effects, e.g. in elderly volunteers (Branconnier and Cole, 1977; Wittenborn, 1981), were indeed due to improved cerebral blood flow or alternatively; the improved cerebral blood flow is more likely to have been secondary to increased brain metabolism. There is no conclusive evidence that *nicotinic acid*, *tocopherol* (vitamin E) or any of the numerous other 'vasodilating agents' improve either cerebral

blood flow or the condition of the Alzheimer patient (Ban, 1978). *Hydergine*, that was developed as a vasodilatator will be discussed in the section on CNS stimulants.

Dicumarol, *warfarin* and other *anticoagulants* have been employed because of the theory that cerebral emboli could contribute to the development of dementia. The studies reported with this therapy were usually uncontrolled and very limited, so that useful conclusions are hard to draw. The risk of bleeding with this therapy is substantial (Ban, 1978; Wittenborn, 1981).

Classical psychotherapeutic drugs

The success of psychotherapeutic drugs in psychiatry has led to their prescription in aging and dementia, where they have to be considered as merely symptomatic agents (Hollister, 1985). Yet, some 36% of the US subjects over 60 years of age have used such drugs (Epstein, 1978). During the last few years, the number of studies on the effect of major tranquilizers on senile patients seems to have diminished (Wittenborn, 1981), presumably because it has become apparent that they have no unequivocally favorable effects on the condition, although the symptomatic improvements may be highly valued by those charged with the care of such patients (cf. Hollister, 1985). On the other hand, this population is certainly at risk for iatrogenic illness secondary to the action of psychotherapeutic drugs.

Antidepressants, neuroleptics and anxiolytic agents

The fact that depression may easily be confused with dementia does of course not mean that *antidepressants* have a favorable action on the clinical condition in Alzheimer's disease. Negative effects have been obtained with such compounds as *neuroleptics*: compounds that even frequently have been the cause of pseudodementia in aged patients (De Beer and Simons, 1977).

Benzodiazepines, *propanediols* and *barbiturates* are frequently used in the elderly and are clearly effective in treating such symptoms as anxiety, tension, restlessness and agitation. However, there is no indication that tranquilizers improve impaired functioning in old people (Wittenborn, 1981). Moreover, benzodiazepines are among the most frequently misused drugs (Epstein, 1978) and may induce similar amnestic performance deficits as found in Alzheimer's disease (Wittenborn, 1981; Bartus et al., 1982). Long-term use of benzodiazepines might possibly even cause some degree of brain atrophy, since it has been reported to be accompanied with an increased ventricle/brain ratio. However, a causal relationship between drug use and brain atrophy in human has not yet been proven (Lader and Petursson, 1983).

Alcohol is most probably the most widely used anxiolytic compound. Wine or beer in modest amounts improved the condition of old subjects, also in chronic brain syndromes, whereas no difference was found when drinks were given either in a pub or a ward setting (Chien, 1971; Chien et al., 1973). Yet, in the long run, alcohol has serious negative effects, e.g. on gnostic functions (Freund, 1982; Freund and Butters, 1982) and may cause brain atrophy (Lader and Petursson, 1983). Therefore, it cannot be recommended as a safe alternative therapy.

Central nervous system stimulants

Because of the changing ideas about the etiology of dementia through the years and the technical improvements that have enabled the measurement of brain metabolism, pharmacotherapeutical interest shifted from the improvement of cerebral circulation to the improvement of brain metabolism in the elderly. This development has led to many claims regarding new gerontopsychiatric drugs. However, only few weakly effective compounds were in fact produced, presumably because the diminished metabolism in the Alzheimer brain is an effect rather than a cause of the condition (Frackowiak, 1986).

Piracetam (2-oxy-1-pyrrolidine acetamide), originally developed as a compound against motion illness, was later claimed to protect the brain against oxygen shortage and to improve learning. It is a GABA-derivate without GABA effects (Cole and Liptzin, 1984). It was considered to be the first compound of a new class of 'nootropic' drugs (Ban, 1978), i.e., able to enhance memory and learning, and thus of possible importance for the treatment of Alzheimer. This idea was confirmed by a number of methodologically imperfect clinical trials. Careful studies, using a standardized factor-analyzed rating scale for elderly patients (BOP), psychometric tests and a double-blind crossover design did not show any significant effect as compared to placebo, upon psychometric performance of Alzheimer patients (Diesfeldt et al., 1978; Wittenborn, 1981). The drug is currently advertized as Nootropil® for transient ischemic attacks and would — according to the advertisement — improve the disturbed microcirculation and the oxygen and glucose utilization. It has been claimed to be effective in Alzheimer's disease in combination with choline (see below).

Magnesium pemoline (Cylert®) was originally introduced as a compound that would increase the synthesis of ribonucleic acid and, consequently, the consolidation of memory. This finding was, however, shown to be in error (Eisdorfer et al., 1968). The favorable results on memory could not be confirmed in subsequent clinical investigations using tests involving learning, memory, and performance. The compound is now marked for use in children suffering from minimal brain dysfunction and/or hyperkinetic behavior (Branconnier and Cole, 1977; Ban, 1978; Wittenborn, 1981).

Yeast RNA taken orally was supposed to affect memory but — perhaps not too surprisingly — had no better effect than did placebo in old impaired or demented patients (Wittenborn, 1981).

Anabolic agents, such as fluoxymesterone, isoprinosine and related hormone preparations, have been administered to gerontopsychiatric patients in the hope of correcting the disturbance of protein synthesis encountered in aging, however, without any clear-cut effect on memory function (Ban, 1978).

Pentylenetetrazole and *methylphenidase* do not

seem to have an apparent value in improving mental functions (Ban, 1978; Wittenborn, 1981; Cole and Liptzin, 1984). The results with *pipradol* seem to be favorable only in the first weeks of the treatment, but not at subsequent assessment periods (Wittenborn, 1981).

Procaine was introduced in 1956 as 'a new method for prophylaxis and treatment of aging' by Dr. A. Aslan from Roumania supposedly having 'eutropic and rejuvenating effects'. In 1958 she started treatment with *Gerovital H3* (2% procaine-HCl combined with a preservative plus an antioxidant) a preparation which she called *Aslavital*® and for which novel pharmacological properties were claimed. Expensive trips to Roumania are still advertized emphasizing the "remarkable value of Dr. Aslan's cure" that "is efficient in the prophylaxis and cure of the phenomena that appear in the affections of the central nervous system...". In addition, "...it has a favorable effect in...memory, attention and concentration capacity troubles...in the decline of intellectual and physical ability". However, most studies provide little support for the claim that this drug improves the mental status of geriatric patients (Wittenborn, 1981; Millard, 1984). An exception is a study by Hall et al. (1983), that reported an effect on consolidation of new learning and muscle strength, but also documented several adverse reactions. Gerovital H3 probably acts, however, as a mild antidepressant drug, because it is a weak, reversible and competitive inhibitor of MAO (Zung et al., 1974; Branconnier and Cole, 1977).

Hydergine® is composed of the methylates of four dihydrogenated ergot derivates. In the period that the decline of cognitive function in aging and Alzheimer's disease was thought to be due to vascular changes, hydergine was developed and advertized as a vasodilator. Evidence for such an effect is totally lacking. Yet, it is still used in various countries even for the treatment of hypertension (Hollister and Yesavage, 1984) in the belief that it possesses a vasodilatory action. Hydergine was subsequently classified as 'a metabolic enhancer', since in some pharmacological tests it induced a changing in cyclic-AMP levels. How such effects relate to Alzheimer's disease is not at all clear (Hollister and Yesavage, 1984). Recently, the action of hydergine has been explained by its binding to dopamine, serotonin and noradrenaline receptors, or was simply called 'a rational approach' (cf. Ermini and Markstein, 1984). This clearly illustrates how time after time the commercial machinery gets its hand on whatever neurobiological approach is in fashion at the moment. It is no less than amazing that the interesting observation of Nandy and Schneider (1978) that hydergine causes a decrease in lipofuscin content as well as an increase in neurite formation in mouse neuroblastoma cells kept in culture, has not been used in advertisements, since on theoretical grounds such a general effect might prove to be beneficial in the treatment of Alzheimer's disease (cf. Coleman and Flood, 1986). This observation may point to a non-specific metabolic activation of neurons and might as such be an alternative explanation for its effects (see below). Regardless of the validity of the various explanatory proposals, double-blind studies of hydergine versus papaverine-hydrochloride or other controls indeed favored the former, also in cognitive tests, although the improvements were relatively modest. Alzheimer patients were those who benefited the most, provided their condition was not too far advanced, while patients with multi-infarct dementia improved less (Loew and Weil, 1982). The generally reported improved mood and feeling of well-being resulting from hydergine are more pronounced than are the reported cognitive improvements. One may wonder, therefore, whether its effects might not best be explained by an antidepressive action (Fliers, 1982), although some correlations plead against this possibility. As an alternative mechanism of action the induction of decreasing prolactin levels by hydergine are mentioned (Loew and Weil, 1982). Although statistically present, the reported improvements with hydergine are clinically marginal and lacunar, while great improvement in memory has never been observed (e.g., Pomara et al., 1983; Cole and Liptzin, 1984). This consider ation puts question marks to the clinical usefulness of this drug in the treatment of Alzheimer's disease (Meier-Ruge, 1983; Hollister and Yesavage, 1984). The combination of hydergine with lecithin was not effective in Alzheimer's disease (see below).

Nafronyl, a new compound that would increase metabolic activity and was claimed to have beneficial clinical effects on dementia patients, is currently under further investigation (Yesavage et al., 1982).

Neurotransmitter substitution therapies

At present, the study of specific neurotransmitter systems is a hot topic in neurobiology. No wonder, thus, that various neurotransmitter substitution therapies are currently being proposed for Alzheimer's disease. Neurotransmitters may be subdivided into acetylcholine, monoamines, amino acids and neuropeptides. All four classes of transmitter systems undergo changes during aging and in Alzheimer's disease; findings that have stimulated clinical trials aimed at their substitution in Alzheimer's disease.

Cholinergic system

The 'cholinergic hypothesis' concerning the etiology for the decrease of cognition in the elderly and in Alzheimer's disease has gained considerable attention during the last years (for review see Bartus et al., 1982). Indeed, choline acetyltransferase (CAT) activity and acetylcholine production is markedly reduced in Alzheimer's disease. Moreover, a severe loss of neurons was found in this condition in the nucleus basalis of Meynert, the main source of neocortical cholinergic innervation. Yet it is questionable whether this is indeed an adequate explanation for the etiology of Alzheimer's disease, since disruption of this cholinergic system in the rat causes only a temporary cognitive impairment (Bartus, 1986), whereas lesions in the rat cerebral cortex induce degenerative changes in Meynert's nucleus (Sofroniew et al., 1986). In addition, many other transmitter systems are affected in Alzheimer's disease (Gottfries, 1986; Swaab et al., 1985, 1986; Fliers and Swaab, 1986; Francis et al., 1985).

Clinical studies, aimed at substituting the cholinergic deficit in Alzheimer, have attempted (1) to enhance the synthesis and release of acetylcholine by providing abundant amounts of precursor substances, such as *lecithin* and *choline*, and (2) to enhance cholinergic activity by giving drugs that interfere at the synaptic or postsynaptic site or (3) by inhibiting acetylcholine breakdown of the endogenous transmitter using *physostigmine*. The reported effects of precursors on cognition are generally far from impressive or sometimes even completely negative. There are, however, a few more optimistic reports (Bartus et al., 1982; Drachman et al., 1982; Hollister, 1985). In addition, the dose range seems to be very narrow and to vary considerably among individual subjects (Bartus et al., 1982). The muscarinic agonist *arecoline* may enhance performance on a memory task in Alzheimer's disease, although not to the extent of achieving any significance (Palacios and Spiegel, 1986). Combinations with central nervous system stimulants have also been tried: *choline-piracetam* and *lecithin-piracetam* combinations were reported to be effective in an open trial and in preliminary results of a double-blind cross-over study, respectively (Bartus et al., 1981; Samorajski et al., 1985), but a *hydergine-lecithin* combination was not (Pomora et al., 1983).

In conclusion, although "some clinical improvement can occasionally be seen" (Barbeau, 1978), a satisfactory treatment of the cognitive impairment of Alzheimer's disease by means of pharmacological substitution for deficits in the cholinergic system seems, at present, not to be feasible.

Amines

Recent evidence for considerable cell loss in the locus ceruleus with normal aging and in Alzheimer's disease (Bondareff, 1982), and data on monoamines in brain and CSF, point to catecholamine impairment in the cognitive disturbances

(Gottfries, 1986). Noradrenaline concentrations in the temporal cortex of Alzheimer patients are reduced, as is the serotonin concentration in the frontal cortex, temporal cortex and limbic areas (Francis et al., 1985).

Bromocryptine, a dopamine agonist, has no demonstrable effect on intellectual functioning in Alzheimer patients (Smith et al., 1979). L-*Dopa*, *tyrosine*, *5-hydroxy-tryptophan* and L-*tryptophan* have all been tried in small samples of patients, occasionally leading to a mild improvement (Cole and Liptzin, 1984). In general, however, compounds influencing the aminergic system have not shown any beneficial effect on cognition or mood superior to that of antidepressants (Reisberg et al., 1983a). For a discussion of the proposal that hydergine is effective by virtue of its action on aminergic systems the reader is referred to Ermini and Markstein (1984) and to p. 418 of the present paper.

Amino acids

Drugs influencing this class of transmitters, e.g. the *benzodiazepines*, do not seem to have a favorable action on cognitive functions (see above). Recently, the Japan Economic Journal reported that Chugai Pharmaceutical Co. researchers are testing dibenzoxazepine. It would improve learning in aged rats. They predict that this substance will be effective against Alzheimer's disease. We shall wait and see.

Neuropeptides

Various neuropeptides were first known as hypothalamic hormones (vasopressin, oxytocin, LHRH, TRH, CRF) or pituitary hormones (peptides of the opiomelanocortin family). Their endocrine history and the data on their central effects have led to the concept that the brain, like the peripheral endocrine glands, is an endocrine target organ. Many of the peptides in the brain show changes with aging (De Wied and Van Ree, 1982; Swaab, 1982; Facchinetti et al., 1984; Fliers and Swaab, 1986).

Moreover, since functions that are influenced by neuropeptides such as motivational, attentional and memory processes tend to decline during aging (Jolles, 1986a), it was postulated that a decreased bioavailability of neuropeptides in the brain of elderly people is associated with specific disturbances in their mental performance (De Wied and Van Ree, 1982). However, neuropeptides appeared not to act centrally as hormones but rather to be transported throughout the brain by extensive fiber systems which terminate on other neurons by means of synapses that cannot be distinguished from those containing the classical neurotransmitters (Buijs and Swaab, 1979; Swaab, 1982). In spite of the relatively short period of research devoted to them, many neuropeptides already fulfill quite some of the accepted transmitter criteria (Buijs, 1982).

Because of the presumed effects of *vasopressin* on memory consolidation in animal studies, the memory disorders commonly observed in the elderly, and a presumed deficiency of neurohypophyseal hormone release into the periphery during aging, Legros (1975; Legros et al., 1978) studied the influence of vasopressin in men aged 50–65 years and reported a positive effect in memory tests. In later studies, however, less favorable results were obtained (cf. Jolles, 1986b).

From our measurements at the hypothalamic sites of production of vasopressin, the supraoptic (SON) and paraventricular nucleus (PVN), and from the recently reported increased vasopressin blood levels in the aged (cf. Fliers et al., 1985b; Hoogendijk et al., 1985), it has become clear that the vasopressin 'substitution' therapy in elderly, and maybe even in Alzheimer patients, has probably been given to subjects in whom neurohypophyseal function was not deficient at all. On the contrary, vasopressin cells were found to be activated in these conditions, probably by way of compensation for decreased renal sensitivity to vasopressin (E. Goudsmit et al., personal communication; Swaab et al., 1986). This might at least partly explain the inconsistent results obtained using this therapy (see Jolles, 1986b).

There are also some general considerations that make 'neurotransmitter substitution' an enterprise with only a limited chance of success, one of them being the heterogeneous way cells of a given transmitter type change during aging and in Alzheimer's disease. As has been reported for other putative neurotransmitter systems, the vasopressin 'system' in the brain does not react as a unity: homogeneous while the SON and PVN are activated under these conditions (Fliers et al., 1985b; Hoogendijk et al., 1985), the suprachiasmatic nucleus (SCN) cells degenerate to a large extent after the age of 80 and even more strongly in Alzheimer's disease (Swaab et al., 1985). Also in 34-months-old rats, the different extrahypothalamic sites of vasopressin-fiber terminations do not show overall changes with age. Areas of termination that have the bed nucleus of the stria terminalis as a source show diminished fiber densities, while other areas remain unaltered (Fliers et al., 1985a). Such differential changes in the vasopressin innervation make it very difficult to substitute vasopressin levels in one area without interfering with normal vasopressin levels in other areas. In addition, deficits have been found in many different transmitter systems in Alzheimer's disease (see above; also Francis et al., 1985), so that normalization of all the different deficits of all the different neurotransmitters throughout the brain would not seem to be a simple task to accomplish.

Apart from the above-mentioned considerations, it is not realistic to expect that one can mimic the complex and naturally occurring spatial-temporal fluctuations of a local transmitter release by means of global administration of chemical substances. In addition, one can never replace the complete integrating function of a neuron by straightforward administration of transmitter. These are some of the considerations (e.g. Swaab et al., 1986) which call for skepticism regarding the potentialities of neurotransmitter 'replacement' therapy, whether in the case of neuropeptides or for other putative neurotransmitters.

In spite of the theoretical reservations which we have concerning neurotransmitter substitution therapies, we should realize that neuropeptides may act by different mechanisms and that some positive results have been reported in Alzheimer's disease following manipulating peptidergic systems. This holds true for trials with vasopressin or its analogs, analogs of *ACTH* (cf. Jolles, 1986b) and the opiate antagonist *naloxone*, that appears to improve cognition (Reisberg et al., 1983b). On the other hand, other peptide trials have turned out negative (cf. Jolles, 1986b) and the possibility of side-effects can not be excluded. For instance, an excited state characterized by paranoid delusions, agitation, elevated pulse rate and blood pressure was induced by *DDAVP* in a young woman with profound Alzheimer's disease (Collins et al., 1981). The interesting observation that *oxytocin* increases life-span in rats (Bodanszky and Engel, 1966) has, so far, not been followed up in the literature.

Miscellaneous therapies

Numerous investigations deal with the possible effects of vitamin preparations in the treatment of geriatric patients with mental impairment.

Nicotinic acid has not proved to be of value (Wittenborn, 1981).

On the basis of the presumptions that zinc deficiency would result in a vitamin B12 deficiency, which in turn would lead to dementia, a combined parenteral therapy of *vitamin B12* with *zinc*-DL-*aspartate* has been administered to Alzheimer patients and has been claimed to be effective in preventing senile dementia (Van Tiggelen et al., 1983). There is at present neither a theoretical framework for such a presumption nor any well-designed clinical trial giving support to this idea (Wittenborn, 1981; WHO, 1981; Ned. T. Geneesk., 1983). However, sellings of the vitamin preparations have gone up following Van Tiggelen's claim.

Vitamin E (alpha-tocopherol) would lower lipofuscin concentration in the mouse brain (Kruk and Enesco, 1981). There is, however, no indication that this compound, that also would act as vasodilator, is effective against dementia (Ban, 1978).

Assuming a causal relationship between Pick's disease, Alzheimer's disease and a disturbance of zinc metabolism, *EDTA* has been given to demented patients (Richard et al., 1978). This therapy is also of interest since aluminum has been implicated in the etiology of Alzheimer's disease (Crapper McLachlan and Van Berkum, 1986). However, aluminum is tightly bound to DNA in neuronal nuclei, a binding that cannot readily be reversed. Anti-aluminum treatments should thus ideally be directed towards coupling aluminum before it gains access to neuronal nuclei in the first place. There are, in addition, at present no compounds that specifically bind aluminum. Although some practitioners claim beneficial effects of 'chelation' in Alzheimer patients, these have been anecdotal reports (with one exception), which may therefore be misleading (Shore and Wyatt, 1982). We thus have to wait for some methodologically sound studies.

Conclusion

In conclusion, 'therapeutic' drugs are at present more often the cause of pseudodementia than they are the cure of Alzheimer's disease. Consequently, there seems to be some truth in the cynical point of view concerning the treatment of old, mentally impaired patients in Shem's 'The House of God' (1984): "the cure is the disease" and that "to deliver *no* medical care is the most important thing you can do". If a patient develops symptoms of dementia, the doctor should first see whether he is not prescribing something that in fact may be causing it. A subsequent thorough clinical investigation should reveal possible pseudodementia (Millard, 1984; Van Crevel, 1986). It is characteristic for the current state of therapeutics that the only dementias for which clinically significant therapeutic results can be obtained, are the pseudodementias. For Alzheimer's disease the conclusion, surely, must be that although some of the available pharmacological therapies may im-

prove the condition a little, there is no indication that any of these treatments can really stop or reverse the disease process. If (as has often been claimed, but so far never proven) a treatment were merely to slow down the progressive deterioration rather than 'cure' the patient, one might even ask if a prolonged suffering is really what we should aim for. Changes in the nutrition and social environment of the Alzheimer patient may be just as effective as pharmacological therapies (Held et al., 1984; Mirmiran et al., 1986). Indeed, beneficial effects from mere participation in the clinical trials are often found, but never emphasized in the placebo group of a clinical trial (e.g. Chierichetti et al., 1981). Pharmacological therapies may, in addition, produce considerable side-effects (cf. Millard, 1984) that have not been scrutinized so far.

A specific strategy for developing therapeutic tools in the Alzheimer's disease treatment has not been available until now. On the contrary, new insights and developments in brain research have simply been applied to Alzheimer patients. Many such therapies have statistically significant but clinically insignificant effects. One may wonder whether the small effects produced by quite different drugs and non-pharmacological therapies cannot best be explained, not so much by specific effects, but rather by a generalized stimulation of the brain. Recent observations, both from our own group and from others give support for such a possibility. The vasopressin neuron in the SON and PVN, probably osmotically stimulated secundary to a loss of binding sites in the kidney, remains capable of increased neurosecretion in senescence, both in rats and in human subjects (Fliers and Swaab, 1983; 1986). In contrast, the vasopressin cells of the SCN degenerate after the age of 80, and even more pronounced in Alzheimer's disease (Swaab et al., 1985).

The idea that symptoms of aging (and dementia) may be due to a decrease in neuronal stimulation, is not a new one. Lorand (1913) already stated: "work of any kind, even mental work alone, is means of preventing precocious senility". Dietary restriction, an effective way to increase the lifespan of rodents, might also work by stimulating the animals in a generalized way (Zoler, 1984). 'Compensatory' dendritic outgrowth is normally occurring in senescence (Buell and Coleman, 1979, 1981). A similar process is stimulated by environmental factors in the adult rat (Uylings et al., 1978; Mirmiran et al., 1986). Since no such 'compensatory' dendritic outgrowth occurs in Alzheimer's disease, a key-question for an effective prevention or therapy in Alzheimer's disease may thus be how to effectively stimulate the various neuronal systems that are most vulnerable in this condition. On the other hand, if Maurice Ravel really had Alzheimer's disease (Dalessio, 1984), then neither a productive life, nor a family stimulating him (e.g., by taking him on frequent trips) prevented or cured him from the disease. Moreover, not every change in environment needs to be beneficial for the Alzheimer patient. These patients may, in fact, be so vulnerable to changes in the environment that the effects of the preparatory workup before

inclusion of such patients in a trial might already have adverse effects on them (Etienne et al., 1981).

For the time being, Millard's advice (1984) might be the best: "Until better evidence is available I think I shall tell my mother to go on doing the crossword: like other organs may not brains deteriorate with disuse?" The lack of therapeutic success clearly underlines the need for fundamental research on aging of the brain and on Alzheimer's disease. At present, this seems to be the only way ever to arrive at a rational strategy for the treatment of this condition.

Acknowledgements

The authors wish to thank Dr. M. A. Corner for revising the English and Mrs. W. Chen-Pelt for preparing the manuscript. This work was supported by The Foundation for Medical Research (FUNGO; project 13-51-30).

References

Ban, T. A. (1978) Vasodilators, stimulants and anabolic agents in the treatment of geropsychiatric patients. In M. A. Lipton, A. DiMascio and K. F. Killam (Eds.), *Psychopharmacology: A Generation of Progress*, Raven Press, New York, pp. 1525–1533.

Barbeau, A. (1978) Emerging treatments: replacement therapy with choline or lecithin in neurological diseases. *J. Can. Sci. Neurol.*, 5: 157–160.

Bartus, R. T., Dean, R. L., Sherman, K. A., Friedman, E. and Beer, B. (1981) Profound effects of combining choline and piracetam on memory enhancement and cholinergic function in aged rats. *Neurobiol. Aging*, 2: 105–111.

Bartus, R. T., Dean, R. L., Beer, B. and Lippa, A. S. (1982) The cholinergic hypothesis of geriatric memory dysfunction. *Science*, 217: 408–417.

Bartus, R. T., Flicker, C., Dean, R. L., Fisher, S., Pontecorvo, M. and Figueiredo, J. (1986) Behavioral and biochemical effects of nucleus basalis magnocellularis lesions: implications and possible relevance to understanding or treating Alzheimer's disease. In D. F. Swaab, E. Fliers, M. Mirmiran, W. A. Van Gool and F. Van Haaren (Eds.), *Aging of the Brain and Alzheimer's Disease, Progress in Brain Research, this volume*, Elsevier, Amsterdam, pp. 345–361.

Bodanszky, M. and Engel, S. L. (1966) Oxytocin and the life-span of male rats. *Nature*, 210: 751.

Bondareff, W., Muntjoy, C. Q. and Roth, M. (1982) Loss of neurons of origin of the adrenergic projection to cerebral cortex (nucleus locus ceruleus) in senile dementia. *Neurology*, 32: 164–168.

Branconnier, R. and Cole, J. O. (1977) Senile dementia and drug therapy. In K. Nandy and I. Sherwin (Eds.), *The Aging Brain and Senile Dementia*, Plenum Press, New York, pp. 271–283.

Brown-Séquard, M. (1889) Des effets produits chez l'homme par des injections sous-cutanées d'un liquide retiré des testicules frais de cobaye et de chien. *CR Soc. Biol.*, 41: 415–419.

Buell, S. J. and Coleman, P. D. (1979) Dendritic growth in the aged human brain and failure of growth in senile dementia. *Science*, 206: 854–856.

Buell, S. J. and Coleman, P. D. (1981) Quantitative evidence for selective dendritic growth in normal human aging but not in senile dementia. *Brain Res.*, 214: 23–41.

Buijs, R. M. (1982) The ultrastructural localization of amines, amino acids and peptides in the brain. In R. M. Buijs, P. Pévet and D. F. Swaab (Eds.), *Chemical Transmission in the Brain. The Role of Amines, Amino Acids and Peptides, Progress in Brain Research Vol. 55*, Elsevier Biomedical Press, Amsterdam, pp. 167–183.

Buijs, R. M. and Swaab, D. F. (1979) Immuno-electron microscopical demonstration of vasopressin and oxytocin synapses in the limbic system of the rat. *Cell Tiss. Res.*, 204: 355–365.

Chien, C.-P. (1971) Psychiatric treatment of geriatric patients: 'pub' or drug? *Am. J. Psychiat.*, 127: 1070–1074.

Chien, C.-P., Stotsky, B. A. and Cole, J. O. (1973) Psychiatric treatment for nursing home patients: drug, alcohol, and milieu. *Am. J. Psychiat.*, 130: 543–548.

Cole, J. O. and Liptzin, B. (1984) Drug treatment of dementia in the elderly. In D. W. K. Kay and G. D. Burrows (Eds.), *Handbook of Studies on Psychiatry and Old Age*, Elsevier Science Publishers BV, pp. 169–179.

Coleman, P. D. and Flood, D. G. (1986) Dendritic proliferation in the aging brain as a compensatory repair mechanism. In D. F. Swaab, E. Fliers, M. Mirmiran, W. A. Van Gool and F. Van Haaren (Eds.), *Aging of the Brain and Alzheimer's Disease, Progress in Brain Research, this volume*, Elsevier, Amsterdam, pp. 227–237.

Collins, G. B., Marzewski, D. J. and Rollins, M. B. (1981) Paranoid psychosis after DDAVP therapy for Alzheimer's dementia. *The Lancet*, October 10: 808.

Crapper McLachlan, D. R. and Van Berkum, M. F. A. (1986) Aluminum: a role in degenerative brain disease associated with neurofibrillary degeneration. In D. F. Swaab, E. Fliers, M. Mirmiran, W. A. Van Gool and F. Van Haaren (Eds.), *Aging of the Brain and Alzheimer's Disease, Progress in Brain Research, this volume*, Elsevier, Amsterdam, pp. 399–410.

Dalessio, D. J. (1984) Maurice Ravel and Alzheimer's disease. *J. Am. Med. Assoc.*, 252: 3412–3413.

De Beer, J. M. M. and Simons, C. H. (1977) Psychopharmaca als oorzaak van pseudodementie. *Ned. T. Geneesk.*, 121: 664–666.

Deslypere, J. P. and Vermeulen, A. (1984) Leydig cell function in normal men: effect of age, life style, residence, diet and activity. *J. Clin. Endocrinol. Metab.*, 59: 955–962.

De Wied, D. and Van Ree, J. M. (1982) Neuropeptides, mental performance and aging. *Life Sci.*, 31: 709–719.

Diesfeldt, H. F. A., Cahn, L. A. and Cornelissen, A. J. E. (1978) Over onderzoek naar het effect van piracetam (Nootropil®) in psychogeriatrie. *Ned. T. Gerontol.*, 9: 81–89.

Drachman, D. A., Glosser, G., Fleming, P. and Longenecker, G. (1982) Memory decline in the aged: treatment with lecithin and physostigmine. *Neurology*, 32: 944–950.

Eisdorfer, C., Conner, J. F. and Wilkie, F. L. (1968) The effect of magnesium pemoline on cognition and behavior. *J. Gerontol.*, 23: 283–288.

Epstein, L. J. (1978) Anxiolytics, antidepressants, and neuroleptics in the treatment of geriatric patient. In M. A. Lipton, A. DiMascio and K. F. Killam (Eds.), *Psychopharmacology: A Generation of Progress*, Raven Press, New York, pp. 1517–1523.

Ermini, M. and Markstein, R. (1984) Pharmacological rationale for a treatment of senile dementia with codergocrine mesylate. In J. T. Hutton and A. D. Kenny (Eds.), *Senile Dementia: Outlook for the Future*, A. R. Liss, Inc., New York, pp. 365–379.

Etienne, P. E., Dastoor, D., Goldapple, E., Johnson, S.,

Rochefort, E. and Ratner, J. (1981) Adverse effects of medical and psychiatric workup in six demented geriatric patients. *Am. J. Psychiat.*, 138: 520–521.

Facchinetti, F., Nappi, G., Petraglia, F., Martignoni, E., Sinforiani, E. and Genazzani, A. R. (1984) Central ACTH deficit in degenerative and vascular dementia. *Life Sci.*, 35: 1691–1697.

Fliers, E. (1982) Aging brain and ergot alkaloids. *Sandorama*, 1: 34–36.

Fliers, E. and Swaab, D. F. (1983) Activation of vasopressinergic and oxytocinergic neurons during aging in the Wistar rat. *Peptides*, 4: 165– 170.

Fliers, E. and Swaab, D. F. (1986) Neuropeptide changes in aging and Alzheimer's disease. In D. F. Swaab, E. Fliers, M. Mirmiran, W. A. Van Gool and F. Van Haaren (Eds.), *Aging of the Brain and Alzheimer's Disease, Progress in Brain Research, this volume*, Elsevier, Amsterdam, pp. 141–152.

Fliers, E., De Vries, G. J. and Swaab, D. F. (1985a) Changes with aging in the vasopressin and oxytocin innervation of the rat brain. *Brain Res.*, 348: 1–8.

Fliers, E., Swaab, D. F., Pool, C. W. and Verwer, R. W. H. (1985b) The vasopressin and oxytocin neurons in the human supraoptic and paraventricular nucleus; changes with aging and in senile dementia. *Brain Res.*, 342: 45–53.

Foley, J. M. (1956) Hypertensive and arteriosclerotic vascular disease of the brain in the elderly. In J. E. Moore et al. (Eds.), *The Neurologic and Psychiatric Aspects of the Disorders of Aging*, The Williams and Wilkins Company, Baltimore, pp. 171–197.

Frackowiak, R. S. J. (1986) Measurement and imaging of cerebral function in ageing and dementia. In D. F. Swaab, E. Fliers, M. Mirmiran, W. A. Van Gool and F. Van Haaren (Eds.), *Aging of the Brain and Alzheimer's Disease, Progress in Brain Research, this volume*, Elsevier, Amsterdam, pp. 69–85.

Francis, P. T., Palmer, A. M., Sims, N. R., Bowen, D. M., Davison, A. N., Esiri, M. M., Neary, D., Snowden, J. S. and Wilcock, G. K. (1985) Neurochemical studies of early-onset Alzheimer's disease. Possible influence on treatment. *N. Engl. J. Med.*, 313: 7–11.

Freund, G. (1982) The interaction of chronic alcohol consumption and aging on brain structure and function. *Alcoholism: Clin. Exper. Res.*, 6: 12–21.

Freund, G. and Butters, N. (1982) Alcohol and aging: challenges for the future. *Alcoholism: Clin. Exper. Res.*, 6: 1–2.

Gottfries, C. G. (1986) Monoamines and myelin components in aging and dementia disorders. In D. F. Swaab, E. Fliers, M. Mirmiran, W. A. Van Gool and F. Van Haaren (Eds.), *Aging of the Brain and Alzheimer's Disease, Progress in Brain Research, this volume*, Elsevier, Amsterdam, pp. 133–140.

Hall, M. R., Briggs, R. S., MacLennan, W. J. Marcer, D., Robinson, M. J. and Everett, F. M. (1983) The effects of procaine/haematoporphyrin on age-related decline: a double-blind trial. *Age Aging*, 12: 302–308.

Held, M., Ransohoff, P. M. and Goehner, P. (1984) A comprehensive treatment program for severely impaired geriatric patients. *Hosp. Commun. Psychiat.*, 35: 156–160.

Hollister, L. E. (1985) Alzheimer's disease. Is it worth treating? *Drugs*, 29: 483–488.

Hollister, L. E. and Yesavage, J. (1984) Ergoloid mesylates for senile dementias: unanswered questions. *Ann. Int. Med.*, 100: 894–898.

Hoogendijk, J. E., Fliers, E., Swaab, D. F. and Verwer, R. W. H. (1985) Activation of vasopressin neurons in the human supraoptic and paraventricular nucleus in senescence and senile dementia. *J. Neurol. Sci.*, 69: 291–299.

Jolles, J. (1986a) Cognitive, emotional and behavioral dysfunctions in aging and dementia. In D. F. Swaab, E. Fliers, M. Mirmiran, W. A. Van Gool and F. Van Haaren (Eds.), *Aging of the Brain and Alzheimer's Disease, Progress in Brain Research, this volume*, Elsevier, Amsterdam, pp. 15–39.

Jolles, J. (1986b) Neuropeptides and the treatment of cognitive deficits in aging and dementia. In D. F. Swaab, E. Fliers, M. Mirmiran, W. A. Van Gool and F. Van Haaren (Eds.), *Aging of the Brain and Alzheimer's Disease, Progress in Brain Research, this volume*, Elsevier, Amsterdam, pp. 429–441.

Kruk, P. and Enesco, H. E. (1981) alpha-Tocopherol reduces fluorescent agent pigment levels in heart and brain of young mice. *Experientia*, 37: 1301–1302.

Lader, M. and Petursson, H. (1983) Long-term effects of benzodiazepines. *Neuropharmacology*, 22: 527–533.

Legros, J. J. (1975) The radioimmunoassay of human neurophysins: contribution to the understanding of the physiopathology of neurohypophyseal function. *Ann. NY Acad. Sci.*, 248: 281–303.

Legros, J. J., Gilot, P., Seron, Z., Claessens, J., Adam, A., Moeglen, J. M., Audibert, A. and Berchier, P. (1978) Influence of vasopressin on learning and memory. *Lancet*, 1: 41–42.

Lieberman, H. R. and Abou-Nader, T. M. (1986) Possible dietary strategies to reduce cognitive deficits in old age. In D. F. Swaab, E. Fliers, M. Mirmiran, W. A. Van Gool and F. Van Haaren (Eds.), *Aging of the Brain and Alzheimer's Disease, Progress in Brain Research, this volume*, Elsevier, Amsterdam, pp. 461–471.

Loew, D. M. and Weil, C. (1982) Gerontology, 28: 54–74.

Lorand, A. (1913) *Old Age Deferred. The Causes of Old Age and its Postponement by Hygienic and Therapeutic Measures*, F. A. Davis Co., Publ., Philadelphia.

McFarland, R. A. (1963) Experimental evidence of the relationship between aging and oxygen want: in search of a theory of ageing. *Ergonomics* 6, 339– 366.

Meier-Ruge, W. (1983) Medicamenten ter behandeling van beginnende dementie. *Ned. Tijdschr. Geneesk.*, 127: 977–978 and editorial, in Dutch.

Millard, P. H. (1984) Treatment for aging brains. *Br. Med. J.*, 289: 1094.

Mirmiran, M., Van Gool, W. A., Van Haaren, F. and Polak, C. E. (1986) Environmental influences on brain and behavior in aging and dementia. In D. F. Swaab, E. Fliers, M. Mirmiran, W. A. Van Gool and F. Van Haaren (Eds.), *Aging of the Brain and Alzheimer's Disease, Progress in Brain Research, this volume*, Elsevier, Amsterdam, pp. 443–459.

Ned. T. Geneesk. (1983) Is dementie met vitaminen en spoorelementen te behandelen? Editorial, Vol. 127: 2250.

Nandy, K. and Schneider, F. H. (1978) Effects of hydergine on aging neuroblastoma cells in culture. *Pharmacology*, 16, Suppl. 1: 88–92, in Dutch.

Palacios, J. M. and Spiegel, R. (1986) Muscarinic cholinergic agonists; pharmacological and clinical perspectives. In D. F. Swaab, E. Fliers, M. Mirmiran, W. A. Van Gool and F. Van Haaren (Eds.), *Aging of the Brain and Alzheimer's Disease, Progress in Brain Research, this volume*, Elsevier, Amsterdam, pp. 485–498.

Pomora, N., Block, R., Abraham, J., Domino, E. F. and Gershon, S. (1983) Combined cholinergic precursor treatment and dihydroergotoxine mesylate in Alzheimer's disease. *IRCS Med. Sci.*, 11: 1048–1049.

Reisberg, B., London, E., Ferris, S. H., Anand, R., and De Leon, M. J. (1983a) Novel pharmacologic approaches to the treatment of senile dementia of the Alzheimer's type (SDAT). *Psychopharmacol. Bull.*, 19, 220–224.

Reisberg, B., Ferris, S., Anand, R., Mir, P., Geibel, V. and De Leon, M. J. (1983b) Effects of naloxone in senile dementia: a double-blind trial. *N. Engl. J. Med.*, 308: 721–722.

Richard, J., Constantinidis, J. and Tissot, R. (1978) Traitement de la maladie de PICK par l'EDTA calcique. *Nouv. Presse Med.*, 7, 15.

Roth, G. S., Henry, J. M. and Joseph, J. A. (1986) The striatal dopaminergic system as a model for modulation of altered neurotransmitter action during aging: effects of dietary and neuroendocrine manipulations. In D. F. Swaab, E. Fliers, M. Mirmiran, W. A. Van Gool and F. Van Haaren (Eds.), *Aging of the Brain and Alzheimer's Disease, Progress in Brain Research, this volume*, Elsevier, Amsterdam, pp. 473–484.

Samorajski, T., Vroulis, G. A. and Smith, R. C. (1985) Piracetam plus lecithin trials in senile dementia of the Alzheimer type. In: Memory Dysfunctions: an Integration of Animal and Human Research from Preclinical Perspectives. *Ann. NY Acad. Sci.*, 444: 478–481.

Shem, S. (1984) The House of God. Dell Publ. Co., Inc., New York.

Shore, D. and Wyatt, R. J. (1982) Research design issues: antialuminum drug studies in Alzheimer's disease. *Clin. Neuropharmacol.*, 5: 337–343.

Smith, A. H. W., Kay, D. S. G., Johnson, K. and Ballinger, B. R. (1979) Bromocriptine in senile dementia — a placebo controlled double blind trial. *IRCS Med. Sci.*, 7: 463.

Sofroniew, M. V., Pearson, R. C. A., Isacson, O. and Björklund, A. (1986) Experimental studies on the induction of retrograde degeneration of basal forebrain cholinergic neurons. In D. F. Swaab, E. Fliers, M. Mirmiran, W. A. Van Gool and F. Van

Haaren (Eds.), *Aging of the Brain and Alzheimer's Disease, Progress in Brain Research, this volume*, pp. 363–389.

Steinach, E. and Leobel, J. (1940) *Sex and Life. Forty Years of Biological and Medical Experiments*, Faber and Faber Ltd., London.

Swaab, D. F. (1982) Neuropeptides. Their distribution and function in the brain. In R. M. Buijs, P. Pévet and D. F. Swaab (Eds.), *Chemical Transmissions in the Brain. The Role of Amines, Amino Acids and Peptides, Progress in Brain Research, Vol. 55*, Elsevier Biomedical Press, Amsterdam, pp. 97–123.

Swaab, D. F., Fliers, E. and Partiman, T. S. (1985) The suprachiasmatic nucleus of the human brain in relation to sex, age and dementia. *Brain Res.*, 342: 37–44.

Swaab, D. F., Fliers, E. and Van Gool, W. A. (1986) Immunocytochemical localization of vasopressin in the human brain; its possible consequences for therapeutic strategies in aging and dementia. In J. M. Van Ree and S. Matthysse (Eds.), *Psychiatric Disorders: Neurotransmitters and Neuropeptides, Progress in Brain Research, Vol. 65*, Elsevier, Amsterdam, pp. 105–113.

Tausk, M. (1976) A brief endocrine history of the german-speaking peoples. In J. Kracht, A. von zur Mühlen and P. C. Scriba (Eds.), *Endocrinology Guide*, Bruhlschen Universität, Gieszen, FRG, pp. 1–34.

Uylings, H. B. M., Kuypers, G., Diamond, M. C. and Veltman, W. A. M. (1978) Effects of differential environments on plasticity of dendrites of cortical pyramidal neurons in adult rats. *Exp. Neurol.*, 62: 658–677.

Van Crevel, H. (1986) Clinical approach to dementia. In D. F. Swaab, E. Fliers, M. Mirmiran, W. A. Van Gool and F. Van Haaren (Eds.), *Aging of the Brain and Alzheimer's Disease, Progress in Brain Research, this volume*, Elsevier, Amsterdam, pp. 3–13.

Van Tiggelen, C. J. M., Peperkamp, J. P. C. and Tertoolen, J. F. W. (1983) Vitamin B12 levels of cerebrospinal fluid in patients with organic mental disorder. *J. Orthomolec. Psychiat.*, 12: 305–311.

Vermeulen, A. (1976) Leydig-cell function in old age. In A. V. Everitt and J. A. Burgess (Eds.), *Hypothalamus, Pituitary and Aging*. C. C. Thomas, Springfield, Il., pp. 458–463.

Voronoff, S. (1925) Etude sur la Vieilesse et la Rajeunissement par la Greffe. Librairie Octave Doin, Paris.

Warner, B. A., Dufau, M. L. and Santen, R. J. (1985) Effects of aging and illness on the pituitary testicular axis in men: qualitative as well as quantitative changes in luteinizing hormone. *J. Clin. Endocrinol. Metab.*, 60: 263–268.

White, L., Crovello, J. N., Rosenberg, S. N. and Neiditch, J. A. (1975) Evaluation of isobaric oxygenation for the aged with cognitive impairment: pilot study. *J. Am. Geriat. Soc.*, 23: 80–85.

Wittenborn, J. R. (1981) Pharmacotherapy for age-related behavioral deficiencies. *J. Nerv. Ment. Dis.*, 169: 139–156.

World Health Organization (1981) Neuronal aging and its implications in human neurological pathology. *Report of a WHO Study Group*. WHO Technical Report Series, No. 665, Geneva.

Yesavage, J. A., Tinklenberg, J. F., Hollister, L. E. and Berger, P. A. (1979) Vasodilatators in senile dementias. *Arch. Gen. Psychiat.*, 36: 220–223.

Yesavage, J. A., Tinklenberg, J. R., Hollister, L. E. and Berger, P. A. (1982) Effect of natronyl on lactate and pyruvate in the cerebrospinal fluid of patients with senile dementia. *J. Am. Geriat. Soc.*, 30: 105–108.

Zoler, M. L. (1984) Diet restriction: new clues to slow the aging process? *Geriatrics*, 39(2): 130–144.

Zung, W. W. K., Gianturco, D., Pfeiffer, E., Wang, H-S., Whanger, A., Bridge, T. P. and Potkin, S. G. (1974) Pharmacology of depression in the aged: evaluation of Gerovital H3 as an antidepressant drug. *Psychosomatics*, 15: 127–131.

Discussion

J. M. RABEY: It still needs to be established if the dying system of the brain works by the principle of all or nothing or there is still a period when the cells are still alive but sick and therefore can be helped by manipulation at the presynaptic level. A good example is the treatment of Parkinson's disease. For years we may have succeeded in treating Parkinson patients, improving their performance until there is a complete failure of the system.

ANSWER: That is true, but I think that also these therapeutic effects in Parkinson's disease are in support of my thesis that little may be expected if transmitters are used to substitute for cell loss. Therapy in Parkinson's disease, although initially effective, becomes at a certain moment ineffective. That means that the precursor (L-dopa) cannot replace the death neurons. It can only help the surviving neurons. However, the biochemistry of the dopaminergic neuron has the advantage of being able to profit from precursor that is administered. This cannot be expected to a similar degree from other transmitter systems (e.g. peptides). Cell loss is the hallmark of dementia and it affects many different brain neurotransmitters, so that I am sceptical about the substitution potentialities.

F. BROWN: Please clarify the statement about neuroleptic therapy causing 'dementia'.

ANSWER: Quite frequently old subjects are brought into the clinics with the diagnosis 'dementia'. The condition appears, however, to be due to misuse of medicines. When the various medicines they got, often from different physicians, are stopped, they are cured within a short time. Neuroleptics are often the cause of such pseudodementias (De Beer and Simons, 1977).

D. M. GASH: In trying to interpret the significance of the loss of small vasopressin neurons in the suprachiasmatic nucleus (SCN) in human aging as compared to the relative stability of large magnocellular supraoptic and paraventricular neurons (SON and PVN) could other principles be operating than those suggested? For example, could those neurons generated earlier in development be more stable during aging? One could also suggest other possibilities, such as the phylogenetically older neurons being the last to undergo aging. Have you evaluated these alternate explanations?

R. M. TERRY: *Comment*: Dr. Gash suggested small neurons particularly lost in normal aging neocortex. Although Brody claimed that in 1955, data from Haug's lab. and my own are quite opposite (cf. Terry, 1986). Large neurons decrease, small neurons are preserved.

ANSWER: Our own work shows also that one cannot simply predict cell death from cell size. In the human hypothalamus the SON and PVN cells are the largest and the most stable (Fliers et al., 1985; Fliers and Swaab, 1986). The SCN cells start to degenerate after the age of 80. These cells are the smallest. However, intermediate in size, the cells of the sexual dimorphic nucleus of the preoptic area (SDN) show the earliest degeneration. A cell loss was found from the age of 40 onwards in this nucleus (Swaab and Fliers, 1985). But, concerning the cause of cell death and cell stability all possibilities are still open. The only way to give a real answer to Dr. Gash's questions is to do the type of experiments we plan to do in the near future, i.e., activate or inhibit the neurons for a long time during aging and see whether we will influence in that way cell stability or degeneration.

A. GOWER: Could you comment further on the use of the 'nootropic' piracetam in Alzheimer's disease, particularly as several drug companies are busy developing similar compounds.
ANSWER: In controlled studies it was inactive in Alzheimer patients (Diesfeldt et al., 1978; Wittenborn, 1981) and it is currently marketed for use in transient ischemic attacks.

J. E. PISETSKY: Have antiviral agents been used? Has nicotinic acid not been used as vasodilator but to reduce cholesterol?

ANSWER: To my knowledge nobody has used antiviral drugs in Alzheimer patients, and there is no positive effect on dementia reported from nicotinic acid (Ban, 1978; Wittenborn, 1981).

References

Ban, T. A. (1978) Vasodilators, stimulants and anabolic agents in the treatment of geropsychiatric patients. In M. A. Lipton, A. DiMascio and K. F. Killam (Eds.), *Psychopharmacology: A Generation of Progress*, Raven Press, New York, pp. 1525–1533.

De Beer, J. M. M. and Simons, C. H. (1977) Psychopharmaca als oorzaak van pseudodementie. *Ned. T. Geneesk.*, 121: 664–666.

Diesfeldt, H. F. A., Cahn, L. A. and Cornelissen, A. J. E. (1978) Over onderzoek naar het effect van piracetam (Nootropil (R)) in psychogeriatrie. *Ned. T. Gerontol.*, 9(2): 81–89.

Fliers, E. and Swaab, D. F. (1986) Neuropeptide changes in aging and Alzheimer's disease. In E. Fliers, M. Mirmiran, D. F. Swaab, W. A. Van Gool and F. Van Haaren (Eds.), *Aging of the Brain and Alzheimer's Disease, Progress in Brain Research, this volume*, Elsevier, Amsterdam, pp. 141–152.

Fliers, E., Swaab, D. F., Pool, C. W. and Verwer, R. W. H. (1985) The vasopressin and oxytocin neurons in the human supraoptic and paraventricular nucleus; changes with aging and in senile dementia. *Brain Res.*, 342: 45–53.

Swaab, D. F. and Fliers, E. (1985) A sexually dimorphic nucleus in the human brain. *Science*, 228: 1112–1115.

Terry, R. D. (1986) Interrelations among the lesions of normal and abnormal aging of the brain. In E. Fliers, M. Mirmiran, D. F. Swaab, W. A. Van Gool and F. Van Haaren (Eds.), *Aging of the Brain and Alzheimer's Disease, Progress in Brain Research, this volume*, Elsevier, Amsterdam, pp. 41–48.

Wittenborn, J. R. (1981) Pharmacotherapy for age-related behavioral deficiencies. *J. Nerv. Ment. Dis.*, 169: 139–156.

D. F. Swaab, E. Fliers, M. Mirmiran, W. A. Van Gool and F. Van Haaren (Eds.)
Progress in Brain Research, Vol. 70.
© 1986 Elsevier Science Publishers B.V. (Biomedical Division)

CHAPTER 27

Neuropeptides and the treatment of cognitive deficits in aging and dementia

J. Jolles

Department of Clinical Psychiatry, State University of Limburg, P.O. Box 616, 6200 MD Maastricht, The Netherlands

Introduction

Neuropeptides have recently been suggested to be potentially useful in the treatment of cognitive deficits in man. This suggestion has been based primarily upon animal experiments in which peptides derived from the pituitary hormones ACTH and vasopressin appeared to improve performance in several experimental paradigms, designed to measure learning and memory. These data have been interpreted in terms of peptide effects on attentional, motivational and memory processes (see De Wied, 1969; De Wied and Jolles, 1983; De Wied, 1983, for references). Clinical researchers have become interested in the laboratory findings in view of the potential use of the neuropeptides to alleviate symptoms which accompany many neuropsychiatric diseases. Unfortunately, the results obtained in clinical trials up till now are difficult to evaluate because of differences in patient populations and treatment parameters. ACTH-like peptides have been used extensively with human volunteers before clinical trials were done with elderly people and demented patients. The reverse is true for vasopressin-like peptides: many different types of patients have been treated with vasopressin before studies with volunteers were carried out. The present paper will review the current knowledge with respect to the clinical studies with ACTH and vasopressin in elderly and (senile) demented subjects. A brief overview will

also be given of the peptide studies which have been performed with other patient groups and rodents. A more detailed description of the clinical effectiveness of vasopressin in other patient populations can be found in Jolles (1983, 1987).

Cognitive dysfunctions in aging and dementia

Complaints of memory and other cognitive functions accompany many neuropsychiatric diseases. The disturbance in the brain processes which underlie these complaints can be very different because of the fact that the etiological and pathogenetic factors are quite varied (see Luria, 1976; Newcombe, 1980; and Russell, 1981, for reviews). It is therefore important to specify the action of the drugs in terms of actions on different aspects of memory and cognition (e.g. Squire and Davis, 1981). This may especially be true because patients suffering from different diseases may have similar complaints. This similarity in the nature of the complaints may result in a wrong impression with respect to drug specificity: it is not to be expected that one drug will have a beneficial effect on all kinds of cognitive (e.g. memory-) deficits in all types of diseases. A brief summary of the nature of the complaints and the cognitive dysfunctions in aging and (pre)senile dementia may illustrate this point. A more thorough description may be found elsewhere (Jolles, 1987; Jolles, 1985; Botwinnick, 1981; Jolles and Hijman, 1983).

Cognitive dysfunctions in aging

Elderly subjects are characterized by an age-associated decline in nearly all cognitive functions (intellectual functioning, memory, language functions, problem solving and perception, Botwinnick, 1981; Jolles and Hijman, 1983; Jolles, 1985). Those behavioral functions seem to be preserved in which the person can rely on well-trained skills and knowledge. Thus, well-learned motor skills are preserved as well as expressive language. In addition, passive recognition of old and newly learnt information does not deteriorate significantly, but active encoding in and retrieval from memory does. An increasing inefficiency in the use of new information is observed. Kral (1962) introduced the term 'senescent forgetfulness' distinguishing benign (BSF) and malignant (MSF) forms. BSF is a deficit in the recollection of relatively minor details of an episode while the episode as such can be recalled. This retrieval deficit is not permanent and is situation-dependent. MSF on the other hand is characterized by the loss of the episode itself. The nature of the memory deficit in BSF may be partly related to a decreased speed of information processing in the elderly subject. It may also be a secondary consequence of a decreased effectiveness of behavioral organization, evidenced by a tendency towards inflexibility, cautiousness and conservatism (Botwinnick, 1981). 'Stimulus persistence' and the fact that more effort is needed to change opinions and beliefs are taken to be an indication of a deficient behavioral planning and organization. There is some evidence suggesting that frontal neocortical structures are involved (Jolles and Hijman, 1983; Jolles, 1985).

Cognitive dysfunctions in (pre)senile dementia

The pattern of cognitive deficits in dementia of Alzheimer type (AD) appears to be qualitatively similar to normal aging (see Jolles and Hijman, 1983; Jolles, 1985). There are also similarities between the presenile and the senile forms of AD (Sulkava and Amberla, 1981). The early stages of AD are difficult to discriminate from 'normal aging' and depression, although a clear-cut consolidation deficit (in AD) seems to differentiate different types of patients (Branconnier and DeVitt, 1984; Jolles, 1985). There seems to be a clearly definable progression in Alzheimer's disease; different functions of the brain are affected in a certain order (Strub and Black, 1981; Reisberg et al., 1982; Jolles, 1985). Symptoms such as a general decrease in activity and deterioration of short-term memory and awareness appear first, followed by behavioral dysfunctions such as disorientation and paranoid delusions. Still later, apraxic, aphasic and agnosic deficits appear. In addition, deterioration of logical reasoning and loss of control over complex and simpler behavioral functions appear. In the final stages of the disease, only some basic autonomic functions are still preserved.

AD clearly differs from other types of dementia. For instance, the (pre)senile dementia of Pick's type especially is characterized by behavioral disturbances and deficits in the planning and organization of behavior which are characteristic for dysfunctions of the frontal lobe. Likewise, those dementias which depend primarily upon vascular disorders ('multiinfarct dementia') are defined by a different profile of cognitive dysfunctions due to its focal deficits (e.g. complex visual deficits and disorientation without a memory deficit for verbal material is characteristic for involvement of right-hemispheric structures; Jolles and Hijman, 1983; Jolles, 1985).

ACTH and cognitive disorders

The notion that neuropeptides like ACTH and vasopressin might affect cognitive disorders in patients and elderly persons has been derived primarily from animal studies by De Wied and coworkers (De Wied, 1969, 1976, 1977; De Wied and Jolles, 1983). A brief description of the major preclinical findings serves to illustrate the similarities and differences which can be expected in the effects of the peptides between rodents and man.

Animal studies

Neuropeptides related to the pituitary hormones ACTH and vasopressin affect animal behavior in a number of different test situations. Twenty years of research have indicated that peptides related to ACTH play a central role in the cerebral organization of adaptive behavior (De Wied, 1969; De Wied and Jolles, 1983; Jolles et al., 1982). It has been shown that hypophysectomized rats perform badly in tests which measure conditioned avoidance behavior. That is, in test situations in which the rat has to learn to avoid a mild electric foot shock by climbing into a pole or by jumping over a small fence mounted in the testcage. This behavioral deficit could be normalized by treatment with adrenocorticotrophic hormone (ACTH). It turned out later that a similar treatment effect could be observed in intact rats. Fragments of the hormone without corticotrophic activity appeared to have a similar effect, suggesting that the peptide might act directly on the brain. Support for this notion came from experiments in which the dosage of the peptide needed to produce a particular behavioral effect was much lower after central than after peripheral administration (De Wied, 1976). In addition, several peptides have been synthetized which have a potentiated behavioral action, but lack the peripheral side effects of the parent compounds. For instance, the synthetic peptide Org 2766 is an ACTH4–9 analog. It has no steroidogenic action but its behavioral action is one thousand times stronger than that of ACTH4–10. It is also reasonably resistant towards enzymatic degradation and thus can be administered orally (Pigache, 1982). The duration of the ACTH effect is relatively short compared to the effect of vasopressin (days). Some consensus exists with respect to the hypotheses concerning the mechanisms of action of the peptide: ACTH-like peptides affect processes that are sometimes described as 'arousal', 'attention' and/or 'motivation' (De Wied and Jolles, 1983; Pigache, 1982). Squire and Davis (1981) summarize these effects in terms of an action on 'extrinsic aspects of memory'. De

Wied has suggested that the peptide temporarily increases the motivational value of environmental stimuli, by selectively inducing a state of arousal in certain limbic structures in the midbrain. This hypothesis is based upon both electrophysiological and neurochemical findings (De Wied and Jolles, 1983).

Human studies, acute or short-term administration

The finding that ACTH-like peptides have an influence on behaviors interpreted in terms of attention and motivation has stimulated similar studies in man. Consistent effects of ACTH4–10 and Org 2766 on memory task performance have not been found: according to Pigache (1982; Pigache and Rigter, 1981) those positive findings which have been published are most probably due to methodological shortcomings (e.g. statistical methods which have not been used correctly, and the use of wrong tests). These authors evaluated the properly performed studies and concluded that ACTH4–10 and Org 2766 do not have clear effects on memory processes (Pigache and Rigter, 1981). This absence of significant effects on memory processes has been observed in healthy young subjects, in patients treated with electroconvulsant therapy, children with minimal brain dysfunction, alcoholics and others with signs of cognitive deficits (Tinklenberg and Thornton, 1983).

Initial trials with both healthy subjects and patients have used either a single dose of the peptide ('acute' treatment) or a relatively short period of administration (several days). Generally, consistent effects have not been found with respect to cognitive functions and memory measured in information processing tasks (for review, see Gaillard, 1981; Pigache and Rigter, 1981). Single doses of ACTH4–10 or Org 2766 appear to enhance human performance on behavioral tasks under certain conditions. For instance, Org 2766 has been found to enhance performance in visual perception and discrimination tasks (e.g. Beckwith and Sandman, 1982). Likewise, significant peptide effects have been found during tasks which required sustained attention or vigilance during long and monotonous sessions. Gaillard (1981) has, thus, suggested that ACTH does not influence 'selective attention', but 'task-directed motivation'. This specific motivation cannot be explained as a change in general motivation or activation, because the peptide did not affect the basal heart frequency. Studies with elderly subjects did not produce the clear-cut effects which had been found in younger subjects (Pigache, 1982).

The human vigilance studies are not of immediate clinical importance because the degree of improvement in the individual subjects was too small. However, the studies do provide relevant theoretical information. For instance, consensus has been reached on the hypothesis that the ACTH effects are not on intrinsic, information-containing memory functions per se, but instead on extrinsic memory modulating processes or other factors that affect task performance, especially during prolonged testing sessions (Gaillard, 1981; Tinklenberg and Thornton, 1983; Squire and Davis, 1981).

Human studies: subchronic administration

Recent findings with subchronically administered Org 2766 (i.e. for more than 1 week) appear to have positive effects in elderly patients. Ferris and coworkers (1980) treated 50 elderly subjects who suffered mild cognitive impairment but lived in the community. These subjects were not depressed or anxious. Ferris et al. observed a significant decrease in 'depression' and an increase in self-rated 'competence' on the 'mood-scales-elderly' (M-SE). Anxiety was also significantly decreased. In another study, with 35 more severely impaired geriatric inpatients, an observer rating scale was used to evaluate the Org 2766 effect on different behaviors: significant treatment effects were found with respect to 'ward behavior' and 'social behavior' (Braverman et al., 1980). Other double blind studies in which 5, 10 or 20 mg Org 2766 per day was administered reported significant effects with respect to 'anxiety' and 'social behavior' (Pigache and Rigter, 1981). In yet another study in which the peptide effect was evaluated by a self-rating scale (Profile of Mood-Scales, POMS), significant peptide effects were not found (Branconnier and Cole, 1977). In addition, Org 2766 did not affect hyperkinetic children (cf. Pigache and Rigter, 1981). In contrast to these effects obtained with subchronic administration, there has never been any effect of this peptide given only once (Pigache, 1982).

These findings suggest that ACTH peptides, especially if given repeatedly for a longer period of time, can affect human behavior under certain conditions. With respect to their mechanism of action, an action on extrinsic memory processes is most probable. It remains to be seen whether the positive effects on mood and social behavior can be explained by the fact that there is an anatomical correlation with respect to the cerebral substrate involved: ascending fibers (noradrenergic and serotonergic fibers) which are known to be involved in the behavioral effects of the ACTH peptides in animals (De Wied and Jolles, 1983) are also involved in mood and depression in man (Van Praag, 1982) and in AD (Rossor, 1982). Clinical trials in depressed subjects or in very early dementia could be more promising than studies with more deteriorated subjects in whom more extensive neuroanatomical degeneration has taken place.

Vasopressin and cognitive disorders

Animal studies

Vasopressin-like peptides appear to improve the performance of normal rats in a variety of behavioral paradigms which measure the acquisition and retention of aversively motivated behavior (De Wied, 1983; Van Wimersma Greidanus et al., 1985). In addition, rats characterized by a decrease or lack of endogenous vasopressin have an impaired performance of particular learning and memory tasks. This phenomenon was observed under three different conditions of vasopressin-deficiency (De Wied, 1983; Van Wimersma Greidanus et al., 1975), namely neurohypophysectomy, hereditary deficits in the production of vasopressin (the Brattleboro rat), and vasopressin antiserum treatment. Interestingly, under these conditions, the impaired behavior could be restored by treatment with vasopressin or its congeners. Similar treatment effects were found in animals with impaired performance due to treatment with CO_2, electroconvulsive shock, or inhibitors of protein synthesis.

There are several arguments which suggest that there is a direct effect of the peptide on the central nervous system (CNS): it appears that the dosage of the peptide which is needed to elicit a particular behavioral effect is much less after central than after peripheral administration (see De Wied, 1983). Secondly, vasopressin fragments exist which have been reported to be practically devoid of classical peripheral-endocrine effects (e.g. desglycinamide-lysine[8]-vasopressin, DGLVP; De Wied, 1983). Incidentally it appears that desglycinamide-arginine[8]-vasopressin (DGAVP) binds to vasopressin receptors in the kidney in in vitro experiments (Ravid et al., 1985). This suggests that the desglycinamide peptides may also have some peripheral effects in vivo; however, effects of DGAVP and DGLVP on blood pressure and/or water retention have until now not been found in normal rats, whereas the behavioral effects seem to be similar to those of the parent compound. Finally, extensive systems of vasopressinergic fibers have been demonstrated in the brain (Buys, 1978), suggesting that central peptidergic mechanisms do exist. However, there is some dispute on the relative importance of peripheral versus central factors in the mechanism of action of the peptide (Gash and Thomas, 1983, 1984; see De Wied, 1984).

The behavioral effect of vasopressin is longer-lasting than that of ACTH (days instead of hours). In addition, the peptide improved both the initial acquisition of the information and the retention of the material, whereas no clear-cut effects of ACTH on acquisition processes have been reported (see De Wied, 1983). Generally, the data with respect to the nature of the vasopressin effect are more in line with a hypothesis in terms of memory processes than those on ACTH.

Research which has interpreted the behavioral action of vasopressin in terms of 'memory processes' has led to the application of the peptide in the treatment of human memory disorders. Unfortunately, there are many differences between the studies with respect to the aspect(s) of memory affected, the type of patient, the severity of the defects and the methods used for treatment evaluation (see Jolles, 1983 and 1986, for an extensive elaboration on these parameters). In addition, the studies differ with respect to the dose, route, frequency and duration of peptide administration and the experimental design used (open, blind, etc.). Furthermore, vasopressin congeners have been used which differ with respect to the peripheral side effects: the mother hormone lysine[8]-vasopressin (LVP) has antidiuretic, vasopressor and behavioral effects; its congener desamino-D-arginine[8]-vasopressin (DDAVP) has antidiuretic and behavioral effects and DGAVP has been claimed to have only the behavioral effects (Jolles, 1983, 1987, but also see above).

Aging and senile dementia

Twelve patients (aged 50–64 years) who were hospitalized with somatic complaints were treated with LVP applied intranasally (Legros et al., 1978). The peptide-treated patients performed better than control subjects on certain tests of attention and memory. The same investigators reported subsequently that the scores on one of these memory tests correlated with the levels of neurophysin-1 in the blood (Legros and Gilot, 1979). Effects of LVP were also found in patients with senile dementia (average age 80 years, Delwaide et al., 1980): a single administration of LVP improved the performance of nine out of ten patients on a word list retention task, and these effects were still present after 48 h. Others have also found that a single administration of DDAVP can improve memory for semantic structures (i.e. word memory) in patients suffering from progressive dementia

(Weingartner et al., 1981b). This was also found in a later study in which seven patients suffering from primary degenerative dementia were treated with gradually increasing doses of DDAVP for 10 days. The demented patients were better able to generate appropriate words to verbal stimuli than controls. The authors suggested that the peptide helps facilitate access to semantic memory (Kaye et al., 1982). In addition, they noted that these patients showed enhanced arousal with increased motor and speech activity.

Ferris (1983; Ferris et al., 1986) treated 20 patients suffering from mild to moderate dementia with LVP for periods of 7 days in a placebo-controlled cross-over study. Consistent but small improvements on memory tests were noted. However, in another study in which carefully diagnosed Alzheimer patients were treated with LVP, effects on tests of memory, learning and visual perception were not observed. The only detectable effect concerned an improved performance in a reaction-time test. These authors concluded that vasopressin might have a 'non-specific activating effect' (Durso et al., 1982). A similar suggestion was made by Tinklenberg et al. (1981, 1982, 1986), who treated patients suffering from a primary degenerative disorder (Alzheimer type). Neither DDAVP nor DGAVP had measurable effects on the tests used. These authors suggested that some patients had more energy and less depression after administration of the compound. This was especially the case in patients with comparatively mild dysfunctions. These same authors later observed some changes on a word-learning test indicating improvement (Peabody et al., 1985). Preliminary data from another study are suggestive of a 'significant improvement in cerebral function' in five out of 20 parkinsonian patients with incipient dementia. These patients had been treated with LVP in an open design (Legros and Lancranjan, 1984).

Improved memory has been reported in five out of 11 patients suffering from multiinfarct dementia, treated in a double-blind placebo-controlled design (Bucht et al., 1986). Social behavior improved in eight out of 11 subjects. Several studies have been published with negative results. Jenkins and coworkers (1982) treated three patients suffering from 'early dementia of the Alzheimer type' (aged 58–65 years) with DDAVP. They observed that none of their patients showed significant improvement with the peptide on any of the test procedures used. Similarly, Franceschi et al. (1982) did not find statistically significant changes in a mixed population of patients suffering from Alzheimer's disease ($n = 10$) and multiinfarct dementia ($n = 8$). These patients had been treated with intranasal LVP for 7 days. Intranasal LVP treatment has been equally ineffective in a double-blind study with parkinsonian patients (Jensen, 1980) in which peptide effects were studied on neurological and psychiatric variables. Evidence is thus available in favor of the hypothesis that vasopressin treatment may be more effective in patients with less extensive degeneration in the brain than in patients with very extensive damage.

Depression

Disturbances in mood, 'energy' and initiative are frequently encountered in elderly subjects and in (pre)senile dementia (e.g. Strub and Black, 1981; Botwinnick, 1981). Several authors have noted that the peptide effects which they observed in dementing persons seemed to be restricted to these 'general' psychological functions. It was thus hypothesized that the — possible — antiamnesic effect of vasopressin-like peptides might be a manifestation of an antidepressant action.

In a study in which patients with endogenous depression and cognitive disorders were treated with DDAVP (Weingartner et al., 1981a; Gold et al., 1979), three out of four patients showed a significant improvement in cognitive functioning. However, upon discontinuation they were back at their pretreatment level after 4 weeks. In a follow-up study in two depressed patients, DDAVP appeared to counteract the amnesia which is a characteristic side effect of electroconvulsive shock therapy. Others have reported that LVP improved memory processes in three depressive patients

(Drago et al., 1981). Likewise, Legros and Lancranjan (1984) cite a preliminary study by Vranckx and coworkers, who reported a beneficial effect of LVP treatment in moderately depressed patients. According to these authors, there was no therapeutical action in more severely depressed patients who did not respond to classical treatment.

Clinical studies in other patients and in healthy volunteers

The observation that vasopressin affects the performance of laboratory animals in tests that are presumed to imply aspects of learning and memory processes, has stimulated clinical trials with the peptide in many different types of patients. The common denominator in all of these patients was the presence of memory complaints and/or deficits. Clinical trials have thus been performed with patients suffering from brain trauma, chronic alcoholism, schizophrenia, diabetes insipidus and attentional deficits (see Jolles, 1983, 1987, for a review). Several of these findings with patients and healthy volunteers deserve attention. For instance, studies in both brain trauma patients and chronic alcoholic/Korsakoff subjects suggest that the treatment only has a measurable effect in patients with relatively mild cognitive deficits and minimal brain damage (Jolles, 1983, 1986, for references). In schizophrenic subjects, vasopressin appeared to induce the reappearance of positive psychotic symptoms such as delusions and hallucinations (first) and a more social and interested attitude (later). A decrease in thinking disorder, blunted affect and emotional withdrawal was noted, accompanied by an increase in energy and activity. These studies point — again — to a peptide effect on those psychological functions which are associated with energy, activity and interest.

Studies in human volunteers especially are important for our understanding of the nature of the peptide effects. In a series of studies with information processing tasks, Beckwith and coworkers showed DDAVP effects on learning a concept shifting-task. There were no effects on visual memory, anxiety, blood pressure and heart rate, which excluded a 'general arousal' explanation (Beckwith et al., 1982, 1983, 1984). Similar findings were obtained by others: Nebes and coworkers (1984) reported peptide effects on memory comparison time and perceptual-motor time in short-term memory and retrieval time in long-term memory. As other aspects were unaffected, these data seem to show that the peptide has a more or less specific influence.

Cognitive disorders and changes in CSF vasopressin levels

There is an increasing number of studies which report that cerebrospinal fluid (CSF) levels of vasopressin (VP) are abnormal in several types of patients suffering from cognitive deficits. Legros (1975) found a decrease in the CSF levels of neurophysin (the vasopressin transport protein) in patients of 50 and older. Moreover, there was a relationship between the circulating neurophysin and some psychometric memory tests. In addition, a reduced vasopressin response to the water deprivation test in old age has been observed (Legros and Gilot, 1979; see also Legros and Lancranjan, 1984). More recently, Sundquist and coworkers (1983) found a slight decrease of the CSF-VP levels with increasing age in neurological patients. The VP values were significantly higher in patients with cerebrovascular disease, whereas lower CSF values were found in patients with dementia and Parkinson's disease. On the other hand, vasopressin levels in the CSF of 10 elderly normal subjects, nine patients with multiinfarct dementia and five patients with AD were all in the same range (Legros and Lancranjan, 1984). A decrease of vasopressin levels with age was not observed either by Jenkins et al. (1981) and Luerssen and Robertson (1980). Swaab et al. (1986) provide a critical evaluation of the data on VP levels and aging.

Changes in AVP levels have been found in several psychiatric populations characterized by cognitive deficits: elevated levels of AVP in spinal

436

fluid were found in anorexia nervosa patients (Strupp et al., 1983), whereas oxytocin levels were depressed in these patients. AVP levels were also elevated in mania, again with oxytocin being decreased (Strupp et al., 1983). The relation between these changed levels and the cognitive deficits remains to be established, but the findings as such may prove to be of importance.

Conclusions and suggestions for future research

The clinical studies with peptides related to ACTH and vasopressin are different with respect to many treatment parameters and other variables. It is therefore not possible to draw definite conclusions as to whether these peptides are clinically effective or not. However, results which have been obtained up till now do allow a set-up of research strategies which are potentially more promising than others. For instance, when vasopressin-like peptides appear to have more clear-cut effects in particular patient populations under certain treatment conditions, clinical trials can be planned in which these variables are systematically controlled. The following variables are potentially relevant in this respect:

The nature of the population. It could be concluded that neuropeptides related to ACTH and vasopressin have behavioral effects in humans: most studies report something, be it a clinical impression of improvement, or objective test results. Those published studies in which the peptide was ineffective were performed on patients with a complex pattern of neuropsychological deficits or other symptoms of profound brain degeneration. This observation should then not be surprising, because degeneration of the relevant brain structures may well destroy the sites of action of the peptide. More positive effects have been found in early versus late stage senile dementia and in light compared to severe trauma subjects. The same seems to be true for the alcoholic/Korsakoff patients. In addition, nine out of 10 studies in volunteers have reported significant effects of the peptide treatment. Taken together, these data may

indicate that future studies should focus on those patients who have mild deficits without pronounced anatomical destruction.

The subjects of choice for peptide studies are elderly people with mild senescent forgetfulness, very early dementia, depression and patients with after-effects of light brain trauma (e.g. concussion). This implies that the patient groups should be better neuropsychologically defined, to assess a specific influence on different types or aspects of memory. We suggest that information-processing tasks which measure the processes underlying both consolidation and retrieval and other aspects of memory may be the most relevant to study. Better, and more specific methods of treatment evaluation (including parallel test versions) should therefore be used (Jolles, 1985).

The nature of the drug. Both animal studies and human studies with ACTH4–10 and the ACTH4–9 analog (Org 2766) have shown that the analog is behaviorally more potent (De Wied and Jolles, 1983; Pigache, 1982). This increased behavioral activity can possibly be explained by an increased resistance towards metabolic degradation (Witter et al., 1975) which effectively prolongs the bio-availability of the peptide. This point is of particular relevance because the route of administration does not favor the penetration of the drug into the CNS, where it is supposed to act: Org 2766 is administered orally, and the vasopressin-like peptides are usually administered via nasal spray. Unfortunately, there is as yet no indication that administration via the nasal route provides better access to the CNS. In addition there is as yet no indication of the mechanism(s) by which peptides might pass the blood–brain barrier (Ang and Jenkins, 1982). Intramuscular administration which will — theoretically — increase the effective amount of peptide in the body will — for obvious reasons — never become a routine method of administration.

A research strategy which may be particularly important is concerned with development and use of peptide congeners that are chemically modified so as to resist enzymatic breakdown. In addition, use of peptide fragments with increased behavioral potency deserves attention. This is especially the case for vasopressin4–9 which has recently been shown to be behaviorally potentiated compared to the parent compound and its desglycinamide fragment (Burbach et al., 1983).

Finally, in addition to ACTH and vasopressin, other (neuro)peptides, such as somatostatin deserve attention as there appears to be a fairly selective decrease in the brain content of this substance in aged and demented subjects. Combination therapy of neuropeptides with drugs related to the classical neurotransmitters deserves attention because of findings in animal experiments that the peptides may modulate ongoing activity in classical — e.g. monoaminergic — synapses (e.g. De Wied and Jolles, 1983).

Other treatment parameters. Longer treatment periods with both ACTH and vasopressin seem to produce more clear-cut results. This is the case for subchronic administration of Org 2766 in elderly and dementing subjects but also for vasopressin. The studies with human volunteers are an exception in that acute administration did produce significant effects: it may be the case that these latter studies produced such effects because more homogenous groups were employed and because potentially interfering variables were more rigidly controlled. Clinical studies may thus need at least 2–4 weeks of peptide administration before a treatment effect develops which is strong enough to be observed. A related point concerns the amount of active peptide which may be administered. The amount of LVP or DDAVP which can be used in humans is limited due to peripheral effects on blood pressure and water retention. DGAVP, which lacks (at least most of) the peripheral effects, is therefore favored over the other congeners. DGAVP can be employed in a higher dose, and this may increase the amount of active principle that eventually reaches its site of action in the CNS. This is especially important in view of the blood–brain barrier which is difficult to pass for

peptides. However, it must be kept in mind that biphasic dosage effects have been reported for ACTH- and vasopressin-like peptides in animal studies (e.g. Jolles et al., 1972). This suggests that some optimal dose level may exist for vasopressin (Jolles, 1987) as has already been shown for other psychoactive drugs.

Some methodological issues. It is beyond discussion that future studies must be controlled (e.g. double-blind placebo-controlled or cross-over with a sufficient number of cases per group). However, it must be acknowledged that studies which are methodologically sound from a scientific point of view may not be clinically relevant. It is, of course, important that group means for peptide-treated groups and placebo groups are statistically different. Such an observation, however, does not teach us very much about the potential clinical effectiveness of the peptide. It is, therefore, important to know more about the number of subjects per group that have responded favorably. Given the recently growing interest in single case methodology, use of multiple single case designs must be initiated.

Combination with non-biological treatment. On the basis of observation in electrophysiological and neurochemical experiments De Wied (1977) proposed that neuropeptides like ACTH can increase the motivational value of environmental stimuli by creating a temporary state of arousal in certain limbic midbrain structures.

It has been suggested for many years that the action of pituitary hormones on peripheral organs causes the organism to be optimally prepared for the effect of a changing environment. These hormones may thus play a role in adaptive behavior. It seems quite probable that the neuropeptides act upon the central nervous system in ways similar to peripherally acting mother hormones (e.g. 'stress hormones'). One common denominator of all the studies with ACTH and vasopressin in animals and humans is that the peptides change the effectiveness with which the organism processes environmental (sensory) stimuli and organizes its behavior in accordance with these stimuli: the peptides may thus improve the manner in which the organism copes with environmental demands. If this is the case, it may be that environmental stimulation is important for the expression of the peptide effects. This suggestion implies that a combination of drug therapy (e.g. neuropeptides) and environmental stimulation (e.g. training the deficient cognitive deficits) deserves consideration in the treatment of maladaptive behavior. A thorough evaluation of the impact

of all variables which appear to influence the treatment effects of neuropeptides is not only relevant with respect to the neuropeptides. These studies, if properly performed, may also help us to define the optimal way to test the possible effects of other biological or non-biological methods of intervention. In addition, when the nature of the treatment effects is carefully considered, they may add to our insight into the cognitive deficits in aging, depression, or early beginning dementia as well as into the relevant etiological and pathogenetic factors.

References

Ang, V. T. Y. and Jenkins, J. S. (1982) Blood CSF barrier to arginine vasopressin desmopressin and desglycinamide arginine-vasopressin in the dog. *J. Endocrinol.*, 93: 319–325.

Beckwith, B. E. and Sandman, C. A. (1982) Central nervous system and peripheral effects of ACTH, MSH and related neuropeptides. *Peptides*, 3: 411–420.

Beckwith, B. E., Petros, T., Kanaan-Beckwith, S., Couk, D. I. and Haug, R. J. (1982) Vasopressin analog (DDAVP) facilitates concept learning in human males. *Peptides*, 3: 627–630.

Beckwith, B. E., Couk, D. I. and Till, T. S. (1983) Vasopressin analog influences the performance of males on a reaction time task. *Peptides*, 4: 707–709.

Beckwith, B. E., Till, R. E. and Schneider, V. (1984) Vasopressin analog (DDAVP) improves memory in human males. *Peptides*, 5: 819–822.

Botwinnick, J. (1981) Neuropsychology of aging. In S. B. Filskov and T. J. Boll (Eds.), *Handbook of Clinical Neuropsychology*, Wiley, New York, pp. 135–171.

Branconnier, R. J. and Cole, J. O. (1977) The effects of Org 2766 on mild senile organic brain syndrome. *Report to Organon*, Oss, The Netherlands.

Branconnier, R. J. and DeVitt, D. R. (1984) Early detection of incipient Alzheimer's disease. In B. Reisberg (Ed.), *Alzheimer's Disease*, pp. 214–227.

Braverman, A., Hamdy, R., Hendrickson, E., Mersner, P., Perrera, J. and Pigache, R. M. (1980). *Report to Organon*, Oss, The Netherlands.

Bucht, G., Adolfsson, R., Lancranjan, I. and Winblad, B. (1986) Vasopressin in multiinfarct dementia and other neuropsychiatric disorders. In J. M. Ordy, J. R. Sladek and B. Reisberg (Eds.), *Neuropeptide and Hormone Modulation of Brain Function and Homeostasis*, Raven Press, New York, in press.

Burbach, P., Kovacs, G. L., De Wied, D., Nispen, J. W. and

Greve, H. M. (1983) A major metabolite of arginine vasopressin in the brain is a highly potent neuropeptide. *Science*, 221: 1310–1312.

Buijs, R. M. (1978) Intra- and extrahypothalamic vasopressin and oxytocin pathways in the rat: pathways to the limbic system, medulla oblongata and spinal cord. *Cell Tiss. Res.*, 192: 423–435.

Delwaide, P. J., Devoitille, J. M. and Ylieff, M. (1980) Acute effects of drugs upon memory of patients with senile dementia. *Acta Psychiat. Belg.*, 80: 748–754.

De Wied, D. (1969) Effects of peptide hormones on behavior. In W. F. Ganong and L. Martini (Eds.), *Frontiers in Neuroendocrinology*, Oxford University Press, London, pp. 97–140.

De Wied, D. (1976) Behavioral effects of intraventricularly administered vasopressin and vasopressin fragments. *Life Sci.*, 19: 685–690.

De Wied, D. (1977) Behavioral effects of neuropeptides related to ACTH, MSH and β-LPH. *Ann. NY Acad. Sci.*, 297: 263–274.

De Wied, D. (1983) Central actions of neurohypophysial hormones. In B. A. Cross and G. Leng (Eds.), *The Neurohypophysis: Structure, Function and Control, Progress in Brain Research, Vol. 60*, Elsevier, Amsterdam, pp. 155–169.

De Wied, D. (1984) The importance of vasopressin in memory. *Trends Neurosci.*, 7: 62–63.

De Wied, D. and Jolles, J. (1983) Neuropeptides derived from pro-opiomelanocortin: Behavioral, physiological and neurochemical effects. *Physiol. Rev.*, 62: 976–1059.

Drago, F., Rapisarda, V., Calandra, A., Filetti, S. and Scapagnini, U. (1981) A clinical evaluation of vasopressin effects on memory disorders. *Acta Ther.*, 7: 345–352.

Durso, R., Fedio, P., Brouwers, P., Cox, C., Martin, A. J., Ruggieri, S. A., Tamminga, C. A. and Chase, T. N. (1982) Lysine vasopressin in Alzheimer's disease. *Neurology*, 32: 674–677.

Ferris, S. H. (1983) Neuropeptides in the treatment of

Alzheimer's disease. In B. Reisberg, (Ed.), *Alzheimer's Disease*. Free Press/Macmillan, New York, pp. 369–373.

Ferris, S. H., Reisberg, B. and Gershon, S. (1980) Neuropeptide modulation of cognition and memory in humans. In L. Poon (Ed.), *Aging in the 1980's: Selected Contemporary Issues in the Psychology of Aging*, American Psychological Association, Washington DC, pp. 212–220.

Ferris, S. H., Reisberg, B., Schneck, M. K., Mir, P. and Geibel, V. H. (1986) Effects of vasopressin on primary degenerative dementia. In J. M. Ordy, J. R. Sladek and B. Reisberg (Eds.), *Neuropeptide and Hormone Modulation of Brain Function and Homeostasis*, Raven Press, New York, in press.

Franceschi, M., Tancredi, O., Savio, G. and Smirne, S. (1982) Vasopressin and physostigmine in the treatment of amnesia. *Eur. Neurol.*, 21: 388–391.

Gaillard, A. W. K. (1981) ACTH analogs and human performance. In J. L. Martinez, R. A. Jensen, R. B. Messing, H. Rigter and J. L. McGaugh (Eds.), *Endogenous Peptides and Learning and Memory Processes*, Academic Press, New York, pp. 181–196.

Gash, D. M. and Thomas, G. T. (1983) What is the importance of vasopressin in memory processes? *Trends Neurosci.*, 6: 197–198.

Gash, D. M. and Thomas, G. T. (1984) The importance of vasopressin in memory: Reply. *Trends Neurosci.*, 7: 64–65.

Gold, P. W., Ballenger, J. C., Weingartner, H., Goodwin, F. K. and Post, R. M. (1979) Effects of 1-desamino-8-D-arginine vasopressin on behavior and cognition in primary affective disorders. *Lancet*, I: 992–994.

Jenkins, J. S., Mather, H. M. and Coughlan, A. K. (1982) Effects of desmopressin in normal and impaired memory. *J. Neurol. Neurosurg. Psychiat.*, 45: 830–831.

Jenkins, J. S., Mather, H. M., Coughlan, A. K. and Jenkins, D. G. (1981) Desmopressin and desglycinamide vasopressin in posttraumatic amnesia. *Lancet*, I: 39.

Jensen, J. P. A. (1980) Vasopressin therapy in Parkinson's disease. *Acta Neurol. Scand.*, 62: 197–199.

Jolles, J. (1983) Vasopressin-like peptides and the treatment of memory disorders in man. In B. A. Cross and G. Leng (Eds.), *The Neurohypophysis: Structure, Function and Control, Progress in Brain Research, Vol. 60*, Elsevier, Amsterdam, pp. 169–182.

Jolles, J. (1985) Early diagnosis of dementia: possible contributions from neuropsychology. In W. H. Gispen and J. Traber (Eds.), *Aging of the Brain*. Springer-Verlag, Berlin, pp. 84–100.

Jolles, J. (1986) Neuropeptides and cognitive disorders. In J. M. Van Ree and S. Matthysse (Eds.), *Psychiatric Disorders: Neurotransmitters and Neuropeptides, Progress in Brain Research, Vol. 65*, Elsevier, Amsterdam, pp. 177–192.

Jolles, J. (1987) Vasopressin and human behavior. In D. M. Gash and G. J. Boer (Eds.), *Vasopressin: Principles and Properties*. Plenum Press, New York, in press.

Jolles, J. and Hijman, R. (1983) The neuropsychology of aging and dementia. *Dev. Neurol.*, 7: 227–250.

Jolles, J., Aloyo, V. J. and Gispen, W. H. (1982) Molecular correlates between pituitary hormones and behavior. In J. R. Brown (Ed.), *Molecular approaches to neurobiology*, Academic Press, New York, pp. 285–316.

Kaye, W. H., Weingartner, H., Gold, P., Ebert, M. H., Gillin, J. C., Sitaram, N. and Smallberg, S. (1982) Cognitive effects of cholinergic and vasopressin-like agents in patients with primary degenerative dementia. In S. Corkin, K. I. Davis, J. H. Growdon, E. Usdin and R. J. Wurtman (Eds.), *Alzheimer's Disease: A Report of Progress in Research*. Raven Press, New York, pp. 433–442.

Kral, V. A. (1962) Senescent forgetfulness: benign and malignant. *Can. Med. Assoc. J.*, 86: 257–260.

Legros, J. J. (1975) The radioimmunoassay of human neurophysins: Contribution to the understanding of the physiopathology of neurohypophysial function. *Ann. NY Acad. Sci.*, 248: 281.

Legros, J. J. and Gilot, P. (1979) Vasopressin and memory in the human. In A. M. Gotto, Jr., E. J. Peck, Jr. and A. E. Boyd, III (Eds,), *Brain Peptides, a New Endocrinology*, Elsevier/North-Holland, Amsterdam, pp. 347–363.

Legros, J. J. and Lancranjan, I. (1984) Vasopressin in neuropsychiatric disorders. In N. S. Shah and A. G. Donald (Eds.), *Psychoneuroendocrine Dysfunction*, Plenum Press, New York, pp. 255–278.

Legros, J. J., Gilot, P., Seron, X., Claessens, J., Adam, A., Moeglen, J. M., Audibert, A. and Berchier, P. (1978) Influence of vasopressin on learning and memory. *Lancet*, I: 41–42.

Luersson, T. G. and Robertson, G. L. (1980) Cerebrospinal fluid vasopressin and vasotocin in health. In J. H. Wood (Ed.), *Neurobiology of Cerebrospinal Fluid*, Plenum Press, New York, pp. 613–625.

Luria, A. R. (1976) *The Neuropsychology of Memory*. Winston, Washington, D. C.

Nebes, R. D., Reynolds, C. F., III and Horn, L. C. (1984) The effect of vasopressin on memory in the healthy elderly. *Psychiat. Res.*, 11: 49–59.

Newcombe, F. (1980) Memory: a neuropsychological approach. *Trends Neurosci.*, 3: 179–182.

Peabody, C. A., Thiemann, S., Pigache, R., Miller, T., Yesavage, J. and Tinklenberg, J. (1985) Desglycinamide-9-Arginine-8-Vasopressin (DGAVP, Organon 5667) in patients with dementia. *Neurobiol. Aging*, 6: 95–100.

Pigache, R. M. (1982) A peptide for the aged? Basic and clinical studies. In D. Wheatley (Ed.), *Psychopharmacology of Old Age*, Oxford University Press, Oxford, pp. 67–97.

Pigache, R. M. and Rigter, H. (1981) Effects of peptides related to ACTH on mood and vigilance in man. *Front. Horm. Res.*, 8: 193–207.

Ravid, R., Swaab, D. F. and Pool, Chr. W. (1985) Immunocytochemical localization of vasopressin-binding sites in the rat kidney. *J. Endocrinol.*, 105: 133–140.

Reisberg, B., Ferris, S. H. and Crook, T. (1982) Signs, symptoms and course of age-associated cognitive decline. In S. Corkin, K. I. Davis, J. H. Growdon, E. Usdin and R. J. Wurtman (Eds.), *Alzheimer's Disease: A Report of Progress*, Raven Press, New York, pp. 463–469.

Rossor, M. N. (1982) Neurotransmitters and CNS disease: dementia. *Lancet*, II: 1200–1204.

Russell, E. W. (1981) The pathology and clinical examination of memory. In S. B. Filskov and T. J. Boll (Eds.), *Handbook of Clinical Neuropsychology*, Wiley, New York, pp. 287–319.

Squire, L. R. and Davis, H. P. (1981) The pharmacology of memory: a neurobiological perspective. *Ann. Rev. Pharmacol. Toxicol.*, 21: 323–356.

Strub, R. I. and Black, F. W. (1981) Alzheimer's/senile dementia. In R. I. Strub and F. W. Black (Eds.), *Organic Brain Syndromes*, F. A. Davis Co., Philadelphia, pp. 119–164.

Strupp, B., Weingartner, H., Goodwin, F. K. and Gold, P. W. (1983) Neurohypophyseal hormones and cognition. *Pharmacol. Ther.*, 23: 267–279.

Sulkava, R. and Amberla, K. (1981) Alzheimer's disease and senile dementia of Alzheimer type: a neuropsychological study. *Acta Neurol. Scand.*, 65: 541–552.

Sundquist, J., Forsling, M. L., Olsson, J. E. and Åkerlund, M. (1983) Cerebrospinal fluid arginine vasopressin in degenerative disorders and other neurological diseases. *J. Neurol. Neurosurg. Psychiat.*, 46: 14–17.

Swaab, D. F., Fliers, E. and Van Gool, W. A. (1986) Immunocytochemical localization of vasopressin in the human brain; its possible consequences for therapeutic strategies in aging and dementia. In: J. M. Van Ree and S. Matthysse (Eds.), *Psychiatric Disorders: Neurotransmitters and Neuropeptides, Progress in Brain Research, Vol. 65*, Elsevier, Amsterdam, pp. 105–113.

Tinklenberg, J. R. and Thornton, J. E. (1983) Neuropeptides in geriatric psychopharmacology. *Psychopharmacol. Bull.*, 19: 198–211.

Tinklenberg, J. R., Pfefferbaum, A. and Berger, P. A. (1981) 1-Desamino-D-arginine-vasopressin in cognitively impaired patients. *Psychopharmacol. Bull.*, 17: 206–207.

Tinklenberg, J. R., Peabody, C. A. and Berger, P. A. (1986) Vasopressin effects on cognition and affect in the elderly. In J. M. Ordy, J. R. Sladek and B. Reisberg (Eds.), *Neuropeptide and Hormone Regulation of Brain Function and Homeostasis*, Raven, New York, in press.

Tinklenberg, J. R., Pigache, R., Pfefferbaum, A. and Berger, P. A. (1982) Vasopressin peptides and dementia. In S. Corkin, K. I. Davis, J. H. Growdon, E. Usdin and R. J. Wurtman (Eds.), *Alzheimer's Disease, a Report of Progress in Research*, Raven Press, New York, pp. 463–469.

Van Praag, H. M. (1982) Depression. *Lancet*, II: 1259–1264.

Van Wimersma Greidanus, Tj. B., Dogterom, J. and De Wied, D. (1975) Intraventricular administration of anti-vasopressin serum inhibits memory consolidation in rats. *Life Sci.*, 16: 637–644.

Van Wimersma Greidanus, Tj. B., Jolles, J. and De Wied, D. (1985) Hypothalamic neuropeptides and memory. *Acta Neurochir.*, 75: 99–105.

Weingartner, H., Gold, P., Ballenger, J. C., Smallberg, S. A., Summers, R., Rubinow, D. R., Post, R. M. and Goodwin, F. K. (1981a) Effects of vasopressin on human memory functions. *Science*, 211: 601–603.

Weingartner, H., Kaye, W., Gold, P., Smallberg, S., Peterson, R., Gillin, J. C. and Ebert, M. (1981b) Vasopressin treatment of cognitive dysfunction in progressive dementia. *Life Sci.*, 29: 2721–2726.

Witter, A., Greven, H. M. and De Wied, D. (1975) Correlation between structure, behavioral activity and rate of biotransformation of some ACTH4–9 analogs. *J. Pharmacol. Exp. Ther.*, 193: 853.

Discussion

J. H. CHRISTINA: (1) What kind of psychometric or clinical tests do you perform to assess the degree of dementia?

(2) Why do you ask for a better patient differentiation (for clinical trials) taking into consideration that the population you are going to treat is a very heterogeneous one?

ANSWERS: (1) The methods that were used by all authors that I have reviewed in the present paper were psychiatric in nature (for details see Jolles, 1986). Especially the earlier papers are usually based upon DSM-III criteria and/or clinical impression. The differentiation between mild, moderate and severe is always based upon clinical criteria and not upon psychometric tests.

(2) Your second question must be based upon a small misunderstanding. In my opinion, nearly all studies performed up till now used heterogeneous patient groups. Strong arguments favor the foundation of groups that are more homogeneous with respect to etiology and cognitive deficits; to decrease intra group variability and characterize those patients who benefit most from the peptide or potential other treatments.

E. FLIERS: In view of the fact that effects of VP and ACTH (analogs) have been found in so many different conditions, could you speculate on their mode of action in the brain? Is there indeed evidence for your hypothesis that these peptides act via the midbrain?

ANSWER: An answer to this question requires more space than is present in this discussion. The hypothesis of De Wied, that ACTH-like peptides increase a state of arousal in limbic midbrain structures, has been based upon electrophysiological experiments in which changes in hippocampal theta rhythms have been found. In addition, neurochemical experiments investigating the influence of the peptides on ascending catecholaminergic fibers point into the same direction.

D. M. GASH: Given the propensity for only clinical studies reporting positive results to be published, careful consideration must be given to those studies which have found no beneficial effects of vasopressin treatment. Is it accurate to conclude that the clinical effects of vasopressin on cognition are rather modest and only affect a subpopulation of the cognitively impaired patient population? Is it also possible to explain the effects of vasopressin in terms of altering mood or a general effect on the level of arousal?

ANSWER: The treatment effects reported in the clinical studies up till now are indeed rather modest. It must be taken into consideration however, that the studies which have been performed correctly, were based upon a group-comparison design in which group means were statistically evaluated. Given the fairly strong arguments which favor the notion that particular population(s) of patients may respond better than others (e.g. patients with only mild deficits without gross lesions), this may mean that patients who are a 'responder' in the clinical sense are not characterized as such due to the design used. Future studies must, in my opinion, use a multiple single-case design to allow statements of treatment effects in individual subjects.

With respect to the possibility that the vasopressin effects might be described in terms of altered mood and a general arousing effect, it seems to me that the discussion in the literature on this topic is confounded by semantic problems. The notion of what constitutes 'memory', 'arousal', 'attention', etc., seems to me to depend upon the discipline and/or the paradigm used. I tend to agree with you that vasopressin does not affect memory per se. However, an effect on more general mechanisms which are necessary for memory processes seems reasonably well established in animal experiments. The methodology in human studies, in my opinion, does not yet allow any conclusions as to the possible mechanisms and aspect(s) of cognition involved.

References

Jolles, J. (1986) Cognitive, emotional and behavioral dysfunctions in aging and dementia. In: D. F. Swaab, E. Fliers, M. Mirmiran, W. A. Van Gool and F. Van Haaren (Eds.), *Aging of the Brain and Alzheimer's Disease, Progress in Brain Research, this volume*, Elsevier, Amsterdam. pp. 15–39.

D. F. Swaab, E. Fliers, M. Mirmiran, W. A. Van Gool and F. Van Haaren (Eds.)
Progress in Brain Research, Vol. 70.
© 1986 Elsevier Science Publishers B.V. (Biomedical Division)

CHAPTER 28

Environmental influences on brain and behavior in aging and Alzheimer's disease

M. Mirmiran[a], W. A. Van Gool[a], F. Van Haaren[a] and C. E. Polak[b]

[a]*Netherlands Institute for Brain Research, Meibergdreef 33, 1105 AZ Amsterdam ZO, The Netherlands and* [b]*Deptartment of Psychology, University of Amsterdam, Weesperplein 8, 1018 XA Amsterdam, The Netherlands*

Introduction

It is well established that environmental factors influence brain and behavior throughout life. The importance of the interaction between the organism and its environment has been demonstrated by both deprivation and stimulation experiments in humans as well as in animals. Classical experiments with kittens and monkeys have shown that monocular deprivation during a critical period of development induces a rewiring of the cerebral cortex as exemplified by a shift in binucolarity of light-responsive neurons (Hubel and Wiesel, 1970; Hubel et al., 1976). Binocular vision also does not develop normally in humans if only one eye is functioning during the first 5 years of life or if both eyes do not perceive congruent visual fields (e.g. Swindale, 1982). Studies on rearing kittens in environments in which they could only perceive either vertical or horizontal lines showed long-lasting changes in cortical neurons and visual receptive fields (Hirsch and Spinelli, 1970; Blackemore and Cooper, 1970). Social deprivation reduces learning and exploration, increases stress reactivity and aggression, disturbs sexual behavior, and leads to inappropriate behavior and withdrawal in later social contacts (Mason, 1968). Recent studies in rats have even suggested that social deprivation reduces life span (Menich and Baron, 1984).

Environmental stimulation has also been shown to influence brain and behavior. The germinal experiments by Hebb showed that daily training in solving different tasks in mazes improved performance of animals in other experimental procedures as well. This observation was followed by several investigators at Berkeley who assigned rats to live in standard, complex or enriched conditions (Rosenzweig and Bennett, 1978). These and many subsequent studies showed that environmental enrichment induced various changes in the anatomy and biochemistry of the brain in addition to behavioral changes. Environmental enrichment was shown to induce: an increase of the weight of the cerebral cortex (Rosenzweig et al., 1972), increased cortical thickness (Diamond, 1967; Diamond et al., 1972), increased dendritic branching of neurons (Volkmar and Greenough, 1972; Greenough, 1976), increased number of glial cells (Diamond et al., 1976), enhanced protein synthesis in the brain (Rosenzweig et al., 1972), increased activity of the cholinergic system as exemplified by higher levels of acetyl cholinesterase in the brain (Rosenzweig and Bennett, 1978), increased number of synapses per neuron (Greenough et al., 1985; Turner and Greenough, 1985), and a superior performance in complex mazes as compared with controls (Greenough, 1976). Improved performance of 'enriched' animals in complex mazes could thus be related to structural and functional changes in the brain.

The aged brain is generally considered to

represent some kind of disease-like state, in which structure and function irrevocably decline at rates which vary between individuals (Greenough and Green, 1984). However, evidence exists to support the notion that the environment may continue to affect the brain even in older age. Some effects of environmental stimulation in animals are opposite to the changes observed in old age. Studies in aging and senile dementia have shown a reduction in brain size due to degeneration of the cerebral cortex, reduced cholinergic activity and protein synthesis, and cognitive impairments (see Terry and Gershon, 1976; Terry, 1986; Candy et al., 1986; Bartus et al., 1986). It is, therefore, interesting to consider the possibility that environmental manipulations may beneficially influence brain and behavior of the aged subject. In the present review, we will describe normal age-related changes of various physiological, behavioral and morphological parameters in the rat and discuss the effects of environmental stimulation on these parameters in animals. Finally, we will summarize the empirical findings in human subjects with respect to the effects of environmental manipulations on behavior in senescence and Alzheimer's disease (AD).

The enriched environment paradigm: methodological issues

In assessing the effects of environmental manipulations on brain and behavior a number of variables have to be taken into account. First of all, a distinction should be made between environmental enrichment in which (1) a subject is passively exposed to numerous repetitive stimuli of one or more modalities and (2) situations in which environmental stimulation is achieved in such a way that the subject actively interacts with the environment and is involved in the selection, perception and integration of the stimuli. The different effects of passive and active environmental enrichment are exemplified by the results of Held's (1965) germinal study, in which the development of visual acuity in kittens was tested. Two kittens, both reared in total darkness, were allowed

to explore a round cylinder painted with stripes of different colors. Both kittens were connected to one another and to the center of the cylinder. One kitten was allowed to move around at will (though connected to the center of the cylinder) and to inspect any visual field, whereas the other one was restrained to a wooden gondola and forced to watch only the visual field presented by the other kitten. Although both kittens received a comparable amount of visual stimulation, the kitten which had actively observed and experienced its visual environment performed better than the other kitten on tests of visual performance in adulthood.

In most studies on environmental enrichment rodents — mostly rats — were used. Different levels of environmental complexity were produced by rearing animals in enriched, standard or isolated conditions (reviewed in Rosenzweig and Bennett, 1978). The enriched environment usually consists of large cages in which several animals are exposed to different objects including ropes, brushes, ladders and plexiglass tubes of various shapes. In addition, the pattern of the enriched environment is usually changed every day. In the original studies, mentioned above, a short daily training in a Hebb-Williams maze was also included (Rosenzweig and Bennett, 1978).

Environmental enrichment can be practised in two ways. First of all, animals may live in the same environment (for 24 h a day) except when the environment is being changed. Secondly, all animals may live in standard large laboratory cages except for 2 h a day during which enriched rats are moved into enriched cages while controls move to a standard laboratory cage. Thus, depending on the controls which are used, effects of sensory deprivation of control rats, daily handling, social housing or excess locomotor activity of enriched rats, rather than effects of environmental enrichment per se may be assessed. Although many investigators have emphasized the drawbacks of considering isolated animals as a control for the effects of an enriched environment (Greenough, 1976), numerous studies used isolated undisturbed rats (e.g. Greenough and Green, 1984). This

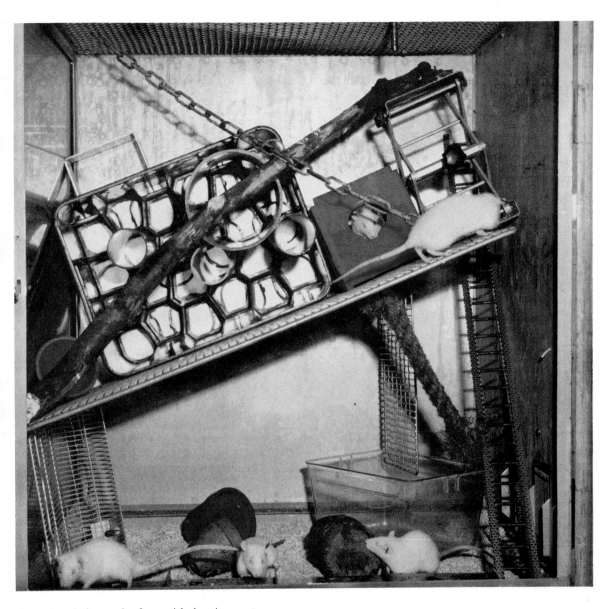

Fig. 1. A typical example of an enriched environment.

practice renders the interpretation of different studies problematic. In our studies the brain and behavioral plasticity of 'enriched' rats was compared with standard rats, which were handled frequently and were housed in group (3–5) cages. The 'enriched' rats were housed in environments differing in degree of complexity; they were moved daily to different cages; once they had visited all of them, the objects were rearranged or new objects were put in the cages, thus introducing new patterns of enrichment. In addition, food and water were situated at the bottom or the top of the cage to encourage exploration. In order to avoid overcrowding and to facilitate comparisons with standard rats, only 3–5 rats were kept in each cage at one time (Mirmiran et al., 1982, Fig. 1).

Rosenzweig and Bennett (1978) have suggested that the effects of environmental manipulations can be best considered to be a consequence of differential experiences rather than environmental stimulation. It has previously been shown that environmental stimulation per se will not induce morphological or behavioral changes in 'enriched' rats. In 'observer' rat experiments in which the animals are individually put into small wire-mesh boxes within enriched cages, these rats were allowed to see the environment and to smell other rats in the enriched cage but were not allowed to actively interact with the environment or their cage-mates (Ferchmin et al., 1975). 'Observer' rats did not differ from controls with respect to brain development, whereas rats that could explore the environment at will showed enhanced brain growth. In addition, neither excess background noise ('auditory enrichment') (Rosenzweig and Bennett, 1976) nor enforced activity (Ferchmin and Eterović, 1977) as such turned out to be effective in inducing a stimulating effect upon brain development. Walsh and Cummins (1975) have proposed that the effect of an enriched environment may be mediated by non-specific arousal of the cerebral cortex. However, a combination of activation of specific and non-specific sensory and reticular systems cannot be the only important factor, because 'observer' rats, 'enforced active' rats, and rats which were hyperexcited by long-term amphetamine treatment (Bennett et al., 1973) failed to show changes in the brain similar to those observed in 'enriched' rats. Overaroused or stressed animals reared in an enriched environment will become unsociable and less active. These rats do not show cortical weight increase in comparison to control rats (Eterović and Ferchmin, 1974). The effect of increased environmental complexity and novelty on development of brain and behavior appears to be the result of differential learning experiences (Greenough, 1976; Rosenzweig and Bennett, 1978; Cummins et al., 1979) and is independent of genetical background of the animal (Ferchmin et al., 1980). Active interaction with a daily changing environment requires continuous

perception, integration and consolidation of information. This process may initiate a sequence of events, which precedes and ultimately results in the enriched environment effects on biochemical, physiological and morphological parameters in the brain.

Effects of environmental manipulations on senescent animals

Physiological and behavioral parameters

Animal studies using aged rats have demonstrated changes in sleep-wake patterns which are to some extent comparable to those observed in elderly humans (Feinberg, 1974; Miles and Dement, 1980; Rosenberg et al., 1979; Ingram et al., 1982; Van Gool and Mirmiran, 1983, 1986b). In two different strains of rats (Wistar and Brown-Norway), 24-h continuous sleep-wake registrations were carried out in young and old rats. The results demonstrated that (1) the amount of time spent in slow wave sleep (SWS) and desynchronized sleep (DS) is reduced, (2) the sleep-cycle length is shortened, and (3) that there are significantly more short awakenings during sleep in old rats. Furthermore, circadian rhythmicity of wakefulness, SWS and DS is reduced in aged rats (Van Gool and Mirmiran, 1986a).

It has been demonstrated by several investigators that environmental enrichment influences the sleep-wake pattern of rodents in a way opposite to the age-related changes observed in senescent animals. Young 'enriched' rats and mice show increased amounts of sleep (both SWS and DS), have longer DS periods and sleep-cycles as compared to age-matched control groups (Tagney, 1973; Gutwein and Fishbein, 1980a, b; Mirmiran et al., 1982; Kiyono et al., 1981). These changes in sleep pattern of 'enriched' rodents have been implicated in the mediation of the enrichment effect upon the cerebral cortex (Mirmiran et al., 1982; Mirmiran and Uylings, 1983; Pearlman, 1983). In an attempt to determine the extent to which environmental enrichment can still influence the sleep-wake pattern in senescence, sleep was monitored in rats of 4–7 and 29–31 months of age, before and after a 4–5 weeks period of housing in an enriched environment. The enriched condition significantly increased both the amount of SWS and DS in old rats to the same extent that was found in young rats (Table I).

It is interesting to note that after 1 month of enrichment the amounts of sleep and wakefulness in old enriched rats were no longer significantly different from those of standard young animals (cf. columns 1 and 4 in Table I). The period of differential housing thus alleviated a number of age-related changes in the old rats' sleep pattern. However, the changes in amplitude of the circadian sleep-wakefulness rhythm was not affected by the environmental enrichment. Of course it was already known that this parameter is not changed, even in young 'enriched' rats (Kiyono et al., 1981; Gutwein and Fishbein, 1980b). Overall, it is clear from these results that a certain amount of 'behavioral plasticity' is preserved even in very old rats and that environmental influences may affect certain behavioral characteristics of aging.

Olton and Samuelson (1976) have developed an animal experimental task which is suitable for testing short-term memory functions. This spatial task is carried out in a radial maze in which eight or more arms radiate from a central platform. The rat is confined to the center with the doors of the arms closed while food pellets are placed at the end of each arm. The optimal strategy for food-deprived animals is to obtain pellets from each arm by visiting each arm once. This task does not require specific motor activity and it is specifically aimed at memory for recent events; it is therefore very suitable for memory testing in old animals. Old rats make significantly more mistakes in this task than young ones, although both young and old rats initially behave slightly above chance level (Van Gool et al., 1985). However, old rats unlike young rats do not show any improvement of performance above their initial level as a function of repeated training and they perform significantly poorer than the young ones, as can be seen in Fig. 2. Moreover, analysis of the type of errors revealed that old rats were more likely than young rats, to repeat a choice of an arm they had just visited.

Analysis of the radial maze data showed no indication of superior performance either in old (30–33 months) or in young (7–8 months) 'en-

TABLE I

Mean (SEM) of wakefulness, slow-wave sleep, and desynchronized sleep in young and old rats, before and after housing in the enriched condition

		Young ($n = 11$)		Old ($n = 9$)	
		before EC (4–5 months)	after EC (6–7 months)	before EC 27–29 months	after EC 29–31 months
Wakefulness	L	22.9 (0.7)	20.0 (0.9)[b]	26.3 (1.5)	23.7 (0.9)[a]
(min/h)	D	37.6 (1.7)	37.4 (0.5)	35.6 (1.7)	34.2 (1.3)
Slow-wave sleep	L	29.5 (0.7)	31.9 (0.8)[b]	27.4 (1.5)	29.4 (0.7)[a]
(min/h)	D	19.5 (1.5)	19.7 (0.5)	22.0 (1.5)	22.7 (1.5)
Desynchronized sleep	L	7.6 (0.3)	8.3 (0.3)[b]	6.3 (0.4)	7.3 (0.4)[b]
(min/h)	D	2.9 (0.3)	2.9 (0.3)	2.9 (0.2)	3.0 (0.4)

L, light period; D, dark period; EC, enriched condition. [a]$p < 0.05$; [b]$p < 0.01$, Lam and Longnecker modification of the Wilcoxon test, one-tailed. (From Van Gool and Mirmiran, 1986b)

riched' rats (Fig. 2, Van Gool et al., 1985). However, before taking these results as negative indication of environmental influences on learning performance in rats, it has to be realized that in this study, in which young and old rats (the same as used for the sleep recordings) were subjected to differential housing conditions for 1–2 months prior to testing, all animals were subsequently housed in a standard environment throughout the shaping and testing period. This procedure, though preventing any bias due to housing condition during testing, apparently prevents the observation of performance improvement attributable to exposure to an enriched environment. Moreover, Juraska et al. (1984) have reported that young enriched rats use a different strategy than isolated rats: they choose adjacent arms more frequently. By confining the rats for several seconds on the central platform between subsequent choices, such strategy no longer influenced the performance, and did not affect the assessment of performance differences between 'enriched' and control rats. Other experiments, however, have shown that environmental enrichment improves performance if environmental complexity plays a role in the testing situations. It has frequently been shown, for instance, that enriched rats are superior to impoverished rats in Hebb-Williams and Lashley Type III mazes (reviewed in Greenough, 1976). However, interpretation of these studies is hampered by the fact that in most cases enriched rats were compared with isolated animals. Thus, the influence of environmental enrichment cannot be separated from the deleterious effects of isolation.

Doty's (1972) finding that 1-year-old rats, who lived in an enriched environment during their second year, performed better than age-matched controls on reversal of a discriminated avoidance task at 2 years of age, suggests that behavior in older age can still be influenced by the environment. This is consistent with a study by Warren et al. (1982) in which 20-months-old mice subjected to enriched environment for a period of 5 months performed better than controls on an incidental learning and a food-seeking task. However, in the

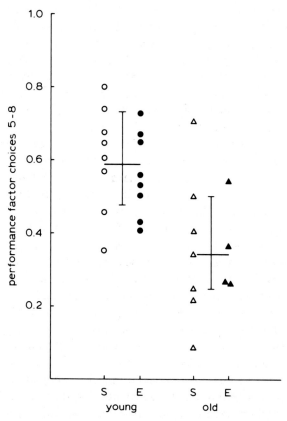

Fig. 2. Performance in the 8-arm radial maze on the choices 5–8 of young and old, standard (S) and enriched (E) rats, as represented by the overall performance factor (cf. Olton and Samuelson, 1976). The median and the interquartile range of the pooled standard and enriched age-groups are indicated; the difference between the young and old groups is significant ($p < 0.02$, Mann-Whitney test, two-tailed). (From Van Gool et al., 1985)

same study effects were not found in either Lashley type III maze or in brightness discrimination. It has, furthermore, been shown that environmental characteristics influence the rate of recovery of brain dysfunction in disabled animals or even humans (for review see Walsh and Greenough, 1976; Feuerstein, 1980). Recovery from septal lesions associated with performance deficits — particularly in reversal water-maze — has been shown to be improved to the level of sham-operated rats by environmental enrichment (Engel-lenner et al., 1982). Moreover, Bartus et al. (1986)

have presented data to suggest that recovery of damage to the basal forebrain cholinergic system in young adult rats can be facilitated by elaborate post-lesion behavioral testing, which may perhaps be considered an analog of environmental enrichment. Finally, recent data on reversal of a discrimination task after brain damage challenge the common notion that recovery of function is decreased in elderly rats after brain damage (LeVere, 1983). Taken together these results tentatively suggest that environmental factors, being either enrichment or isolation, may affect levels of performance even in old age.

The enriched environment has also been reported to affect the characteristics of visual evoked responses (Edwards et al., 1969; Mailloux et al., 1974). In our own studies we focused on recovery cycles of visual evoked potentials by presenting two visual stimuli at different, but short, interstimulus intervals (Van Gool et al., 1985). The ratio of the amplitudes of the second relative to the first evoked potential was taken as a dependent variable. This ratio did not differ between young (9–10 months) and old (32–35 months) rats at an interstimulus interval of 400 ms, whereas as the interstimulus interval decreased the amplitude ratio was consistently smaller in old compared to young rats. At 100 ms interstimulus interval none of the old rats responded to the second stimulus whereas most of the young ones did. This observation was taken to reflect an age-related change in the speed of the recovery of the visual system. Similar results have been recently demonstrated in the recovery cycle of auditory evoked potentials in elderly humans (Papanicolaou et al., 1984). However, differential environmental housing conditions did not influence the recovery cycles in young or old rats (Van Gool et al., 1985).

Morphological parameters

Diamond et al. (1977) compared brains of 108- and 650-days-old Long Evans rats and reported a significant 6% reduction of cortical thickness of the medial occipital cortex and a non-significant

4% decrease in the number of neurons and glial cells. However, recent studies by Peters et al. (1983) have shown that a change in cortical size (length, width and thickness), or in the number of neurons in rat cortical area 17 does not occur as a result of aging. On the other hand, the influence of environmental enrichment on cortical morphology in juvenile and adult rats has been shown in many different studies (Rosenzweig et al., 1972; Rosenzweig and Bennett, 1978; Uylings et al., 1978a, b). This effect seems to be limited to the occipital cortical area even in blinded rats. The magnitude of the effect was not always comparable and, unfortunately, in most cases enriched rats were compared with isolated animals. Recent studies by Connor et al. (1981a, 1982a) have shown the presence of environmentally induced plasticity even in middle-aged rats. Male Sprague-Dawley rats that had been reared socially for 20 months were divided into two groups: a group spending their final month in an enriched environment was compared with litter mates which continued to live in standard laboratory conditions. This experiment showed a significant increase in the length of terminal segments of layer II and III pyramidal neurons, in both the somatosensory and occipital cortex in enriched rats. Other studies of the same group (Connor et al., 1981b, 1982b) in which the effects of social and isolated housing conditions were compared, showed a higher order of dendritic branching in the socially reared group in old rats. However, an earlier study (Connor et al., 1980) had failed to show a change in dendritic patterns after differential housing, even though a non-significant environmental increase of cortical thickness was reported both in young and in old rats. Greenough (1984) also observed increased dendritic branching of layer IV pyramidal neurons in 450-days-old female hooded rats housed socially since weaning and later on transferred to either an enriched or an isolated condition for another 50 days. These findings are consistent with results from an early study of Cummins et al. (1973). In the latter study, cerebral dimensions were shown to be dependent on the amount of differential experience in 530-days-old Wistar albino rats. Moreover, results from studies on regeneration after knife-cut lesions of the medial forebrain bundle are also consistent with preserved plasticity in the aged brain. Vigorous regrowth of catecholaminergic fibers in the hypothalamus was observed after such lesion in both young and old rats (Phelps and Sladek, 1983), and the time course for synapse replacement in the denervated zone of the molecular layer of the dentate gyrus was similar in young and old rats.

In our own studies we have compared thickness of different cortical areas in young (7–8 months) and old (32–33 months) male Brown-Norway rats which lived either in an enriched or social environment and were used in sleep studies (Van Gool and Mirmiran, 1986b). In serial sections a significant 10–15% decrease in cortical thickness and total cortical volume could be demonstrated in old rats in all cortical areas, whereas the effect of environmental enrichment was similarly small in young and in old rats. Only one of the parameters relating to cortical size was significantly increased in both age groups. This observation could of course be due to several variables among which frequent handling, increased level of social interaction and higher baseline level of cortical thickness in controls can be mentioned. Furthermore, dendritic outgrowth may have been changed as a consequence of environmental enrichment without any changes in cortical size.

Taken together it appears that a certain amount of plasticity in brain morphology is preserved in old age, although environmental influences upon behavioral parameters (e.g. sleep) are not necessarily accompanied by dramatic morphological changes.

Effects of environmental manipulations on elderly humans

General considerations

In humans, aging induces regressive changes in a number of different functions. Especially demented patients are suffering from devastating functional impairments. At present, there is no effective pharmacological treatment to influence brain and behavior in Alzheimer's disease (AD) (Swaab and Fliers, 1986). Studies on the effects of environmental manipulations upon mental well-being of healthy elderly or demented subjects are scarce. There is, therefore, little experimental support for the intuitively appealing contention that a stimulating environment may beneficially influence behavioral functioning in the elderly. In the following two sections it will be attempted to review studies into the effects of non-pharmacological intervention in aged and demented subjects. First the effects of physical activation will be discussed and finally the results of behavioral programs will be reviewed.

Physical activation

In the general population adequate levels of physical activity are considered to be beneficial for the health status of its members. This notion has also stimulated physical training programs in aged and even in demented subjects. At present there is little, but indeed intriguing experimental support for the thesis that stimulation of physical activity is beneficial for self-respect as well as for neuropsychological test-performance in the elderly. Health improvements which can be expected to result from increased physical activity such as increased muscle strength, reduced body weight and blood pressure will not be reviewed here. Instead, we will focus on the effects of training programs on various measures of subjective well-being or neuropsychological performance in the elderly.

Low levels of activity correlate with a negative body image (Kreitler and Kreitler, 1970), whereas 5–6 weeks of treadmill activity of varying intensities resulted in improved subjective well-being in 70–81-years-old men (Benestad, 1965). These data are consistent with the observation that the elderly sleep better, and become less concerned about health problems and more sociable as a result of physical training (Laerum and Laerum, 1982). Blumenthal et al. (1982) reported positive effects on endurance as a consequence of an 11-week training program on a bicycle ergometer, but these effects were not accompanied by changes in mood, temperament, activity, or general health in their 70–85-years-old subjects. Spirduso's (1975) results, showing that both simple and choice reaction times are more strongly affected by degree of physical activity rather than by age *per se*, support the general idea that deficits in physical and cognitive abilities may be related to changes in general 'activity' measures. Even a discrete effect on reaction times may have an important functional impact, since improved reaction times may reduce the risk of morbidity resulting from injuries sustained during every-day activities (Wulp and Huijing, 1981).

Effects of increased physical activity on measures of cognitive performance have been ambiguous. Stanford (1975) described improvements on the 'General Information' subtest of the WAIS, but no changes on the 'Digit Span'. Similarly, Barry (1966) reported improved vigilance and visual discrimination but no effects on short-term memory and reasoning. After exposing institutionalized geriatric mental patients to a 12-week exercise program Powell (1974) reported significant changes in performance on 'Raven's Progressive Matrices' test and the 'Wechsler's Memory Scale'. Significant positive changes on a test sensitive to organic brain damage were not observed in this study. Interestingly, improved performance on the two tests mentioned above was accompanied by an apparent increase in restlessness and irritability. Powell (1974) interpreted this observation as a possible indication of awakened antagonism towards hospitalization or institutional routine, essentially reflecting increased self-independence and reduced apathy as a consequence of training. Elderly persons aged 82 years on average and suffering from mental and physical handicaps showed changed test scores compatible with improved cognitive performance after a gymnastic program (Diesfeldt and Diesfeldt-Groenendijk, 1977). Free recall and recognition improved in comparison with non-trained age-matched elderly in this study, but visuomotor

abilities did not change as a result of the training program. Papaspiroutous is reported to have found similar results in a Norwegian study (Ingebretsen, 1982).

Recently, Dustman et al. (1984) assessed the effects of a 4-month aerobic exercise program in 55–70-years-old healthy subjects. Depression scores, sensory thresholds and visual acuity did not change in comparison with controls, but the conditioning program resulted in improved neuropsychological test performance and increased physical fitness. It was speculated that improved test performance was promoted by increased cerebral metabolic activity, since maximum minute ventilation and oxygen uptake increased in trained subjects (Dustman et al., 1984), which is consistent with data from other studies (cf. De Vries, 1970). Currently a well-designed study into the effects of activation therapy in demented subjects is being carried out in Holland (Droës, 1984).

Behavioral programs

A number of vital functions may change as a function of age. It is therefore not surprising that elderly people may find themselves in a situation in which previously appropriate behavioral repertoires are no longer accessible, due to either an inappropriate arrangement of the immediate environment, or simply because of the fact that previously appropriate behavior can no longer be physically executed. Whatever the reason, restructuring of the elderly's environment or shaping new behavioral repertoires may contribute to the solution of the problem.

In an early report by Cosin et al. (1951), for instance, rearranging the furniture resulted in improved socialization in a geriatric ward. A variety of approaches of behavioral intervention has been applied in elderly subjects. As summarized by Woods and Holden (1981) the following strategies can be distinguished: (1) reality orientation, (2) global changes in the environment or institutional routine, and (3) intervention based on the principles of learning and reinforcement.

Reality orientation (RO) was first introduced in the Winter Veterans Administration Hospital, Topeka, Kansas, 1959. Folsom then started a program attempting to reorient elderly patients with respect to time, place and person (Taulbee and Folsom, 1966). RO is aimed at stimulating isolated elderly patients into reusing neglected functions or into developing new behavioral strategies in order to compensate for deficits (Stephens, 1969). RO can be either formalized into daily classroom sessions or it can be presented informally if the ward staff continuously conveys information related to the patients' orientation. Powell-Proctor and Miller (1982) described an outline of formal RO programs in which classrooms were equipped with clocks, calendars, weather cards, etc. During the sessions, information with respect to orientation is presented or, depending on the degree of impairment, subjects themselves may suggest topics to be discussed. Recent reviews on the effectiveness of RO conclude that this procedure has modest positive effects, which may exceed only slightly the non-specific effects of merely instituting any form of intervention (Miller, 1977; Woods and Holden, 1981; Leng, 1982; Powell-Proctor and Miller, 1982).

Severely invalidated subjects appear to benefit less from RO than mildly impaired subjects, in which an improvement on a rating behavior scale was found by Brook et al. (1975). Interestingly, reinforcement given by the therapist appeared to play a crucial role in achieving the beneficial effect; a control group having access to all facilities in the RO classroom, without receiving active encouragement, tended to slip back to initial levels of functioning after only a slight improvement (Brook et al., 1975). A similarly interesting control group was used by Woods (1979) showing that if RO sessions were run as unstructured discussion groups, participants benefited less than the patients in the RO groups, who attained superior scores on a cognitive test.

In contrast to Brook et al.'s results (1975), Hanley et al. (1981) showed that a 12-week RO program may induce cognitive improvements irrespective of the degree of dementia. Furthermore, this study also revealed a significant improvement in ward orientation as a result of specific training. Signs posted around the ward were not sufficient to improve ward orientation; the patients had to be trained to pay attention to the notices in order to benefit from the environmental change (Hanley, 1981). Similarly, Bergert and Jacobson (1976) concluded that improved orientation primarily results from learning where and how to obtain the necessary information rather than from just encountering the information.

Significant effects of formal RO training were not obtained in studies by Hogstel (1979) and Holden and Sinebruchow (1978). In various other studies, however, questionnaires and rating scales revealed improvements of orientation in experimental groups without convincing effects on general or specific behavioral scores (Citrin and Dixon, 1977; Harris and Ivory, 1976; Zepelin et al., 1981). Johnson et al. (1981) showed that these improvements are not dependent on the frequency (once or twice daily) of the RO training in the demented patients.

Greene et al. (1983) argued that RO might be of greater value to elderly demented patients who are not yet hospitalized. Patients still living in the community who received about 30 half-hour sessions of RO in a 6-week period while attending a geriatric psychiatry day hospital indeed showed significant improvement on tests of orientation and mental impairment (Greene et al., 1983). Ratings of behavior and mood disturbances revealed only improvement of mood as a result of RO (Greene et al., 1983). Interestingly, self-ratings of mood were improved in relatives of the patients as well, even though the behavior of the patients at home was still disturbed. The importance of this effect on the patients' relatives cannot be underestimated since this group is suffering considerably from the consequences of the patients' disorder and the relatives have, furthermore, been identified as a group which has the potential to markedly reduce the frequency of admissions to geriatric wards (Sanford, 1975).

Global changes in the environment may also beneficially affect well-being in institutionalized elderly as was exemplified in the study of Cosin et al. (1951) mentioned above. Shultz (1976) showed, furthermore, that predictability and controllability of positive events (in this study: a social visit by a college student) positively affected physical and psychological status as measured by several health, medication, and activity ratings. Emphasizing and giving opportunities to practise self-responsibility appeared to increase alertness, activity, and well-being in elderly healthy residents, suggesting that apathy and depression, although frequently observed, may not be inevitable consequences of aging but rather side effects of specific living conditions (Langer and Rodin, 1976). This notion is also exemplified by Liberman et al. (1968) who studied the effects of institutionalization on various psychological and cognitive measures. The results indicated that cognitive performance of institutionalized patients was inferior to the community dwelling and the waiting list groups. Davis (1967) emphasized the importance of motivations on function and well-being in older people. A mild degree of frustration may even be beneficial, since a continuous reassurance of having accomplished everything in life obviating the need to be actively involved, may promote a passive and depressive attitude.

In a recent study by Reeve and Ivison (1985) two of the approaches mentioned above, RO and more global changes in the environment, were combined. Both cognitive and behavioral measures were improved after the combined 1-month intervention. The particular combination was effective in maintaining the positive result throughout the 12 weeks of the study, whereas the effects of RO alone are usually reported to be short-lasting (Miller, 1977).

Systematic behavioral analysis of a specific symptom found in senility was introduced by Cameron (1941). He showed that patients suffering from nocturnal confusion, could show similar disorganized behavior during daytime merely by placing the patient in a darkened room. Miller (1977) labeled this observation as the first and important indication of an environmental control of behavioral disturbances in senescence. Social (appraisal) and material (candies, cigarettes) reinforcement, however, did not alter the frequency of incontinence in hospitalized patients (Pollock and Liberman, 1974). The negative results were partially attributed to methodological difficulties such as the exact determination of incontinence rate, and perhaps more significantly to the memory defects in the demented patients. Amnesia may prohibit strengthening of the link between the behavior and its reinforcer, and thus hamper severely demented subjects from benefiting from reinforcement techniques (Pollock and Liberman, 1974). Interestingly, the youngest and best oriented subject was the only one responding to the reinforcement, illustrating that environmental contingencies may control undesirable behavior at least in mildly impaired patients. This is consistent with data showing that verbal interaction or socialization in regressed, socially isolated elderly increased as a function of reinforcers such as sweets, tokens, and social reinforcement (Mueller and Atlas, 1972; MacDonald, 1978).

Several factors should be taken into account in evaluating rehabilitative interventions in aging and dementia as discussed above. Psychogeriatrics is usually surrounded by therapeutic nihilism (Miller, 1977) because the effects of the various approaches are small and mostly short-lasting. However, an approach towards elderly and demented patients, which aims at doing more to the patients than just supplying the basic needs, requires a continuous and motivated effort on the part of the therapists and nursing staff. Even small intra-individual improvement may be of great functional significance in a disorder which is usually progressive. Interventions should, furthermore, be tailored to the needs of the individual patient. Assessment of their efficacy should, therefore, also be aimed at specific abilities of the individual, rather than at group scores on an abstract rating scale with little or no practical relevance.

Summary and conclusions

Environmental factors play an important role in the development and plasticity of brain structure and function. It is generally accepted that various functions of the brain as well as its plasticity deteriorate with age. Experimental research in animals, however, shows that a certain amount of behavioral and structural plasticity is preserved even into old age. Research in elderly healthy and demented subjects suggests that some measures of brain function in senescent humans can, at least in part, be influenced by environmental factors. In contrast to pharmacological treatments, which cannot be rational as yet, because little is known about the mechanism(s) underlying malfunctioning in aging and dementia, physical training programs, reality orientation, changed institutional approaches of geriatric patients, or behavior modification can be expected to have few side effects. Even if the effects of these paradigms of intervention turn out to be small, they can be considered to be improvements of the standard of general 'care' rather than means for 'cure' (Bandera et al., 1984). These minor changes may have great impact on the quality of life in geriatric institutions (Gloag, 1985).

Effective drug treatment in Alzheimer disease is at present not available. The search for environmental contingencies which maximize performance levels given the degree of dementia, deserves as much scientific attention as the search for pharmacological treatment. It has been argued (Fliers et al., 1983) that the former kind of research cannot reasonably be expected to be initiated by pharmaceutical companies. This puts a specific scientific responsibility on the shoulders of those working at universities or other governmental institutions. They should seriously consider to investigate the environmental factors which may influence brain and behavior in aging and dementia.

References

Bandera, R., Cotecchia, S., De Blasi, A., Di Mascio, R., Pirone, F., Spagnoli, A. and Tognoni, G. (1984) Drug trials in the elderly. In D. L. Knook, G. Calderini and L. Amaduci (Eds.), *Proceedings of the EURAGE-workshop 'Aging of the brain and senile dementia: the inventory of EEC potentialities'*, EURAGE, Rijswijk, pp. 141–161.

Barry, A. J. (1966) The effects of physical conditioning on older individuals. II. Motor performance and cognitive function. *J. Gerontol.*, 21: 192–199.

Bartus, R. T., Flicker, C., Dean, R. L., Fisher, S., Pontecorvo, M. and Figueiredo, J. (1986) Behavioral and biochemical effects of nucleus basalis magnocellularis lesions: implications and possible relevance to understanding or treating Alzheimer's disease. In D. F. Swaab, E. Fliers, M. Mirmiran, W. A. Van Gool and F. Van Haaren (Eds.), *Aging of the Brain and Alzheimer's Disease, Progress in Brain Research, this volume*, Elsevier, Amsterdam, pp. 345–361.

Benestad, A. M. (1965) Trainability of old men. *Acta Med. Scand.*, 178: 321–327.

Bennett, E. L., Rosenzweig, M. R. and Wu, S. Y. C. (1973) Excitant and depressant drugs modulate effects of environment on brain weight and cholinesterase. *Psychopharmacology*, 33: 309–328.

Blackemore, C. and Cooper, G. F. (1970) Development of brain depends on the visual environment. *Nature*, 228: 477–478.

Blumenthal, J. A., Schocken, D. D., Needels, T. L. and Hindle, P. (1982) Psychological and physiological effects of physical conditioning on the elderly. *J. Psychosom. Res.*, 26: 505–510.

Brook, P., Degun, G. and Mather, M. (1975) Reality orientation, a therapy for psychogeriatric patients: a controlled study. *Br. J. Psychiat.*, 127: 42–45.

Candy, J. M., Perry, E. K., Perry, R. H., Court, J. A., Oakley, A. E. and Edwardson, J. A. (1986) The current status of the cortical cholinergic system in Alzheimer's disease and Parkinson's disease. In D. F. Swaab, E. Fliers, M. Mirmiran, W. A. Van Gool and F. Van Haaren (Eds.), *Aging of the Brain and Alzheimer's Disease, Progress in Brain Research, this volume*, Elsevier, Amsterdam, pp. 105–132.

Citrin, R. S. and Dixon, D. N. (1977) Reality orientation: a milieu therapy used in an institution for the aged. *Gerontologist*, 17: 39–43.

Connor, J. R., Diamond, M. C. and Johnson, R. E. (1980) Occipital cortical morphology of the rat: alterations with age and environment. *Exp. Neurol.*, 68: 158–170.

Connor, J. R., Melone, J. H., Yuen, A. R. and Diamond, M. C. (1981a) Dendritic length in aged rats' occipital cortex: an environmentally induced response. *Exp. Neurol.*, 73: 827–830.

Connor, J. R., Diamond, M. C., Connor, J. A. and Johnson, R. E. (1981b) A Golgi study of dendritic morphology in the occipital cortex of the socially reared aged rats. *Exp. Neurol.*, 73: 525–533.

Connor, J. R., Wang, E. C. and Diamond, M. C. (1982a) Increased length of terminal dendritic segments in old adult rats' somatosensory cortex: an environmentally induced response. *Exp. Neurol.*, 78: 466–470.

Connor, J. R., Bedan, S. E., Melone, J. H., Yuen, A. and Diamond, M. C. (1982b) A quantitative Golgi study in the occipital cortex of the pyramidal dendritic topology of old adult rats from social or isolated environments. *Brain Res.*, 251: 39–44.

Cosin, L. S., Mort, M., Post, F., Westroop, C. and Williams, M. (1951) Persistent senile confusion: study of 50 consecutive cases. *Int. J. Soc. Psychiat.*, 3: 195–202.

Cummins, R. A., Walsh, R. N., Budtz-Olsen, O. E., Konstantinos, T. and Horsfall, C. R. (1973) Environmentally-induced changes in the brains of elderly rats. *Nature*, 243: 516–518.

Cummins, R. A., Livessey, P. J., Evans, J. G. M. and Walsh, R. N. (1977) A developmental theory of environmental enrichment. *Science*, 197: 692–694.

Cummins, R. A., Livessey, P. J., Evans, J. G. M. and Walsh, R. N. (1979) Mechanism of brain growth by environmental stimulation. *Science*, 205: 522.

Davis, R. W. (1967) Activity therapy in a geriatric setting. *J. Am. Geriatr. Soc.*, 13: 1144–1152.

De Vries, H. A. (1970) Physiological effects of an exercise training regimen upon men aged 52 to 88. *J. Gerontol.*, 25: 325–336.

Diamond, M. C. (1967) Extensive cortical depth measurements and neuron size increase in the cortex of environmentally enriched rats. *J. Comp. Neurol.*, 131: 357–364.

Diamond, M. C. and Connor, J. R. (1982) Plasticity of the aging cerebral cortex. *Exp. Brain Res.*, 5: 36–44.

Diamond, M. C., Rosenzweig, M. R., Bennett, E. L., Linder, B. and Lyon, L. (1972) Effects of environmental enrichment and impoverishment on rat cerebral cortex. *J. Neurobiol.*, 3: 47–64.

Diamond, M. C., Ingham, C. A., Johnson, R. E., Bennett, E. L. and Rosenzweig, M. R. (1976) Effects of environment on morphology of rat cerebral cortex and hippocampus. *J. Neurobiol.*, 7: 75–85.

Diamond, M. C., Johnson, R. E. and Gold, M. W. (1977) Changes in neuron number and size and glia number in the young, adult, and aging rat medial occipital cortex. *Behav. Biol.*, 20: 409–418.

Diesfeldt, H. F. A. and Diesfeldt-Groenendijk, H. (1977) Improving cognitive performance in psychogeriatric patients: the influence of physical exercise. *Age Ageing*, 6: 58–64.

Doty, B. A. (1972) The effects of cage environment upon avoidance responding of aged rats. *J. Gerontol.*, 27: 358–360.

Droës, R. M. (1984) Bewegingsaktivering bij demente bejaarden. *Bewegen Hulpverlening*, 2: 135–147, in Dutch.

Dustman, R. E., Ruhling, R. O., Russell, E. M., Shearer, D. E., Bonekat, H. W., Shigeoka, J. W., Wood, J. S. and Bradford, D. C. (1984) Aerobic exercise training and improved neuropsychological function of older individuals. *Neurobiol. Aging*, 5: 35–42.

Edwards, H. P., Barry, W. F. and Wyspianski, J. P. (1969) Effect of differential rearing on photic evoked potentials and brightness discrimination in the albino rat. *Dev. Psychobiol.*, 2: 133–138.

Engellenner, W. J., Goodlett, C. R., Burright, R. G. and Donovick, P. J. (1982) Environmental enrichment and restriction: effects on reactivity, exploration and maze learning in mice with septal lesions. *Physiol. Behav.*, 29: 885–893.

Eterović, V. A. and Ferchmin, P. A. (1974) Interaction of environment and injections on brain weight in rats. *Dev. Psychobiol.*, 7: 515–517.

Fiala, B. A., Joyce, J. N. and Greenough, W. T. (1978) Environmental complexity modulates growth of granule cell dendrites in developing but not adult hippocampus of rats. *Exp. Neurol.*, 59: 372–383.

Feinberg, I. (1974) Changes in sleep cycle patterns with age. *J. Psychiat. Res.*, 10: 283–306.

Ferchmin, P. A. and Eterović, V. A. (1977) Brain plasticity and environmental complexity: role of motor skills. *Physiol. Behav.*, 18: 455–461.

Ferchmin, P. A., Bennett, E. L. and Rosenzweig, M. R. (1975) Direct contact with enriched environment is required to alter cerebral weight in rats. *J. Comp. Physiol. Psychol.*, 88: 360–367.

Ferchmin, P. A., Eterović, V. A. and Levin, L. E. (1980) Genetic learning deficiency does not hinder environment-dependent brain growth. *Physiol. Behav.*, 24: 45–50.

Feuerstein, R. (1980) *Instrumental Enrichment*, University Park Press, Baltimore.

Fliers, E., Lisei, A. and Swaab, D. F. (1983) *Dementia. Some Current Concepts and Research in The Netherlands*. A report at the request of the Netherlands Institute for Gerontology.

Gloag, D. (1985) Rehabilitation of the elderly. 2. Mind and body. *Br. Med. J.*, 290: 542–544.

Greene, J. G., Timbury, G. C., Smith, R. and Gardiner, M. (1983) Reality orientation with elderly patients in the community: an empirical evaluation. *Age Ageing*, 12: 38–43.

Greenough, W. T. (1976) Enduring brain effects of differential experience and training. In M. R. Rosenzweig and E. L. Bennett (Eds.), *Neural Mechanisms of Learning and Memory*, MIT Press, Massachusetts, pp. 255–278.

Greenough, W. T. and Green, E. J. (1984) Experience and the changing brain. In J. L. McGaugh, J. G. March and S. B. Kiesler (Eds.), *Aging: Biology and Behavior*, Academic Press, New York, pp. 159–200.

Greenough, W. T., Hwang, H. M. F. and Gorman, C. (1985) Evidence for active synapse formation or altered postsynaptic metabolism in visual cortex of rats reared in complex environments. *Proc. Natl. Acad. Sci. USA*, 82: 4549–4552.

Gutwein, B. M. and Fishbein, W. (1980a) Paradoxical sleep and memory. I. Selective alterations following enriched and impoverished environmental rearing. *Brain Res. Bull.*, 5: 9–12.

Gutwein, B. M. and Fishbein, W. (1980b) Paradoxical sleep and memory. II. Sleep circadian rhythmicity following enriched and impoverished environmental rearing. *Brain Res. Bull.*, 5: 105–109.

Hanley, I. G., McGuire, R. J. and Boyd, W. D. (1981) Reality orientation and dementia: a controlled trial of two approaches. *Br. J. Psychiat.*, 138: 10–14.

Harris, C. S. and Ivory, P. B. C. B. (1976) An outcome evaluation of reality orientation therapy with geriatric patients in a state mental hospital. *Gerontologist*, 16: 496–503.

Held, R. (1965) Plasticity in sensory-motor systems. *Scient. Am.*, 213: 84–94.

Hirsch, H. V. and Spinelli, D.N. (1970) Visual experience modifies distribution of horizontally and vertically oriented receptive fields in cats. *Science*, 168: 869–871.

Hogstel, M. O. (1979) Use of reality orientation with ageing confused patients. *Nurs. Res.*, 28: 161–165.

Holden, V. P. and Sinebruchow, A. (1978) Reality orientation therapy: a study investigating the value of this therapy in the rehabilitation of elderly people. *Age Ageing*, 7: 83–90.

Hubel, D. H. and Wiesel, T. N. (1970) The period of susceptibility to the physiological effects of unilateral eye closure in kittens. *J. Physiol.*, 206: 419–436.

Hubel, D. H., Wiesel, T. N. and Le Vay, S. (1976) Functional architecture of area 17 in normal and monocularly deprived macaque monkeys. *Cold Spring Harbour Symposia on Quantitative Biology*, 40: 581–589.

Ingebretsen, R. (1982) The relationship between physical activity and mental factors in the elderly. *Scand. J. Soc. Med.*, Suppl. 29: 153– 159.

Ingram, D. K., London, E. D. and Reynolds, M. A. (1982) Circadian rhythmicity and sleep: effects of aging in laboratory animals. *Neurobiol. Aging*, 3: 287–297.

Johnson, C. H., McLaren, S. M. and McPherson, F. M. (1981) The comparative effectiveness of three versions of 'classroom' reality orientation. *Age Ageing*, 10: 33–35.

Juraska, J. M., Henderson, C. and Müller, J. (1984) Differential rearing experience, gender and radial maze performance. *Dev. Psychobiol.*, 17: 209–215.

Kiyono, S., Seo, MN. L. and Shibagaki, M. (1981) Effects of rearing environments upon sleep-wake patterns in rats. *Physiol. Behav.*, 26: 391–394.

Kreitler, H. and Kreitler, S. (1970) Movement and aging: a psychological approach. *Med. Sport*, 4: 302–306.

Laerum, M. and Laerum, O. D. (1982) Can physical activity counteract ageing? *Scand. J. Soc. Med.*, Suppl. 29: 147–152.

Langer, E. J. and Rodin, J. (1976) The effects of choice and enhanced personal responsibility for the aged: a field experiment in an institutional setting. *J. Personal. Soc. Psychol.*, 34: 191–198.

Leng, N. (1982) Behavioural treatment of the elderly. *Age Ageing*, 11: 235–243.

LeVere, N. D. (1983) Recovery of function after brain damage: differences in aged rats? *Neurobiol. Aging*, 4: 181–185.

Liberman, M. A., Prock, V. N. and Tobin, S. S. (1968) Psychological effects of institutionalization. *J. Gerontol.*, 23: 343–353.

MacDonald, M. L. (1978) Environmental programming for the socially isolated aging. *Gerontologist*, 18: 350–354.

Mailloux, J. G., Edwards, H. P., Barry, W. F., Rowsell, H. C. and Achorn, E. G. (1974) Effects of differential rearing on cortical evoked potentials of the Albino rats. *J. Comp. Physiol. Psychol.*, 87: 475–480.

Mason, W. A. (1968) Early social deprivation in the nonhuman primates: implications for human behavior. In D. C. Glass (Ed.), *Environmental Influences*, Rockefeller University Press, New York, pp. 70–101.

Menich, S. R. and Baron, A. (1984) Social housing of rats: lifespan effects on reaction time, exploration, weight, and longevity. *Exp. Aging Res.*, 10: 95–100.

Miles, L. E. and Dement, W. C. (1980) Sleep and aging. *Sleep*, 3: 119–220.

Miller, E. (1977) The management of dementia: a review of some possibilities. *Br. J. Soc. Clin. Psychol.*, 16: 77–83.

Mirmiran, M. and Uylings, H. B. M. (1983) The environmental enrichment effect upon cortical growth is neutralized by concomitant pharmacological suppression of active sleep in female rats. *Brain Res.*, 261: 331–334.

Mirmiran, M., Van den Dungen, H. and Uylings, H. B. M. (1982) Sleep patterns during rearing under different environmental conditions in juvenile rats. *Brain Res.*, 233: 287–298.

Mueller, D. J. and Atlas, L. (1972) Resocialization of regressed elderly residents: a behavioral management approach. *J. Gerontol.*, 27: 390–392.

Olton, D. S. and Samuelson, R. J. (1976) Remembrance of place passed: spatial memory in rats. *J. Exp. Psychology: Animal Behavior Processes*, 2: 97–116.

Papanicolaou, A. C., Loring, D. W. and Eisenberg, H. M. (1984) Age related differences in recovery cycle of auditory evoked potentials. *Neurobiol. Aging*, 5: 291–295.

Pearlman, C. (1983) Impairment of environmental effects of brain weight by adrenergic drugs. *Physiol. Behav.*, 30: 161–163.

Peters, A., Feldman, M. L. and Vaughan, D. W. (1983) The effect of aging on the neuronal population within area 17 of adult rat cerebral cortex. *Neurobiol. Aging*, 4: 273–282.

Phelps, C. J. and Sladek, J. R. (1983) Regeneration of central catecholamine fibers in young and aged rat brain. *Brain Res. Bull.*, 11: 735–740.

Pollock, D. D. and Liberman, R. P. (1974) Behavior therapy of incontinence in demented inpatients. *Gerontologist*, 14: 488–491.

Powell, R. R. (1974) Psychological effects of exercise therapy upon institutionalized geriatric mental patients. *J. Gerontol.*, 29: 157–161.

Powell-Proctor, L. and Miller, E. (1982) Reality orientation: a critical appraisal. *Br. J. Psychiat.*, 140: 457–463.

Reeve, W. and Ivison, D. (1985) Use of environmental

manipulation and classroom and modified informal reality orientation with institutionalized, confused elderly patients. *Age Ageing*, 14: 119–121.

Rosenberg, R. S., Zepelin, H. and Rechtschoffen, A. (1979) Sleep in young and old rats. *J. Gerontol.*, 34: 525–532.

Rosenzweig, M. R. and Bennett, E. L. (1976) Enriched environments: facts, factors and fantasies. In L. Petrinovich and J. McGaugh (Eds.), *Knowing, Thinking and Believing*. Plenum Press, New York, pp. 179–213.

Rosenzweig, M. R. and Bennett, E. L. (1978) Experimental influences on brain anatomy and brain chemistry in rodents. In C. Gottlieb (Ed.), *Studies on the Development of Behavior and the Nervous System, Vol. 4: Early Influences*, Academic Press, New York, pp. 289–327.

Rosenzweig, M. R., Love, W. and Bennett, E. L. (1968) Effects of a few hours a day of enriched experience on brain chemistry and brain weights. *Physiol. Behav.*, 3: 819–825.

Rosenzweig, M. R., Bennett, E. L. and Diamond, M. C. (1972) Chemical and anatomical plasticity of brain: replications and extensions, 1970. In J. Gaito (Ed.), *Macromolecules and Behavior*, Appelton, New York, pp. 205–277.

Rosenzweig, M. R., Bennett, E. L., Hebert, M. and Morimoto, H. (1978) Social grouping cannot account for cerebral effects of enriched environments. *Brain Res.*, 153: 563–576.

Sanford, J. R. A. (1975) Tolerance of debility in elderly dependants by supporters at home: its significance for hospital practice. *Br. Med. J.*, 3: 471–473.

Scheff, S. W., Anderson, K. and De Kosky, S. T. (1984) Morphological aspects of brain damage in aging. In: S. W. Scheff (Ed.) *Aging and Recovery of Function in the Central Nervous System*, Plenum Publishing Corporation, New York, London, pp. 57–85.

Schulz, R. (1976) Effects of control and predictability on the physical and psychological well-being of the institutionalized aged. *J. Personal. Soc. Psychol.*, 33: 563–573.

Spirduso, W. W. (1975) Reaction and movement time as a function of age and physical activity level. *J. Gerontol.*, 30: 435–440.

Stephens, L. P. (Ed.) (1969) *Reality Orientation*. American Psychiatric Association Hospital and Community Psychiatric Service, Washington D. C.

Swaab, D. F. and Fliers, E. (1986) Clinical strategies in the treatment of Alzheimer's disease. In D. F. Swaab, E. Fliers, M. Mirmiran, W. A. Van Gool and F. Van Haaren (Eds.), *Aging of the Brain and Alzheimer's Disease, Progress in Brain Research, this volume*, Elsevier, Amsterdam, pp. 413–427.

Swindale, N. V. (1982) The development of columnar systems in the mammalian visual cortex. The role of innate and environmental factors. *Trends Neurosci.*, 5: 235–241.

Taulbee, L. R. and Folsom, J. C. (1966) Reality orientation for geriatric patients. *Hosp. Commun. Psychiat.*, 17: 133–135.

Terry, R. D. (1986) Interrelations among the lesions of normal and abnormal aging of the brain. In D. F. Swaab, E. Fliers, M. Mirmiran, W. A. Van Gool and F. Van Haaren (Eds.), *Aging of the Brain and Alzheimer's Disease, Progress in Brain Research, this volume*, Elsevier, Amsterdam, pp. 41–48.

Terry, R. D. and Gershon, S. (Eds.) (1976) *Neurobiology of Aging*, Raven Press, New York.

Turner, A. M. and Greenough, W. T. (1985) Differential rearing effects on rat visual cortex synapses. I. Synaptic and neuronal density and synapses per neuron. *Brain Res.*, 329: 195–203.

Uylings, H. B. M., Kuypers, K. and Veltman, W. A. M. (1978a) Environmental influences on the neocortex in later life. In: M. A. Corner, R. E. Baker, N. E. Van de Poll, D. F. Swaab and H. B. M. Uylings (Eds.), *Maturation of the Nervous System, Progress in Brain Research, Vol. 48*, Elsevier/North-Holland, Amsterdam, pp. 261–272.

Uylings, H. B. M., Kuypers, K., Diamond, M. C. and Veltman, W. A. M. (1978b) Effects of differential environments on plasticity of dendrites of cortical pyramidal neurons in adult rats. *Exp. Neurol.*, 62: 658–677.

Van Gool, W. A. and Mirmiran, M. (1983) Age-related changes in the sleep pattern of male adult rats. *Brain Res.*, 279: 394–398.

Van Gool, W. A. and Mirmiran, M. (1985) Housing in an enriched environment: changes in the sleep pattern of young and old rats. In W. P. Koella, E. Rüther and H. Schulz (Eds.), *Sleep '84*, Gustav Fischer Verlag, Stuttgart, New York, pp. 207–209.

Van Gool, W. A. and Mirmiran, M. (1986a) Aging and circadian rhythms. In D. F. Swaab, E. Fliers, M. Mirmiran, W. A. Van Gool and F. Van Haaren (Eds.), *Aging of the Brain and Alzheimer's Disease, Progress in Brain Research, this volume*, Elsevier, Amsterdam, pp. 255–277.

Van Gool, W. A. and Mirmiran, M. (1986b) Effects of aging and housing in an enriched environment on sleep-wake patterns in rats. *Sleep*, 9: 335–347.

Van Gool, W. A., Mirmiran, M. and Van Haaren, F. (1985) Spatial memory and visual evoked potentials in young and old rats after housing in an enriched environment. *Behav. Neur. Biol.*, 44: 454–469.

Volkmar, F. R. and Greenough, W. T. (1972) Rearing complexity affects branching of dendrites in the visual cortex of the rat. *Science*, 176: 1445–1447.

Walsh, R. N. and Cummins, R. A. (1975) Mechanisms mediating the production of environmentally induced brain changes. *Psychol. Bull.*, 82: 986–1000.

Walsh, R. N. and Greenough, W. T. (1976) *Environment as Therapy for Braindysfunction*. Plenum Press, New York, London.

Warren, J. M., Zerweck, C. and Anthony, A. (1982) Effects of environmental enrichment on old mice. *Dev. Psychobiol.*, 15: 13–18.

Woods, R. T. (1979) Reality orientation and staff attention: a controlled study. *Br. J. Psychiat.*, 134: 502–507.

Woods, R. T. and Holden, U. P. (1981) Reality orientation. In B. Isaacs (Ed.), *Recent Advances in Geriatric Medicine*, Churchill-Livingstone, Edinburgh, pp. 181–199.

458

Wulp, M. A. and Huijing, P. A. J. B. M. (1981) Het effect van bewegingsprogramma's bij ouderen. *Gerontologie*, 12: 202–211, in Dutch.

Zepelin, H., Wolfe, C. S. and Kleinplatz, F. (1981) Evaluation of a yearlong reality orientation program. *J. Gerontol.*, 36: 70–77.

Discussion

P. D. COLEMAN: I feel somewhat uncertain about the meaning of enriched environment studies in rats. On the one hand, it is emotionally appealing to think that it may be possible to influence the course of age-related declines. In addition, there are studies that do not depend on the enriched environment paradigm that show plasticity in the adult aged brain. Rutledge (1978) showed dendritic growth resulting from electrical stimulation; Scheff et al. (1984) have shown residual (but reduced) axonal plasticity in response to lesions in the aged rat brain; and our work certainly suggests dendritic plasticity in the aged human brain (Coleman and Flood, 1986). On the other hand, it has long been suggested that 'environmental complexity' studies are really deprivation studies in which the EC condition is similar to the natural environment of the rat, and the standard and isolated conditions represent varying degrees of deprivation. With regard to environmental complexity for Alzheimer patients, many care givers for these people believe that they can function best if their environment is kept simple and constant. I would be interested in your thoughts about the uncertainties regarding the role of environment in the aged and Alzheimer brain.

ANSWER: I think that uncertainties are present with regard to the role of the environment, particularly in the human. But let me discuss a couple of important points that you have raised in your remarks.

First of all, the presence of plasticity in the old brain. This is clear from your own data (Coleman and Flood, 1986) as well as from Greenough and Green (1984) on dendritic outgrowth in the aged human and rat. Secondly, in relation to the work of Rutledge (1978) and also Bloch (1976), it has even been suggested that one of the mechanisms underlying plasticity of the brain as a result of differential experiences is non-specific reticular formation activation. Therefore, the Rutledge data is not contradictory to environmental enrichment. Similar mechanisms have been suggested for consolidation of learning and memory which is the basic mechanism underlying environmental plasticity (Bloch, 1976). In relation to the work of Scheff et al. (1984) we should also consider better recovery of function in socially reared vs. isolated in basal forebrain cholinergic lesion experiments (Bartus et al., 1986). I agree with your remark that our 'enriched' environment is more similar to natural rat environment and other 'standard' or 'isolated' conditions are a sort of deprivation. This matter has been discussed by Rosenzweig and Bennett (1978). I only like to emphasize the fact that for standardization of procedure and having a better control over the outcome of data in animal studies, we have to use these paradigms.

With regard to environmental manipulations in AD patients, I do not agree with you that AD patients' environment should be kept constant. I believe that these patients are deprived of beneficial stimulations. I do not mean that we should take an AD patient out of his single room to Manhattan, but leaving him/her undisturbed, even if this makes them live longer, would be a sort of longevity in hibernation. We do not simply want to live longer, but indeed we want to have a successful, enjoyable aging.

R. D. TERRY: Are there epidemiological studies of Alzheimer's disease taking occupation into account? I have the impression that, coming to our clinics and autopsy rooms, there are as many lawyers as laborers, as many physicians as farmers and as many writers as wreckers. I doubt therefore that environmental enrichment in anyway prevents Alzheimer's disease.

ANSWER: By referring to environmental management, particularly in elderly and AD patients, we are not talking about the life history or genetical background of the subject. These are facts which might be interesting for people studying causality in aging and senile dementia. What I emphasize here is that, once the patient is aged or demented and particularly when he is institutionalized, environmental manipulations help in improving or at least slowing down the degeneration processes which are already there. Once again, I emphasize the fact that although many people wrongly use the term environmental therapy, we mean 'care' giving by environmental changes.

K. L. BICK (*comment* on Terry's remark): In the Italian multicentre study of risk factors in AD, there were no differences in social status and/or educational level of patients versus hospital or community controls. However, earlier visits to physicians for dementia were reported for patients with higher educational levels (e.g. a young mathematician who came to a medical doctor because he could no longer do square roots). Politicians and older housewives came to medical attention later in the course of the disease.

J. HAGAN: Does reality training alter post-mortem pathology?

ANSWER: There has been no systematic study carried out on this matter. If you want to know my point of view, I guess any improvement at the behavioral level should not necessarily express itself in neuropathological examinations. As I said in answer to Dr. Terry's question, we are not curing cortical plaques; we prevent deterioration of the residual functioning of the CNS by exciting it rather than further frustrating it.

R. NIEUWENHUYS: Have studies been carried out on the beneficial effect of 'reality orientation' or 'environmental enrichment' on specific subsets of dementing patients, e.g., on a group of true Alzheimer patients in the age of 55–60?

ANSWER: Unfortunately, most of the reality orientation studies have not been followed by post-mortem pathology. Most of the patients were diagnosed on the basis of psychological tests. There are several studies which were carried out in senile dementia (age at the time of study ranged from 70–90). These are: Brook et al. (1975); Woods (1979); Johnson et al. (1981) and Hanley et al. (1981). But I am afraid none of these were pre-senile dementia of the Alzheimer type within the age range you mentioned. Although they might have been included without being notified.

J. E. PISETSKY: Experience of anxiety or reaction to stress in the demented patients — it is likely that enrichment is helpful in re-establishing contact and interaction by decreasing anxiety.

ANSWER: Certainly anxiety and feelings of hopelessness might play an important role a priori of deterioration of function of elderly people. I agree with your suggestion that one way in which environmental enrichment might influence behavioral performances (even at the level of cognition) is by decreasing anxiety. In animal studies we have noticed that enriched rats are easier to handle and they seem more familiar with testing conditions than standard rats and far less anxious than isolated animals.

References

Bartus, R. T., Flicker, C., Dean, R. L., Fisher, S., Pontecorvo, M. and Figueiredo, J. (1986) Behavioral and biochemical effects of nucleus basalis magnocellular lesions: implications and possible relevance to understanding or treating Alzheimer's disease. In D. F. Swaab, E. Fliers, M. Mirmiran, W. A. Van Gool and F. Van Haaren (Eds.), *Aging of the Brain and Alzheimer's Disease, Progress in Brain Research, this volume*, Elsevier, Amsterdam, pp. 345–361.

Bloch, V. (1976) Brain activation and memory consolidation. In M. R. Rosenzweig and E. L. Bennett (Eds.), *Neural Mechanisms of Learning and Memory*, MIT Press, Massachusetts, pp. 583–590.

Brook, P., Degun, G. and Mather, M. (1975) Reality orientation, a therapy for psychogeriatric patients: a controlled study. *Br. J. Psychiat.*, 127: 42–45.

Coleman, P. D. and Flood, D. G. (1986) Dendritic proliferation in the aging brain as a compensatory repair mechanism. In D. F. Swaab, E. Fliers, M. Mirmiran, W. A. Van Gool and F. Van Haaren (Eds.), *Aging of the Brain and Alzheimer's Disease, Progress in Brain Research, this volume*, Elsevier, Amsterdam, pp. 227–237.

Greenough, W. T. and Green, E. J. (1984) Experience and the changing brain. In J. L. McGaugh, J. G. March and S. B. Kiesler (Eds.), *Aging: Biology and Behavior*, Academic Press, New York, pp. 159–200.

Hanley, I. G., McGuire, R. J. and Boyd, W. D. (1981) Reality orientation and dementia: a controlled trial of two approaches. *Br. J. Psychiat.*, 138: 10–14.

Johnson, C. H., McLaren, S. M. and McPherson, F. M. (1981) The comparative effectiveness of three versions of 'classroom' reality orientation. *Age Ageing*, 10: 33–35.

Rosenzweig, M. R. and Bennett, E. L. (1978) Experimental influences on brain anatomy and brain chemistry in rodents. In C. Gottlieb (Ed.), *Studies on the Development of Behavior and the Nervous System, Vol. 4, Early Influences*, Academic Press, New York, pp. 287–327.

Rutledge, L. T. (1978) Effects of cortical denervation and stimulation on axons, dendrites and synapses. In C. W. Cotman (Ed.), *Neuronal Plasticity*, Raven Press, New York, pp. 273–289.

Scheff, S. W., Anderson, K. and De Kosy, S. T. (1984) Morphological aspects of brain damage in aging. In S. W. Scheff (Ed.), *Aging and Recovery of Function in the Central Nervous System*, Plenum Publ. Corp., New York, pp. 57–85.

Woods, R. T. (1979) Reality orientation and staff attention: a controlled study. *Br. J. Psychiat.*, 134: 502–507.

D. F. Swaab, E. Fliers, M. Mirmiran, W. A. Van Gool and F. Van Haaren (Eds.)
Progress in Brain Research, Vol. 70.
© 1986 Elsevier Science Publishers B.V. (Biomedical Division)

CHAPTER 29

Possible dietary strategies to reduce cognitive deficits in old age

H. R. Lieberman[a,b] and T. M. Abou-Nader[b]

Departments of [a]Brain and Cognitive Sciences and [b]Applied Biological Sciences, E20-138, Massachusetts Institute of Technology, Cambridge, MA 02139, USA

Introduction

Currently most treatment-oriented neurobiological research on aging is, quite appropriately, focused on specific neurological and psychiatric diseases such as Alzheimer's, stroke, parkinsonism and depression. However, many age-related changes in mental abilities seem to be the consequence of the 'normal' aging process. It is possible, however, that this process is less than totally inevitable. Age-related declines in organ systems other than the brain have been shown to sometimes be sensitive to external factors and specific interventions. For example, until recently bone demineralization in elderly females, and to a lesser extent males, was considered to be the normal consequence of aging, but it is now clear that specific interventions can limit this process. One such intervention is nutritional, i.e. supplementation of the normal dietary calcium intake with substantial quantities of additional calcium. We suggest here that dietary supplementation with appropriate food constituents — in particular neurotransmitter precursors — should be considered as one potential intervention strategy for ameliorating or at least slowing some of the so called 'inevitable' consequences of central nervous system (CNS) aging. Some evidence in support of such dietary interventions will be discussed below. We will first review some of the data on age-related decrements in certain neurotransmitter systems. The focus of this brief discus-

sion will be on those systems known to be affected by specific food constituents. We will then discuss the food constituents that are known to affect these same neurotransmitter systems.

Changes in certain neurotransmitter systems with aging

Deterioration of certain mental functions is well documented in elderly people (Birren and Schaie, 1977; Corkin et al., 1982). Such changes are accompanied by, and possibly caused by, the alterations in brain function that occur with aging. The functioning of various neurotransmitter systems both in aging humans and animals has been extensively investigated and impaired function is often reported.

Acetylcholine

Considerable evidence suggests that the cholinergic neurotransmitter system is important in the formation of memory, a function which often deteriorates during aging (Bartus et al., 1982; Kubanis and Zornetzer, 1981). To examine changes in the cholinergic neurotransmitter system with aging, investigators have measured the levels of enzymes involved in the synthesis and breakdown of acetylcholine. These enzymes, choline acetyltransferase (CAT) and acetylcholinesterase (AChE), have been used because acetylcholine levels are difficult to measure reliably. Studies using human autopsy material have found age-related declines in CAT levels in various areas of the brain. McGeer and McGeer (1975) reported a 40–66% decrease in the level of cortical CAT between the ages of 20 and 50, while Perry et al. (1977) found large decreases in CAT in the hippocampus. Animal studies have found no changes in cortical CAT in aging rats (Meek et al., 1977; Timiras and Vernadakis, 1972), but decreases in CAT have been found in the nucleus accumbens, caudate nucleus, nucleus interpeduncularis, locus ceruleus, septum and hippocampus (Meek et al., 1977).

Conflicting results have been reported with respect to age-related changes in AChE. While McGeer and McGeer (1975) reported significant decreases in cortical AChE with aging (similar to those they reported for CAT), Perry (1980) found no such changes. One study with rats also found age-related decreases in AChE in the striatum and cerebellum of these animals (Morin and Wasterlain, 1980).

In addition to changes in cholinergic enzymes, age-related decreases in cholinergic muscarinic binding in the human temporal cortex have been reported (Perry, 1980). It has also been suggested that the blood–brain barrier transport system for choline may become impaired with age (Hicks et al., 1979).

Changes in cholinergic function like those reported could be associated with the 'normal' deterioration of memory with age (Bartus et al., 1982). This hypothesis is, of course, also consistent with the severe deterioration of the cholinergic system seen in Alzheimer's disease (AD) and the corresponding severe memory deficits (Bartus et al., 1982).

Catecholamines

Levels of catecholamines (CAs), dopamine (DA) and norepinephrine (NE), in the brain have been examined in several animal species and in humans of different ages. No change in whole brain levels was found (Finch, 1973; McGeer et al., 1971),

however, regional alterations have been consistently reported. Significant decreases in DA as a function of increasing age have been reported in human caudate, globus pallidus, midbrain and hippocampus (Adolfsson et al., 1979). Striatal DA has been reported to decline in adult humans at the rate of about 1% per year (Carlsson and Winblad, 1976; Riederer and Wuketich, 1976). NE levels in human hindbrain from subjects 65 years and older were 40–50% lower than levels of 20-years-old subjects (Robinson, 1975; Robinson et al., 1972). Significant decreases with aging in NE concentrations in brain stem and hypothalamus were also reported in the rhesus monkey (Samorajski and Rolsten, 1973). Corresponding decreases in CA turnover also seem to occur in specific brain regions (Finch, 1973; Ponzio et al., 1978).

Tyrosine hydroxylase (TH) is the rate-limiting enzyme for CA synthesis. Therefore, it is possible that age-related changes in CA function could result from declines in activity of this enzyme. Several investigators (Cote and Kremzner, 1974; McGeer and McGeer, 1975, 1976) have reported substantial age-related declines in TH activity in certain regions of human brains (especially striatum), in some cases by as much as 50%.

Other findings relating to CA function include an increase in the activity of monoamine oxidase (MAO), a catabolic enzyme for CAs (Robinson et al., 1972) and a decrease in the uptake of DA and NE in specific brain regions (Haycock et al., 1977; Jonec and Finch, 1975). Also, a significant decline in receptor concentrations with increasing age has been noted (Severson and Finch, 1980; Maggi et al., 1979).

In AD, cell losses in the locus ceruleus have been frequently documented (Bondareff et al., 1981; Mann et al., 1980) while reductions in NE and DA β-hydroxylase have been repeatedly reported (Adolfsson et al., 1979; Gottfries et al., 1983; Yates et al., 1983).

Several laboratories have recently been investigating age-associated changes in the response of CA systems to experimentally induced stress. Significant differences in response to stress, resulting in a greater depletion of NE in old as compared to young animals, have been observed (Ritter and Pelzer, 1978).

The generalized nature of these CA deficits in normal animals and humans suggests that these transmitter systems may be functionally impaired in old age. For example, data from rodents suggest that the ability to respond to acutely stressful situations is reduced in older animals concomitant with reductions in NE or DA levels or turnover (Brady et al., 1981; Thurmond and Brown, 1984). Treatments which augment CA function can mitigate to a greater extent the behavioral impairments seen in acutely stressed older animals than in younger animals (Brady et al., 1981; Thurmond and Brown, 1984).

Serotonin

Few correlations between age and serotoninergic systems have been found in any of the brain regions studied to date, except perhaps in the mesencephalon (Gottfries et al., 1974; Bucht et al., 1981). In AD however, reduced cell counts and increased numbers of tangles were found in the raphe nucleus (Mann and Yates, 1983; Ishii, 1966) along with decreased serotonin and 5-HIAA concentrations (Adolfsson et al., 1979; Gottfries et al., 1983).

Intervention strategies based on nutrition

It is apparent from the evidence discussed above that substantial biochemical and physiological alterations occur in the brain as a consequence of normal aging, although many details remain to be resolved. It is likely that many of the behavioral impairments seen as a consequence of aging can be attributed to these physiological deficits. Many of these changes are probably inevitable; however, some may be, if not correctable, at least partially preventable. It is certainly unlikely, at least in the foreseeable future, that any intervention will be discovered which will stop the normal progression of brain aging and the resulting adverse consequences. However, it may be possible to develop treatments which at least are able to partially retard this aging process in some individuals.

Data from a number of research areas suggest that relatively minor long-term dietary manipulations or interventions may have substantial long-term beneficial health consequences. For example, there is now little doubt that calcium supplementation can prevent some of the bone loss that occurs in elderly women. Also, there is considerable evidence that a variety of vascular and cardiovascular diseases (e.g. hypertension, arteriosclerosis, stroke) may be associated with dietary patterns in a manner totally unrelated to essential dietary requirements. Even in such areas as these, only the most obvious relationships have been explored. It is not completely unexpected that increased calcium availability improves bone calcium deposition or that plasma lipid concentration affects the formation of plaques in blood vessels. Other dietary interventions, with less obvious connections to specific diseases, probably remain to be discovered. We suggest that long-term differences in the consumption of specific foods, or pure nutrients administered as dietary supplements, could chronically affect brain function. This hypothesis can be advanced because definitive, acute relationships between brain function and various dietary neurotransmitter precursors have recently been recognized (Wurtman et al., 1981; Growdon and Gibson, 1982). A variety of CNS neurotransmitter systems have, within the last 15 years, been shown to be affected by consuming an ordinary meal or by administration of a specific food constituent in pure form. Such data provide a solid biochemical and physiological basis for the more speculative hypotheses advanced here. The various food constituents that have been shown to alter brain composition will be discussed in detail below. The known functions of these substances provide the basis upon which initial hypotheses relating chronic dietary manipulations and age-related deficits in brain functions have been or could be formulated.

464

Neurotransmitter precursors and aging

One type of nutritional intervention could involve the use of compounds which modify neurotransmitter synthesis — either neurotransmitter precursors or foods which modify the availability of precursors. The foods or food constituents which affect the brain may act in a variety of ways. They may increase their own levels in the brain if they are neurotransmitter precursors. They may also diminish neurotransmitter precursor levels in the brain, thus suppressing neurotransmission, if they compete with a precursor for transport across the blood–brain barrier. Alternatively, the appropriate food constituents could restore putative 'reservoirs' for neurotransmitter precursors in the brain (specifically choline, present within membrane phosphatidylcholine) that are constituents of both neurotransmitters and brain membranes. One neurotransmitter precursor, tryptophan, can apparently always increase the production of its neurotransmitter product serotonin, when taken orally (Wurtman et al., 1981; Growdon and Gibson, 1982; Young, 1986). A given dose of tryptophan can be potentiated by co-administering it with enough carbohydrate to cause insulin secretion, which can lower plasma levels of the other large neutral amino acids that compete with tryptophan for blood–brain barrier transport (Wurtman et al., 1981; Growdon and Gibson, 1982). Treatments that are as subtle as administration of a protein versus a carbohydrate meal can affect brain serotonin concentration. In fact, it appears that a single protein or carbohydrate meal can have measurable behavioral effects, and these are consistent with the differential effects the meals have on brain serotonin (Lieberman et al., 1986).

Other neurotransmitter precursors like tyrosine or choline may or may not enhance the synthesis of their neurotransmitter products, depending upon the physiological activity of each neuron. When particular neurons are firing frequently they are very responsive to supplemental choline or tyrosine; when they are quiescent they are unresponsive. This property allows the physiological and behavioral effects of tyrosine and choline to be very selective, i.e. the precursor will work only in neurons that continue to fire frequently (Wurtman et al., 1981; Milner and Wurtman, 1986).

Neurotransmitter precursors have already been used in research studies to attempt to treat a variety of CNS disorders such as insomnia, schizophrenia, affective disorders, AD and tardive dyskinesia (Wurtman et al., 1981; Growdon and Gibson, 1982; Hartmann, 1983; Young, 1986). They appear to be effective in certain instances. We are aware of few published studies where precursors have been chronically administered to animals and the neurochemical and behavioral consequences determined (Wurtman et al., 1981; Growdon and Gibson, 1982; Young, 1986). We are not aware of any study conducted with healthy humans where long-term precursor treatment has been given to mitigate age-related deterioration in mental performance.

Cholinergic precursors: choline and lecithin

Choline and lecithin, because they are the substrates for acetylcholine synthesis, are the precursors which have attracted the greatest interest with respect to various CNS deficits associated with aging. Although acetylcholine is involved in the regulation of numerous brain functions, of particular interest with respect to aging is its well-documented role in memory (Bartus et al., 1982; Kubanis and Zornetzer, 1981). Brain choline is derived from at least three sources: a small amount is synthesized in the brain itself, some is derived from the breakdown of phosphatidylcholine in membranes and some is transported into the brain from the plasma (Growdon and Gibson, 1982). Plasma choline fluctuates as a function of dietary intake of lecithin, which is the primary source of choline in the diet. When plasma choline does vary, for example after a meal high in choline or after a dose of choline or lecithin, there is a subsequent increase in brain choline (Cohen and Wurtman, 1976; Wurtman et al., 1981; Growdon and Gibson, 1982). When cholinergic neurons are firing frequently, the increased availability of this precursor increases the release of acetylcholine. Lecithin is the preferred form of choline supplementation because it elevates plasma choline more efficiently and because choline causes food to taste bitter, as well as imparting a fishy odor to the patient. However, the lecithin must be the specific phospholipid phosphatidylcholine, not the common form of lecithin used as a food emulsifier. This commercial form of lecithin may contain as little as 10% phosphatidylcholine (Growdon and Gibson, 1982).

As noted above the most thoroughly documented neurochemical deficit in AD is the loss of cholinergic activity in the hippocampus. Since cholinergic terminals in the hippocampus are believed to be critical for memory formation, it has been suggested that some of the cognitive deficits seen in AD are a direct result of impaired cholinergic function (Bartus et al., 1982). Therefore, a number of investigators have attempted to restore cognitive function in patients with AD by administering choline or lecithin. Although some initial reports were positive, they have not been replicated (Growdon and Gibson, 1982; Gauthier et al., 1981; Wurtman, 1985). However, almost all of the studies conducted to date have used relatively brief periods (typically a few weeks in duration) of lecithin or choline treatment (Wurtman, 1985). One study where lecithin was administered for a longer period of time (6 months) did find a subgroup of patients who responded positively, as measured by a psychological test battery, to the treatment (Little et al., 1985). The responders were actually somewhat older on the average than the non-responders. This suggests that the responders may have had a different form of the disease with later onset, and with a more purely cholinergic character.

AD is usually characterized by very severe and generalized brain deterioration. Numerous transmitter systems are known to be severely impaired, and in later stages of the disease generalized pathology is seen throughout the brain (Gottfries et al., 1983). It is hardly surprising that a few days of lecithin or choline supplementation, even in the intermediate stages of the disease, have no detectable effect. Even long-term treatments should not be expected to have unrealistic benefits, given the severity of the underlying pathology. Perhaps therapy needs to begin in the earliest stages of the disease, before obvious symptoms are recognized.

In any case, the difficulties in demonstrating unequivocal benefits of treatment with acetylcholine precursors in Alzheimer's disease could have little to do with the likelihood of observing positive effects of long-term dietary supplementation in normal individuals treated either with cholinergic or other precursors.

Studies of aged but otherwise healthy animals using cholinergic precursors have been more promising, especially when sufficient doses of a precursor are given chronically. For example, Bartus et al. (1980) found that administration of a choline-rich diet (about 1 g/kg/day) for several months mitigated the age-related decline in passive avoidance retention seen in control animals. Leathwood et al. (1982) found a substantial improvement in passive avoidance performance in old but not young mice after only 4 days of high-dose phosphatidylcholine administration (about 1.2 g/kg/day). Lower doses of this precursor failed to significantly improve performance in the Leathwood et al. (1982) study, and Bartus et al. (1980) also failed to find any improvement in passive avoidance performance in aged rats after short-term choline chloride supplementation of only 100 mg/kg/day. Additional studies with animals receiving high-dose, long-term lecithin supplements would therefore be appropriate, both to confirm the initial positive finding and to extend them to other behavioral paradigms and other species. Of special importance would be studies where supplementation is given throughout the life of the animals. Long-term studies with healthy humans should also be contemplated.

Tryptophan

Tryptophan, an essential amino acid found in most protein-containing foods, is the dietary precursor of the brain neurotransmitter serotonin. Like all the large neutral amino acids it is actively transported across the blood–brain barrier. Serotoninergic neurons have been implicated in numerous psychiatric diseases (e.g. depression, mania) and the regulation of a variety of important central nervous system functions (e.g. sleep, pain sensitivity and aggression) (Growdon and Gibson, 1982; Lieberman et al., 1983; Young, 1986). Tryptophan has therefore already been evaluated for a variety of therapeutic uses in various patient populations. For example, many studies have demonstrated that tryptophan, when administered in doses of one gram or greater, increases human sleepiness (Hartmann, 1983; Lieberman et al., 1983) and, in patients with insomnia, decreases latency to fall asleep (Hartmann, 1983). Although tryptophan does not appear to be as potent a hypnotic as prescription medications used for this purpose, it may be clinically useful as a mild hypnotic. Tryptophan's effects on sleep are consistent with one of the functions associated with serotonin — this transmitter appears to participate in the induction and maintenance of sleep. It is well documented that certain aspects of sleep deteriorate with aging. For example, increased wakefulness is observed during the usual sleep period, Stage 4 sleep is greatly reduced and subjective complaints increase in elderly people (Kripke et al., 1983; Zepelin, 1983). Administration of tryptophan could be considered as a potential sleep aid in this population, either on an acute, as-needed basis in higher doses, or perhaps in chronic low doses administered regularly before bedtime. Since, unlike lecithin or choline, tryptophan has definite acute effects, it would probably not be advisable to administer it — even in lower doses — at times when optimal alertness is desirable (Lieberman et al., 1983). However, it might be of interest to examine the chronic effects of tryptophan administration on sleep and daytime alertness (if sleep quality is enhanced then daytime alertness and circadian rhythms might also be improved) in animals and humans. Tryptophan should be administered just prior to the normal sleep period

of the species being tested. Møller et al. (1980), have demonstrated a significant inverse correlation between plasma tryptophan ratio (which determines tryptophan's access to the brain) and age in normal volunteers and so, as a consequence of normal aging, less tryptophan may be available to the brain.

Another common problem that is seen more frequently in elderly people is depression. The highest first incidence of depression, particularly of a severe attack, occurs between the ages of 55 and 65 in men and 50 and 60 in women (Kaplan and Sadock, 1981). Since many of the drugs used to treat depression increase serotoninergic activity, many investigators have tested tryptophan as a treatment for this disorder. The results have been mixed, with numerous positive as well as negative findings reported in the literature (Young, 1986). There is some evidence that there are subgroups of depressed patients who are more likely to respond positively to tryptophan treatment. These responders tend to have lower plasma tryptophan ratios prior to treatment, as do elderly people in general (Møller et al., 1980). (The plasma ratio of tryptophan to the other large neutral amino acids (LNAA) determines the rate of entry of tryptophan into the brain (Wurtman et al., 1981).) Tryptophan has actually been tested in elderly demented patients (for 1 month, given as a single dose of 3 g in the evening) with no overall benefit observed (Smith et al., 1984). However, such severely impaired patients are likely to be among the most difficult to treat with any intervention.

Given the potential beneficial effects of tryptophan on sleep and mood state, additional studies, both human and animal, would seem appropriate.

Tyrosine

The LNAA tyrosine, like tryptophan, is a common constituent of nearly all protein foods. It is readily transported across the blood–brain barrier by the same carrier system that carries all the large neutral amino acids, including tryptophan, into the brain. Tyrosine is the precursor of the brain neurotransmitters DA, NE and epinephrine (E). Although little is known of the function of epinephrine there is considerable evidence, from both animal and clinical studies, that DA and NE have important functions in the brain. DA neurons participate in the regulation of motor activity and various mood states. Norepinephrine neurons also seem to participate in the regulation of mood, especially with regard to anxiety and stress (Gray, 1982). When catecholaminergic neurons are firing frequently the availability of tyrosine, their precursor, can be rate-limiting (Milner and Wurtman, 1986). To date, only a few behavioral studies have been conducted with tyrosine in either animals or humans. Most of the animal studies have focused on the possible beneficial effects of tyrosine when animals are acutely stressed. When animals are subjected to a variety of stressors, brain NE stores, and also turnover, decline (Stone, 1975). Under these same conditions substantial alterations in a number of behaviors are observed: exploration, learning, eating, drinking and sleep are all disturbed (Stone, 1975). When single doses of tyrosine are given to animals that are acutely stressed by tail-shock, it appears to antagonize both the neurochemical and the behavioral consequences of this very stressful treatment. Animals pretreated with tyrosine do not exhibit shock-induced impairments in exploratory behavior (locomotion and hole-poking). In addition, in pretreated animals brain NE is not depleted and its turnover appears to increase (Reinstein et al., 1984). Adding supplemental tyrosine to the diet has similar positive effects on the neurochemical and behavioral response of animals to tail-shock induced stress (Lehnert et al., 1984). The effects also appear to generalize to other forms of stress (Brady et al., 1981). Moreover, in the latter study, greater effects of tyrosine were seen in older animals that were stressed (Brady et al., 1981). Short-term (1 week) dietary tyrosine supplementation has also been shown to facilitate motor activity seen in old mice (Thurmond and Brown, 1984), an effect the authors attribute to increased DA activity. Few behavioral studies have been conducted to examine the effects of tyrosine on humans. Although when administered acutely it appears to have little effect on young, unstressed volunteers (Lieberman et al., 1983), there is some evidence it does have beneficial effects on mood (vigor) in older subjects (Leathwood and Pollet, 1983). These results are consistent with the reports of substantial deficits in catecholaminergic function present in elderly or stressed animals and people noted above. Further studies, animal and human, would certainly be appropriate at this time. For example, the effects of tyrosine, administered either acutely prior to stress or as a long-term dietary supplement, should be studied in both young and old humans who are either acutely stressed in the laboratory, or are under considerable stress in their daily lives. Although such studies will be difficult to perform, the potential benefits could be substantial.

Summary and conclusions

Attempting to slow the decline in cognitive functioning that seems inevitably to occur as humans age by using nutritional interventions is hardly a new idea. Many unproven nutritional supplements have been, or are currently, marketed as anti-aging nostrums. However, recent advances have demonstrated that the brain is not isolated from systemic, diet-related changes in some of its key components. Therefore, there is some scientific merit to considering nutritional variables (especially the availability of neurotransmitter precursors) as a relevant variable in studies of brain aging.

If neurotransmitter precursors or other nutrients with known neurochemical effects turn out to be effective in treating various behavioral consequences of aging, these compounds will probably have certain significant advantages over 'classic drugs'. They have always been consumed by humans. They are well tolerated and very rapidly metabolized to known non-toxic compounds, using enzyme systems that have fulfilled this function throughout man's history. Therefore side effects, particularly serious chronic ones, like carcinogenic or teratogenic risk, are less likely to be a problem.

Precursors may also act synergistically when administered in combination, although some, notably tryptophan and tyrosine, compete for access to the brain. If these precursors were to be given concurrently, it would have to be at different times of the day. A different pattern of administration of these two amino acids would also be advisable because any acute effects of tyrosine would be desirable during waking, and of tryptophan during sleep. These compounds may also have utility in combination with drugs: for example it might be advantageous to combine a compound that enhances a neurotransmitter's synthesis (i.e. its precursor) with one that slows its uptake or enzymatic inactivation, or accelerates firing of neurons that release it. Studies on such combinations are in their infancy.

It should be noted that detecting positive effects of such treatments on humans is certain to be quite difficult. Nutrients, even when administered in large, long-term doses are likely to have subtle effects on the brain and behavior. Detecting the behavioral effects of food constituents, even under optimal, well-controlled conditions when rigorous psychometric tests are used, is difficult (Lieberman and Wurtman, 1984; Lieberman et al., 1986). The increased variability in behavior which occurs as humans age is also certain to contribute to the difficulty of such studies. Precedents for very large scale studies to measure the effects of nutritional interventions on healthy population groups already exist. For example, in one study with beta-carotene a sample size of 20 000 was deemed appropriate to ensure sufficient statistical power to detect a 30% reduction in cancer incidence (Hennekens et al., 1983). For a variety of reasons, including the fact that age-related cognitive changes in behavior are much more common than cancer, such a large sample size would not be necessary for behavioral studies.

Finally, it should be noted that aging is obviously a heterogeneous process. It clearly proceeds at different rates in different individuals and, in all probability, differentially affects specific neurotransmitter systems. Therefore, precursor treatments are likely to be effective in some people but not in others. Detailed data on individual pretreatment status, both cognitive and when possible neurochemical, would be important covariates in any studies where neurotransmitter precursors are to be administered. These data might be useful for distinguishing responding from non-responding subgroups of patients.

Acknowledgements

The authors wish to gratefully acknowledge the valued advice and collaboration of Dr. Richard J. Wurtman. This research was supported by NASA Grant NAG 2-210 and NIH Grants 1 R01-AG/AM04591, 2R01-HD11722 and 5M01-RR00088.

References

Adolfsson, R., Gottfries, C. G., Roos, B. E. and Winblad, B. (1979) Postmortem distribution of dopamine and homovanillic acid in human brain, variations related to age, and a review of the literature. *J. Neur. Transm.*, 45: 81–105.

Bartus, R. T., Dean, R. L., Goas, T. A. and Lippa, A. F. (1980) Age related changes in passive avoidance retention: modulation with dietary choline. *Science*, 209: 301–303.

Bartus, R. T., Dean, R. L., Beer, B. and Lippa, A. S. (1982) The cholinergic hypothesis of geriatric memory dysfunction. *Science*, 217: 408–417.

Birren, J. E. and Schaie, K. W. (1977) *Handbook of the Psychology of Aging.* Van Nostrand Reinhold, New York.

Bondareff, W., Mountjoy, C. Q. and Roth, M. (1981) Selective loss of neurons of origin of adrenergic projection to cerebral cortex (nucleus locus coeruleus) in senile dementia. *Lancet*, 1: 783–784.

Brady, K., Brown, J. W. and Thurmond, B. (1981) Behavioral and neurochemical effects of dietary tyrosine in young and aged mice following cold swim stress. *Pharmacol. Biochem. Behav.*, 12: 667–674.

Bucht, G., Adolfsson, R., Gottfries, C. G., Roos, B. E. and Winblad, B. (1981) Distribution of 5-hydroxytryptamine and

5-hydroxyindoleacetic acid in human brain in relation to age, drug influence, agonal status and circadian variation. *J. Neural Transm.*, 51: 185–203.

Carlsson, A. and Winblad, B. (1976) The influence of age and time interval between death and autopsy on dopamine and 3-methoxytyramine levels in human basal ganglia. *J. Neural Transm.*, 83: 271–276.

Cohen, E. L. and Wurtman, R. J. (1976) Brain acetylcholine: control by dietary choline. *Science*, 191: 561–562.

Corkin, S., Davis, K., Growdon, J., Usdin, E. and Wurtman, R. (1982) *Alzheimer's Disease: A Report of Progress in Research, Aging, Vol. 19*, Raven Press, New York.

Cote, L. J. and Kremzner, L. T. (1974) Changes in neurotransmitter systems with increasing age in human brain. In *Transactions of the American Society for Neurochemistry*, 5th Annual Meeting, New Orleans, La., p. 83.

Finch, C. (1973) Catecholamine metabolism in the brains of aging male mice. *Brain Res.*, 52: 261–276.

Gauthier, S., Etienne, P., Dastoor, D., Collier, B. and Ludwick, R. (1981) Lack of an effect of a 3 month treatment with lecithin in Alzheimer's disease. *Neurology (NY)*, 31: 89.

Gottfries, C. G., Oreland, L., Wiberg, A. and Winblad, B. (1974) Letter: Brain-levels of monoamine oxidase in depression. *Lancet*, 2: 360–361.

Gottfries, C. G., Adolfsson, R., Aquilonius, S. M., Carlsson, A., Eckernas, S. A., Nordberg, A., Oreland, L., Svennerholm, L., Wiberg, A. and Winblad, B. (1983) Biochemical changes in dementia disorders of Alzheimer type (AD/S-DAT). *Neurobiol. Aging*, 4: 261–271.

Gray, J. A. (1982) *The Neuropsychology of Anxiety: An Enquiry Into the Functions of the Septo-hippocampal System*. Clarendon Press, Oxford.

Growdon, J. H. and Gibson, C. J. (1982) Dietary precursors of neurotransmitters: treatment strategies. In S. H. Appel (Ed.), *Current Neurology, Vol. 4*, Wiley and Sons, Inc., New York.

Hartmann, E. (1983) Effects of L-Tryptophan on sleepiness and on sleep. *J. Psychiat. Res.*, 17(2): 107–113.

Haycock, J. W., White, W. F., McGaugh, J. L. and Cotman, C. W. (1977) Enhanced stimulus-secretion coupling from brains of aged mice. *Exp. Neurol.*, 57: 873–882.

Hennekens, C. H. and Physicians Health Study Research Group (1983) Strategies for a primary prevention trial of cancer and cardiovascular disease among U.S. physicians (Abstract). *Am. J. Epidemiol.*, 118: 453–454.

Hicks, P., Rolsten, C., Hsu, L., Schoolar, J. and Samorajski, T. (1979) Brain uptake index for choline in aged rats. *Society for Neuroscience Abstracts*, 5: 6.

Ishii, T. (1966) Distribution of Alzheimer's neurofibrillary changes in the brain stem and hypothalamus of senile dementia. *Acta Neuropathol.*, 6: 181–187.

Jonec, V. J. and Finch, C. E. (1975) Senescence and dopamine uptake by subcellular fractions of the C57BL/6J male mouse brain. *Brain Res.*, 91: 197–215.

Kaplan, H. I. and Sadock, B. J. (1981) *Modern Synopsis of a Comprehensive Textbook of Psychiatry/III, 3rd edn.*, Williams and Wilkins, Baltimore MD, p. 1018.

Kripke, D. F., Ancoli-Israel, S., Mason, W. and Messin, S. (1983) Sleep related mortality and morbidity in the aged. In M. Chase and E. D. Weitzman (Eds.), *Sleep Disorders Basic and Clinical Research*. SP Medical and Scientific Books, New York, pp. 415–429.

Kubanis, P. and Zornetzer, S. F. (1981) Age related behavioral and neurobiological changes: a review with an emphasis on memory. *Behav. Neur. Biol.*, 31: 115–172.

Leathwood, P. D. and Pollet, P. (1983) Diet-induced mood changes in normal populations. *J. Psychiat. Res.*, 17: 147.

Leathwood, P. D., Heck, E. and Mauron, J. (1982) Phosphatidylcholine and avoidance performance in 17 month-old SEC/1ReJ mice. *Life Sci.*, 30: 1065–1071.

Lehnert, H., Reinstein, D. K., Strowbridge, B. W. and Wurtman, R. J. (1984) Neurochemical and behavioral consequences of acute, uncontrollable stress: effects of dietary tyrosine. *Brain Res.*, 303: 215–223.

Lieberman, H. R. and Wurtman, R. J. (1984) Techniques for evaluating the behavioral effects of food constituents. *J. Am. Coll. Nutr.*, 3(3): 247, abstract.

Lieberman, H. R., Corkin, S., Spring, B. S., Growdon, J. H. and Wurtman, R. J. (1983) Mood, performance and pain sensitivity: changes induced by food constituents. *J. Psychiat. Res.*, 17: 135–145.

Lieberman, H. R., Spring, B. J. and Garfield, G. S. (1986) The behavioral effects of food constituents: Strategies used in studies of amino acids, proteins, carbohydrate and caffeine, In *Diet and Behavior: A Multidisciplinary Evaluation, Nutr. Rev.*, Suppl. 44: 61–70.

Little, A., Levy, R., Chuaqui-Kidd, P. and Hand, D. (1985) A double-blind, placebo controlled trial of high-dose lecithin in Alzheimer's disease. *J. Neurol. Neurosurg. Psychiat.*, 48: 736–742.

Maggi, A., Schmidt, M. J., Ghetti, B. and Enna, S. J. (1979) Effect of aging on neurotransmitter receptor binding in rat and human brain. *Life Sci.*, 24: 367–374.

Mann, D. M. A. and Yates, P. O. (1983) Serotonin nerve cells in Alzheimer's disease. *J. Neurol. Neurosurg. Psychiat.*, 46: 96.

Mann, D. M. A., Lincoln, J., Yates, P. O., Stamp, J. E. and Toper, S. (1980) Changes in monoamine containing neurons of the human CNS in senile dementia. *Br. J. Psychiat.*, 136: 533–541.

McGeer, E. G. and McGeer, P. L. (1975) Age changes in the human for some enzymes associated with metabolism of catecholamines, GABA, and acetylcholine. In J. M. Ordy and K. R. Brizzee (Eds.), *Neurobiology of Aging*, Plenum Press, New York, pp. 287–305.

McGeer, E. G., Fibiger, H. C., McGeer, P. L. and Wickson, V. (1971) Aging and brain enzymes. *Exp. Gerontol.*, 6: 391–396.

McGeer, P. L. and McGeer, E. G. (1976) Enzymes associated with the metabolism of catecholamines, acetylcholine and GABA in human controls and patients with Parkinson's disease and Huntington's chorea. *J. Neurochem.*, 26: 65–76.

Meek, J. L., Bertilsson, L., Cheney, D. L., Zsilla, G. and Costa, E. (1977) Aging-induced changes in acetylcholine and serotonin content of discrete brain nuclei. *J. Gerontol.*, 32: 129–131.

Milner, J. and Wurtman, R. J. (1986) Catecholamine synthesis: physiological coupling to precursor supply. *Biochem. Pharmacol.*, 35: 875–881.

Møller, S. E., Kirk, L. and Honore, P. (1980) Relationship between plasma ratio of tryptophan to competing amino acids and the response to L-tryptophan treatment in endogenously depressed patients. *J. Affect. Disorders*, 2: 47–59.

Morin, A. M. and Wasterlain, C. G. (1980) Aging and rat brain muscarinic receptors as measured by quinuclidinyl benzilate binding. *Neurochem. Res.*, 5: 301–308.

Perry, E. K. (1980) The cholinergic system in old age and Alzheimer's disease. *Age Aging*, 9: 1–8.

Perry, E. K., Perry, R. H., Gibson, P. H. Blessed, G. and Tomlinson, B. E. (1977) A cholinergic connection between normal aging and senile dementia in the human hippocampus. *Neurosci. Lett.*, 6: 85–89.

Ponzio, F., Brunello, N. and Algeri, S. (1978) Catecholamine synthesis in brain of aging rats. *J. Neurochem.*, 30: 1617–1620.

Reinstein, D. K., Lehnert, H., Scott, N. A. and Wurtman, R. J. (1984) Tyrosine prevents behavioral and neurochemical correlates of an acute stress in rats. *Life Sci.*, 34: 2225–2231.

Riederer, P. and Wuketich, S. T. (1976) Time course of nigrostriatal degeneration in Parkinson's disease. *J. Neural Transm.*, 38: 277–301.

Ritter, S. and Pelzer, N. L. (1978) Magnitude of stress-induced brain norepinephrine depletion varies with age. *Brain Res.*, 152: 170–175.

Robinson, D. S. (1975) Changes in monoamine oxidase and monoamines with human development and aging. *Fed. Proc.*, 34: 103–107.

Robinson, D. S., Davis, J. N., Nies, A., Colburn, R. W., Davis, J. M., Bourne, H. R., Bunney, W. E., Shaw, D. M. and Coppen, A. J. (1972) Aging monoamines and monoamine-oxidase levels. *Lancet*, 1: 290–291.

Samorajski, T. and Rolsten, C. (1973) Age and regional differences in the chemical composition of brains of mice, monkeys and humans. In D. H. Ford (Ed.), *Neurobiological aspects of maturation and aging, Progress in Brain Research, Vol. 40*, Elsevier, Amsterdam, pp. 253–265.

Severson, J. A. and Finch, C. E. (1980) Age changes in human basal ganglion dopamine receptors. *Fed. Proc.*, 39: 508.

Smith, D. F., Stromgren, E., Petersen, H. N., Williams, D. G. and Sheldon, W. (1984) Lack of effect of tryptophan treatment in demented gerontopsychiatric patients: a double-blind, crossover-controlled study. *Acta Psychiat. Scand.*, 70: 470–477.

Stone, E. A. (1975) Stress and Catecholamines. In A. J. Friedhoff (Ed.), *Catecholamines and Behavior*, Plenum Press, New York, pp. 31–72.

Thurmond, J. B. and Brown, J. W. (1984) Effect of brain monoamine precursors on stress induced behavioral and neurochemical changes in aged mice. *Brain Res.*, 296: 93–102.

Timiras, P. S. and Vernadakis, A. (1972) Structural, biochemical, and functional aging of the nervous system. In P. S. Timiras (Ed.), *Developmental Physiology and Aging*, Macmillan, New York, pp. 502–526.

Wurtman, R. J. (1985) Alzheimer's disease. *Sci. Am.*, 252(1): 62–74.

Wurtman, R. J., Hefti, F. and Melamed, E. (1981) Precursor control of neurotransmitter synthesis. *Pharmacol. Rev.*, 32: 315–335.

Yates, C. M., Simson, J., Gordon, A., Maloney, A. J. F., Allison, Y., Ritchie, I. M. and Urquhart, A. (1983) Catecholamines and cholinergic enzymes in pre-senile and senile Alzheimer-type dementia and Down's syndrome. *Brain Res.*, 280: 119–126.

Young, S. N. (1986) The clinical psychopharmacology of tryptophan. In R. J. Wurtman and J. J. Wurtman (Eds.), *Nutrition and the Brain, Vol. 7*, Raven Press, New York, pp. 49–88.

Zepelin, H. (1983) Normal age related change in sleep. In M. Chase and E. D. Weitzman (Eds.), *Sleep Disorders Basic and Clinical Research*, SP Medical and Scientific Books, New York.

Discussion

D. F. SWAAB: We have got mechanisms to deal with the enormous daily fluctuations in precursor intake, otherwise we should have greater psychic changes throughout the day. Do you have epidemiological data with regard to different cultures or different cultural groups and the frequency in the symptoms of aging and dementia, supporting your hypothesis that dietary circumstances are essential?

ANSWER: It is certainly true that we have mechanisms to deal

with fluctuations in precursors' availability. However, it is also true that changes in the plasma concentration of certain precursors, for example tryptophan, tyrosine and choline acutely alter brain levels of these same substances. Tryptophan availability appears to directly affect the activity of brain serotoninergic neurons. Under certain circumstances (e.g. when the affected neurons are firing frequently) tyrosine and choline availability can affect brain levels of dopamine and norepinephrine (tyrosine) and acetylcholine (choline). We do not know if changes such as these have chronic consequences with respect to brain aging. However, precursors and foods which alter precursor levels in the brain can have acute effects on behavior, as I briefly discussed, so they apparently are not as well regulated as one might expect.

I am aware of no recent epidemiological studies that have directly addressed the question of lifelong nutritional habits and the preservation of CNS function in old age; I would certainly hope that such issues would be investigated in the future.

R. N. KALARIA: I wonder if you would like to make a comment on an in vitro observation we made. We measured the percentage of choline transported that is acetylated into ACh in striated slices from lesioned and control rats. As expected, although CAT and choline transport were impaired (by > 50%) in the lesioned tissue, the percentage of choline transported and converted to ACh was the same in both controls and experimental rats. Could choline replacement in AD patients significantly affect overall ACh synthesis?

ANSWER: I suspect that your very interesting observations reflect the particular dose you used, i.e., a dose in which most of the choline uptake would have involved a transport system that delivered it preferentially to surviving cholinergic terminals. Unlabeled circulating choline enters brain neurons by high-and-low affinity transport systems, such that even the total destruction of cholinergic terminals (which totally block acetylcholine synthesis) would not block some choline uptake. Coyle's laboratory some years ago showed that animals with a unilateral striatal lesion, destroying a large fraction of ipsilateral cholinergic neurons, were especially sensitive to supplementary choline; it markedly increased acetylcholine levels on the lesioned side without affecting those on the unlesioned side. These data again suggest the importance of increased neuronal firing as would probably occur among 'surviving' cholinergic neurons, for demonstrating choline dependence.

J. KORF: How critical do you think that precursor availability (such as tyrosine or choline) is for central neuron transmission? Several authors have reported essentially negative effects in 'rest' conditions. Also after stimulation of, e.g., ascending dopaminergic fibers in the rat brain loading with tyrosine did not influence dopamine metabolite formation (e.g. Korf et al., 1976). Several others observed that, e.g., striatal ACh levels, either with or without neuroleptic treatment (thus stimulating ACh release) were unable to be compensated by dietary Ch or

other precursors (such as lecithin). Can you explain the discrepancies?

ANSWER: The response of cholinergic or catecholaminergic neurons to their precursors, tyrosine and choline, differ from those of serotonin to tryptophan in one important way: in order for the former neurons to respond to supplemental precursor, they must be physiologically active, e.g. firing frequently. Virtually any treatment that accelerates firing of particular neurons causes them to make and release more of their transmitter when provided with more tyrosine. The list includes physiological manipulations (hypotension on sympathetic neurons; hypertension on brain-stem noradrenergic neurons; light on retinal amacrine cells, etc.) and various drug treatments (haloperidol, reserpine, etc.). Almost all investigators have observed this relationship as reviewed by Milner and Wurtman (1986). The relationship between neuronal firing and tyrosine dependence apparently derives both from the firing-induced activation of tyrosine hydroxylase and from an actual depletion of pre-synaptic tyrosine (Milner and Wurtman, 1986). The mechanism of the relationship between the firing of choline neurons and choline availability awaits discovery.

R. RAVID: (1) Do you have information on central effects of glutamic acid and MSG on the normal and aging brain?

(2) Is there any known correlation between vegetarian dietary habits and lifespan?

ANSWER: (1) There is no evidence to suggest that oral monosodium glutamate (MSG) has any effect on the human brain at any age. Massive parenteral doses can damage brain cells in newborn rodents, but even these doses have never been shown to be neurotoxic in primates.

(2) I am not aware of any good studies on this question.

References

Korf, J., Grasdijk, E. G. and Westerink, B. H. C. (1976) Effects of electrical stimulation of the nigrostriatal pathway of the rat on dopamine metabolism. *J. Neurochem.*, 26: 579–584.

Milner, J. and Wurtman, R. J. (1986) Catecholamine synthesis: physiological coupling to precursor supply. *Biochem. Pharmacol.*, 35: 875–881.

D. F. Swaab, E. Fliers, M. Mirmiran, W. A. Van Gool and F. Van Haaren (Eds.)
Progress in Brain Research, Vol. 70.
© 1986 Elsevier Science Publishers B.V. (Biomedical Division)

CHAPTER 30

The striatal dopaminergic system as a model for modulation of altered neurotransmitter action during aging: effects of dietary and neuroendocrine manipulations

G. S. Roth[a], J. M. Henry[a] and J. A. Joseph[b]

[a]*Molecular Physiology and Genetics Section, Laboratory of Cellular and Molecular Biology, Gerontology Research Center, National Institute on Aging, Francis Scott Key Medical Center, Baltimore, MD 21224, USA* and [b]*Lederle Laboratories of American Cyanamid, Pearl River, NY 10965, USA*

Introduction

The dopaminergic system provides a prime example of an impaired ability to regulate physiological and biochemical functions during the aging process. These include dopaminergic control of neurotransmitter release (Thompson et al., 1984), cyclic nucleotide (Puri and Volicer, 1977; Walker and Boas-Walker, 1973; Schmidt and Thornberry, 1978) and energy (Pizzolato et al., 1983) metabolism, and motor behavior (Joseph et al., 1978; Cubells and Joseph, 1981). Because of the obvious relevance of the latter dysfunction to many overt psychomotor problems of the elderly, much recent interest has been focussed on the mechanisms by which such dopaminergic regulation deteriorates with age.

Within the past few years, there have been attempts to explore the link between changes in the nigrostriatal dopaminergic system and motor behavior seen in aged animal models. It appears that the more complex the motor tests, the greater the observed deficit in the aged animal. Tasks that require greater psychomotor coordination and muscle strength, such as walking the length of a stationary horizontal rod (Dean et al., 1981; Wallace et al., 1980), show greater deficits in aged animals. It is difficult, however, in these tasks to

rule out the involvement of other neuronal areas, such as cerebellum (Zornetzer and Rogers, 1981). Thus, the dopamine (DA) receptor-motor behavior link might be difficult to examine using these tasks. We have chosen instead to confine our research to rotational behavior. This behavior shows a decline in the aged animal and seems to be controlled by the nigrostriatal system. More recently we have begun to examine other stereotypes (sniffing, grooming, gnawing) that are known to have nigrostriatal involvement.

Several years ago Ungerstedt and his co-workers developed a model to examine and quantify motor behavior (Ungerstedt et al., 1969; Ungerstedt, 1971). They found that if a unilateral lesion is made in the substantia nigra (A-9) of the rodent (Hodge and Butcher, 1979), striatal DA stores on the side ipsilateral to the lesion will be depleted, creating an imbalance in dopamine levels between the intact and lesioned hemispheres. If an agent is administered which causes DA to be released from the intact striatum, (such as amphetamine) the animal rotates toward the lesioned side. Through the use of a rotometer, which counts complete clockwise and counterclockwise rotations, the direction and magnitude of the rotations can be accurately assessed. In our initial experiments

(Joseph et al., 1978) young (6 months) and old (25–29 months) male and female Wistar rats were unilaterally lesioned in the left substantia nigra, and rotational behavior was examined following graded doses of amphetamine (AMPH). It was clear that the old animals, following the lesions, showed a lowered baseline turning with vehicle injections (distilled water), thus a strength of response measure was computed by dividing the left turns by the right turns (L/R). The results showed that the old animals exhibited decided decrements in the L/R index which increased in magnitude as the dose of AMPH was increased. Thirty-five percent (6 out of 17) of the old animals showed either a potentiation of responses in both directions or a selective increase in contralateral (to the lesion) turning until the maximal dose of 5 mg/kg of AMPH was given. Neither bidirectional potentiation nor contralateral turning was seen in any of the young animals at the lower dose. Moreover, the results showed that while the lesion may have lowered activity in the old animal, the degree of potentiation of overall turning to AMPH (2 left turns baseline to 45 left turns overall to AMPH old; 13 to 137 young) was actually greater than in the young. In addition, the selective increase in left as opposed to right turns was far lower in the senescent animals. These experiments revealed for the first time in a defined animal model, motor behavioral changes occurring with senescence in the neostriatal DA regulatory system. However, the specific mechanistic lesion remained to be elucidated.

It was thought that the decrements in amphetamine-induced rotation seen in the senescent animals might be due to an age-related decline in DA release following AMPH. However, a recent experiment showed that ^{3}H-dopamine release from striatal slices following incubation in KCl or amphetamine did not show any age-related differences. It appears, then, that although there may be small reductions in tyrosine hydroxylase and some loss of ability to convert L-dopa to DA in aged animals, presynaptic DA release potentialities remain relatively intact in senescence.

In order to further investigate the mechanism of this loss of rotational behavior, a study was carried out in which DA (50 μg) was applied directly through cannulas chronically implanted in the right (intact) striatum in rats unilaterally lesioned in the left substantia nigra (Cubells and Joseph, 1981). Results showed that the L/R index was essentially the same in the two age-groups following intrastriatal vehicle (distilled water) administration. However, following intrastriatal DA administration, the young animals showed increases in rotational behavior significantly greater than those of old animals. Subsequent replication and elaboration of this model using several doses of intrastriatally administered dopamine (0, 10, 25, 50 μg) or amphetamine (1, 2.5, 5, 7, 10 μg), indicated that old animals failed to increase their L/R index even to the highest doses of the compounds. The deficits in the dopaminergic system therefore, appear to be at least partially post-synaptic, and reflect direct impairment in responsiveness to DA.

Dopamine effects on sniffing behavior were also age-related. There were greater increases in sniffing behavior in the young animals than in the senescent animals. Similar findings were seen for AMPH effects on sniffing behavior. Amphetamine and dopamine effects on grooming behavior were inconsistent. However, it is believed that since the animals were lesioned, the turning behavior took precedence over the grooming behavior and the latter was suppressed. Thus, it would appear that age differences persist following direct striatal injection.

Having established an age-associated decrement in dopaminergic regulation of psychomotor behavior, it became necessary to determine the precise biochemical changes responsible. This required utilization of various pharmacological and neurochemical techniques; initially and primarily those involving DA receptor methodology.

Attempts to elucidate the mechanisms of impaired striatal dopaminergic responsiveness during aging (changes in dopamine receptors)

Dopaminergic agents initiate their actions by attaching to specific cell membrane receptors

TABLE I

Analysis of young and old rat striatal DA receptors by ^{3}H-haloperidol-specific binding

Age (months)	n	Receptor concentration	
		(fmoles/mg protein)	K_d (mM)
6	6	228 ± 18[a]	2.3 ± 0.7[b]
25	6	146 ± 22[a]	2.0 ± 0.4[b]

Values represent the means ± SE for the indicated numbers of experiments (n).
[a]Age difference significant to $p < 0.002$ by Student's t test.
[b]No significant age difference.

(Kebabian and Kalne, 1979; Seeman, 1980). Since many reductions in hormone/neurotransmitter responsiveness during aging have been attributed to receptor loss (Roth and Hess, 1982), it was initially decided to examine striatal DA receptors in young and old Wistar rats. Table I summarizes the results of our earliest experiments using ^{3}H-haloperidol to analyze these receptors as a function of age (Joseph et al., 1978). An approximately 35% reduction in concentration, with no loss of binding affinity, was observed. This was the first evidence suggesting that loss of DA receptors might be responsible for loss of DA responsiveness during aging.

This observation has subsequently been repeated under a variety of experimental conditions and in various experimental models including humans, and is probably the best documented loss of a hormone/neurotransmitter receptor during aging (Joseph et al., 1981; Levin et al., 1981, 1983; Roth et al., 1984; Wong et al., 1984; DeBlasi et al., 1982; DeBlasi and Mennini, 1982; Hirschhorn et al., 1982; Memo et al., 1980; Misra et al., 1980; Severson and Finch, 1980; Severson et al., 1982; Thal et al., 1980; Morgan et al., 1984; Severson, 1984; O'Boyle and Waddington, 1984; Roy et al., 1982; Henry and Roth, 1984).

In light of the general agreement among various laboratories as to the age-related loss of striatal DA receptors, it became necessary to determine whether fluctuations in receptor levels on the order

of those observed during aging could result in altered rotational responsiveness. Young and old rats of both sexes were lesioned in the left substantia nigra with 6-hydroxydopamine to induce striatal receptor supersensitivity (increase in receptor levels) and allow assessment of rotational response to AMPH. The resultant degrees of responsiveness and receptor alteration varied within and among groups over the range of normal age change. The correlation between receptor-specific binding of ^{3}H-spiperone or spiroperidol (a DA antagonist which became available for radioreceptor analysis shortly after haloperidol) and rotational responsiveness of the various groups is indicated in Table II. This relationship is positive and highly significant (Joseph et al., 1981). Although correlations alone are not sufficient to prove causality, it certainly appears that essentially every manipulation used to date to modulate striatal DA receptor levels (see also below) results in concomitant alteration in behavioral response. Thus, we believe that receptor loss during aging is most likely the cause of dopaminergic psychomotor impairments.

Differential changes in dopamine receptor subtypes

Having established this relationship, efforts next focussed on the mechanisms of the age-associated loss of striatal DA receptors. Another aspect of the study cited above (Joseph et al., 1981) was an

TABLE II

Correlations between rotational responsiveness and rat striatal DA receptor specific binding of ^{3}H-spiperone

Group	n	r value
Males	12	0.94[c]
Females	9	0.68
Young	10	0.93[b]
Old	11	0.75[a]
All	21	0.93[c]

Partial r values were determined as previously described (Joseph et al., 1983). [a]$p < 0.05$; [b]$p < 0.01$; [c]$p < 0.001$.

476

attempt to distinguish between differential changes in dopamine receptor subtypes with age. While some confusion exists as to the exact number of classes and putative function of the striatal DA receptors, there seems to be some consensus that there are at least three of these subtypes, i.e., D1, D2, D3 (Creese, 1982; McGeer et al., 1971). D1 receptors are linked to stimulation of adenylate cyclase activity, have low (in the μM range) ^{3}H-agonist (e.g., 6,7-amino-6,7-dihydroxy-1,2,3,4-tetrahydronapthalene, ^{3}H-ADTN), as well as butyrophenone (^{3}H-spiperone) affinity, are lost following striatal kainate lesions and may be located on intrinsic striatal neurons (Creese, 1982). D2 receptors are believed to be identical to the majority of the ^{3}H-butyrophenone binding sites previously identified in the striatum. They (D2) demonstrate guanine nucleotide regulation of agonist binding and may be located on intrinsic striatal neurons (Creese, 1982). D3 receptors demonstrate high affinity (nM range) to ^{3}H-agonists (e.g., ^{3}H-ADTN), low affinity (nM range) to butyrophenones, and may be located on intrinsic striatal nerve terminals and nigrostriatal terminals (Creese, 1982). It is generally agreed that aside from the involvement of cyclic AMP in D1 receptor mediated actions and the existence of so-called second messengers, the nature of other intermediate events have not been established for D2 and D3 receptors. It is believed, however, that the D2 receptors may be most closely associated with the behavioral effects of DA antagonists in animals (Creese, 1982; Seeman, 1980).

We were somewhat surprised to observe good correlations between ^{3}H-spiperone binding and both rotational behavior and adenylate cyclase stimulation (Joseph et al., 1981). To date we cannot explain the relationship to the latter, especially in light of recent reports utilizing ^{3}H-spiperone as a primarily D2-selective ligand (Leff et al., 1984; Hyttel, 1981). We also had occasion to compare agonist binding (^{3}H-ADTN) with the ^{3}H-antagonists in striata of Wistar rats of various ages (Levin et al., 1981, 1983). The number of specific binding sites (displaceable by 10^{-5} or 10^{-6}M (+)

butaclamol) for all of these ligands decreases with increasing age. The absolute decrease for all ligands represents about 80 fmoles per mg of protein between 3–6 months and 22–25 months. However, on a percentage basis the decrease in ADTN binding sites is greatest (about 40%) since young animals possess 10–20% fewer sites for ADTN than for the antagonists. At the concentration of ^{3}H-ADTN generally utilized for these studies, the D3 receptor subtypes which have a high affinity for ^{3}H-agonists, may be the sites that are being assessed. Thus, it appears that ADTN-binding sites sensitive to nM concentrations of ^{3}H-ADTN are being lost from the striatal intrinsic neurons during aging. Additionally, striatal D2 receptor sites as assessed with ^{3}H-butyrophenones appear to be lost as well.

Further support for an age-related loss of D3 as well as D2 receptors comes from several other laboratories. Makman's group (Thal et al., 1980) have reported that D2 receptors as measured by ^{3}H-spiroperidol-specific binding are lost from striatum, frontal cortex and anterior limbic cortex as rabbits age from 15 to 65 months. The relative reductions are approximately 30%, 30%, and 20% for the three regions, respectively. Binding affinity remains constant over this period. When binding measurements were repeated with ^{3}H-ADTN, (0.625–10 nM concentrations) (D3), the age-related reduction in striatal concentration was greater than 50%. Young rabbits possess about three times as many spiroperidol binding sites as those for ADTN.

Similar observations have been made by Severson, Finch and coworkers (Severson and Finch, 1980; Severson et al., 1982) in striata of C57BL/6J mice and in caudate nucleus, substantia nigra, putamen and nucleus accumbens obtained from post-mortem human brains. In mice, ^{3}H-spiroperidol-specific binding sites progressively decrease about 50% between 3 and 28 months of age, while binding affinity remains unaltered. ^{3}H-Spiroperidol binding sites also decrease about 35% in hypothalamus between 8 and 28 months of age while no change was observed in olfactory bulbs.

ADTN binding sites decrease about twice as much as spiroperidol sites over comparable age ranges. Significant age-related reductions in both ADTN and spiroperidol sites were also observed in human caudate nucleus and substantia nigra. The magnitude of the loss is about three times as great for the ADTN sites. No age differences in binding affinity were observed in any of the human brain regions.

One interesting difference between the studies of our own laboratory using rats and those of Finch using mice and humans and Makman using rabbits is the relative ratio of ADTN to spiroperidol binding sites in the striatum. Our findings reveal between 20 and 75% more spiroperidol sites than those for ADTN in young rats (Joseph et al., 1978, 1981; Levin et al., 1981, 1983; Roth et al., 1984). In contrast, Makman's group reports about three times as many spiroperidol sites as ADTN sites in young rabbits. Finally, Finch's laboratory (Severson and Finch, 1980; Severson et al., 1982) finds more ADTN sites in both mice and humans, about twice the number of spiroperidol sites. It is possible, but not extremely likely that these discrepancies are due to strain differences. The actual explanation awaits further experimentation.

Very recently, apparently truly selective ligands have become available for the D1 and D2 sites (Stoop and Kebabian, 1984). Initial studies using such methodology have revealed a preferential loss of D2 receptors during aging in rats and humans (O'Boyle and Waddington, 1984; Morgan et al., 1984). D1 receptor levels remain constant in aged rats while actually appearing to increase in aged humans (O'Boyle and Waddington, 1984; Morgan et al., 1984). Such evidence would seem to localize age-associated deficits in stimulation of adenylate cyclase at the postreceptor level and to rule out any direct relationship of D1 receptors or adenylate cyclase to impaired psychomotor function.

Although affinity of striatal DA receptors for antagonists and for the agonist ADTN does not appear to change with age, subtle alterations may occur in the proportion of D2 receptors in a 'high affinity' form (Severson and Randall, 1985). There appears to be a major loss of this form before midlife in mice, while total receptor decline is progressive over the entire lifespan.

Biosynthesis of dopamine receptors

In addition to attempting to distinguish between differential age-associated loss of DA receptor subtypes and affinity states, studies have examined receptor biosynthetic rates. Male Wistar rats young (3–6 months) and old (24–25 months) were injected intraperitoneally with the irreversible dopamine receptor alkylating agent N-ethoxycarbonyl-2-ethoxy-1,2-dihydroquinoline (EEDQ). All animals received 6 mg/kg body weight and were sacrificed at 0, 6, 24, 48, 96 and 192 h after injection. We observed that the rate of reappearance of striatal dopamine receptors is slower (25–35%) in old rats when compared with young counterparts. The results summarized in Table III clearly show that control B_{max} is about 30% higher in young animals, then decreases markedly 6 h after drug administration (Henry and Roth, 1984). B_{max} values increase thereafter, with younger animals reaching higher levels at later times. When receptor concentrations are expressed as a percentage of control values, however, no age differences are observed, suggesting that recovery from EEDQ proceeds at equal relative rates in young and old rats. Furthermore, no significant differences in K_d are seen (Henry and Roth, 1984). These results suggest that a possible cause of reduced striatal dopamine receptor levels during aging might be a decreased rate of biosynthesis. An identical conclusion was recently drawn in a similar study using younger rats (Leff et al., 1984). Such decrement might be due to altered regulation of receptor synthesis; either impaired maintenance or stimulation of this process or possible down regulation by inhibitory factors in aged animals. Similar biosynthetic deficits have been reported for several other receptor systems during aging (Chang et al., 1981; Pitha et al., 1982; Greenberg and Weiss, 1979).

Although EEDQ is not selective for dopamine receptors since it also binds to α-adrenergic

TABLE III

Effect of age and time after EEDQ administration on striatal dopamine receptors

	0 hours	6 hours	24 hours	48 hours	96 hours	192 hours
3–6 months						
n	10	10	2	3	3	6
B_{max} (fmol/mg protein)	352 ± 14[a]	69 ± 9	73 ± 5	107 ± 27	157 ± 24	261 ± 21
% control B_{max}	100 ± 4	19 ± 2	20 ± 1	30 ± 7	44 ± 7	73 ± 6
K_d (nm)[b]	0.07 ± 0.03	0.19 ± 0.05	0.11 ± 0.05	0.06 ± 0.02	0.08 ± 0.01	0.09 ± 0.01
24–25 months						
n	11	13	2	3	4	4
B_{max} (fmol/mg protein)	268 ± 9[a]	76 ± 13	77 ± 17	64 ± 18	141 ± 21	205 ± 10
% control B_{max}	100 ± 3	27 ± 4	28 ± 7	24 ± 6	52 ± 7	75 ± 3
K_d (nM)[b]	0.09 ± 0.02	0.19 ± 0.04	0.24 ± 0.03	0.20 ± 0.03	0.14 ± 0.03	0.05 ± 0.02

Values represent the means $\pm$ SE for the indicated numbers of experiments (n).
[a]Significantly different from each other ($p < 0.01$) as determined by one-way analysis of variance as determined by Duncan's Multiple Range Test.
[b]No significant differences among age or time groups.

receptors (Belleau et al., 1968), its use as a tool for blocking available dopamine receptor seems reasonably valid (Hamblin and Creese, 1983). Moreover, several groups have indicated that EEDQ exerts pharmacological effects on the dopaminergic system *in vivo* as influenced by altered stereotypy, catalepsy, and avoidance behavior (Hamblin and Creese, 1983; Belleau et al., 1968; Martel et al., 1969; Muren and Weissman, 1971). Our results are similar to those of Hamblin and Creese (Hamblin and Creese, 1983) for control B_{max} and K_d as well as for about 80% receptor blockade 6 h after EEDQ injection and recovery to 70–80% of control levels by 7–8 days.

Although DA receptor biosynthetic rates appear to decline during aging, we cannot rule out the possibility that some receptors become non-functional, masked or hidden with age. S-adenosyl-L-methionine (SAM) stimulation of phospholipid methylation failed to reveal additional ^{3}H-spiperone-specific binding sites and/or dopamine-stimulated adenylate cyclase in either young or old rat striata (Cimino et al., 1984). Under the same conditions, hidden β-adrenergic receptors were

unmasked. These results suggest that cryptic dopamine receptors may be so tenaciously embedded in the membrane that mechanical manipulation by fluidizing agents is incapable of detaching them.

Solubilization of young and old rat striatal membranes with the detergent 3-(3-cholamidopropyl)-dimethylammonio-2-hydroxy-1-propanesulfonate (CHAPSO), allowed detachment of essentially all of the receptor proteins without affecting age differences in concentration (Henry and Roth, 1986). Approximately 80–90% of the receptors recovered were detected in the supernatant fraction with a small percentage remaining membrane-bound in both age groups. A ten-fold reduction in binding affinity for ^{3}H-spiperone was observed for solubilized receptors of young and old rats following Scatchard analyses (Henry and Roth, 1986). The reduced binding affinity may be attributed to a change in the solubilized receptor protein configuration after release from the intact membrane. These results are consistent with those of Cimino and his co-workers in that they suggest that dopamine receptors are not sequestered in the membrane with advancing age (Cimino et al., 1984). Taken together with our previous findings (Henry and Roth, 1984), and with those of Leff and co-workers (Leff et al., 1984), it appears that a decreased biosynthetic rate (or receptor inactivation or malformation) rather than membrane sequestration, accounts for loss of dopamine receptors with age.

One other possible explanation for the observed reductions in striatal DA receptor concentrations and biosynthetic rates is simple loss of receptor-containing neurons. Early attempts to examine this possibility cited evidence for decreased choline acetyltransferase activity in this brain region in rats, suggesting possible neuronal loss (Severson and Finch, 1980). More recently, however, it has been pointed out that dopamine-sensitive adenylate cyclase in striatum is substantially decreased before 12 months in rats (Schmidt and Thornberry, 1978), an age when supersensitization responses to chronic haloperidol are not altered in mice (Randall et al., 1981). Thus, subsequent impairments in supersensitization may derive from loss of different striatal cells or may require more extensive loss. The failure of generalized cell loss to account for striatal receptor loss is also supported by the data of Makman et al. (1980), who found no evidence for neuronal loss in striatum, anterior limbic cortex, or frontal cortex as assessed by dopamine and norepinephrine concentrations, choline acetylase activity and ^{3}H-quinuclidinyl benzilate binding.

More recently, it has been suggested that D1 and D2 receptor subtypes exist on the same cells (Stoop and Kebabian, 1984; Onali et al., 1984). Since the former have now been reported not to decrease during aging (O'Boyle and Waddington, 1984; Morgan et al., 1984), loss of D2-containing neurons seems less likely but direct measurement is still necessary.

Attempts to delay and/or reverse age deficits in dopamine receptors/response

Attention has been recently focussed on the ability to regulate DA receptor levels in response to various manipulations. Randall et al. (1981) observed that senescent C57BL/6J mice were unable to proliferate striatal dopamine receptors following chronic haloperidol treatment even though young counterparts increased receptors by 25–30%. In contrast, we have employed 6-hydroxydopamine (6-OHDA) to induce denervation of Wistar rats and detected no age difference in the relative ability to develop receptor supersensitivity (Joseph et al., 1981). Both mature and senescent animals showed increases of 40–50% in ^{3}H-spiroperidol-specific binding, although the absolute levels of receptors were always 40% lower in the aged group. These data were subsequently supported by Hirschhorn et al. (1982) who showed increases in ^{3}H-ADTN binding in the striatum of the senescent rat following unilateral 6-hydroxydopamine lesions. Since a 2-nM concentration of ^{3}H-ADTN was used for these determinations, D3 receptors were probably being assessed. Thus, both D2 and D3 striatal DA receptors can proliferate in the senescent animal following 6-hydroxydopamine lesions. Indications of D1 receptor proliferation were also seen in these studies since DA stimulated adenylate cyclase activity increased in these animals as well (Hirschhorn et al., 1982).

Conceivably, differences between these two studies and that of Finch are due to the type of manipulation used to attempt induction of supersensitivity. Snyder's group (Burt et al., 1977; Creese et al., 1977) has reported that 6-hydroxydopamine may be more effective than haloperidol in inducing DA receptor proliferation. Possibly older animals require a more severe challenge to enable them to proliferate striatal DA receptors.

Another manipulation which we recently employed to 'up-regulate' striatal dopamine receptors was prolactin administration (Levin et al., 1983). Such treatment had previously been reported to induce ^{3}H-spiroperidol receptor supersensitivity in young rats (Hruska et al., 1982). Since prolactin levels are often elevated in senescent counterparts, yet dopamine receptor content is low, it was possible that old rats lose responsiveness to this postulated control mechanism. Surprisingly, however, 7 days after implantation of osmotic mini-pumps releasing 150 ng of highly purified rat prolactin per hour, striatal receptor concentrations increased in both mature and senescent animals (Levin et al., 1983). In fact, the prolactin effect was much greater in the old group, elevating receptors to levels comparable to that of young control animals (mature controls, 250 ± 23 fm/mg protein; mature treated, 285 ± 14 fm/mg protein; senescent controls, 178 ± 17 fm/mg protein, senescent treated, 245 ± 21 fm/mg protein). Thus, loss of rat striatal dopamine receptors during aging does not appear to be a consequence of insensitivity to maintenance by prolactin.

Concomitant with the prolactin-induced increase in receptors in the aged rats, DA-stimulated rotational behavior was enhanced nearly to the levels of young untreated animals (Joseph et al., 1986). Thus, administration of low levels of homologous prolactin offers a more physiological manipulation than neuroleptic injections or nigral lesioning with which to acutely modulate DA receptors and response.

Finally, we have examined the effects of dietary restriction on the age-associated loss of DA receptors from the rat corpus striatum. If rats receive food only on alternative days, lifespan is extended by 40% and receptor concentrations, as measured by both ³H-ADTN and specific ³H-spiroperidol binding (Table IV) are maintained at young levels into middle age before declining (Levin et al., 1981; Roth et al., 1984). Table IV also shows that acute (2 weeks) dietary restriction has no effect on receptor levels of 24-months-old animals.

As with the prolactin-treated old rats, 24-months-old dietarily restricted animals exhibited DA-stimulated rotational behavior comparable to ad libitum fed young counterparts (Joseph et al., 1983).

Our observation that an age-related biochemical alteration in the rat brain can be retarded through dietary restriction is consistent with numerous other reports of the beneficial effects of similar regimens on biochemical variables in other organ

TABLE IV

Effect of dietary restriction on age-related loss of striatal dopamine receptors

Group	n	Receptor concentration (fm/mg protein)
3-months-old C	15	376 ± 18
3-months-old R	8	370 ± 36
12-months-old C	8	288 ± 18
13-months-old R	7	352 ± 23[a]
24-months-old C	14	246 ± 10
24-months-old R	7	294 ± 19[a]
24-months-old CR	11	242 ± 14[b]
30-months-old R	7	233 ± 27

Values represent the means $\pm$ SE for the indicated numbers of experiments (n).

C, animals fed ad libitum; R, animals fed every other day; CR, animals fed ad libitum until 24 months, then every other day for 2 weeks.

[a]Restricted animals are significantly above control counterparts as analyzed by one-way analysis of variance ($p < 0.001$).

[b]Not significantly different from 24 mo. C animals.

and physiological systems (Barrows and Kokkonen, 1977; Gerbase-DeLima et al., 1975; Masoro et al., 1980; Ross, 1959; Young, 1979; Yu et al., 1980). Whether other parameters of brain function are affected remains to be investigated. Furthermore, whether the effect of dietary restriction is a general phenomenon with widespread effects in brain or is selective for certain parameters has yet to be determined completely. Preliminary analysis suggests that in 24-months-old male Wistar rats the effects are selective in brain. For example, the activity of choline acetyltransferase, the synthetic enzyme for acetylcholine, was higher in the striatum, hippocampus, and cerebellum of 24-months-old rats on EOD diets compared to AL-fed counterparts (London et al., 1983). In contrast, there appeared to be few significant diet effects on the activity of glutamic acid decarboxylase, the synthetic enzyme for γ-amino butyric acid, in brain regions examined (London et al., 1983).

Thus, the beneficial effects of dietary restriction do not appear at this stage of research to represent a universal retardation of brain aging. Moreover, in spite of these dramatic biochemical and behavioral effects, past and current research has yet to identify a mechanism that can account for the beneficial effects of dietary restriction. Mechanisms that have been proposed include: (1) enhanced immunological functioning (Gerbase-DeLima, 1975; Weindruch et al., 1982; Weindruch, 1979); (2) modification of disease patterns (Barrows and Kokkonen, 1977; Ross, 1959); (3) reduced utilization of those molecular components required for gene expression (Barrows and Kokkonen, 1977); and (4) reduced production or increased protection against toxic products of oxidative metabolism (Chipalkatti et al., 1983; Enesco and Kruk, 1981; Noda et al., 1982). Furthermore, we cannot rule out the possibility of modulation by a dietary-neuroendocrine link, if not through prolactin then possibly other hormone/neurotransmitter systems. Our observations may yield a reliable assay for testing hypotheses bearing on these proposed mechanisms.

Summary and conclusions

Dopaminergic regulation of certain motor functions, neurotransmitter release, and cyclic nucleotide metabolism deteriorates during the aging process. Attempts to elucidate the mechanisms of such changes have focussed on the nigro-striatal system, a major center of dopaminergic control.

Early studies revealed loss of striatal dopamine receptors with age in various animal species as well as in man. These have been reconfirmed many times, indicating no loss of binding affinity but an apparently quantitative reduction in concentration. A close relationship was established between receptor levels and the degree of dopaminergic response. Recent studies suggest a preferential age-related loss of the D2 receptor subtype, the species most closely linked to control of motor function.

Decreases in the available concentration of this receptor appear to be due to biosynthetic deficits, rather than membrane sequestration. Loss of neurons remains a plausible explanation for receptor disappearance. However, current investigations suggesting the presence of D1 and D2 subtypes on the same neurons seem to rule out this possibility, since D1 receptors have been reported to persist in the aged striatum.

Attempts to delay or reverse the deterioration of the dopaminergic system in rodents have included dietary restriction as well as administration of 6-hydroxydopamine, chronic haloperidol, and prolactin. The former retards the loss of both receptor and psychomotor responsiveness in conjunction with an approximately 40% lifespan extension. The latter treatments all acutely elevate striatal receptor levels concomitant with restoration of responsiveness. Although the precise relationships of these modulations to the normal mechanisms of age-related loss of dopaminergic responsiveness remain to be elucidated, this model offers a unique opportunity to attempt controlled amelioration of a defined biochemical deficit in physiological responsiveness during aging.

Acknowledgements

Thanks are due to Rita Wolferman for typing of the manuscript.

References

Barrows, C. H. and Kokkonen, G. C. (1977) Relationship between nutrition and aging. In H. Draper (Ed.), *Advances in Nutritional Research, Vol. 1*, Plenum, New York, pp. 253–298.

Belleau, B., Marlet, R., Lacasse, G., Menard, M., Weinberg, N. L. and Kerron, Y. G. (1968) *N*-Carboxylic acid esters of 1,2-and 1,4-dihydroquinolines. A new class of irreversible inactivators of the catecholamine α receptors and potent central nervous system depressants. *J. Am. Chem. Soc.*, 90: 823–824.

Burt, D. R., Creese, I. and Snyder, S. H. (1977) Antischizophrenic drugs: chronic treatment elevates dopaminergic receptor binding in the brain. *Science*, 196: 326–327.

Chang, W. C., Hoopes, M. T. and Roth, G. S. (1981) Biosynthetic rates of proteins having the characteristics of glucocorticoid receptors in adipocytes of mature and senescent rats. *J. Gerontol.*, 36: 386–390.

Chipalkatti, S., De, A. K. and Aiyar, A. S. (1983) Effect of diet restriction on some biochemical parameters related to aging. *Mech. Ageing Dev.*, 21: 37–48.

Cimino, M., Vantini, G., Algeri, S., Curatola, G., Pezzoli, C. and Stramentinoli, G. (1984) Age-related modification of dopaminergic and β-adrenergic receptor systems: restoration to normal activity by modifying membrane fluidity with S-adenysyl-methionine. *Life Sci.*, 34: 2029–2039.

Creese, I. (1982) Dopamine receptors explained. *Trends Neurosci. Res.*, Feb., 40–43.

Creese, I., Burt, D. R. and Snyder, S. H. (1977) Dopamine receptor binding enhancement accompanies lesion induced behavioral supersensitivity. *Science*, 197: 596–598.

Cubells, J. F. and Joseph, J. A. (1981) Neostriatal dopamine receptor loss and behavioral deficits in the senescent rat. *Life Sci.*, 28: 1215–1220.

Dean, R. L., Scozzafava, J., Goas, J. A., Regan, B., Beer, B. and Bartus, R. T. (1981) Age-related differences in behavior across the lifespan of the C57BL/6J mouse. *Exp. Aging Res.*, 7: 427–433.

DeBlasi, A. A. and Mennini, T. (1982) Selective reduction of one class of dopamine receptor binding sites in the corpus striatum of aged rats. *Brain Res.*, 242: 361–364.

DeBlasi, A. A., Cotecchia, S. and Mennini, T. (1982) Selective changes of receptor binding in brain regions of aged rats. *Life Sci.*, 31: 335–340.

Enesco, H. E. and Kruk, P. (1981) Influence of dieting restriction and accumulation of fluorescent age pigment. *Gerontologist*, 21: 87–88.

Gerbase-DeLima, M., Lu, R. K., Cheney, K. E., Mickey, R. and Walford, R. L. (1975) Immune function and survival in a long-lived mouse strain subjected to undernutrition. *Gerontologia*, 21: 184–202.

Greenberg, L. H. and Weiss, B. (1979) Ability of aged rats to alter beta adrenergic receptors of brain in response to repeated administration of reserpine and desmethylimipromine. *J. Pharmacol. Exp. Ther.*, 211: 309–316.

Hamblin, M. W. and Creese, J. (1983) Behavioral and radioligand binding evidence for irreversible dopamine receptor blockade by N-ethoxycarbonyl-2-ethoxy-1,2-dihydroquinoline. *Life Sci.*, 32: 2247–2255.

Henry, J. M. and Roth, G. S. (1984) Effect of aging on recovery of striatal dopamine receptors following N-ethoxycarbonyl-2-ethoxy-1,2-dihydroquinoline (EEDQ) blockade. *Life Sci.*, 35: 899–904.

Henry, J. M. and Roth, G. S. (1986) Solubilization of striatal dopamine receptors: evidence that apparent loss is not due to membrane sequestration. *J. Gerontol.*, 41: 129–135.

Hirschhorn, I. D., Makman, M. H. and Sharpless, N. S. (1982) Dopamine receptor sensitivity following nigrostriatal lesion in the aged rat. *Brain Res.*, 234: 357–368.

Hodge, G. K. and Butcher, L. L. (1979) Role of the pars compacta of the substantia nigra in circling behavior. *Pharmacol. Biochem. Behav.*, 10: 695–702.

Hruska, R. E., Pitman, K. T., Silbergeld, E. K. and Ludner, L. M. (1982) Prolactin increases the density of striatal dopamine receptors in normal and hypophysectomized male rats. *Life Sci.*, 30: 547–553.

Hyttel, J. (1981) Flupentixol and dopamine receptor selectivity. *Psychopharmacology*, 75: 217.

Joseph, J. A., Roth, G. S. and Lippa, A. S. (1986) Effect of prolactin on restoration of dopamine stimulated rotational behavior in aged rats. *Neurobiol. Aging*, 7: 31–35.

Joseph, J. A., Berger, R. E., Engel, B. T. and Roth, G. S. (1978) Age-related changes in the nigrostriatum: a behavioral and biochemical analysis. *J. Gerontol.*, 33: 643–649.

Joseph, J. A., Filburn, C. R. and Roth, G. S. (1981) Development of dopamine receptor deviation supersensitivity in the neostriatum of the senescent rat. *Life Sci.*, 29: 575–584.

Joseph, J. A., Whitaker, J., Roth, G. S. and Ingram, D. K. (1983) Life-long dietary restriction affects striatally-mediated behavioral responses in aged rats. *Neurobiol. Aging*, 4: 191–199.

Kebabian, J. W. and Calne, D. B. (1979) Multiple receptors for dopamine. *Nature*, 277: 93–96.

Leff, S. E., Gariano, R. and Creese, J. (1984) Dopamine receptors turnover rates in rat striatum are age dependent. *Proc. Natl. Acad. Sci. USA*, 81: 3910–3914.

Levin, P., Janda, J. K., Joseph, J. A., Ingram, D. K. and Roth, G. S. (1981) Dietary restriction retards the age associated loss of rat striatal dopaminergic receptors. *Science*, 214: 561–562.

Levin, P., Haji, M., Joseph, J. A. and Roth, G. S. (1983) Effect of aging on prolactin regulation of rat striatal dopamine receptor concentrations. *Life Sci.*, 32: 1743–1749.

London, E. D., Ingram, D. K. and Waller, S. B. (1983) Effects of dietary restriction on neurotransmitter synthetic enzymes and binding in aging rat brain. *Soc. Neurosci. Abstr.*, 9: 98.

Makman, M. H., Ahn, H. S., Thal, L. J., Sharpless, N. S., Dvorkin, B., Horowitz, S. G. and Rosenfeld, M. (1980) Evidence for selective loss of brain dopamine and histamine stimulated adenylate cyclase activities in rabbits with aging. *Brain Res.*, 192: 177–183.

Martel, K. K., Berman, K. and Belleau, B. (1969) Pharmacology of EEDQ (N-ethoxycarbonyl-2-ethoxy-1,2-dihydroquinoline). *Can. J. Physiol. Pharmacol.*, 47: 909–912.

Masoro, E. J., Yu, B. P., Bertrand, H. A. and Lynd, F. T. (1980) Nutritional probe of the aging process. *Fed. Proc.*, 39: 3178–3182.

McGeer, E. G., Fibiger, H. C., McGeer, P. L. and Wickson, V. (1971) Aging and brain enzymes. *Exp. Gerontol.*, 6: 391–400.

Memo, M., Lucchi, L., Spano, P. F. and Trabucchi, M. (1980) Aging process affects a single class of dopamine receptors. *Brain Res.*, 202: 488–492.

Misra, C. H., Shelat, H. S. and Smith, R. C. (1980) Effect of age on adrenergic and dopaminergic binding in rat brain. *Life Sci.*, 27: 521–526.

Morgan, D. G., Marcusson, J. O., Winblad, B. and Finch, C. E. (1984) Reciprocal changes in D-1 and D-2 dopamine binding sites in human caudate nucleus and putamen during normal aging: $\pm$ [3]H1 fluphenazine as a dopamine receptor ligand. *Abstracts of the Soc. for Neuroscience, Vol. 10,* p. 445.

Muren, J. F. and Weissman, A. (1971) Depressant 1,2-dihydroquinolines and related derivatives. *J. Med. Chem.,* 14: 49–53.

Noda, Y., McGeer, P. L. and McGeer, E. G. (1982) Lipid peroxides in brain during aging and vitamin E deficiency; possible relations to changes in neurotransmitter indices. *Neurobiol. Aging,* 3: 173–178.

O'Boyle, K. M. and Waddington, J. L. (1984) Loss of rat striatal dopamine receptors with ageing is selective for the D-2 but not D-1 sites: association with increased non-specific binding of the D-1 ligand, $\pm$ ^{3}H-piflutixol. *Eur. J. Pharmacol.,* 105: 171–174.

Onali, P., Olianas, M. C. and Geara, G. L. (1984) Selective blockade of dopamine D-1 receptors by SCH 23390 discloses striatal dopamine D-2 receptors mediating the inhibition of adenylate cyclase in rats. *Eur. J. Pharmacol.,* 99: 127–128.

Pitha, J., Hughes, B. A., Kusiak, J. W., Dax, E. M. and Baker, S. P. (1982) Regeneration of β-adrenergic receptors in senescent rats: a study using an irreversible binding antagonist. *Proc. Natl. Acad. Sci. USA,* 79: 4424–4427.

Pizzolato, G., Soncrant, T. T. and Rapoport, S. I. (1983) Age-associated decline in effect of haloperidol on local cerebral glucose utilization in rats. *J. Am. Aging Assoc.,* 6: 131–134.

Puri, S. K. and Volicer, L. (1977) Effect of aging on cyclic AMP levels and adenylate cyclase and phosphodiesterase activities in rat corpus striatum. *Mech. Ageing Devel.,* 6: 53–58.

Randall, P. K., Severson, J. A. and Finch, C. E. (1981) Aging and the regulation of striatal dopaminergic mechanisms in mice. *J. Pharmacol. Exp. Ther.,* 219: 695–705.

Ross, M. H. (1959) Proteins, calories and life expectancy. *Fed. Proc.,* 18: 1190–1207.

Roth, G. S. and Hess, G. D. (1982) Changes in the mechanisms of hormone and neurotransmitter action during aging: current status of the role of receptor and post-receptor alterations. *Mech. Ageing Dev.,* 20: 175–194.

Roth, G. S., Ingram, D. K. and Joseph, J. A. (1984) Delayed loss of striatal dopamine receptors during aging of dietarily restricted rats. *Brain Res.,* 300: 27–32.

Roy, E. J., Sheinkop, S. and Wilson, M. A. (1982) Age alters dopaminergic responses to estradiol. *Eur. J. Pharmacol.,* 83: 73–75.

Schmidt, M. J. and Thornberry, J. F. (1978) Cyclic AMP and cyclic GMP accumulation in vitro in brain regions of young, old and aged rats. *Brain Res.,* 139: 169–177.

Seeman, P. (1980) Brain dopamine receptors. *Pharmacol. Rev.,* p. 229.

Severson, J. A. (1984) D-2 dopamine receptors in aging mouse striatum: determination of high and low affinity agonist binding sites. *J. Pharmacol. Exp. Ther.,* 233: 361–368.

Severson, J. A. and Finch, C. E. (1980) Reduced dopaminergic binding during aging in the rodent striatum. *Brain Res.,* 192: 147–162.

Severson, J. A., Marcusson, J., Winblad B. and Finch, C. E. (1982) Age related changes in dopaminergic binding sites in human basal ganglia. *J. Neurochem.,* 39: 1623–1631.

Stoop, J. C. and Kebabian, J. W. (1984) Two dopamine receptors: biochemistry and pharmacology. *Life Sci.,* 35: 2281–2296.

Thal, L. J., Horowitz, S. G., Dvorkin, B. and Makman, M. H. (1980) Evidence for loss of brain ^{3}H-ADTN binding sites in rabbit brain with aging. *Brain Res.,* 192: 185–194.

Thompson, J. M., Makino, C. L., Whitaker, J. R. and Joseph, J. A. (1984) Age-related decrease in apomorphine modulation of acetylcholine release from rat striatal slices. *Brain Res.,* 299: 169–173.

Ungerstedt, U. (1971) Post synaptic supersensitivity after 6 hydroxydopamine induced degeneration of the nigrostriatal dopamine system. *Acta Physiol. Scand.,* Suppl. 367: 69–93.

Ungerstedt, U., Britcher, L. L., Butcher, S. G., Anden, N. E. and Fuxe, K. (1969) Direct chemical stimulation of dopaminergic mechanisms in the nigrostriatum of the rat. *Brain Res.,* 14: 461–473.

Walker, J. P. and Boas-Walker, J. (1973) Properties of adenylate cyclase from senescent rat brains. *Brain Res.,* 54: 391–396.

Wallace, J. E., Krauter, E. E. and Campbell, B. A. (1980) Motor and reflexive behavior in the aging rat. *J. Gerontol.,* 35: 364–371.

Weindruch, R., Kristie, J. A., Cheney, K. E. and Walford, R. L. (1979) Influence of controlled dietary restriction on immunologic function and aging. *Fed. Proc.,* 38: 2007–2016.

Weindruch, R., Gottesman, S. R. S. and Walford, R. L. (1982) Modification of age-related immune decline in mice dietarily restricted from or after mid-adulthood. *Proc. Natl. Acad. Sci. USA,* 79: 898–902.

Wong, D. F., Wagner, H. N., Dannals, R. F., Links, J. M., Frost, J. J., Rovert, H. T., Wilson, A. A., Rosenbaum, A. E., Gjedde, A., Douglas, K. H. Petronis, J. D., Folstein, M. F., Toung, J. K. T., Burns, H. D. and Kuhar, M. J. (1984) Effects of age on dopamine and serotonin receptors measured by positron tomography in the living human brain. *Science,* 226: 1391–1395.

Young, V. R. (1979) Diet as a modulator of aging and longevity. *Fed. Proc.,* 38: 1994–2000.

Yu, B. P., Bertrand, A. and Masoro, E. J. (1980) Nutrition-aging influence of catecholamine promoted lipolysis. *Metabolism,* 29: 438–444.

Zornetzer, S. F. and Rogers, J. (1931) Animal models for assessment of geriatric mnemonic and motor deficits. In T. Crook, S. Ferris and R. Bartus (Eds.), *Behavioral Assessments in Geriatric Pharmacology,* Pawley, Assoc., New London, CT, pp. 301–322.

484

Discussion

R. RAVID: (1) To which receptor subgroup does the antagonist bind?

(2) How do you explain the correlation between the supersensitivity and cyclase formation?

ANSWER: (1) Spiperone is now believed to bind primarily to the D2 receptor subtype in striatum (List and Seeman, 1981).

(2) In our Wistar rat strain we observe a good correlation between the concentrations of D1 and D2 receptor subtypes in striata (Roth et al., 1986). Thus, the correlation between supersensitivity and cyclase activity may be due to the correlation between receptor subtype concentrations.

C. F. HOLLANDER: I would like to challenge your statement on life prolongation in the dietary manipulation experiment for the following reasons: (1) the survival curve of the restricted animals was hardly rectangular; (2) the maximum observed age in this group was around 120 weeks, which is far below the 50% survival of 30 months observed in most other rat strains used for aging research; (3) no pathological data were presented so your data might also be explained by a shift in disease load between the two groups.

ANSWER: We certainly agree that pathological characterization is needed, and we plan to begin this shortly. With reference to lifespan, our outbred Wistar strain has a mean lifespan of 24 months and we seldom see ad libitum fed animals beyond 27 months of age. In this particular experiment, all our controls died by 28 months of age, although 80% of the restricted rats lived longer (up to 42 months).

A. KEYSER: Can you please comment on the mechanism of action for the increase in life expectancy of Parkinson patients as obtained by the use of monoamine oxidase type B inhibitors?

ANSWER: Although we have not worked in this area, I believe some groups have examined the effects of MAO inhibitors and other general antioxidants on lifespan (Armstrong et al., 1984).

Results have been somewhat conflicting. Possibly this is due to the postulated net level of antioxidant protection which, by compensatory mechanisms, may remain relatively constant despite endogenous administration of these agents.

D. F. SWAAB: Is it possible that prolactin works by activating, e.g. spontaneous behavior and might be, therefore, more comparable in its mechanism of action to restricted feeding and enriched environment than we would expect at first glance?

ANSWER: That is an interesting idea. In fact, some investigators have proposed that dietary restriction exerts its effects on lifespan and function through a neuroendocrine mechanism (P. Segal, personal communication). Similar effects can be elicited through reduction of the intake of certain amino acids essential for neurotransmitter metabolism.

H. SWANSON: Was there a sex difference in the lifespan of rats fed either ad lib or with dietary restriction?

ANSWER: Unfortunately, we did not use females in our dietary restriction experiments. In our strain, females tend to outlive males by about 1 month (mean lifespan), but I don't believe this is statistically significant.

References

Armstrong, D., Cutler, R. G. and Sohal, R. (1984) *Free Radicals in Molecular Biology and Aging*, Raven Press, New York.

List, S. J. and Seeman, P. (1981) Resolutions of dopamine and serotonin receptor components of [3H]spiperone binding to rat brain regions. *Proc. Natl. Acad. Sci. USA*, 78: 2620–2624.

Roth, G. S., Henry, J. M. and Joseph, J. A. (1986) The striatal dopaminergic system as a model for modulation of altered neurotransmitter action during aging: effects of dietary and neuroendocrine manipulations. In: D. F. Swaab, E. Fliers, M. Mirmiran, W. A. Van Gool and F. Van Haaren (Eds.), *Aging of the Brain and Alzheimer's Disease, Progress in Brain Research, this volume*, Elsevier, Amsterdam, pp. 473–484.

D. F. Swaab, E. Fliers, M. Mirmiran, W. A. Van Gool and F. Van Haaren (Eds.)
Progress in Brain Research, Vol. 70.
© 1986 Elsevier Science Publishers B.V. (Biomedical Division)

CHAPTER 31

Muscarinic cholinergic agonists: pharmacological and clinical perspectives

J. M. Palacios[a] and R. Spiegel[b]

[a]*Preclinical Research and* [b]*Clinical Research, Sandoz Ltd., CH-4002 Basle, Switzerland*

Introduction

A wealth of experimental data supports a role for central cholinergic mechanisms in the consolidation and expression of learning and memory, both in human and in experimental animals. Based on the behavioral effects of the administration of inhibitors of the enzyme acetylcholinesterase and of muscarinic receptor antagonists, Deutsch proposed in the early 70's that cholinergic synapses were involved in memory processes (Deutsch, 1971). In recent years this work has been extended and confirmed in different animal species, including primates, aging animals and animals with lesions of cholinergic pathways (Squire and Davis, 1981; Bartus et al., 1982; Coyle et al., 1983). These animal studies have demonstrated the effects of cholinergic drugs on memory processes and stressed that the effects are largely dependent upon the dose of the drug used, the route of administration and the age that memory is studied (Flood et al., 1981). Also in healthy human volunteers the effects of cholinergic drugs on aspects of memory are now well established (Drachman, 1977). Thus, amnesia is produced by administration of scopolamine and can be reversed by the administration of physostigmine, an acetylcholinesterase inhibitor, or the muscarinic agonist arecoline, but not by the catecholaminergic drug amphetamine.

The consistent finding of a characteristic and dramatic decrease of presynaptic cholinergic markers in the brains of patients with Alzheimer's disease has corroborated the suggestion of a predominant role of acetylcholine in human memory processes (Bartus et al., 1982; Rossor, 1982; Coyle et al., 1983). Although acetylcholine is not the only neurotransmitter altered in AD, it is the one which is found to be decreased most consistently (Rossor, 1982). Taken together with the previously mentioned literature on the influence of cholinergic activity in memory, this has led to the formulation of the 'cholinergic hypothesis of AD' which states that drugs which increase cholinergic neurotransmission should be therapeutically useful in the treatment of memory disorders.

The goal of the present paper is to review the current status of the human and animal pharmacology of the cholinergic system, particularly regarding the use of cholinergic agonists as therapeutic agents for the treatment of diseases such as senile dementia of Alzheimer.

'Classic' and 'new' muscarinic cholinergic agonists

Many, probably up to several hundreds of molecules with agonistic activity on the muscarinic cholinergic receptor (MChR) have been synthesized or isolated from natural sources in the past century (cf. e.g. Brimblecombe, 1974; Taylor, 1980). This concerns in particular cholinesters or alkaloids such as muscarin, arecoline or pilocarpine. Only few of these compounds have reached extensive clinical use, particularly in psychopharmacology. The chemical structures of some of

486

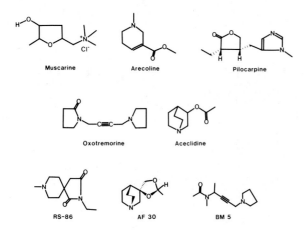

Fig. 1. Chemical structures of three 'classic' and some 'new' muscarinic agonists.

these cholinergic agonists are illustrated in Fig. 1. More recently, some new agonists with novel features have been synthesized and studied in animal models as potential therapeutic tools. Examples are the compounds AF 30 (2-methyl-spiro-1,3-dioxolane-4,3-quinuclidine) (Fisher et al., 1976), the oxotremorine analog BM-5 (N-methyl-N-[1-methyl-4-pyrrolidino-2-butynyl]acetamide) (Nordström et al., 1983) and RS 86 (2-ethyl-8-methyl-2,8-diazospiro-[4,5]-decan-1,3-dion hydrobromide) (Palacios et al., 1985). The chemical structures of these compounds are also shown in Fig. 1. Of these compounds only RS 86 has been extensively tested in man (see below).

Central and peripheral effects of the administration of muscarinic agonists to the experimental animal

Acetylcholine acting through nicotinic and MChR's plays an important role not only in the central nervous system but also in peripheral synapses. Cholinergic mechanisms are involved in the physiological regulation of many body functions. In the brain MChR's appear to play a predominant role in the mediation of cholinergic effects. It is, therefore, not surprising that the direct activation of MChR's results in both central and peripheral effects. One of the most characteristic central effects of muscarinic agonists is the induc-

tion of a typical pattern of arousal of the cortical electrical activity and the induction of a rhythmic slow activity (theta waves) in the hippocampal electroencephalogram (Robinson, 1980; Bevan, 1984). The action of muscarinic agonists on central MChR's results, in addition, in a number of behavioral and physiological effects. In mice, for example, administration of oxotremorine is followed by episodes of what is called 'alert non-mobile behavior', decreased locomotor activity, catalepsy and tremors. Muscarinic agonists can also affect sleep patterns (Karczmar, 1978 for review). Agonists' actions on central MChR's may produce a decrease in body temperature (hypothermia) and have effects on cardiovascular mechanisms, respiratory control and nociception (analgesia) in some species (Taylor, 1980; Brimblecombe, 1974).

Muscarinic agonists elicit a variety of effects on smooth muscle, exocrine glands and the cardiovascular system by stimulating peripheral MChR's. Readily observable in the experimental animal is the increase in lacrimation, salivation, sweating, urination and gastrointestinal transit. Muscarinic agonists also affect gastric acid secretion and have important direct effects in the heart and in vascular beds. Peripheral effects are blocked by atropine or scopolamine and their N-methyl derivatives, while central effects are less sensitive to the latter, because of the lower ability of the N-methyl derivatives to penetrate the blood–brain barrier (Taylor, 1980; Brimblecombe, 1974). Both peripheral and central effects of MChR agonists are dose-dependent. Fig. 2 illustrates this dose-dependency of central and peripheral effects for several muscarinic agonists. Differences in dose-dependency for the different compounds reflect differences in potency of these compounds at the MChR, different metabolism and tissue distribution and, more interestingly, differences in the dose requirements for different effects. For example, some central effects, such as electrophysiological or behavioral effects, are maximal at doses at which some other central or peripheral effects (tremor, salivation) are not yet detectable. Due to their wide

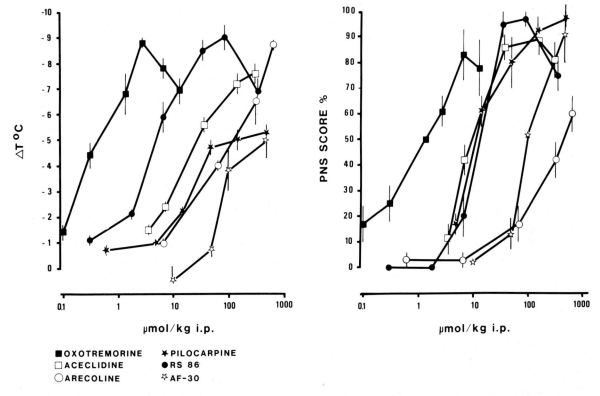

Fig. 2. Dose-dependency of central and peripheral effects after the systemic administration of several muscarinic agonists. Hypothermia, a central effect, was determined by measuring the rectal temperature. Data represent the mean maximal effect (±SD) from four animals. Lacrimation, salivation and diarrhea were scored as absent (0) present (1) or intense (2). Data are the mean (±SD) of the sum of maximal effects for four animals. Note that the rank order of activity of the agonists is different with respect to central and peripheral effects. For example, RS 86 elicits more central than peripheral effect while aceclidine and pilocarpine elicit stronger peripheral effects.

range of effects, none of the 'classical' muscarinic agonists appear suitable for the treatment of diseases such as AD. What, then are the characteristics of an 'ideal' muscarinic agonist for the treatment of AD? Evidently, such ideal muscarinic agonists should act on brain receptors and should also have an adequate duration of action without any major side effect, particularly not on the cardiovascular system.

Theoretical basis for the development of organ-, tissue- or function-specific muscarinic agonists

The development of a muscarinic agonist with an optimal pharmacological profile for the treatment

of memory disorders would be impossible if all muscarinic receptors distributed throughout the body were the same. Until recently such a similarity was generally assumed. At present, however, advances in the understanding of the MChR have provided a theoretical framework for the development of organ-, tissue- or function-specific or selective muscarinic agonists. The main features of this framework are summarized in Table I and have recently been critically reviewed by Jenden and Ehlert (1984). The starting point was the realization that MChR's are most probably heterogeneous, based upon pharmacological experiments with compounds such as gallamine (Riker and Wescoe, 1951) or the atypical agonist

TABLE I

Theoretical basis for the development of organ/tissue/function specific muscarinic agonists

---

Muscarinic receptor multiplicity
Differences in receptor reserve
  (partial agonists)
Receptor coupling differences
Allosteric mechanisms

McN A 343 (4-[m-chlorophenylcarbamoyloxy]-2-butynyltrimethylammonium chloride) (Roszkowski, 1961) (Fig. 3). These compounds have selective effects in the heart or in the sympathetic ganglia without affecting other muscarinic responses. The recent development of the tricyclic compound pirenzepine (Gastrozepine, LS 519; Fig. 3), an antimuscarinic drug useful in the clinical treatment of peptic ulcers, and lacking other unwanted antimuscarinic, particularly cardiovascular effects (Hammer et al., 1980; Hammer and Giachetti, 1982; Eltze et al., 1985), was mainly responsible for the now generally accepted concept of multiple MChR's. Analysis of MChR's by radioligand binding techniques has added further support to this concept. Binding studies have revealed that

both muscarinic agonists and antagonists interact with more than one population of sites (Birdsall et al., 1978; Watson et al., 1983; Vickroy et al., 1984).

Based upon these experimental data and on the use of the selective antagonist pirenzepine, two subtypes of the MChR have been postulated. The following terminology was proposed by Hirschowitz et al. (1984): M_1-receptors are those exhibiting high sensitivity to pirenzepine and are labeled with high affinity by this compound in binding assays; M_2-receptors show low sensitivity to pirenzepine in functional assays and bind this drug with low affinity. According to some authors M_2-receptors are probably heterogeneous, those in smooth muscle, for example, being different from receptors in cardiac muscle (Birdsall and Hulme, 1983), thus a further subdivision may be necessary.

The subtypes of the MChR appear to be very heterogeneously distributed throughout the body. Nervous tissue both centrally and peripherally is rich in receptors of the M_1 type, while M_2 receptors are predominant in exocrine glands or smooth muscles. Both subtypes are present in the brain where they present a differential regional distribution. An illustration of this differential distribution of M_1 and M_2 subtypes of the MChR in the rat brain is presented in Fig. 4. MChR's can be visualized autoradiographically using, for example, [^{3}H]N-methylscopolamine, a ligand with the same affinity for both M_1 and M_2 sites (Fig. 4A). By adding to the incubation medium low concentrations of carbachol (Fig. 4B) or pirenzepine (Fig. 4C) one can mask selectively M_2 or M_1 sites, allowing the visualization of the brain areas rich in the different subtypes. M_1 sites predominate in forebrain areas such as the nucleus caudatus-putamen and the hippocampus. The neocortex is also rich in M_1 sites. Brain stem, midbrain and

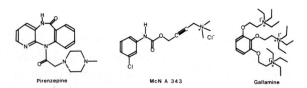

Pirenzepine   McN A 343   Gallamine

Fig. 3. Muscarinic compounds differentiating M_1 and M_2 receptor subtypes, such as the selective M_1 agonist McN-A-343 or the M_1 antagonist pirenzepine, and/or recognizing the allosteric site associated with the muscarinic receptor, such as the compound gallamine.

Fig. 4. The distribution of M_1 and M_2 subtypes in the rat brain. (A) is a photomicrograph from an autoradiogram showing the distribution of MChR (both M_1 and M_2) in a sagittal section, as labeled with [^{3}H]N-methylscopolamine. High densities of MChR (dark areas) were seen in forebrain areas such as the nucleus caudatus putamen (cp) or the hippocampal formation (Hi) and in some brain-stem areas such as the nucleus tractus solitarius. In (B) M_2 sites have been blocked, in a consecutive section, by adding to the incubation medium a low concentration of carbachol (10^{-4} M). The picture illustrates the areas enriched in M_1 sites. In (C) pirenzepine (2 μM) was added to block preferentially M_1 sites. Note the sensitivity to pirenzepine of forebrain areas (enriched in M_1 sites), as compared to brain-stem and midbrain areas (enriched in M_2 sites).

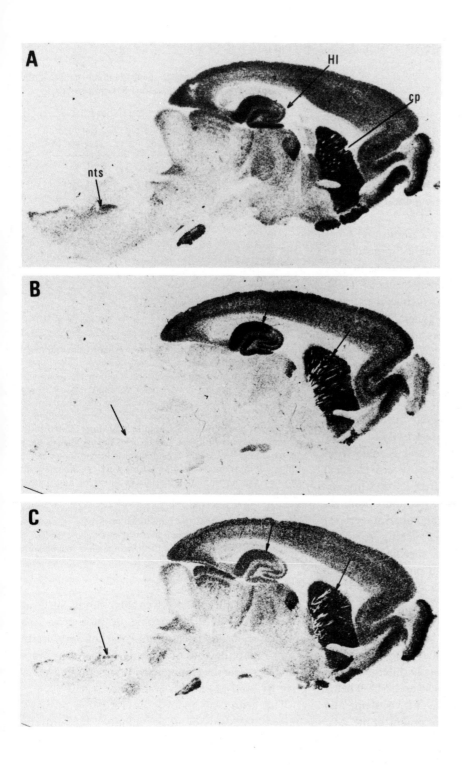

Fig. 4

some thalamic nuclei present MChR's belonging to the M_2 class (Wamsley et al., 1984; Cortés and Palacios, 1986).

Examination of post-mortem tissues has shown that also in the human brain the subtypes of the MChR are present and distributed similarly to that in experimental animals (Cortés et al., 1986). The differential regional distribution suggests that M_1 sites could play a predominant role in higher brain functions such as learning and memory, particularly in view of the enrichment of M_1 sites in areas such as the neocortex, the hippocampus and other limbic areas. M_2 sites are probably important in the central control of vegetative functions in view of their predominance in brain-stem nuclei. However, important forebrain areas such as the septum and the nucleus basalis of Meynert also contain M_2 sites, as does the thalamus, indicating that a role of these sites in memory processes cannot be excluded.

M_1 and M_2 MChR subtypes have been defined mainly on the basis of their sensitivity to the antagonist pirenzepine. However, very few agonists appear to present a clear selectivity for one or the other MChR subtypes. In Table II (data from Palacios et al., 1986) the effects of several classical and new agonists are compared in two preparations which are considered to contain homogeneous populations of M_1 (rat superior cervical ganglion) or M_2 (guinea-pig ileum) receptors (Brown et al., 1980a,b). This specificity is illustrated by the higher potency of pirenzepine in the superior cervical ganglion as compared to the ileum. Of all the agonists tested only the compound McN-A-343 was selective for one of the test systems, i.e. the ganglion. All the other compounds were active in both assays. Interestingly, the rank order of activity of the agonists is different in the two tests, with pilocarpine, RS 86 and AF 30 being somewhat more potent in the 'M_1' system, and aceclidine being relatively more potent in the 'M_2' tests. Similar dissociations in the rank orders of activity of muscarinic agonists have also been observed in in vivo tests of central activity (Palacios et al., 1986; Pazos et al., 1986). However,

TABLE II

The effects of some muscarinic agonists and antagonists in the guinea-pig ileum and the rat superior cervical ganglion

	Guinea-pig ileum	Rat superior cervical ganglion
Agonists, pD_2 values		
RS 86	6.05 ± 0.4	6.7 ± 0.2
oxotremorine	7.1 ± 0.1	8.0 ± 0.2
pilocarpine	5.9 ± 0.2	6.5 ± 0.2
arecoline	6.4 ± 0.1	6.6 ± 0.1
aceclidine	6.0 ± 0.1	5.4 ± 0.4
(cis)AF-30	4.8 ± 0.2	6.0 ± 0.1
McN-A-343	inactive	6.3 ± 0.3
Antagonists, pA_2 values		
Scopolamine	9.6 ± 0.03	10.0 ± 0.1
Atropine	8.9 ± 0.2	9.3 ± 0.2
Pirenzepine	6.8 ± 0.2	8.3 ± 0.1

Data in this Table represent the mean $\pm$ SEM from four to six separate measurements.

Quantification of the ability of several muscarinic agonists to contract the guinea-pig ileum (a tissue rich in M_2-MChR's), and to depolarize sympathetic ganglion cells (an effect mediated by M_1-MChR's). pD_2 values represent the negative logarithm of the agonist concentration eliciting half-maximal effects. Muscarinic antagonists blocked the effect of the agonists in these preparations. pA_2 values for antagonists are an index of the affinity of these antagonists for MChR's. pA_2 values represent the negative logarithm of the concentration of antagonists, which requires doubling of the concentration of agonist to produce the same effect observed in the absence of the antagonists. Note that the rank-order of activity of agonists differs in the two test systems and that pirenzepine exhibits a higher affinity for receptors in the ganglion while scopolamine and atropine have similar affinities in both systems.

the most subtype-selective compounds such as McN-A-343 and pirenzepine do not cross the blood–brain barrier and are thus not very useful to examine the role of M_1 and M_2 sites in brain function. The development of brain-entering selective M_1 and M_2 agents is thus necessary.

The action of agonists on receptors is determined not only by their 'affinity', but also by another property, namely their 'intrinsic activity'. Compounds with intrinsic activity similar to the natural agonists are able to elicit 'maximal' responses comparable to those of the endogenous ligands. Such compounds require the occupancy of only few receptors to elicit the corresponding response. Other compounds do not have the same intrinsic activity as the natural agonists and require the occupancy of more receptors to produce a maximal response, and may elicit only a partial response. Such compounds are called 'partial agonists'. Most of the muscarinic agonists mentioned in this review are in fact partial agonists. Their behavior is determined by the 'receptor reserve' of the effect being studied, a parameter which varies from response to response and from tissue to tissue. This property opens an additional approach in the attempt to develop tissue- or organ-specific agonists. In the case of the muscarinic agonists the effects of differences in intrinsic activity have been examined in detail in series of analogs of several compounds, particularly oxotremorine (Ringdahl and Jenden, 1983). These studies have shown that variations in the intrinsic activity can be used to produce compounds behaving as agonists in some models, e.g., in inducing salivation, but as antagonists in others, e.g. in blocking the tremorogenic effect of oxotremorine (Eicholzer and Oegren, 1977). Similar differences in 'intrinsic activity' and 'receptor reserve' are now postulated to explain the pronounced organ selectivity of α-adrenergic agonists, such as oxymetazoline (Kenakin, 1984) as well as the mixed agonistic and antagonistic behavior of dopaminergic agents such as 3-PPP (Carlsson, 1983).

The differences in intrinsic activity might in fact reflect differences in the capacity of these molecules to induce conformational changes associated with the coupling of the recognition unit to the effector mechanisms. These mechanisms have been examined in detail in a number of tissues and cellular systems for the MChR (McKinney and Richelson, 1984). Two effector systems linked to muscarinic responses are now well characterized: (1) the stimulatory effect of muscarinic receptor agonists on the turnover of the membrane lipid phosphatidylcholine and (2) the inhibitory effect of these compounds on adenylate cyclase. The rank order of activity and the efficacy of several muscarinic agonists is very different in the two systems. While it is not yet certain if the differences reflect a selective association of M_1 and M_2 receptors with one or the other effector system it is clear that the intrinsic activity of the known agonists is very different in the two systems and that these differences could provide a basis for selectivity of action.

Besides their recognition site and their effector mechanism some neurotransmitter receptors have regulatory sites which modulate through an allosteric mechanism the binding of agonists and antagonists. The best characterized example of such a system is the GABA receptor modulatory site where the benzodiazepine anxiolytic drugs act. The MChR appears to contain such a regulatory allosteric site. Pharmacological and radioligand studies have shown that the neuromuscular (nicotinic) blocker gallamine has a selective antimuscarinic effect in heart but not in other tissues such as ileum, bladder or salivary glands (Clark and Mitchelson, 1976; Stockton et al., 1982). Gallamine, as well as other drugs, produce their atypical antimuscarinic effect by binding to a novel site, resulting in a negative heterotropic cooperativity, i.e. reducing the affinity of other ligands for their recognition sites. Most of the compounds acting on these sites are potent nicotinic antagonists and thus without much use in psychopharmacology. The development of a compound acting selectively through this site on brain MChR's is, however, conceivable.

The main conclusions of this brief overview of the current status of the pharmacology of the muscarinic system could be summarized as follows: (1) none of the known muscarinic agonists described until now appears to present an optimal profile for clinical use in AD; (2) there is, however, enough theoretical basis for the development of selective agents based on receptor selectivity, coupling mechanisms or action on regulatory sites; (3) until such selective compounds have been developed and clinically tested it is impossible to predict which mechanism will offer the best way to approach the clinical treatment of AD.

Clinical testing of the cholinergic hypothesis of AD

The social and economic impact of AD in our society is enormous and the necessity of effective medical treatment of this disease does not need to be stressed. Since the formulation of the cholinergic hypothesis of AD, numerous clinical trials have been carried out to test the effects of cholinomimetics on human memory in normal young and elderly volunteers and in patients suffering from AD. The results of a large part of these trials have been comprehensively reviewed (Crook and Gershon, 1982; Corkin et al., 1982; Bartus et al., 1982; Johns et al., 1983; Reisberg, 1983; Wurtman et al., 1984; Sitaram, 1984). While the focus of the present paper is on directly acting muscarinic agonists, we will first briefly review other approaches which have, in fact, been used more extensively than the directly acting postsynaptic agonists.

There are basically three approaches to increase cholinergic neurotransmission in AD. The first one, tailored in analogy to the precursor therapy of Parkinson's disease, is the administration of the acetylcholine precursor choline or its normal dietary source lecithin. This is based on the observation that an increase in brain choline can induce an increase in the synthesis and release of acetylcholine (cf. Wurtman et al., 1984). A second approach consists in the administration of inhibitors of the enzymatic breakdown of acetylcholine by acetylcholinesterase (AChE). The most commonly used AChE inhibitor has been physostigmine, although a second compound, tetrahydroaminoacridine, has also been studied in AD. Finally, a few direct muscarinic agonists have been clinically examined.

The first two approaches rely on the at least partial preservation of the endogenous neuronal machinery for the synthesis and release of acetylcholine, and therefore these approaches must be expected to succeed at best in patients with a moderate cholinergic deficit. The third approach requires the presence of intact functional MChR's which, at least in terms of receptor binding, appear to be unaltered in AD (Bartus et al., 1982). In some clinical trials more than one approach has been combined, e.g. choline or lecithin administration together with an inhibitor of AChE or with a directly acting agonist.

The precursor strategy

Of the 17 studies reviewed by Bartus et al. (1982), where small or large doses of both choline and lecithin were tested for durations of up to 3 months, only one resulted in substantial improvement, while ten others did not report any definite effect of acetylcholine precursor administration on cognitive tasks. Some positive trends were observed in a small proportion of patients in a number of clinical trials. This lack of convincing clinical benefit may be due to the inability of choline or lecithin to increase brain acetylcholine or to many other factors. More recent studies (Little et al., 1984) have been directed at demonstrating 'preventive' rather than 'curative' effects of the precursors, but so far the results do not indicate that this strategy is clinically successful in AD.

Anticholinesterase strategy

The number of therapeutic trials with anticholinesterase agents is smaller than that with acetylcholine precursors. This is mainly due to the fact that AChE inhibitors may have serious peripheral effects, particularly on the cardiovascular system. Most studies have been performed with the AChE inhibitor physostigmine. This compound has been shown to facilitate performance in memory tasks in young and elderly humans and primates (see Bartus et al., 1982). The main drawbacks seen in these studies were: (1) the narrow dose range in which physostigmine can be used, with doses below this range being ineffective and doses above producing impairments in performance; (2) the great variability of the optimal dose from individual to individual; and (3) the short duration of action (about 30 min) of the pharmaceutical preparation so far available. An oral form of physostigmine resulting in a prolonged duration of action became available only recently. Administration of physostigmine to AD patients has produced variable results (Mohs et al., 1985; Sitaram, 1984; and Johns et al., 1983). A perhaps typical example of a clinical trial with physostigmine was reported by Mohs et al. (1985). In this study oral administration of doses from 0.5 to 2 mg of physostigmine every 2 h for 3 to 5 days resulted in repeated clinical improvements in three out of ten patients, four patients showing some marginal effects and the other three responding inconsistently. In analyzing their results, Mohs et al. (1985) propose the following reasons for the inconsistent improvement: (1) some patients may have been misdiagnosed, in spite of the extensive selection criteria used; (2) deficits in other neurotransmitters (noradrenaline, serotonin, somatostatin) are not corrected by physostigmine treatment, which may be particularly important in patients with a presenile onset, as those of their own study; (3) in the non-responsive patients physostigmine failed to increase central cholinergic activity, either because these patients had an extensive cholinergic deficit or because the drug was not absorbed. The latter possibility was also suggested by Thal and colleagues (1983) who examined the degree of inhibition of AChE in the cerebrospinal fluid of patients treated with physostigmine. In this study, a clear correlation between inhibition of the enzyme and clinical improvement was seen. However, none of these possibilities accounts for the fact that, in the study by Mohs et al., all ten cases showed some improvement in the physostigmine dose-finding phase, while only three out of ten had their previous results confirmed in a subsequent replication study.

Directly acting muscarinic agonists

From the animal pharmacological profiles described above it is clear that most of the currently available directly acting muscarinic agonists have, besides their central effects, marked activities on peripheral MChR's which limit their clinical utility, e.g. in AD. In spite of these limitations a number of clinical trials have been done with some of these muscarinic agonists.

Oxotremorine and pilocarpine have been tested on a few occasions, the first one in combination with a peripheral muscarinic blocker (Wettstein, 1983) and the second one together with lecithin (Caine, 1980). No improvement in memory was reported by these investigators. Arecoline has been given to human volunteers and was shown to improve performance in serial learning (Sitaram et al., 1978). It has also been tested in affective disorders, but we know of only one controlled clinical experiment in AD (see Christie et al., 1981): intravenous infusions of 1, 2 and 4 mg were given to 11 patients with early (<65 years) disease onset. The same patients were given physostigmine on a separate occasion. Improvement in a picture recognition test was seen in seven patients with a dosis of 4 mg of arecoline, although the changes were only slight. Compared with physostigmine, arecoline and probably other directly acting agonists could have a wider effective dose range. However, in the opinion of Christie et al., "neither physostigmine nor arecoline offers a practical therapy for Alzheimer's disease".

The most extensively tested direct muscarinic agonist in AD is the compound RS 86 (Spiegel et al., 1984; Wettstein and Spiegel, 1984; Wettstein et al., 1985). First developed in the 60's, this compound has only recently been characterized in preclinical models of cholinergic activity (Palacios et al., 1986) and was found to be a potent centrally acting muscarinic agonist with affinity and activity in models for both M_1 and M_2 subtypes, although with a relatively higher activity in M_1 systems. Central and peripheral cholinergic activity of RS 86 has been demonstrated in man. For example, administration of RS 86 to healthy volunteers resulted in sedation and, more importantly, in reduction of the REM sleep latency and slow-wave sleep (Spiegel, 1984), both changes believed to be mediated by activation of central MChR's (see, for example, Sitaram et al., 1978). Peripheral signs of muscarinic activity were hypersalivation, lacrimation and sweating, observed in both experimental subjects and patients. The cardiovascular effects noted (slight increase in pulse rate and in blood pressure) are probably centrally mediated (Pazos et al., 1986). The minimum effective dose in man was 1 mg. Oral absorption appears to be very good, as almost identical effects were seen after oral and subcutaneous administration of the same dose of RS 86. Preliminary estimates of the biological half-life of this compound gave figures of more than 6 h.

RS 86 had previously been tested in a variety of clinical indications other than AD in almost 500 patients (see Spiegel et al., 1984). A limited research program, started in 1982, has so far (May 1985) included some 80 healthy subjects and 78 patients, whereof 61 with Alzheimer's disease. RS 86 was administered in single doses up to 5.0 mg and in maximal daily doses of 5.0 mg. Treatment duration in therapeutic studies was between 1 and 6 weeks in most cases and exceeded 6 months in a few instances. The main target of RS 86, patients with AD, did not respond to the drug in a uniform way (Fig. 5). A majority of them displayed no or only minimal therapeutic benefit, and only isolated cases, one to two per trial, showed a clinically convincing response (Spiegel et al., 1984; Wettstein and Spiegel, 1984; Wettstein et al., 1985). It was not possible so far to relate clinical response to other (anamnestic, symptomatic) patient characteristics, but efforts are still underway in this respect. An attempt will also be made to reduce peripheral muscarinic effects by concomitant administration of pirenzepine in order to permit the use of higher, and hopefully more therapeutically active, doses of RS 86.

Concluding remarks

The cholinergic hypothesis of AD has not yet undergone a definite test, although a considerable number of clinical studies with various cholinergic drugs has been reported.

A straightforward precursor strategy, i.e. the administration of lecithin or choline, has so far

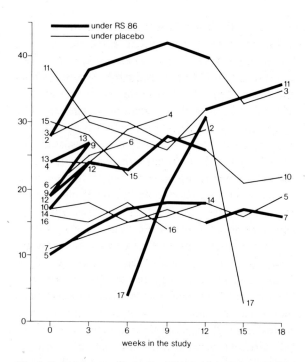

Fig. 5. Performance of AD patients in a test of verbal fluency (producing words with a given first letter). After a 6-week parallel-group trial (50% of patients on RS 86, 50% on placebo) followed a 2 × 6-week crossover trial with 2–3 mg RS 86 per day vs. placebo. There were many drop-outs in this study with 17, mostly very old, patients, but verbal performance was generally improved on the active drug, with some spectacular changes (patients Nos. 17, 10, 3). (From Wettstein et al., 1985)

been the most frequently tried, but least promising approach. Although not limited by side effects or toxicity, administration of even high doses of lecithin has not resulted in clear-cut therapeutic effects, whereas the use of choline has been discouraged by the unpleasant odor it produces in its consumers. What is still open to questions is the effect of chronic administration of lecithin over years, i.e. a long-term therapeutic or even prophylactic administration of this precursor. Whether such a trial is feasible, and whether it should be undertaken at all, is presently discussed by several groups.

Physostigmine has been tested extensively and has shown effects in both experimental and clinical studies. Its practical use is limited by its short biological half-life and poor tolerability, particularly with regard to cardiovascular effects. There is some hope, however, that better results will be obtained, or at least more viable clinical studies can be realized, once a more suitable way of administration — e.g. slow release forms avoiding high drug plasma peaks — becomes available. Evidently, the use of physostigmine and other enzyme inhibitors presupposes at least partly intact presynaptic cholinergic neurons.

Directly acting cholinergic agonists, such as arecoline and oxotremorine have had little applications, the latter drug due to its tremorogenic potential, the first one because of poor tolerability and short biological half-life. Here again, progress may depend on more appropriate forms of drug delivery, which could help to reduce the number of doses per time and to curb unduly high — and toxic — drug plasma peaks.

Modifications of the arecoline or oxotremorine molecules with the same goal in mind may also be a useful approach. RS 86, another directly acting postsynaptic agonist, has undergone a number of experimental and clinical tests and has shown some of the expected effects. At this time it appears to be a suitable tool for testing the cholinergic hypothesis of AD thanks to its longer plasma half-life and better tolerability, although RS 86 is not devoid of side effects either, and although clinical success rates have been low.

What, then, is the outlook for the cholinergic approach in AD? Can one maintain the original optimism which had its origin in the discovery of a specific neuronal degeneration in this condition and the simultaneous success of a replacement therapy in another degenerative brain disorder, i.e. Parkinson's disease? We believe that the very limited success of therapeutic trials with acetylcholine precursors and cholinomimetics so far undertaken should not lead to pessimism and therapeutic nihilism for the following reasons:

(1) AD is probably not a homogeneous disease entity, both on clinical and neuronal/biochemical grounds. Several lines of evidence, including the fact that in most clinical trials with cholinomimetics rather spectacular individual cases of improvement were seen, suggest that the clinical entity AD is heterogeneous and that efforts must be made to identify 'cholinergic responders' as opposed to non-responders. Neurobiochemical and endocrinological studies in patients will be necessary for this purpose (see Johns et al., 1983).

(2) The fact that cholinergic drugs, with the exception of acetylcholine precursors, produce unpleasant or even vital peripheral effects has limited clinical trials and possibly also the administration of doses sufficient to produce therapeutic effects in the brain. Combining cholinergic agonists with specific peripheral blockers, such as antimuscarinics of the pirenzepine type, may improve the results of future trials.

(3) Recent neuropathological studies indicate that cholinergic neuronal deficits in AD are often combined with degeneration of other types of brain cells. A continuum of 'patterns of degeneration', ranging from pure cholinergic deficits to e.g., pure dopaminergic ones, is conceivable, and the necessity of combining different aminergic agonists would be an obvious consequence. Until more is known about a hypothetical continuum of this kind, carefully controlled clinical trials with cholinomimetic drugs, alone and in combination with other compounds, and the development of new agonists with different pharmacodynamic and -kinetic profiles, seems a logical way to proceed, at least for those of us who work with the pharmaceutical industry.

References

Bartus, R. T., Dean, R. L., Beer, B. and Lippa, A. S. (1982) The cholinergic hypothesis of geriatric memory dysfunction. *Science*, 217: 408–417.

Bevan, P. (1984) Effect of muscarinic ligands on the electrical activity recorded from the hippocampus: a quantitative approach. *Br. J. Pharmacol.*, 82: 431–440.

Birdsall, N. J. M. and Hulme, E. C. (1983) Muscarinic receptor subclasses. *Trends Pharmacol. Sci.*, 4: 459–463.

496

Birdsall, N. J. M., Burgen, A. S. V. and Hulme, E. C. (1978) The binding of agonists to brain muscarinic receptors. *Mol. Pharmacol.*, 14: 723–736.

Brimblecombe, R. W. (1974) *Drug Actions on Cholinergic Systems*. The Macmillan Press Ltd., London.

Brown, D. A., Fatherazi, S., Garthwaite, J. and White, R. D. (1980a) Muscarinic receptors in rat sympathetic ganglia. *Br. J. Pharmacol.*, 70: 577–592.

Brown, D. A., Forward, A. and Marsh, S. (1980b) Antagonist discrimination between ganglionic and ileal muscarinic receptors. *Br. J. Pharmacol.*, 71: 362–364.

Caine, E. D. (1980) Cholinomimetic treatment fails to improve memory disorders. *N. Engl. J. Med.*, 303: 585–586.

Carlsson, A. (1983) Dopamine receptor agonists: intrinsic activity vs. state of the receptors. *J. Neural Transm.*, 57: 309–315.

Christie, J. E., Shering, A., Ferguson, J. and Glen, A. I. M. (1981) Physostigmine and arecoline: effects of intravenous infusions in Alzheimer's presenile dementia. *Br. J. Psychiat.*, 138: 46–50.

Clark, A. L. and Mitchelson, F. (1976) The inhibitory effect of gallamine on muscarinic receptors. *Br. J. Pharmacol.*, 58: 323–331.

Corkin, S., Davis, K. L., Growdon, J. H., Usdin, E. and Wurtman, R. J. (Eds.), (1982) *Alzheimer's Disease: A Report on Progress in Research*, Raven Press, New York.

Cortés, R. and Palacios, J. M. (1986) Muscarinic cholinergic receptor subtypes in the rat brain: quantitative autoradiographic studies. *Brain Res.*, 362: 227–238.

Cortés, R., Probst, A., Tobler, H.J. and Palacios, J.M. (1986) Muscarinic cholinergic receptor subtypes in the human brain: quantitative autoradiographic studies. *Brain Res.*, 362: 239–253.

Coyle, J. T., Price, D. L. and DeLong, M. R. (1983) Alzheimer's disease: a disorder of cortical cholinergic innervation. *Science*, 219: 1184–1190.

Crook, Th. and Gershon, S. (1981) *Strategies for the Development of an Effective Treatment for Senile Dementia*. Mark Powley Associates, Inc., Connecticut.

Deutsch, J. A. (1971) The cholinergic synapse and the site of memory. *Science*, 174: 788–794.

Drachman, D. A. (1977) Memory and cognitive function in man: does the cholinergic system have a specific role? *Neurology*, 27: 783–790.

Eicholzer, A. and Oegren, S. O. (1977) The central and peripheral effectiveness of two oxotremorine-antagonists determined using oxotremorine-induced tremor and salivation. *J. Pharm. Pharmacol.*, 29: 609–611.

Eltze, M., Gönne, S., Riedel, R., Schlotke, B., Schudt, C. and Simon, W. A. (1985) Pharmacological evidence for selective inhibition of gastric acid secretion by telenzepine, a new antimuscarinic drug. *Eur. J. Pharmacol.*, 112: 211–224.

Fisher, A., Weinstock, M., Gitter, S. and Cohen, S. (1976) A new probe for heterogeneity in muscarinic receptors: 2-methylspiro-(1, 3-dioxolane-4, 3')quinuclidine. *Eur. J. Pharmacol.*, 37: 329–338.

Flood, J. F., Landry, D. W. and Jarvik, M. E. (1981) Cholinergic receptor interactions and their effects on long-term memory processing. *Brain Res.*, 215: 177–185.

Hammer, R. and Giachetti, A. (1982) Muscarinic receptor subtypes: M_1 and M_2 biochemical and functional characterization. *Life Sci.*, 31: 2991–2998.

Hammer, R., Berrie, C. P., Birdsall, N. J. M., Burgen, A. S. V. and Hulme, E. C. (1980) Pirenzepine distinguishes between different subclasses of muscarinic receptors. *Nature*, 283: 90–92.

Hirschowitz, B. I., Hammer, R., Giachetti, A., Keirns, J. J. and Levine, R. R. (1984) Subtypes of muscarinic receptors. Proceedings of the international symposium on subtypes of muscarinic receptors. *Trends Pharmacol. Sci.*, Suppl. 1.

Jenden, D. J. and Ehlert, F. J. (1984) Heterogeneity of cholinergic receptors. In R. J. Wurtman, S. H. Corkin and J. H. Growdon (Eds.), *Alzheimer's Disease: Advances in Basic Research and Therapies*, Center for Brain Sciences and Metabolism Charitable Trust, Cambridge, USA, pp. 123–144.

Johns, C. A., Greenwald, B. S., Mohs, R. C. and Davis, K. L. (1983) The cholinergic treatment strategy in aging and senile dementia. *Psychopharmacol. Bull.*, 19: 185–197.

Karczmar, A. G. (1978) Exploitable aspects of central cholinergic functions, particularly with respect to the EEG, motor, analgesia and mental functions. In D. J. Jenden (Ed.), *Cholinergic Mechanism and Psychopharmacology*, Plenum Press, New York, pp. 679–708.

Kenakin, T. (1984) The relative contribution of affinity and efficacy to agonist activity: organ selectivity of noradrenaline and oxymetazoline with reference to the classification of drug receptors. *Br. J. Pharmacol.*, 81: 131–141.

Little, A., Chuaqui-Kidd, P. and Levy, R. (1984) Early results from a double-blind, placebo-controlled trial of high dose lecithin in Alzheimer's disease: psychometric test performance, plasma choline levels and the effects of drug compliance. In R. J. Wurtman, S. H. Corkin and J. H. Growdon (Eds.), *Alzheimer's Disease: Advances in Basic Research and Therapies*, Center for Brain Sciences and Metabolism Charitable Trust, Cambridge, USA, pp. 313–331.

McKinney, M. Richelson, E. (1984) The coupling of the neuronal muscarinic receptor to responses. *Ann. Rev. Pharmacol. Toxicol.*, 24: 121–146.

Mohs, R. C., Davis, B. M., Johns, C. A., Mathé, A. A., Greenwald, B. S., Horvath, Th. B. and Davis, K. L. (1985) Oral physostigmine treatment of patients with Alzheimer's disease. *Am. J. Psychiat.*, 142: 28–33.

Nordstrom, B., Alberts, P., Westlind, A., Unden, A. and Bartfai, T. (1983) Presynaptic antagonist — postsynaptic agonist at muscarinic cholinergic synapses. *N*-Methyl-*N*-(1-methyl-4-pyrrolidino-2-butynyl) acetamide. *Mol. Pharmacol.*, 24: 1–5.

Palacios, J. M., Bolliger, G., Closse, A., Enz, A., Gmelin, G. and Malanowski, J. (1986) The pharmacological assessment of RS 86 (2-ethyl-8-methyl-2, 8-diazospiro-[4,5]-decan-1, 3-dion hydrobromide). A potent, specific muscarinic cholinergic agonist. *Eur. J. Pharmacol.*, 125: 45–62.

Pazos, A., Wiederhold, K.-H. and Palacios, J. M. (1986) Central pressor effects induced by muscarinic agonists: evidence for a predominant role of the M_2-receptor subtype. *Eur. J. Pharmacol.*, 125: 63–70.

Reisberg, B. (Ed.) (1983) *Alzheimer's Disease*. The Free Press, New York.

Riker, W. F. and Wescoe, W. C. (1951) The pharmacology of flaxedil with observations on certain analogs. *Ann. N. Y. Acad. Sci.*, 54: 373–394.

Ringdahl, B. and Jenden, D. J. (1983) Pharmacological properties of oxotremorine and its analogues. *Life Sci.*, 32: 2401–2413.

Robinson, T. E. (1980) Hippocampal rhythmical slow activity (RSA; theta): a critical analysis of selected studies and discussion of possible species differences. *Brain Res. Rev.*, 2: 69–101.

Rossor, M. N. (1982) Dementia (neurotransmitters and CNS disease). *Lancet* ii: 1200–1204.

Roszkowski, A. P. (1961) An unusual type of sympathetic ganglion stimulant. *J. Pharmacol. Exp. Ther.*, 132: 156–170.

Sitaram, N. (1984) Cholinergic hypothesis of human memory: review of basic and clinical studies. *Drug Dev. Res.*, 4: 481–488.

Sitaram, N., Weingartner, H. and Gillin, J. C. (1978) Human serial learning: enhancement with arecoline and impairment with scopolamine correlated with performance on placebo. *Science*, 201: 274–276.

Spiegel, R. (1984) Effects of RS 86, an orally active cholinergic agonist, on sleep in man. *Psychiat. Res.*, 11: 1–13.

Spiegel, R., Azcona, A. and Wettstein, A. (1984) First results with RS 86, an orally active muscarinic agonist, in healthy subjects and in patients with dementia. In R. J. Wurtman, S. H. Corkin and J. H. Growdon (Eds.), *Alzheimer's Disease: Advances in Basic Research and Therapies*, Center for Brain Sciences and Metabolism Charitable Trust, Cambridge, USA, pp. 391–405.

Squire, L. R. and Davis, H. P. (1981) The pharmacology of

memory: a neurobiological perspective. *Ann. Rev. Pharmacol. Toxicol.*, 21: 323–356.

Stockton, J. M., Birdsall, N. J. M., Burgen, A. S. V. and Hulme, E. C. (1982) Modification of the binding properties of muscarinic receptors by gallamine. *Mol. Pharmacol.*, 23: 551–557.

Taylor, R. (1980) Cholinergic agonists. In G. A. Goodman, L. L. Goodman and A. Gilman (Eds.), *The Pharmacological Basis of Therapeutics*, MacMillan Publ. Co., New York, pp. 91–99.

Thal, L. J., Fuld, P. A., Masur, D. M. and Sharpless, N. S. (1983) Oral physostigmine and lecithin improve memory in Alzheimer's disease. *Ann. Neurol.*, 13: 491–496.

Vickroy, T. W., Watson, M., Yamamura, H. I. and Roeske, W. R. (1984) Agonist binding to multiple muscarinic receptors. *Fed. Proc.*, 43: 2785–2790.

Wamsley, J. K., Zarbin, M. A. and Kuhar, M. J. (1984) Distribution of muscarinic cholinergic high and low affinity agonist binding sites: a light microscopic autoradiographic study. *Brain Res. Bull.*, 12: 233–243.

Watson, M., Yamamura, H. I. and Roeske, W. R. (1983) A unique regulatory profile and regional distribution of [^{3}H]pirenzepine binding in the rat provide evidence for distinct M_1 and M_2 muscarinic receptor subtypes. *Life Sci.*, 32: 3001–3011.

Wettstein, A. (1983) Ein kasuistischer Beitrag zur kontroversen Hypothese des Morbus Alzheimer als Dysfunktion der frontobasalen cholinergen Zellen. *Schweiz. Arch. Neurol. Neurochirurg. Psychiat.*, 133: 215–216.

Wettstein, A. and Spiegel, R. (1984) Clinical trials with the cholinergic drug RS 86 in Alzheimer's disease (AD) and senile dementia of the Alzheimer type (SDAT). *Psychopharmacology*, 84: 572–573.

Wettstein, A., Köppel-Hefti, A. and Spiegel, R. (1985) Therapeutic trial with the muscarinic agonist RS 86 in patients with senile dementia of Alzheimer type. In G. D. Burrows and T. R. Norman (Eds.), *Clinical and Pharmacological Studies in Psychiatric Disorders*, John Libbey, London, pp. 268–272.

Wurtman, R. J., Corkin, S. H. and Growdon, J. H. (Eds.) (1984) *Alzheimer's Disease: Advances in Basic Research and Therapies*, Center for Brain Sciences and Metabolism Charitable Trust, Cambridge, USA.

Discussion

H. VAN CREVEL: You mentioned 'subpopulations' of AD patients that responded well to your treatment. Could this response be repeated under double-blind conditions?

ANSWER: Yes, in fact the studies I was referring to were double-blind, placebo controlled with different designs, depending on the investigators (see for example Spiegel et al., 1984).

J. HAGAN: Chronic exposure to cholinergic drugs may result in receptor changes. Does not this constitute a serious objection to treatment with agonists?

ANSWER: Animal studies have shown that muscarinic receptors (at least in the brain) do not present marked adaptative response (hyper- or hyposensitivity). One can treat animals with high doses of, for example, atropine or scopolamine and observe only small (10–20%) receptor increases (see for example Yamada et al., 1983).

References

Spiegel, R., Azcona, A. and Wettstein, A. (1984) First results with RS 86, an orally active muscarinic agonist, in healthy subjects and in patients with dementia. In R. J. Wurtman, S. H. Corkin and J. H. Growdon (Eds.), *Alzheimer's Disease: Advances in Basic Research and Therapies*, Center for Brain Sciences and Metabolism Charitable Trust, Cambridge, USA, pp. 391–405.

Yamada, S., Isogai, M., Okudaira, H. and Hayashi, E. (1983) Regional adaptation of muscarinic receptors and choline uptake in brain following repeated administration of diisopropylfluorophosphate and atropine. *Brain Res.*, 268: 315–320.

D. F. Swaab, E. Fliers, M. Mirmiran, W. A. Van Gool and F. Van Haaren (Eds.)
Progress in Brain Research, Vol. 70.
© 1986 Elsevier Science Publishers B.V. (Biomedical Division)

CHAPTER 32

Transplantation of basal forebrain cholinergic neurons in the aged rat brain

A. Björklund and F. H. Gage

Department of Histology, University of Lund, Lund, Sweden and Department of Neuroscience, U.C.S.D., La Jolla, CA, USA

Introduction

Grafts of fetal ventral forebrain, rich in developing cholinergic neurons, are capable of reinnervating large areas of the hippocampal formation or neocortex in young rats with denervating brain lesions (Björklund and Stenevi, 1977; Björklund et al., 1983a,b; Lewis and Cotman, 1983; Fine et al., 1985b; Kromer, 1985). In the hippocampal formation the grafted cholinergic neurons have been shown to establish electrophysiologically and morphologically normal synapses with neuronal elements of the host, including granule cells and pyramidal cells, in the dentate gyrus and the CA1 area (Low et al., 1982; Segal et al., 1985; Clarke et al., 1986b). In addition, biochemical measures of acetylcholine synthesis rates have indicated that the grafted cholinergic neurons are spontaneously active and operate at a fairly normal functional level (Björklund et al., 1983a). In animals with fimbria-fornix lesions which transect the septo-hippocampal projection system, septal grafts have been shown to restore normal hippocampal functional metabolic rates, as assessed by autoradiographic measurements of regional 2-deoxyglucose utilization (Kelly et al., 1985), and they have been shown to promote behavioral recovery in hippocampus-dependent spatial learning in different types of radial maze tasks (Low et al., 1982, 1985; Dunnett et al., 1982). Similarly, grafts of ventral forebrain cholinergic neurons, implanted into the

fronto-parietal cortex of rats with excitotoxic lesions of the nucleus basalis region, have been found to ameliorate both sensorimotor and learning impairments in the lesioned rats (Fine et al., 1985a, Dunnett et al., 1985). The significant correlation between the degree of acetylcholine esterase (AChE) positive fiber ingrowth from the septal grafts and the functional effects, as observed in the maze learning study of Dunnett et al. (1982), in the 2-deoxyglucose study of Kelly et al. (1985) and in the in vitro electrophysiological study of Segal et al. (1985) provide some evidence, albeit circumstantial, that the cholinergic graft-host connections may be important, perhaps even necessary, for the graft-induced functional effects in this model.

The ability of the cholinergic septal grafts to substitute, morphologically and functionally, for the loss of a cholinergic pathway in young brain-damaged rats has raised the question whether similar effects could also be obtained in aged rats, where defects in learning and memory have been associated with an age-dependent decline in different parameters of forebrain cholinergic functions (Strong et al., 1980; Lippa et al., 1980, 1981; Gibson et al., 1981; Sherman et al., 1981; Sims et al., 1982; Bartus et al., 1982). Thus, although there are no data to implicate an actual loss of cholinergic forebrain neurons with age in rodents, similar to that which occurs in Alzheimer's type dementia in man (Hornberger et al., 1985; see

Bartus et al., 1982; Coyle et al., 1983), it seems likely that a functional deterioration of the limbic and cortical cholinergic afferent systems contributes to the age-related spatial learning impairments (Barnes et al., 1983; Ingram et al., 1981; Bartus et al., 1982) also in these species. In the present paper we will review a series of recent studies, conducted in our laboratory, which indicate that grafts of acetylcholine-rich tissue into the brain of aged rats can influence age-dependent learning and memory deficits, perhaps by a cholinergic mechanism.

General principles of intracerebral grafting

Several general principles have been identified as being critical for the survival of neural transplants in the CNS of mammals (See Björklund and Stenevi, 1984, for review). One principle is that grafting of mammalian central nervous tissue is possible only from fetal or early neonatal donors, and that survival of mature (or adult) CNS tissue so far has not been possible to obtain. Though the reason for this time constraint is not known, it has been suggested that fetal neurons are subjected to less damage due to extensive axotomy during dissection since their axons have not yet extended greatly. In addition, fetal tissue may be able to survive anoxia better than mature tissue and has the capacity for continued neurogenesis after transplantation.

A second principle is that the brain is a privileged immunological site, and as long as the CNS grafting is carried out between individuals of the same breeding stock, the grafts should not be rejected as immunologically incompatible. Cross-species grafting of CNS tissue has proven to be substantially less successful (Björklund et al., 1982; Freed, 1983; Low et al., 1983). Though some neurons from cross-species grafts may survive, perhaps due to migration behind the protection of the blood–brain barrier, the bulk of the graft tissue will be rejected unless immunosuppressive treatment is used (Brundin et al., 1985).

A third principle is that in order for intracerebral grafts to survive, there must be a rapid and sufficient integration of the graft into the blood and cerebral spinal fluid circulation of the host brain. All the successful intracerebral grafting methods now in use in adult recipients take advantage of CSF-filled or highly vascularized transplantation sites, either using natural sites, such as the anterior chamber of the eye (Olson et al., 1983), the ventricular system (Freed, 1983), or by surgically exposing richly vascularized surfaces as transplantation cavities (Stenevi et al., 1985), or by surgically inducing a vascular bed some weeks prior to transplantation in sites that are normally poorly vascularized (Stenevi et al., 1985). By contrast, in neonatal recipient rats neural grafts survive well also when they are placed directly into the host brain parenchyma.

The requirement for a suitable vascularized site in adult or aged hosts restricts greatly the number of available transplantation sites. This problem has been overcome by the development of a technique which involves the intracerebral injection of dissociated suspensions of embryonic CNS tissue. The technique is a modification of the standard technique used for dispersed cell cultures, and involves the following steps: (1) dissection of the embryonic donor; (2) collection of tissue pieces; (3) incubation in trypsin; (4) washing; (5) mechanical dissociation of the tissue; and (6) stereotaxic injection of the resultant cell suspension into the host brain. Details of the method and procedure are presented elsewhere (Björklund et al., 1983c). The primary advantage of the suspension grafting technique, not least within the context of grafting in aged rats, is that the dissociated cells can be implanted in direct contact with the host neuropil without the need of access to a special pial surface or to CSF-filled spaces, and that the surgery involves minimal trauma to the host. It is advantageous also in that it allows implantation of fetal CNS neurons into any site in the brain or spinal cord with high survival, and it allows implantation of multiple grafts within a single host brain region, or the implantation of mixtures of different cell populations which have been combined within a single suspension.

The limbic system and cognitive decline with age in rodents

In aged rats, significant cell loss has been reported in the pyramidal layer of the hippocampal formation (Landfield et al., 1977, 1981) as well as a significant reduction in axo-dendritic and axosomatic synapses in the granular cell layer of the dentate gyrus (Bondareff and Geinisman, 1976; Geinisman, 1979, 1981; Hoff et al., 1982). In addition, aged rats show a dramatic astrocytic hypertrophy (Landfield et al., 1977), possibly indicative of an ongoing response to neuronal degeneration. Several reports show significant decrease in muscarinic binding sites (Lippa et al., 1980, 1981), in acetylcholine synthesis (Sims et al., 1982) and in high-affinity choline uptake (Sherman et al., 1981) in the hippocampal formation. These cholinergic deficits are further supported by evidence that pyramidal cells of aged rats show a decrease in responsiveness to iontophoretically applied acetylcholine (Segal, 1982; Lippa et al., 1981). Although no actual cell loss in the basal forebrain cholinergic system has been reported, a recent study has observed significant atrophy of these neurons in aged mice (Hornberger et al., 1985).

It is now well established, by using a variety of behavioral test procedures, that aged rats display a significant impairment in spatial working memory and spatial reference memory (Wallace et al., 1980; Barnes et al., 1980; Ingram et al., 1981; Gage et al., 1984b,c). In addition, data from several laboratories have provided evidence that the age-related deficits in spatial memory are closely related to electrophysiological changes in the aged rat hippocampal formation (Barnes and McNaughton, 1980; Barnes et al., 1980, 1983). We have recently reported that the spatial memory deficits are significantly correlated with decreases in 2-deoxyglucose utilization in the hippocampal formation, prefrontal cortex and the septal area of aged rats (Gage et al., 1984c). Taken together these data strongly suggest that the decreases in memory function observed in the aged animals are dependent at least partly upon altered function in the hippocampal formation and its associated limbic and cortical structures, and that decline in function of the septohippocampal cholinergic system may contribute to decreased cognitive function.

Graft survival and fiber outgrowth in the aged rat brain

Azmitia et al. (1981) were the first to report successful intracerebral neural grafting in aged rodents. They examined the outgrowth of serotonergic fibers from fetal grafts obtained from the brain stem raphe region implanted in the hippocampus of adult and aged (24-months-old) mice. The raphe grafts survived and extended immunocytochemically positive serotonergic processes into the host hippocampus both in the young adult and aged recipients, although the density of innervation was greater in the young than in the aged host hippocampus. Sladek and Gash (1982) grafted fetal hypothalamic neurons to the third ventricle of middle-aged (12-months-old) and aged (25-months-old) Brattleboro rats. No major differences were observed between grafts in the young and middle-aged host brains, though few neurophysin-containing processes were identified as passing through the graft-host border. More recently, Matsumoto et al. (1984) have reported that grafts of newborn medial basal hypothalamus will survive grafting to the third ventricle of 21–30 months old Wistar rats, and Rogers et al. (1984) have reported that fetal medial preoptic area grafts will survive in middle-aged (13–15-months-old) Long-Evans rats. Sladek et al. (1984) have also reported that fetal grafts of the locus ceruleus regions will survive and extend noradrenergic axons in aged rats when grafted to the third ventricle.

In our own studies (Gage et al., 1983a,b, 1984a) we have obtained good survival of grafts of neuronal cell suspensions prepared from the ventral mesencephalon and septal-diagonal band area of rat fetuses into the depths of intact neostriatum and hippocampus of 21–23-months-old female Sprague-Dawley rats of the same strain

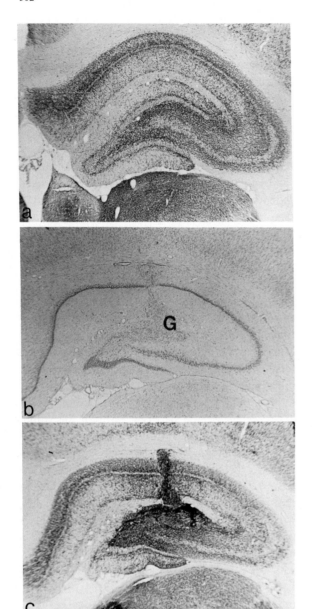

Fig. 1. Graft survival and AChE-positive fiber outgrowth into the host hippocampal formation of an aged rat. The intrinsic AChE-positive innervation had been removed by a fimbria-fornix lesion 7 days before sacrifice. (a) Photomicrograph of the AChE-positive graft-derived fiber plexus in the host dorsal hippocampus rostral to the implantation sites. (b) Photomicrograph of hippocampus stained with cresyl violet at the site of the rostral graft (G) placement. (c) Photomicrograph of an AChE-stained section adjacent to the one in (b), showing the rostral graft placement and the extent of AChE-positive fiber outgrowth into the host hippocampus from the graft. (From Gage et al., 1984a)

(Fig. 1). Graft survival assessed 3–4 months after grafting was comparable to that seen in our previous studies of young adult recipients. Fiber outgrowth into the host brain was evaluated in animals which were subjected to lesions of the intrinsic nigro-striatal or septo-hippocampal pathways 6–10 days before killing. Dense dopaminergic fiber outgrowth was seen within a zone of up to about 1 mm radius around the nigral implants, and the dense outgrowth of AChE-positive fibers occurred up to 2 mm away from the septal implants. In a recent electron microscopical investigation of the ingrowing cholinergic fibers, using choline acetyltransferase immunocytochemistry, we have obtained evidence that the grafts are capable of forming mature synaptic contacts with neurons in the aged host hippocampus (Clarke et al., 1986a). The overall magnitude of fiber outgrowth was less than generally seen in previously *denervated* targets in young adult recipients. The outgrowth seen in the aged rats with intact afferents, however, appeared to be at least as extensive as in young recipients when the grafts are placed in *non-denervated* targets. In addition, the distribution of the AChE-positive fibers from the septal implants in the host hippocampus suggested that the pattern found in the non-denervated target tissue of the aged recipients was more diffuse and partly different from normal. An interesting possibility is that synapse loss in the intrinsic connections of the hippocampus mentioned above may influence the pattern of the graft-derived innervation and in fact improve the implants' ability to terminate in the otherwise intact target of the aged host brain.

Effects of intrahippocampal grafts of fetal basal forebrain cholinergic neurons on learning and memory deficits in aged rats

As summarized in the Introduction, intracerebral grafts of suspensions of embryonic tissue rich in developing cholinergic neurons have been shown to provide a new extensive cholinergic innervation in young rats with surgical lesions of the forebrain cholinergic projection systems, and they have been demonstrated to restore, at least partly, functional deficits associated with destruction of the septo-hippocampal or basalo-cortical cholinergic pathways. Based on these considerations we have studied the behavioral effects of similar suspension grafts, implanted into the hippocampal formation of 21–23-months-old female Sprague-Dawley rats (Gage et al., 1984a; Gage and Björklund, 1986).

The age-dependent learning and memory deficits were assessed in the Morris water maze task (Morris, 1981) 1 week prior and 2½–3 months after transplantation. This test requires that the rat uses spatial cues in the environment to find a platform hidden below the surface of a pool of opaque water. Normal young rats have no trouble learning this task with speed and accuracy (Fig. 2; upper panel). On the final day of testing, the rat's memory of the location of the platform site is tested in the last trial, when the platform is removed from the pool (trial 5:5 in Fig. 2). The strength of the spatial memory is displayed by how well the rat focuses his search over the platform site. Since our initial studies using this task (Gage et al., 1984b,c) showed that only a portion (1/4 to 1/3) of our rats were markedly impaired, a pretransplant test served to identify those impaired individuals in the aged rat group. Based on the performance of the young controls, we set the criterion for impaired performance in the aged rats such that the mean escape latency (i.e., swim time to find the submerged platform) should be above an upper 99% confidence limit of the escape latencies recorded in the young control group. A subgroup of old rats showed mean swim times greater than the criterion and were thus allocated to the 'old impaired' group, which was used for subsequent transplantation. The remaining subgroup of aged rats constituted the 'old non-impaired' group. Fig. 2 shows representative examples of the performance of an impaired aged rat (middle panel) and a non-impaired rat of the same age (21–23-months-old; bottom panel). The aged impaired rat does not find the platform, and in the last trial, when the platform is removed (5:5),

it does not display any search over the previous platform site.

'Old impaired' rats, selected in this way, received bilateral suspension grafts prepared from the septal-diagonal band area obtained from 14- to 16-days-old embryos of the same rat strain. Three implant deposits were made stereotaxically into the hippocampal formation on each side. Other 'old impaired' rats were left unoperated and served as the 'old impaired' control group. On the post-transplantation test, 2½–3 months after grafting, the non-grafted rats remained impaired, while the grafted animals, as a group, showed a significant improvement in performance as indicated by their reduced escape latency (Fig. 3A,B). This improvement of the grafted group was demonstrated by comparisons to its pre-transplantation performance as well as to the performance of the non-grafted old controls in the second test.

The ability of the rats to use spatial cues for the location of the platform in the pool was assessed by analyzing their search behavior after removal of the platform on the 5th day of testing (Fig. 3C,D and Fig. 4). While the young rats and rats in the old non-impaired group (Fig. 4,A and B) focused their search on the 4th quadrant, where the platform had previously been placed, the 'old-impaired' rats failed to do so in the pre-transplant test (left circles in Fig. 4,C and D). In the post-transplantation test the grafted rats, but not the non-grafted 'old-impaired' group, showed significantly improved performance (middle circle). Swim distance in the 4th quadrant was increased by 83% and they swam significantly more in the 4th quadrant than in other quadrants of the pool (Fig. 3,D). By contrast the non-grafted controls showed no significant change over their pre-transplant performance.

In a subsequent study (Gage and Björklund, 1986) we have made some initial attempts to analyze the septal graft effects pharmacologically. In these experiments we used a modified water-maze protocol in which the platform was visible ('cue' trials) and invisible ('place' trials) on alternating trials. In these tests it became clear that the

504

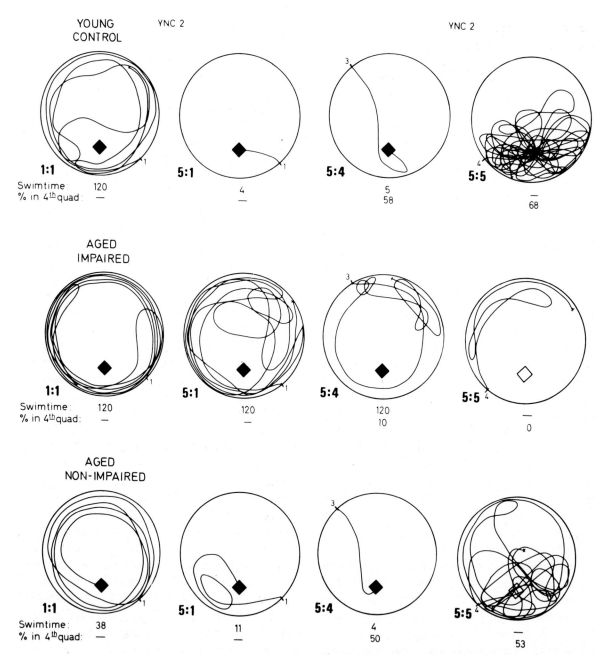

Fig. 2. Tracings of water maze performance of a young control rat, an aged impaired rat and an aged non-impaired rat, on four different trials during the week of testing; 1:1 corresponds to the first trial on day 1, 5:1 corresponds to the first trial on day 5, 5:4 corresponds to the fourth trial on day 5, and 5:5 corresponds to the fifth trial on the fifth day, when the platform had been removed from the pool. The filled square marks the location of the platform in the pool. The empty square marks the location of where the platform had been on the previous trials. Escape latency corresponds to the time required to find the platform on each trial; % in the fourth quadrant is the percentage of the total distance swum in the trial prior to platform removal (5:4) or in the trial following platform removal: 'spatial probe' trial (5:5). The smaller number next to the pool (1, 3 and 4) corresponds to the starting location for the rat on those trials. (From Gage et al., 1985)

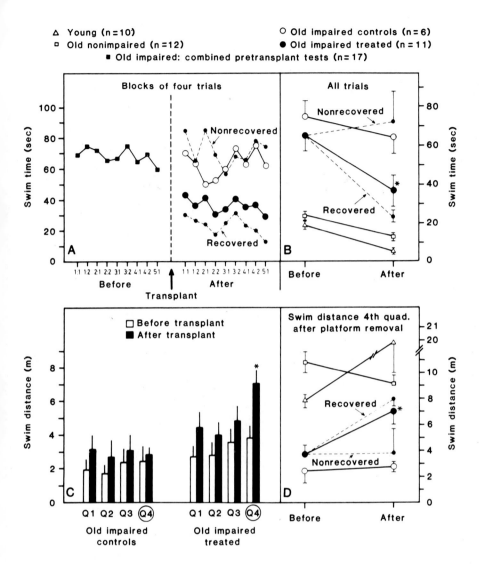

Fig. 3. Water maze performance of the four groups of rats, young controls, old impaired rats, old non-impaired rats, and old impaired rats which received intrahippocampal septal suspension grafts (for symbols, see key above the figure). (A) Escape latency is plotted as nine blocks of four trials, with eight trials presented each day. The left panel represents the performance of all old impaired rats before transplant. The statistical analysis of these data was conducted with the pretransplant performance of the age-impaired group subdivided into their respective categories of old impaired controls and old impaired with grafts. Since no statistical difference existed between the two groups before transplantation, they were combined graphically for simplicity and clarity of presentation. The right panel represents the performance of the two groups of old impaired rats after the one group received transplants. 'Recovered' (in A, B and D) refers to eight of the 11 old impaired rats with grafts that on the posttransplant trials had recovered to within the 99% confidence interval of the young control group performance. 'Nonrecovered' refers to the remaining three that showed no improvement after the transplant. (B) Total mean ($\pm$SEM) escape latency summed over all 36 trials. The asterisk indicates a significant decrease in escape latency by the old impaired rats with grafts compared with their pretransplant performance and compared with the old impaired control rats after transplant. (C) Total distance swum in each quadrant on the last trial when the platform had been removed from the pool. The asterisk indicates a significant increase in distance swum in quadrant 4 (Q4) (where the platform had been located) in the posttransplant test by the old impaired rats with grafts compared with their earlier performance and with the mean of the distances they swam in quadrants 1 to 3 (Q1, Q2, Q3) after transplantation. (D) Total distance swum in Q4. The asterisk indicates a significant increase in swim distance of the old impaired group with grafts compared with its performance before the transplant and with the old impaired control rats after transplant. (From Gage et al., 1984)

506

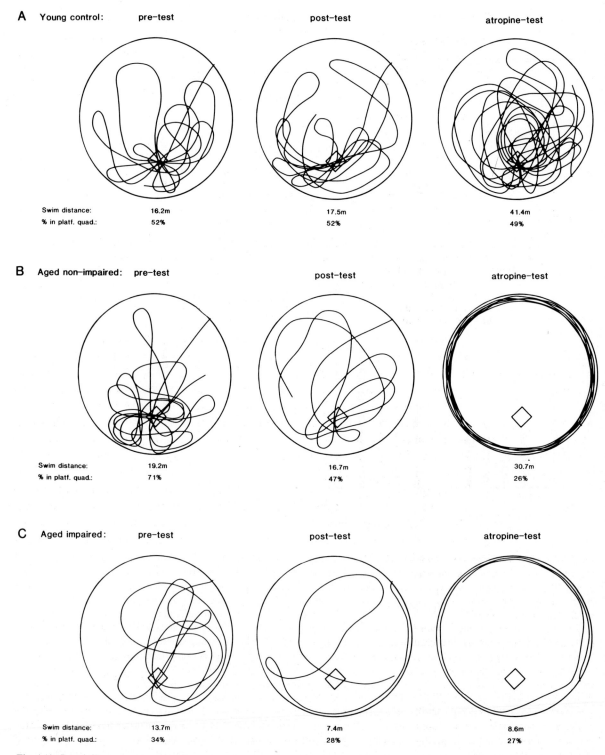

A Young control: pre-test   post-test   atropine-test

Swim distance: 16.2m   17.5m   41.4m
% in platf. quad.:   52%   52%   49%

B Aged non-impaired: pre-test   post-test   atropine-test

Swim distance: 19.2m   16.7m   30.7m
% in platf. quad.:   71%   47%   26%

C Aged impaired: pre-test   post-test   atropine-test

Swim distance: 13.7m   7.4m   8.6m
% in platf. quad.:   34%   28%   27%

Fig. 4 (A, B and C)

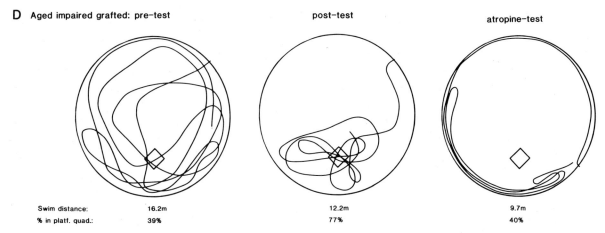

D Aged impaired grafted: pre-test　　　post-test　　　atropine-test

	pre-test	post-test	atropine-test
Swim distance:	16.2m	12.2m	9.7m
% in platf. quad.:	39%	77%	40%

Fig. 4 (A–D). Effect of septal grafts and atropine treatment (50 mg/kg) on spatial memory in the water maze test, showing the swim pattern on the last 'spatial probe' trial, when the platform had been removed. (A) young control rat; (B) aged non-impaired rat; (C) aged-impaired rat; (D) aged-impaired grafted rat. The pretransplant performance is shown to the left, and the posttransplant performance after saline or atropine is shown in the two right circles. The rat with median performance in each group was selected. (From Gage and Björklund, 1986)

'old impaired' rats were severely impaired not only when the platform was hidden (i.e. spatial reference memory), but also in the acquisition of the task when the platform was visible (which can be taken as a measure of non-spatial reference memory). The non-grafted impaired rats remained as impaired on both the 'cue' and the 'place' tasks when re-tested 2½ months after the first test, while the impaired rats with septal suspension implants in the hippocampal formation were significantly improved on both components of the tasks. Moreover, while the non-grafted animals showed worse performance during the first two days of the second test session, as compared to the last days of the first test session, the grafted animals retained their level of performance from the end of the first test session. This indicates that the septal grafts can have an effect not only on acquisition but also on retention of the learned performance.

In the pharmacological test, atropine (50 mg/kg, i.p.) abolished completely the ability to find the platform in the grafted animals, both with visible and non-visible platform (Gage and Björklund, 1986). Consistent with this the ability to locate the platform site ('spatial probe' trial) was also reduced (as illustrated by the right-hand circle in

Fig. 4,D). By contrast, atropine had no significant effect in the 'old-impaired' rats without grafts (Fig. 4,C), and only marginal effect in the young control rats (Fig. 4,A). Moreover, it is interesting to note that the aged non-impaired rats were more sensitive to the effect of atropine (Fig. 4,B). Physostigmine (0.05 mg/kg, i.p.) had no significant effect on either grafted or non-grafted animals when administered during a single day of trials. These observations seem consistent with the idea that the graft-mediated improvements on both spatial and non-spatial learning and memory in the water-maze test are dependent on intact cholinergic neurotransmission.

Discussion

From the studies conducted in young adult rats with lesions of the cholinergic projection systems it appears that implanted embryonic cholinergic nerve cells in some cases can substitute quite well for a lost afferent cholinergic input to a denervated brain region. The intracerebral implants can probably exert their effects in several ways. The functional effects seen with grafts of nigral, hypothalamic or adrenal medullary tissue placed into one of the cerebral ventricles, such as in the studies of Perlow et al. (1980), Freed et al. (1983) and Gash et al. (1980, 1985), can probably be explained on the basis of diffuse release of an active amine or peptide into the host CSF and adjacent brain tissue. In other instances, such as in animals with dopamine-rich grafts reinnervating the previously denervated neostriatum, or acetylcholine-rich grafts reinnervating the previously denervated hippocampus (see Dunnett et al., 1983; Gage et al., 1985, for reviews), we believe that the available data provide quite substantial evidence that behavioral recovery is caused by the ability of the grafted neurons to reinnervate relevant parts of the host brain. This is illustrated, for example, by studies in young rats with lesions of the nigrostriatal dopamine pathway showing that the degree of functional recovery induced by nigral transplants is well correlated with the extent of striatal dopamine reinnervation, and that the 'profile' of functional recovery is dependent on the area of the striatal complex which is reinnervated by the graft. Moreover, recent electron microscopic studies (Freund et al., 1985; Clarke et al., 1986b) on nigral grafts in the caudate-putamen and septal grafts reinnervating the hippocampus, have demonstrated that the ingrowing dopaminergic and cholinergic fibers, respectively, establish abundant mature synaptic contacts with the initially denervated host target neurons.

To what extent the intracerebral implants can be functionally integrated with the host brain is, however, still poorly known and remains therefore an interesting question for further investigation. The chances for extensive integration may be greatest for neuronal suspension grafts implanted as deposits directly into the depth of the brain, but even solid grafts inserted as whole pieces into the brain have in several cases been seen to become reinnervated from the host brain, both in adult and developing recipients (See Björklund and Stenevi, 1979, 1984, for reviews). To what extent this may be the case for basal forebrain neurons implanted into the hippocampal formation has, however, so far not been explored.

Whether these observations on grafts in young adult rats with denervating lesions are valid for the interpretation of the graft-induced functional effects in aged rats (without any preceding experimentally induced brain damage) is unclear. The observations of fiber outgrowth from the graft into the surrounding host brain region seem to support the possibility that also in the non-denervated aged host brain the implanted cholinergic neurons may act via specific efferent connections with the host. Ultrastructural observations, using electron microscopic immunocytochemistry (Clarke et al., 1986b) indicate that the graft-derived cholinergic fibers, growing into the dentate gyrus in the aged recipients, indeed are capable of forming normal synaptic contacts with neuronal elements in the host.

As a working hypothesis we propose, therefore, that the functional effects of implanted neural tissue in aged rats are also exerted by a specific action of selective neuronal elements in the graft on a dysfunctioning surrounding brain region of the host, and that this influence is mediated via the fiber connections established by the implanted neurons. On the assumption that impaired cholinergic neurotransmission contributes to the age-dependent cognitive impairments, we also propose that the ameliorative action of the septal grafts is, at least partly, due to a restoration of neurotransmission in the area. Our results suggest, however, that although cholinergic reinnervation of the target may be *necessary* for the effects of septal grafts in the water maze task, this may not be *sufficient* for graft function. Several neuronal cell types may participate, and the presence or absence of specific afferent connections to the grafts may also be important.

Neuronal replacement by intracerebral implants in aged rats, or in brain-damaged young rats, is a striking example of how the brain can allow new elements to be inserted and linked into its own functional subsystems. Obviously there must be definite limitations as to which types of neurons or functional subsystems can successfully be manipulated in this way. Neural implants would seem most likely to have behaviorally meaningful functional effects with types of neurons that normally do not convey, or link, specific or patterned messages, e.g., in sensoric or motoric input and output systems. Indeed, functional or behavioral recovery in the neuronal replacement paradigm has so far been demonstrated primarily for neurons of the types that normally appear to act as tonic regulatory or level-setting systems.

The basal forebrain cholinergic neurons are commonly conceived of as a modulatory or level-setting system which tonically regulates the activity of the hippocampal neuronal machinery. Removal of the cholinergic control mechanisms seems to result in inhibition or impairment of hippocampal function. Functional recovery seen after reinstatement of impaired cholinergic transmission by drugs or by neural implants can thus be interpreted as a reactivation of an inhibited, but otherwise intact, neuronal machinery.

An interesting implication of this model is that it may be sufficient for the septal grafts to reinstate cholinergic neurotransmission in the reinnervated target in a tonic and relatively non-specific manner in order to compensate for at least part of the lesion-induced or age-dependent behavioral impairments. Temporally or spatially patterned inputs to the grafted neurons may not be necessary for the maintenance of such tonic activity. Indeed, our studies on nigral grafts reinnervating the neostriatum in young animals with nigro-striatal bundle lesion, using biochemical analyses of dopamine synthesis and metabolism (Schmidt et al., 1982, 1983) or in vivo brain dialysis (Zetterström et al., 1986), indicate that grafted dopaminergic neurons can maintain a sufficiently high spontaneous activity even in the absence of any major afferents from the host brain. It is obvious, however, that such a tonic model of action may severely limit the functionality of the grafted neurons, particularly in systems like the septo-hippocampal pathway where rhythmic firing (theta rhythm) is a characteristic feature of the normal cholinergic afferent input. The degree to which intracerebrally implanted neurons can become integrated into the host neuronal networks is, therefore, a highly interesting issue for future research.

Acknowledgement

We thank Siv Carlson for generous assistance in the preparation of the manuscript. Our research was supported by the Swedish MRC and the National Institute of Aging (AG03766).

References

Azmitia, E. C., Perlow, M. J., Brennan, M. J. and Lauder, J. M. (1981) Fetal raphe and hippocampal transplants into adult and aged C57BL/6N mice: a preliminary immunocytochemical study. *Brain Res. Bull.*, 7: 703–710.

Barnes, C. A. and McNaughton, B. L. (1980) Physiological compensation for loss of afferent synapses in rat hippocampal granule cells during senescence. *J. Physiol.*, 309: 473–485.

Barnes, C. A., Nadel, L. and Honig, W. K. (1980) Spatial memory deficits in senescent rats. *Can. J. Psychol.*, 34: 29–39.

Barnes, C. A., McNaughton, B. L. and O'Keefe, J. (1983) Loss of place specificity in hippocampal complex spike cells of senescent rat. *Neurobiol. Aging*, 4: 113–119.

Bartus, R. T., Dean, R. L., Beer, B. and Lippa, A. S. (1982) The cholinergic hypothesis of geriatric memory dysfunction. *Science*, 217: 408–416.

Björklund, A. and Stenevi, U. (1977) Reformation of the severed septohippocampal cholinergic pathway in the adult rat by transplanted septal neurons. *Cell Tiss. Res.*, 185: 289–302.

Björklund, A. and Stenevi, U. (1979) Regeneration of monoaminergic and cholinergic neurons in the mammalian central nervous system. *Physiol. Rev.*, 59: 62–100.

Björklund, A. and Stenevi, U. (1984) Intracerebral neural implants: Neuronal replacement and reconstruction of damaged circuitries. *Ann. Rev. Neurosci.*, 7: 279–308.

Björklund, A., Stenevi, U., Dunnett, S. B. and Gage, F. H. (1982) Cross-species neural grafting in a rat model of Parkinson's disease. *Nature*, 298: 652–654.

Björklund, A., Gage, F. H., Schmidt, R. H., Stenevi, U. and Dunnett, S. B. (1983a) Intracerebral grafting of neuronal cell suspensions. VII. Recovery of choline acetyltransferase activity and acetylcholine synthesis in the denervated hippocampus reinnervated by septal suspension implants. *Acta Physiol. Scand.* Suppl., 522: 59–66.

Björklund, A., Gage, F. H., Stenevi, U. and Dunnett, S. B. (1983b) Intracerebral grafting of neuronal cell suspensions. VI. Survival and growth of intrahippocampal implants of septal cell suspensions. *Acta Physiol. Scand.* Suppl., 522: 49–58.

Björklund, A., Stenevi, U., Schmidt, R. H., Dunnett, S. B. and Gage, F. H. (1983c) Intracerebral grafting of neuronal cell suspensions: I. Introduction and general methods of preparation. *Acta Physiol. Scand.*, Suppl., 522: 1–7.

Bondareff, W. and Geinisman, Y. (1976) Loss of synapses in the dentate gyrus of the senescent rat. *Am. J. Anat.*, 145: 129–136.

Brundin, P., Nilsson, O. G., Gage, F. H. and Björklund, A. (1985) Cyclosporin A increases survival of cross-species intrastriatal grafts of embryonic dopamine-containing neurons. *Exp. Brain Res.*, 60: 204–208.

Clarke, D. J., Gage, F. H., Nilsson, O. G. and Björklund, A. (1986a) Grafted septal neurons from synaptic connections in the dentate gyrus of behaviorally-impaired aged rats. *J. Comp. Neurol.*, in press.

Clarke, D. J., Gage, F. H. and Björklund, A. (1986b) Formation of cholinergic synapses by intrahippocampal septal grafts as revealed by choline acetyl-transferase immunocytochemistry. *Brain Res.*, 369: 151–162.

Coyle, J. T., Price, D. L. and DeLong, M. R. (1983) Alzheimer disease: a disorder of cortical cholinergic innervation. *Science*, 219: 1184–1189.

Dunnett, S. B., Low, W. C., Iversen, S. D., Stenevi, U. and Björklund, A. (1982) Septal transplants restore maze learning in rats with fornix-fimbria lesions. *Brain Res.*, 251: 335–348.

Dunnett, S. B., Björklund, A. and Stenevi, U. (1983) Dopamine-rich transplants in experimental Parkinsonism. *Trends Neurosci.*, 6: 266–270.

Dunnett, S. B., Toniolo, G., Fine, A., Ryan, C. N., Björklund, A. and Iversen, S. D. (1985) Transplantation of embryonic ventral forebrain neurons to the neocortex of rats with lesions of nucleus basalis magnocellularis. II. Sensorimotor and learning impairments. *Neuroscience*, 16: 787–797.

Fine, A., Dunnett, S. B., Björklund, A. and Iversen, S. D. (1985a) Cholinergic ventral forebrain grafts into the neocortex improve passive avoidance memory in a rat model of Alzheimer disease. *Proc. Natl. Acad. Sci. USA*, 82: 5227–5230.

Fine, A., Dunnett, S. B., Björklund, A., Clarke, D. and Iversen, S. D. (1985b) Transplantation of embryonic ventral forebrain neurons to the neocortex of rats with lesions of nucleus basalis magnocellularis: I. Biochemical and anatomical observations. *Neuroscience*, 16: 769–786.

Freed, W. J. (1983) Functional brain tissue transplantation: reversal of lesion-induced rotation by intraventricular substantia nigra and adrenal medulla grafts, with a note on intracranial retinal grafts. *Biol. Psychiat.*, 18: 1205–1266.

Freund, T. F., Bolam, J. P., Björklund, A., Stenevi, U., Dunnett, S. B. and Smith, A. D. (1985) Efferent synaptic connections of grafted dopaminergic neurons reinnervating the host neostriatum: a tyrosine hydroxylase immunocytochemical study. *J. Neurosci.*, 3: 603–616.

Gage, F. H. and Björklund, A. (1986) Cholinergic septal grafts

into the hippocampal formation improve spatial learning and memory in aged rats by an atropine sensitive mechanism. *J. Neurosci.*, in press.

Gage, F. H., Dunnett, S. B., Stenevi, U. and Björklund, A. (1983a) Intracerebral grafting of neuronal cell suspensions. VIII. Survival and growth of implants of nigral and septal cell suspensions in intact brains of aged rats. *Acta Physiol. Scand.*, Suppl., 522: 67–75.

Gage, F. H., Dunnett, S. B., Stenevi, U. and Björklund, A. (1983b) Aged rats: recovery of motor impairments by intrastriatal nigral grafts. *Science*, 221: 966–969.

Gage, F. H., Björklund, A., Stenevi, U., Dunnett, S. B. and Kelly, P. A. T. (1984a) Intrahippocampal septal grafts ameliorate learning impairments in aged rats. *Science*, 225: 533–536.

Gage, F. H., Dunnett, S. B. and Björklund, A. (1984b) Spatial learning and motor deficits in aged rats. *Neurobiol. Aging*, 543–48.

Gage, F. H., Kelly, P. A. T. and Björklund, A. (1984c) Regional changes in brain glucose metabolism reflect cognitive impairments in aged rats. *J. Neurosci.*, 4: 2856–2866.

Gage, F. H., Björklund, A., Stenevi, U. and Dunnett, S. B. (1985) Grafting of embryonic CNS tissue to the damaged adult hippocampal formation. In A. Björklund and U. Stenevi (Eds.), *Neural Grafting in the Mammalian CNS*, Elsevier, Amsterdam, pp. 559–573.

Gash, D. M., Sladek, J. R., Jr. and Sladek, C. D. (1980) Functional development of grafted vasopressin neurons. *Science*, 210: 1367–1369.

Gash, D. M., Notter, M. F. D., Dick, L. B., Kraus, A. L., Okawara, S. H., Wechkin, S. W. and Joynt, R. J. (1985) Cholinergic neurons transplanted into the neocortex and hippocampus of primates: studies on African Green monkeys. In A. Björklund and U. Stenevi (Eds.), *Neural Grafting in the Mammalian CNS*, Elsevier, Amsterdam, pp. 595–603.

Geinisman, Y. (1979) Loss of axosomatic synapses in the dentate gyrus of aged rats. *Brain Res.*, 168: 485–492.

Geinisman, Y. (1981) Loss of axon terminals contacting neuronal somata in the dentate gyrus of aged rats. *Brain Res.*, 212: 136–139.

Gibson, G. E., Peterson, C. and Jensen, D. J. (1981) Brain acetylcholine synthesis declines with senescence. *Science*, 213: 674–676.

Hoff, S. F., Scheff, S. W., Bernardo, L. S. and Cotman, C. W. (1982) Lesion-induced synaptogenesis in the dentate gyrus of aged rats. I. Loss and reacquisition of normal synaptic density. *J. Comp. Neurol.*, 205: 246–252.

Hornberger, J. C., Buell, S. J., Flood, D. G., McNeill, T. H. and Coleman, P. D. (1985) Stability of numbers but not size of mouse forebrain cholinergic neurons to 53 months. *Neurobiol. Aging*, 6: 269–275.

Ingram, D. K., London, E. D. and Goodrick, C. L. (1981) Age and neurochemical correlates of radial maze performance in rats. *Neurobiol. Aging*, 2: 41–47.

Kelly, P. A. T., Gage, F. H., Ingvar, M., Lindvall, O., Stenevi, U. and Björklund, A. (1985) Functional reactivation of the deafferented hippocampus by embryonic septal grafts as assessed by measurements of local glucose utilization. *Exp. Brain Res.*, 58: 570–579.

Kromer, L. F. (1985) Factors in neural transplants which influence regeneration in the mature mammalian central nervous system. In A. Björklund and U. Stenevi (Eds.), *Neural Grafting in the Mammalian CNS*, Elsevier, Amsterdam, 309–318.

Landfield, P. W., Rose, G., Sandles, L., Wohlstadter, T. C. and Lynch, G. (1977) Patterns of astroglial hypertrophy and neuronal degeneration in the hippocampus of aged, memory-deficient rats. *J. Gerontol.*, 32: 3–12.

Landfield, P. W., Braun, L. D., Pitler, T. A., Lindsey, J. D. and Lynch, G. (1981) Hippocampal aging in rats: a morphometric study of multiple variables in semithin sections. *Neurobiol. Aging*, 2: 265–275.

Lewis, E. R. and Cotman, C. W. (1983) Neurotransmitter characteristics of brain grafts: striatal and septal tissues form the same laminated input to the hippocampus. *Neuroscience*, 8: 57–66.

Lippa, A. S., Pelham, R. W., Beer, B., Critchett, D. J., Dean, R. L. and Bartus, R. T. (1980) Brain cholinergic dysfunction and memory in aged rats. *Neurobiol. Aging*, 1: 13–19.

Lippa, A. S., Critchett, D. J., Ehlert, F., Yamamura, H. I., Enna, S. J. and Bartus, R. T. (1981) Age-related alterations in neurotransmitter receptors: an electrophysiological and biochemical analysis. *Neurobiol. Aging*, 2: 3–8.

Low, W. C., Lewis, P. R., Bunch, S. T., Dunnett, S. B., Thomas, S. R., Iversen, S. D., Björklund, A. and Stenevi, U. (1982) Functional recovery following transplantation of embryonic septal nuclei into adult rats with septo-hippocampal lesions: the recovery of function. *Nature*, 300: 260–262.

Low, W. C., Lewis, P. R. and Bunch, S. T. (1983) Embryonic neural transplants across a major histocompatibility barrier: survival and specificity of innervation. *Brain Res.*, 262: 328–333.

Low, W. C., Daniloff, J. K., Bodony, R. P. and Wells, J. (1985) Cross-species transplants of cholinergic neurons and the recovery of function. In A. Björklund and U. Stenevi (Eds.), *Neural Grafting in the Mammalian CNS*, Elsevier, Amsterdam, pp. 575–584.

Matsumoto, A., Kobayashi, S., Muralsami, S. and Arai, Y. (1984) Recovery of declined ovarian function in aged female rats by transplantation of newborn hypothalamic tissue. *Proc. Japn. Acad.*, 60: 73–76.

Morris, R. G. M. (1981) Spatial localization does not require the presence of local cues. *Learn. Motiv.*, 12: 239–260.

Olson, L., Seiger, Å. and Strömberg, I. (1983) Intraocular transplantation in rodents. A detailed account of the procedure and examples of its use in neurobiology with special reference to brain tissue grafting. In S. Fedoroff (Ed.), *Advances in Cellular Neurobiology, Vol. 4*, Academic Press, New York, 407.

Perlow, M. J., Kumakura, K. and Guidotti, A. (1980) Prolonged survival of bovine adrenal chromaffin cells in rat cerebral ventricle. *Proc. Natl. Acad. Sci. USA*, 77: 5278–5281.

Rogers, J., Hoffman, G. E., Zornetzer, S. F. and Vale, W. W. (1984) Hypothalamic grafts and neuroendocrine cascade theories of aging. In J. R. Sladek and D. M. Gash (Eds.), *Neural Transplants: Development and Function*, Plenum Press, New York, 205–222.

Schmidt, R. H., Ingvar, M., Lindvall, O., Stenevi, U. and Björklund, A. (1982) Functional activity of substantia nigra grafts reinnervating the striatum: Neurotransmitter metabolism and [^{14}C]-2-deoxy-D-glucose autoradiography. *J. Neurochem.*, 38: 737–748.

Schmidt, R. H., Björklund, A., Stenevi, U., Dunnett, S. B. and Gage, F. H. (1983) Intracerebral grafting of neuronal cell suspension. III. Activity of intrastriatal nigral suspension implants as assessed by measurements of dopamine synthesis and metabolism. *Acta Physiol. Scand.*, Suppl. 522: 23–32.

Segal, M. (1982) Changes in neurotransmitter actions in aged rat hippocampus. *Neurobiol. Aging*, 3: 121–124.

Segal, M., Björklund, A. and Gage, F. H. (1985) Transplanted septal neurons make viable cholinergic synapses with a host hippocampus. *Brain Res.*, 336: 302–307.

Sherman, K. A., Kuster, J. E., Dean, R. L., Bartus, R. T. and Friedman, E. (1981) Presynaptic cholinergic mechanisms in brain of aged rats with memory impairments. *Neurobiol. Aging*, 2: 99–104.

Sims, N. R., Marek, K. L., Bowen, D. M. and Davison, A. N. (1982) Production of [^{14}C]acetylcholine and [^{14}C]carbon dioxide from [U − ^{14}C]glucose in tissue prisms from aging rat brain. *J. Neurochem.*, 38: 488–492.

Sladek, J. R. and Gash, D. M. (1982) The use of neural grafts as a means of restoring neuronal loss associated with aging. *Anat. Rec.*, 202: 178A.

Sladek, J. R., Gash, D. M. and Collier, T. J. (1984) Noradrenergic neuron transplants into the third ventricle of aged F344 rats improve inhibitory avoidance memory performance. *Sco. Neurosci. Abstr.*, 10: 772.

Stenevi, U., Kromer, L. F., Gage, F. H. and Björklund, A. (1985) Solid neural grafts in intracerebral transplantation cavities. In A. Björklund and U. Stenevi (Eds.), *Neural Grafting in the Mammalian CNS*, Elsevier, Amsterdam, p. 41.

Strong, R., Hicks, P., Hsu, L., Bartus, R. T. and Enna, S. J. (1980) Age-related alterations in the rodent brain cholinergic system and behavior. *Neurobiol. Aging*, 1: 59–63.

Wallace, J. E., Krauter, E. E. and Campbell, B. A. (1980) Animal models of declining memory in the aged: Short term and spatial memory in the aged rat. *J. Gerontol.*, 35: 355–363.

Zetterström, T., Brundin, P., Gage, F. H., Sharp, T., Isacson, O., Dunnett, S. B., Ungerstedt, U. and Björklund, A. (1986) In vivo measurement of spontaneous release and metabolism of dopamine from intrastriatal nigral grafts using intracerebral dialysis. *Brain Res.*, 362: 344–349.

Discussion

G. W. VAN HOESEN: We know that deafferented neurons in the hippocampus often do peculiar things, e.g. they may spike and cause seizure activity. We have preliminary observations in AD that surviving neurons not affected by pathology, but deafferented by pathology elsewhere may produce large quantities of neuropeptides. It is difficult to understand how a transplanted or grafted neuron with no substantial input of its own can ameliorate a behavioral deficit. Is it possible that by reinnervating deafferented neurons they prevent it from doing unusual things that are in fact equally disruptive to behavior?

ANSWER: Yes, this is certainly a possibility. In the hippocampal formation, in particular, fimbria-fornix lesions are known to result in abnormal electrical activity. It is an interesting possibility, therefore, that the graft effect could be due to a normalization of this activity, thus eliminating a disruptive mechanism. Whether any neuropeptides are involved in this is presently unclear.

P. D. COLEMAN: Since the target cell population in the aged rat hippocampus is relatively intact, while it is far less intact in normal human aged hippocampus and even less intact in the Alzheimer hippocampus, you might expect grafts to produce less improvement in humans than in rats.

ANSWER: I think this is likely. The neuropathology is much more widespread in aged humans, and in Alzheimer's disease in particular, than in aged rodents. Cognitive impairments in Alzheimer's disease may therefore have a complex anatomical background. Thus, we will have to learn much more about the mechanisms underlying dementia, and about the role of the cholinergic system in particular, before one can even speculate on the potential of neural grafting in cases of dementia in humans.

R. NIEUWENHUYS: Is anything known concerning the afferents of the implanted dopaminergic and cholinergic cells?

ANSWER: There is one paper by Arbuthnott et al. (1985) that has been able to demonstrate afferent inputs from the host to intrastriatal grafts of nigral dopamine neurons. This was done with electrophysiological technique, and they showed that grafted nigral neurons were responsive to electrical stimulation in a variety of host sites, including cortex, striatum, locus ceruleus and raphe.

J. KORF: Is there a possibility that not only cholinergic neurons but also that non-cholinergic neurons are transplanted? In particular glutamate containing neurons could be of interest in the case of hippocampal dysfunction.

ANSWER: We know that our grafts contain also non-cholinergic neurons, and we think that some of our results indicate that although the cholinergic neurons in the grafts may be necessary for the observed functional effects, they are probably not sufficient. This opens up the possibility that also other transmitter systems are active as well. Whether glutamate is one of them will require further studies.

References

Arbuthnott, G., Dunnett, S. and MacLeod, N. (1985) Electrophysiological properties of single units in dopamine-rich mesencephalic transplants in rat brain. *Neurosci. Lett.*, 57: 205–213.

Subject Index